Oxford American Handbook of
Infectious Diseases

D0814362

About the Oxford American Handbooks in Medicine

The Oxford American Handbooks are pocket clinical books, providing practical guidance in quick reference, note form. Titles cover major medical specialties or cross-specialty topics and are aimed at students, residents, internists, family physicians, and practicing physicians within specific disciplines.

Their reputation is built on including the best clinical information, complemented by hints, tips, and advice from the authors. Each one is carefully reviewed by senior subject experts, residents, and students to ensure that content reflects the reality of day-to-day medical practice.

Key series features

- Written in short chunks, each topic is covered in a two-page spread to enable readers to find information quickly. They are also perfect for test preparation and gaining a quick overview of a subject without scanning through unnecessary pages.
- Content is evidence based and complemented by the expertise and judgment of experienced authors.
- The Handbooks provide a humanistic approach to medicine – it's more than just treatment by numbers.
- A "friend in your pocket," the Handbooks offer honest, reliable guidance about the difficulties of practicing medicine and provide coverage of both the practice and art of medicine.
- For quick reference, useful "everyday" information is included on the inside covers.

Published and Forthcoming Oxford American Handbooks

Oxford American Handbook of Clinical Medicine
Oxford American Handbook of Anesthesiology
Oxford American Handbook of Cardiology
Oxford American Handbook of Clinical Dentistry
Oxford American Handbook of Clinical Diagnosis
Oxford American Handbook of Clinical Examination and Practical Skills
Oxford American Handbook of Clinical Pharmacy
Oxford American Handbook of Critical Care
Oxford American Handbook of Emergency Medicine
Oxford American Handbook of Endocrinology and Diabetes
Oxford American Handbook of Gastroenterology and Hepatology
Oxford American Handbook of Geriatric Medicine
Oxford American Handbook of Hospice and Palliative Medicine
Oxford American Handbook of Infectious Diseases
Oxford American Handbook of Nephrology and Hypertension
Oxford American Handbook of Neurology
Oxford American Handbook of Obstetrics and Gynecology
Oxford American Handbook of Oncology
Oxford American Handbook of Ophthalmology
Oxford American Handbook of Otolaryngology
Oxford American Handbook of Pediatrics
Oxford American Handbook of Physical Medicine and Rehabilitation
Oxford American Handbook of Psychiatry
Oxford American Handbook of Pulmonary Medicine
Oxford American Handbook of Rheumatology
Oxford American Handbook of Sports Medicine
Oxford American Handbook of Surgery
Oxford American Handbook of Urology

Oxford American Handbook of
Infectious Diseases

Aimee K. Zaas, MD, MHS

Associate Professor of Medicine
Division of Infectious Diseases and International Health
Duke University Medical Center
Durham, North Carolina

Deverick J. Anderson, MD, MPH

Chair, Antibiotic Evaluation Team
Assistant Professor of Medicine
Division of Infectious Diseases
Duke University Medical Center
Durham, North Carolina

Kimberly E. Hanson, MD, MHS

Assistant Professor of Medicine
Division of Infectious Diseases
University of Utah School of Medicine
Salt Lake City, Utah

Elizabeth S. Dodds Ashley, PharmD, MHS, FCCP, BCPS

Associate Director for Clinical Pharmacy Services
Infectious Diseases Pharmacist
University of Rochester Medical Center
Rochester, New York

with

Estée Török

Ed Moran

Fiona J. Cooke

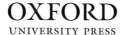

OXFORD
UNIVERSITY PRESS

OXFORD
UNIVERSITY PRESS

Oxford University Press, Inc. publishes works that further
Oxford University's objective of excellence in research, scholarship and education.

Oxford New York

Auckland Cape Town Dar es Salaam Hong Kong Karachi
Kuala Lumpur Madrid Melbourne Mexico City Nairobi
New Delhi Shanghai Taipei Toronto

With offices in

Argentina Austria Brazil Chile Czech Republic France Greece
Guatemala Hungary Italy Japan Poland Portugal
Singapore South Korea Switzerland Thailand Turkey Ukraine Vietnam

Published by Oxford University Press Inc.
198 Madison Avenue, New York, New York 10016

www.oup.com

Oxford is a registered trade mark of Oxford University Press

First published 2012
UK version published: 2009

Library of Congress Cataloging-in-Publication Data

Oxford American handbook of infectious diseases / Aimee Zaas ... [et al.] ;
with Estee Torok, Ed Moran, Fiona J. Cooke.
p. ; cm. — (Oxford American handbooks in medicine)
Handbook of infectious diseases
Includes index.
ISBN 978-0-19-538013-2 (pbk. : alk. paper)
1. Communicable diseases—Handbooks, manuals, etc. I. Zaas, Aimee. II. Title:
Handbook of infectious diseases. III. Series: Oxford American handbooks.
[DNLM: 1. Communicable Diseases—Handbooks. 2. Anti-Infective Agents—
Handbooks. 3. Communicable Disease Control—Handbooks. WC 39]
RC112.5.O94 2012
616.9—dc23
2011012547

10 9 8 7 6 5 4 3 2 1
Printed in China

Preface

Infectious diseases remain a predominant cause of morbidity and mortality worldwide. Current issues facing practitioners include the growing prevalence of drug-resistant organisms, emerging diseases such as pandemic H1N1 influenza, and an increase in the number of immune-compromised hosts. Working knowledge of microbiology and antimicrobial pharmacotherapy are critical to the practice of medicine in the hospital and the clinic setting.

In this Handbook, we attempt to represent the wide range of infectious diseases. Chapters cover basic microbiology, epidemiology, pharmacology, and clinical syndromes. While any book is not a substitute for gaining clinical experience or accessing the primary literature, we hope this book will appeal to trainees, hospitalist physicians, general practitioners, and infectious diseases specialists as a comprehensive rapid reference for infectious diseases.

Aimee Zaas
Dev Anderson
Libby Dodds Ashley
Kimberly Hanson

Acknowledgments

We, the four editors of the *Oxford American Handbook of Infectious Diseases*, would like to express our gratitude to all the contributors. We also acknowledge all involved at Oxford University Press, most notably Andrea Seils, Senior Editor of Clinical Medicine. Most importantly, we want to formally and emphatically display our gratitude to Estée Török, Ed Moran, and Fiona J. Cooke, the authors of the original UK version, *Oxford Handbook of Infectious Diseases*. Much of their extraordinary work has been retained, with adaptations for the U.S. audience. We truly appreciate the groundwork from the UK team and hope for continued success in the practice of medicine and infectious diseases.

Contents

Detailed contents

Symbols and abbreviations

Ab	antibody
ABG	arterial blood gas
ABPA	allergic bronchopulmonary aspergillosis
ABPI	ankle/brachial pressure index
ACIP	(CDC) Advisory Committee on Immunization Practices
ACT	adenylate cyclase toxin
ADH	antidiuretic hormone
ADME	absorption, distribution, metabolism, excretion
ADV	adefovir
AFB	acid-fast bacilli
AFLP	amplified fragment length polymorphism
AFP	alphafetoprotein
Ag	antigen
ALP	alkaline phosphatase
ALT	alanine aminotransferase
AME	aminoglycoside-modifying enzyme
AMP	adenosine monophosphate
ANA	antinuclear antibody
ANCA	antineutrophil cytoplasmic antibody
AO	acridine orange
ap	acellular pertussis (vaccine)
API	Analytical Profile Index
APIC	Association of Professionals in Infection Control
APUA	Alliance for Prudent Use of Antibiotics
ARDS	acute respiratory distress syndrome
ARF	acute renal failure
ART	antiretroviral therapy
ASOT	anti-streptolysin O titer
AST	aspartate transaminase
ATP	adenosine triphosphate
ATN	antiretroviral toxic neuropathy
ATS	American Thoracic Society
AV	atrioventricular
BA	bacillary angiomatosis; blood agar
BAL	bronchoalveolar lavage
BCG	bacillus Calmette–Guérin

BCYE	buffered charcoal yeast extract
BDNA	branched-chain DNA
bid	twice daily
BMT	bone marrow transplant
bp	base pair
BP	bacillary peliosis
BSE	bovine spongiform encephalopathy
BSI	bloodstream infection
BV	bacterial vaginosis
cAMP	cyclic AMP
CA-MRSA	community-acquired MRSA
CAP	community-acquired pneumonia
CAPD	continuous ambulatory peritoneal dialysis
CAUTI	catheter-associated urinary tract infection
CBC	complete blood count
CBD	common bile duct
CCDC	consultant in communicable disease control
CCEY	cefoxitin cycloserine egg yolk
CCFA	cefoxitin cycloserine fructose agar
CCHF	Congo–Crimean hemorrhagic fever
CCR	cassette chromosome recombinase
CDAD	*Clostridium difficile*–associated disease or diarrhea
CDC	Centers for Disease Control and Prevention
CDI	*Clostridium difficile* infection
CEE	central European encephalitis
CF	cystic fibrosis
CFA	colonization factor antigen
CFS	chronic fatigue syndrome
CFT	complement fixation test
CFU	colony-forming unit
CGD	chronic granulomatous disease
CHF	congestive heart failure
CIN	cervical intraepithelial neoplasia
CJD	Creutzfeldt–Jakob disease
CK	creatine kinase
CL	containment level
CLABSI	central line–associated bloodstream infection
CLED	cysteine lactose electrolyte deficient (agar)
CLSI	Clinical Laboratory Standards Institute
CMI	cell-mediated immunity
CMV	cytomegalovirus
CNA	colistin nalidixic acid (agar)

CNS	central nervous system
CO_2	carbon dioxide
CoNS	coagulase-negative staphylococci
COPD	chronic obstructive pulmonary disease
CPE	carbapenemase-producing *Enterobacteriaceae*
CPK	creatine phosphokinase
CrCl	creatinine clearance
CRF	circulating recombinant form
CRP	C-reactive protein
CSF	cerebrospinal fluid
CT	computerized tomography
CTL	cytotoxic T lymphocyte
CVC	central venous catheter
CVS	cardiovascular system
CXR	chest X-ray
CYP	cytochrome P-450
DCA	desoxycholate citrate
DF	dengue fever
DFA	direct immunofluorescence assay
DHF	dengue hemorrhagic fever
DHFR	dihydrofolate reductase
DHHS	Department of Health and Human Services
DIC	disseminated intravascular coagulation
DKA	diabetic ketoacidosis
DNA	deoxyribonucleic acid
DNase	deoxyribonuclease
DNT	dermonecrotic toxin
DSN	distal surgery neuropathy
DSP	dry sterilization process
DVT	deep venous thrombosis
EBNA	Epstein–Barr virus nuclear antigen
EBV	Epstein–Barr virus
ECG	electrocardiogram
EEE	eastern equine encephalitis
EEG	electroencephalogram
EF	edema factor
eGFR	estimated glomerular filtration rate
EI	erythema iinfectiosum
EIA	enzyme immunosorbent assay
EIEC	enteroinvasive *E. coli*
ELISA	enzyme-linked immunosorbent assay
EM	electron microscopy

EMB	ethambutol
ENT	ear, nose, and throat
EPA	Environmental Protection Agency
EPP	exposure-prone procedure
ERCP	endoscopic retrograde cholangiopancreatography
ESBL/ESBL	extended-spectrum β-lactamase
ESR	erythrocyte sedimentation rate
ESRD	end-stage renal disease
ETEC	enterotoxigenic *E. coli*
ETV	entecavir
EVD	external ventricular drain
FAT	fluorescent antibody test
FBC	full blood count
FDA	Food and Drug Administration
FEV_1	forced expiratory volume in 1 second
FFI	fatal familial insomnia
FGF	fibroblast growth factor
FHA	filamentous hemagglutinin
FNA	fine needle aspiration
FTA-Abs	fluorescent treponemal antibody antibody-absorption test
FUO	fever of unknown origin
G6PD	glucose-6-phosphate dehydrogenase
GAS	group A *Streptococcus*
GBS	group B *Streptococcus*
G-CSF	granulocyte-colony-stimulating factor
GDP	guanosine diphosphate
GERD	gastroesophageal reflux disease
GFR	glomerular filtration rate
GGT	gamma-glutamyl transferase
GI	gastrointestinal
GISA	glycopeptide-intermediate *Staphylococcus aureus*
GM-CSF	granulocyte-macrophage-colony-stimulating factor
GNR	Gram-negative rod
GRE	glycopeptide-resistant enterococcus
GSS	Gerstmann–Sträussler–Schenker (syndrome)
GU	genitourinary
GVHD	graft-vs.-host disease
HA	hemagglutinin
HAART	highly active antiretroviral therapy
HAI	hospital-acquired infection
HAP	hospital-acquired pneumonia
HAV	hepatitis A virus
Hb	hemoglobin

HBcAg	hepatitis B core antigen
HBeAg	hepatitis B e antigen
HBIG	hepatitis B immune globulin
HBsAg	hepatitis B surface antigen
HBV	hepatitis B virus
HCC	hepatocellular carcinoma
HCAI	health care–associated infection
HCV	hepatitis C virus
HCW	health care worker
HDV	hepatitis D virus
HEPA	high-efficiency particulate air
HEV	hepatitis E virus
HFM	hand, foot, and mouth disease
HHV	human herpesvirus
Hib	*H. influenzae* type b (vaccination)
HICPAC	Healthcare Infection Control Practices Advisory Committee
HIV	human immunodeficiency virus
HLA	human leukocyte antigen
HNIG	human normal immunoglobulin
HPLC	high-pressure liquid chromatography
HPV	human papillomavirus
HSP	Henoch–Schönlein purpura
HSV	herpes simplex virus
HTLV	human T-cell lymphotropic virus
HUS	hemolytic uremic syndrome
IBD	inflammatory bowel disease
ICC	infection control committee
ICP	intracranial pressure
ICU	intensive care unit
ID	infectious diseases; implanted device
IDSA	Infectious Diseases Society of America
IDU	injecting drug user
IE	infective endocarditis
IFA	immunofluorescence assay; indirect fluorescent antibody
IFAT	immunofluorescence antibody test
IFN	interferon
Ig	immunoglobulin (IgA, IgE, IgG, IgM)
IGRA	interferon-gamma release assay
IHI	Institute for Healthcare Improvement
IL	interleukin
IM	intramuscular
IMP	imipenem

IND	Investigational New Drug (protocol)
INH	isoniazid
INR	International Normalized Ratio
IP	infection preventionist
IPV	inactivated polio vaccine
IS	insertion sequence
ITP	idiopathic thrombocytopenic purpura
IUCD	intrauterine contraceptive device
IUGR	intrauterine growth restriction
IV	intravenous
IVC	intravenous catheter; inferior vena cava
IVDU	intravenous drug user
IVIG	intravenous immunoglobulin
JE	Japanese encephalitis
kbp	kilo base pair
KPC	*Kliebsiella pneumoniae* carbapenemase
KS	Kaposi sarcoma
LAM	lamivudine
LCMV	lymphocytic choriomeningitis virus
LCR	ligase chain reaction
LDH	lactate dehydrogenase
LdT	telbivudine
LF	lethal factor
LFT	liver function test
LGV	lymphogranuloma venereum
LIP	lymphoid interstitial pneumonitis
LOS	lipo-oligosaccharide
LP	lumbar puncture
LPS	lipopolysaccharide
LRTI	lower respiratory tract infection
MAC	*M. avium* complex; membrane attack complex
MAI	*Mycobacterium avium intracellulare*
MALT	mucosa-associated lymphoid tissue
MAT	microagglutination test
MBC	minimum bactericidal concentration
MC&S	microscopy, culture, and sensitivity
MDRAB	multi-drug-resistant *Acinetobacter*
MDRO	multi-drug-resistant organism
MDT	multi-drug therapy
MGE	mobile genetic element
MHC	major histocompatibility complex
MI	myocardial infarction

MIC	minimum inhibition concentration
MLEE	multi-locus enzyme electrophoresis
MLS$_B$	macrolide-lincosamide-streptogramin B (resistance)
MLST	multi-locus sequence typing
MLVA	multiple-loci variable number tandem repeat analysis
MMR	measles, mumps, rubella (vaccination)
MOTT	mycobacteria other than tuberculosis
MRI	magnetic resonance imaging
mRNA	messenger RNA
MRSA	methicillin-resistant *Staphylococcus aureus*
MSM	men who have sex with men
MSSA	methicillin-sensitive *Staphylococcus aureus*
MSU	midstream urine
MTB	*Mycobacterium tuberculosis*
MVA	modified vaccinia Ankara
NA	neuraminidase
NAD	nicotinamide adenine dinucleotide
NADP	NAD phosphate
NADPH	nicotinamide adenine dinucleotide phosphate-oxidase
NARMS	National Antimicrobial Resistance Monitoring System
NASBA	nucleic acid sequence–based amplification
NASH	non-alcoholic steatohepatitis
NCCLS	National Committee on Clinical Laboratory Standards
NEB	nebulized
NG	nasogastric
NGU	nongonococcal urethritis
NHSN	National Healthcare Safety Network
NLF	non-lactose fermenter
NNIS	National Nosocomial Infection Surveillance
NNRTI	non-nucleoside reverse transcriptase inhibitor
NPA	nasopharyngeal aspirate
NRTI	nucleoside/nucleotide analog reverse transcriptase inhibitor
NTM	nontuberculous mycobacteria
NTS	nontyphoidal *Salmonella* spp.
nvCJD	new-variant CJD
NVS	nutritionally variant streptococci
OAP	ova and parasite (exam)
od	once a day
OHS	oral hydration salts
OMP	outer membrane protein
OPAT	outpatient antimicrobial therapy
OPV	oral polio vaccine

ORF	open reading frame
PA	protective antigen
PABA	para-aminobenzoic acid
PAE	post-antibiotic effect
PAIR	puncture, aspiration, injection, and re-aspiration
PaO_2	partial pressure of arterial oxygen
PAS	para-aminosalicylic acid
PAS	periodic acid–Schiff
PBMC	peripheral blood mononuclear cell
PBP	penicillin-binding protein
PCP	Pneumocystis pneumonia
PCR	polymerase chain reaction
PCV	pneumococcal conjugate vaccine
PD	peritoneal dialysis
PDA	patent ductus arteriosis
PDGF	platelet-derived growth factor
PDH	progressive disseminated histoplasmosis
PE	pulmonary embolism
PEA	phenyl ethanol agar
PEG-IFN	pegylated interferon
PEP	post-exposure prophylaxis
PET	post-exposure treatment
PFGE	pulsed-field gel electrophoresis
PGL	persistent generalized lymphadenopathy; phenolic glycopeptide
PI	protease inhibitor
PIA	polysaccharide intracellular adhesin
PICC	peripherally inserted central catheter
PID	pelvic inflammatory disease
PIV	peripheral intravenous catheter
PK	pyruvate kinase
PML	progressive multifocal leukoencephalpathy
PO	orally
POHS	presumed ocular histoplasmosis syndrome
PPD	purified protein derivative
PPE	personal protective equipment
PPI	proton pump inhibitor
ppm	parts per million
PR	per rectum
PRA	PCR restriction enzyme assay
PRCA	pure red cell aplasia
PROM	premature rupture of the membranes
PrP	prion protein

PSA	prostate-specific antigen
PSI	Pneumonia Severity Index
PT	prothrombin time; pertussis toxin
PTLD	post-transplant lymphoproliferative disorder
PTT	partial thromboplastin time
PV	per vagina
PVC	peripheral venous catheter
PVE	prosthetic valve endocarditis
PVL	Panton–Valentine leukocidin
PZA	pyrazinamide
q	every
qid	four times a day
RA	rheumatoid arthritis
RBC	red blood cell
RCT	randomized controlled trial
REA	restriction endonuclease analysis
RFLP	restriction fragment length polymorphism
RIBA	recombinant immunoblot assay
RIDT	rapid influenza diagnostic test
RIF	rifampin
RMAT	rapid micro-agglutination test
RMSF	Rocky Mountain spotted fever
RNA	ribonucleic acid
rRNA	ribosomal RNA
RSSE	Russian spring–summer encephalitis
RSV	respiratory syncytial virus
RT-PCR	reverse transcription polymerase chain reaction
RVF	Rift Valley fever
SaO_2	arterial oxygen saturation
SARS	severe acute respiratory syndrome
SCC	staphylococcal cassette chromosome
SCID	severe combined immunodeficiency disease
SCIP	Surgical Care Improvement Project
sCJD	sporadic CJD
SDD	selective decontamination of the digestive tract
SE	staphylococcal enterotoxin
SENIC	Study on Efficacy of Nosocomial Infection Control
SHEA	Society for Healthcare Epidemiology of America
SIADH	syndrome of inappropriate antidiuretic hormone secretion
SIRS	systemic inflammatory response syndrome
SLE	systemic lupus erythematosus
SM	streptomycin

SNP	single nucleotide polymorphism
SPS	sodium polyanetholsulfonate
ss	single strand
SSA	*Salmonella Shigella* agar
SSI	surgical site infection
SSPE	subacute sclerosing panencephalitis
STI	sexually transmitted infection
SVR	sustained virological response rate
TAC	transient aplastic crisis
TB	tuberculosis
TCBS	thiosulfate citrate bile salts
TCT	tracheal cytotoxin
Td	tetanus, diphtheria (vaccine)
Tdap	tetanus, diphtheria, acellular pertussis (vaccine)
TDF	tenofovir
TEE	transesophageal echocardiography
TGF-β	transforming growth factor beta
tid	three time a day
TIG	tetanus immunoglobulin
TK	thymidine kinase
TMP-SMX	trimethoprim/sulfamethoxazole
TNF	tumor necrosis factor
TOP	topically
TPHA	treponema pallidum hemagglutination assay
TPN	total parenteral nutrition
TQM	total quality management
TP-EIA	treponema enzyme immunoassay
tRNA	transfer RNA
TSE	transmissible spongiform encephalopathy
TSS	toxic shock syndrome
TSST	toxic shock syndrome toxin
TST	tuberculin skin test
TTE	transthoracic echocardiography
TU	tuberculin units
U&E	urea and electrolytes
UICP	universal infection control precautions
UMF	ultramicrofibers
UNOS	United Network for Organ Sharing
URTI	upper respiratory tract infection
USS	ultrasound scan
UTI	urinary tract infection
UTR	untranslated region

UV	ultraviolet
VA	ventriculoatrial
VAP	ventilator-associated pneumonia
VATS	video-assisted thoracoscopic surgery
vCJD	variant CJD
VDRL	Venereal Disease Research Laboratory (test)
VEE	Venezuelan equine encephalitis
VHF	viral hemorrhagic fever
VISA	vancomycin-intermediate *Staphylococcus aureus*
VNTR	multiple-locus variable-number tandem repeats
VP	ventriculoperitoneal
VRE	vancomycin-resistant enterococci
VRSA	vancomycin-resistant *Staphylococcus aureus*
VUR	vesicoureteric reflux
VZIG	varicella zoster immune globulin
VZV	varicella zoster virus
WBC	white blood cell
WCC	white cell count
WEE	western equine encephalitis
WHO	World Health Organization
XDR	extensively drug resistant
XLD	xylose lysine deoxycholate
ZN	Ziehl–Neelsen (stain)

Antimicrobials

Definitions

Antimicrobials/anti-infectives
These are umbrella terms for drugs with activity against microorganisms. They include antibacterials, antivirals, antifungals, and antiparasitic agents.

Antibacterial
Antibacterial agents are anti-infective agents that are effective at treating or preventing bacterial infections.

Antibiotic
This is strictly defined as a chemical compound made by a microorganism that inhibits or kills other microorganisms at low concentrations.[1] This does not include synthetic agents, although in practice it is often used for any antibacterial.

Antifungal
Antifungal agents are used to treat both superficial and invasive fungal infections. They include agents such as amphotericin B, fluconazole, and caspofungin.

Antiparasitic
Antiparasitic agents are used to treat parasitic diseases and include anti-protozoals and anthelmintics.

Antiviral
Antiviral compounds are those agents used to treat viral infections.

Reference
1. Waksman SA (1945). *Microbial Antagonisms and Antibiotic Substances*. The Commonwealth Fund, New York..

Development of antibiotics

Substances with some form of anti-infective action have been used since ancient times. The Chinese used "moldy" soybean curd to treat boils and carbuncles. South American Indians chewed cinchona tree bark (contains quinine) for malaria. They also wore "moldy" sandals for foot infections.

In Europe one of the earliest recorded examples was the use of mercury to treat syphilis in the 1400s.

In 1877, Louis Pasteur showed that injections of extracts of soil bacteria cured anthrax in animals.

In 1908–1910, Paul Erlich, known as the father of chemotherapy and a Nobel Prize winner, synthesized arsenic compounds that were effective against syphilis.

In 1924 the compound actinomycetin, so named because it is produced by Actinomycetes, was discovered.

In 1932, Domagk discovered the dye prontosil, which cured streptococcal infections in animals. The active group turned out to be the sulfonamide attached to the dye, and by 1945 over 5000 sulfonamide derivatives had been developed. However, clinical use of these compounds has been limited by their adverse effects and by drug resistance.

In 1939, Dubos isolated two agents that were active against Gram-positive organisms (gramicidin and tyrocidin) from *Bacillus brevis*.

In 1944–1945, Waksman isolated streptomycin from the soil microbe *Streptomyces griseus*. It was active against *Mycobacterium tuberculosis* and some Gram-negative organisms. For this discovery Waksman was awarded the Nobel Prize.

History of penicillin

In 1928, Alexander Fleming returned to St Mary's Hospital after a weekend away to discover that the mold *Penicillium notatum* had contaminated his culture plates. He observed that the colonies of *S. aureus* nearest the mold had lysed, while those further away had not, and hypothesized that the *Penicillium* had released a product that caused bacterial cell lysis. He called this product *penicillin*.

Although Fleming discovered penicillin, he was unable to purify sufficient quantities for clinical trials. In 1939, Howard Florey, Ernst Chain, and Norman Heatley, working in Oxford, obtained the *Penicillium* fungus from Fleming. They overcame the technical difficulties and conducted clinical trials to demonstrate the efficacy of penicillin.

Mass production soon began in the UK and United States. Initially penicillin was used almost exclusively for soldiers injured during the Second World War. It became widely available by 1946.

As soon as he discovered penicillin, Fleming warned of the development of penicillin resistance. He was right, and resistance was seen almost immediately. Scientists have chemically modified the drug to create derivatives (e.g., ampicillin) less susceptible to enzymatic degradation.

Table 1.1 shows a timeline of the discovery or introduction of many antibiotics.

Table 1.1 Timeline of the discovery/introduction of some anti-infectives

Year	Antibiotic	Class of antibiotic
1928	Penicillin discovered	β-lactam
1932	Prontosil discovered	Sulfonamide
1942	Penicillin introduced	β-lactam
1943	Streptomycin discovered	Aminoglycoside
1945	Cephalosporins discovered	β-lactam
1947	Chloramphenicol discovered	Protein synthesis inhibitor
1947	Chlortetracycline discovered	Tetracycline
1949	Neomycin discovered	Aminoglycoside
1952	Erythromycin discovered	Macrolide
1956	Vancomycin discovered	Glycopeptide
1960	Flucloxacillin introduced	β-lactam

Table 1.1 (Contd.)

Year	Antibiotic	Class of antibiotic
1961	Ampicillin introduced	β-lactam
1963	Gentamicin discovered	Aminoglycoside
1964	Cephalosporins introduced	β-lactam
1964	Vancomycin introduced	Glycopeptide
1966	Doxycycline introduced	Tetracycline
1971	Rifampin introduced	Rifamycin
1974	Co-trimoxazole introduced	Sulfonamide and trimethoprim
1976	Amikacin introduced	Aminoglycoside
1984	Ampicillin/clavulanate introduced	β-lactam/β-lactamase inhibitor
1987	Imipenem/cilastatin introduced	Carbapenem
1987	Ciprofloxacin introduced	Quinolone
1993	Azithromycin and clarithromycin	Macrolide
1999	Quinupristin/dalfopristin introduced	Streptogramin
2000	Linezolid introduced	Oxazolidinone
2003	Daptomycin introduced	Lipopeptide
2004	Telithromycin introduced	Ketolide
2005	Tigecycline introduced	Glycylcycline

Global antibiotic use

The quantity and trends of antibiotic use at the national level are usually difficult to obtain. However, it is generally thought that about 50% of all antimicrobials are used in human medicine and about 50% for animals and crops. The total amount of antimicrobials used varies between countries, with developed countries using proportionately more than developing countries.

Different countries have different antibiotics available, e.g., Japan has a large number of carbapenems, whereas the U.S. has only four (imipenem, meropenem, doripenem, and ertapenem). Just because an antibiotic is widely prescribed in one country does not mean it will be licensed in another, e.g., teicoplanin is widely used in Europe but is not available in the United States, where vancomycin is used predominantly.

Human use of antibiotics

Most infections are treated in the community, by outpatient providers; this accounts for the greatest number of antibiotic prescriptions. However, there is also significant use of anti-infective agents within hospitals. The quantity of antibiotics used varies between hospitals, depending on patient populations cared for at various facilities (e.g., hospitals with large intensive care units, ongology or transplant programs are likely to use more antibiotics).

Sometimes hospitals with similar patient populations have different approaches to prescribing antibiotics, which may be influenced by local antimicrobial susceptibility data. In many institutions, the use of anti-infective agents is driven by an antimicrobial stewardship program, which is a multidisciplinary group consisting of specialists in infectious disease, microbiology, infection prevention, and pharmacy that works together to promote appropriate anti-infective use.

Problems with human use of antibiotics

Overuse of antibiotics has led to rising rates of antimicrobial resistance, with the result that a few organisms have become virtually untreatable (e.g., vancomycin-resistant *S. aureus* and extensively drug-resistant Gram-negative pathogens). The impact of resistance in terms of increased morbidity and mortality and economic and social consequences are considerable. In the United States, the Centers for Disease Control and Prevention (CDC) estimates that one-third of all outpatient antibiotic prescriptions are not required.

Hence, many organizations have been working to reduce inappropriate prescribing, through public education (e.g., most upper respiratory tract infections [URTIs] are caused by viruses, so antibiotics will not work), and changing the practice of health care prescribers (e.g., limiting treatment duration for an uncomplicated urinary tract infection [UTI] to 3 days).

Other problems associated with the overuse of antibiotics include superinfection (e.g., with *Candida albicans, Clostridium difficile*) and the unnecessary risk of adverse effects and drug interactions and expense.

In the developing world, a number of additional problems exist:

- Antibiotics are often available without prescription.
- If the patient does take an appropriate antibiotic, they may take the wrong dose for the incorrect duration.
- Often, patients self-treat with anti-infectives prescribed for others. In these cases, the agent may be inappropriate, so the infection remains untreated and patients may therefore develop a more severe or complicated infection before consulting a doctor.

Nonhuman use of antibiotics

Antimicrobials have been used increasingly for the prevention and treatment of infections in animals (e.g., on farms, in fish factories, and for domestic pets) and in the environment (e.g., crop production). Since the discovery of their growth-promoting abilities, they have also been added to animal feed (particularly for pigs and poultry).

In addition, some antibiotics increase feed efficiency (the amount of feed absorbed by an animal), increasing the chance that the animal reaches its target weight on time.

Other examples of nonhuman use include the following:

- Tetracycline is sprayed on apple plantations to treat fire-blight.

- Oxytetracycline is added to water in commercial fish farms to treat infections.
- Antibiotics are used to eliminate bacterial growth inside oil pipelines.

When farm animals consume antibiotics in their feed, they excrete them into the environment. This pattern may select for antibiotic-resistant organisms that may then infect other animal species. In addition, this practice may also promote colonization of the food chain with drug-resistant pathogens.

Antibiotics in the environment undoubtedly contribute to increasing antibiotic resistance, particularly among food-borne pathogens such as *Salmonella* spp. and *Campylobacter* spp. Many organizations have developed strategies to try to control the nonhuman use of antibiotics (particularly in agriculture and animal husbandry) and thus reduce the development of resistance. These include the Alliance for the Prudent Use of Antibiotics (APUA) and the World Health Organization (WHO).

Table 1.2 gives sources of information on antimicrobial resistance.

Table 1.2 Sources of information on antimicrobial resistance

Information	Web address
Alliance for the Prudent Use of Antibiotics	http://www.tufts.edu/med/apau
World Health Organization	http://www.who.int/foodborne_disease/resistance/en/
National Antimicrobial Resistance Monitoring System (NARMS)	http://www.cdc.gov/narms/
Get Smart: Know When Antibiotics Work on the Farm (CDC)	http://www.cdc.gov/narms/get_smart.htm
Food and Drug Administration (FDA): NARMS	http://www.fda.gov/AnimalVeterinary/ SafetyHealth/AntimicrobialResistance/ NationalAntimicrobialResistanceMonitoringSystem/ ucm209496.htm
Drug resistance updates	http://health.surfwax.com/files/Antibiotic Resistance. html
History of antibiotic resistance	http://www.fda.gov/fdac/features/795_antibio.html
The Alexander project	http://www.ncbi.nlm.nih.gov/pubmed/12865398
The MYSTIC program	http://www.blackwellpublishing.com/eccmid17/ abstract.asp?id=57603

Mechanisms of action

Antimicrobial agents are classified by their specific mechanisms of action against bacterial cells. The mechanisms of action of antimicrobial agents against Gram-positive and Gram-negative bacteria are very similar and can be divided into five categories:

• Inhibition of cell wall synthesis
• Inhibition of protein synthesis
• Inhibition of nucleic acid synthesis
• Inhibition of folate synthesis
• Disruption of the cytoplasmic membrane.

Inhibition of cell wall synthesis

Antimicrobial agents that interfere with cell wall synthesis block pepti-doglycan synthesis. They are active against growing bacteria and are bactericidal.

• *Gram-negative bacteria:* β-lactam antimicrobials enter the cell through porin channels in the outer membrane and bind to penicillin-binding proteins (PBPs) on the surface of the cytoplasmic membrane. This blocks their function, causing weakened or defective cell walls and leads to cell lysis and death.
• *Gram-positive bacteria* lack an outer membrane, so β-lactam antimicrobials diffuse directly through the cell wall and bind to PBPs, which results in weakened cell walls and cell lysis.

Inhibition of protein synthesis

• *Tetracyclines* bind to the 30S ribosomal subunit and block attachment of transfer RNA (tRNA) and addition of amino acids to the protein chain. Tetracyclines are bacteriostatic.
• *Aminoglycosides* also bind to the 30S ribosomal subunit and prevent its attachment to messenger RNA (mRNA). They can also cause misreading of the mRNA, resulting in insertion of the wrong amino acid or interference in the ability of amino acids to connect with each other. The combined effect of these two mechanisms is bactericidal.
• *Macrolides and lincosamides* attach to the 50S ribosomal subunit causing termination of the growing protein chain. They are bacteriostatic.
• *Chloramphenicol* also binds to the 50S ribosomal subunit and interferes with binding of amino acids to the growing chain. It is also bacteriostatic.
• *Linezolid* (an oxazolidinone) binds to the 23S ribosomal RNA of the 50S subunit and prevents formation of a functional 70S initiation complex, which is necessary for protein synthesis. It is bacteriostatic.

Inhibition of nucleic acid synthesis

• *Fluoroquinolones* interfere with DNA synthesis by blocking the enzyme DNA gyrase. This enzyme binds to DNA and introduces double-stranded breaks that allow the DNA complex to unwind. Fluoroquinolones bind to the DNA gyrase–DNA complex and allow

broken DNA strands to be released into the cell, resulting in cell death.
- *Rifampin* binds to DNA-dependent RNA polymerase, which blocks synthesis of RNA and results in cell death.

Inhibition of folate synthesis
- For many organisms, para-aminobenzoic acid (PABA) is an essential metabolite that is involved in the synthesis of folic acid, an important precursor to the synthesis of nucleic acids.
- *Sulfonamides* are structural analogs of PABA and compete with PABA for the enzyme dihydropteroate synthetase.
- *Trimethoprim* acts on the folic acid synthesis pathway at a point after the sulfonamides, inhibiting the enzyme dihydrofolate reductase.
- Both trimethoprim and the sulfonamides are bacteriostatic. When they are used together (e.g., co-trimoxazole), they produce a sequential blockade of the folic acid synthesis pathway and have a synergistic effect.

Disruption of the cytoplasmic membrane
- *Polymyxin* molecules diffuse through the outer membrane and cell wall of susceptible cells to the cytoplasmic membrane. They bind to the cytoplasmic membrane and disrupt and destabilize it. This causes the cytoplasm to leak out of the cell, resulting in cell death.
- *Daptomycin* exhibits activity by destroying membrane potential. It is believed that the mechanism of this activity is a two-step process by which daptomycin inserts itself into the cell membrane causing membrane depolarization followed by a halt of protein synthesis resulting in bacterial cell death. Daptomycin is bactericidal.

Mechanisms of resistance

There are a number of ways by which microorganisms become resistant to antimicrobial agents:
- Production of enzymes
- Alteration in outer membrane permeability
- Alteration of target sites
- Efflux pumps
- Alteration of metabolic pathways

Production of enzymes
β-*lactamases* are enzymes that hydrolyse β-lactam drugs. In Gram-negative bacteria, the β-lactam drug enters the cell through the porin channels and encounters β-lactamases in the periplasmic space. This results in hydrolysis of the β-lactam molecules before they reach their PBP targets.

There are several different types of β-lactamases that confer resistance to different Gram-negative pathogens.

In Gram-positive bacteria, the β-lactamases are secreted extracellularly into the surrounding medium and destroy the β-lactam molecules before they enter the cell.

- *Aminoglycoside-modifying enzymes:* Gram-negative bacteria may produce adenylating, phosphorylating, or acetylating enzymes that modify an aminoglycoside so that it is no longer active.
- *Chloramphenicol acetyl transferase:* Gram-negative bacteria may produce an acetyl transferase that modifies chloramphenicol so that it is no longer active.

Alteration in outer-membrane permeability

- Gram-negative bacteria may become resistant to β-lactam antibiotics by developing permeability barriers.
- Mutations resulting in the loss of porin channels in the outer membrane no longer allow the entrance and passage of antibiotic molecules into the cell.
- Alterations in proton motive force may result in reduced inner-membrane permeability.

Alteration of target sites

- PBPs in Gram-positive and Gram-negative bacteria may be altered through mutation so that β-lactams can no longer bind to them.
- Methylation of ribosomal RNA confers resistance to macrolides, linconsamides, and streptogramins.
- Mutations in the chromosomal genes for DNA gyrase and topoisomerase IV confer quinolone resistance.

Efflux pumps

A wide variety of efflux pumps produce antimicrobial resistance in both Gram-positive and Gram-negative bacteria. Active efflux of antibiotics is mediated by transmembrane proteins which form channels that actively export an antimicrobial agent out of the cell as fast as it enters. This is the main mechanism of resistance to tetracyclines.

Alteration of metabolic pathways

Some microorganisms develop an altered metabolic pathway that bypasses the reaction inhibited by the antimicrobial. Mutations that inactivate thymidylate synthetase block the conversion of deoxyuridylate to thymidylate. These mutants use exogenous thymine or thymidine for DNA synthesis and therefore are resistant to folate synthesis antagonists.

Molecular genetics of resistance

Genetic variability is essential for microbial evolution and may occur by a variety of mechanisms:
- Point mutations
- Rearrangements of large segments of DNA from one location of a bacterial chromosome or plasmid to another
- Acquisition of foreign DNA from other bacteria, via a mobile genetic element (MGE)

Acquisition of resistance, in the presence of the antibiotic, confers a survival advantage on the host, thus leading to the emergence of resistant clones. The overuse, incorrect use, or injudicious use of antibiotics contributes to this problem and explains why new resistance patterns tend to emerge in areas of the hospital with the greatest antibiotic consumption (e.g., intensive care units).

This antibiotic resistance may be passed vertically to future generations through clonal expansion, resulting in a bacterial population that is resistant to an antibiotic.

Point mutations

These are often referred to as *single nucleotide polymorphisms* (SNPs). The bacterial genome is dynamic, in that bacteria are constantly undergoing mutations. Some of these mutations will (by chance) result in a survival advantage to the organism, e.g., due to increased virulence or antibiotic resistance.

In certain environments, these will be preferentially selected for, thus the mutation that arose by chance will be preferentially retained and passed to future generations. Examples of point mutations include the generation of β-lactamases and fluoroquinolone resistance.

Mobile genetic elements (MGE)

These are pieces of DNA that can move around between genomes. They may thus be involved in the horizontal transfer of resistance genes between bacteria, in contrast to the vertical transfer of resistance by clonal expansion (see list following). Bacterial genomes consist of core genes and accessory genes—the latter are defined by acquisition and loss.

There are several different MGEs, described in the following list.

Plasmids

These are extrachromosomal pieces of circular DNA, which vary in size from 10 kilobase pairs (kbp) to over 400 kbp. In addition to carrying resistance genes, they may determine other functions, e.g., virulence factors and metabolic capabilities.

They are autonomous self-replicating genetic elements that possess an origin for replication and genes that facilitate their maintenance in the host bacteria. Conjugative plasmids require additional genes to initiate self-transfer.

Insertion sequences (IS)

These are short DNA sequences that are usually only 700 to 2500 base pairs (bp) long. They encode for an enzyme needed for transposition (i.e., to excise a segment of DNA from one position in the chromosome and insert it elsewhere) and a regulatory protein, which either stimulates or inhibits the transposition activity.

They are thus different from transposons, which also carry accessory genes, such as antibiotic resistance genes. The coding region in an insertion sequence is usually flanked by inverted repeats.

Transposons

These are often called "jumping genes" and may contain insertion sequences. They cannot replicate independently but can move between one replicating piece of DNA to another, e.g., from a chromosome to a plasmid. Conjugative transposons mediate their own transfer between bacteria, whereas non-conjugative transposons need prior integration into a plasmid to be transferred.

Integrons

These may be defined as a genetic element that possesses a site (*att*1) at which additional DNA in the form of gene cassettes can be integrated by site-specific mutation. They also encode a gene, integrase, that mediates these site-specific recombination events.

Gene cassettes normally consist of an antibiotic resistance gene and a 59 base element that functions as a site-specific recombination site. The largest integrons (e.g., in *V. cholerae*) can contain hundreds of gene cassettes.

Bacteriophages

A bacteriophage is a virus that infects bacteria and may become integrated into the bacterial chromosome (and is then called a *prophage*). They typically consist of an outer protein enclosing genetic material (which may be single- or double-stranded DNA or RNA).

Bacteriophages may be considered MGEs, but are rarely involved in the transfer of resistance genes. They have been used as an alternative to antibiotics (phage therapy) in Eastern Europe and the former USSR for ~60 years.

Clonal expansion

Clonal expansion refers to the multiplication of a single "ancestor" cell. This may result in the propagation of antibiotic resistance into daughter cells. The antibiotic resistance genes will be passed from one generation of bacteria to the next, which is also called *vertical transfer of resistance*.

If an organism becomes resistant to an antibiotic, either by mutation or acquisition of a mobile genetic element, it will have a survival advantage in an environment where that antibiotic is present. Thus the daughter cells that are generated will be positively selected for over daughter cells from another antibiotic sensitive strains of the bacteria, and future generations will be resistant to that agent.

A *bacterial clone* (see Box 1.1) refers to all organisms that are likely to have arisen from a common ancestor. This may not be immediately obvious—e.g., in the case of *S. typhi*, the common origin has been estimated by molecular techniques (multiple locus sequence typing [MLST]) to have existed 50,000 years ago.

Examples of more recent clonal expansion relating to the spread of antibiotic resistance genes are methicillin-resistant *Staphylococcus aureus* (MRSA) and penicillin-resistant pneumococci.

> **Box 1.1 Important definitions for anti-infective therapy**
> - *Isolate* refers to a pure culture. It says nothing about typing.
> - *Clone* refers to bacterial cultures that have been isolated independently, from different sources, in different places, and maybe at different times, but are so similar phenotypically and genotypically that the most likely explanation is that they arose from a common ancestor.
> - *Strain* refers to a phenotypically and/or genotypically distinctive group of isolates. It is dependent on the typing scheme used, and some experts suggest avoiding the use of this term.
> - *Type* refers to organisms with the same pattern or set of markers displayed by a strain, when the bacteria are subject to a particular typing system.

Breakpoints

Definition

Breakpoints are antibiotic concentrations that have been established for most antimicrobial–organism combinations to interpret the results of susceptibility testing. Thus strains are categorized as susceptible, resistant, or intermediate (or susceptible dose-dependent in the case of azole susceptibility testing against yeast) to each drug tested. When new breakpoints are set, clinical, microbiological, and pharmacological factors must be considered.

Practical aspects

Each isolate cultured in the microbiology laboratory that is deemed significant (rather than a likely contaminant) is tested against a panel of appropriate antibiotics. This panel may vary between hospitals, depending on local antibiotic policies, available testing systems, and microbiologist preferences.

Many methods exist for susceptibility testing. These include Stoke's method, Kirby–Bauer disk diffusion, and minimum inhibition concentration (MIC) determination by broth microdilution, E-Test,® or automated testing methods. Methods for conducting susceptibility testing, including interpretive criteria, are established by the Clinical and Laboratory Standards Institute (CLSI), formerly National Committee on Clinical Laboratory Standards (NCCLS). The FDA also establishes breakpoints for antibiotic susceptibility testing; however, since CLSI is the accrediting body for clinical laboratories in the United States, the CLSI standards are more commonly followed.

Because of differences in the testing methods, MIC breakpoints are established for each anti-infective agent as well as a zone of inhibition breakpoints if disk diffusion testing is conducted. If the diameter of clearance is greater than or equal to the susceptible breakpoint, the isolate is classified as sensitive to that antibiotic. If there is no zone of clearing, or the diameter of the zone is less than or equal to the resistant breakpoint, the isolate is classified as resistant to that antibiotic. While zone of inhibition and MIC are often related, the correlation is not perfect, thus the zone of inhibition cannot be used to estimate MIC.

Each isolate is reported as *sensitive*, *intermediate*, or *resistant* to each antibiotic tested. Some microbiologists only report certain sensitivity results (usually consistent with the hospital antibiotic policies) to encourage use of certain drugs, a practice also referred to as *cascade reporting*.

It is worth remembering that susceptibility data not reported in the initial results may be readily available, so if none of the sensitivity results available are suitable, contact a microbiologist. Also, when an organism is "fully sensitive" this only means fully sensitive to the antibiotics tested, not to all agents.

Heteroresistance

Heteroresistance occurs when one bacterial subpopulation has a higher MIC than that of the rest of the bacterial population. Often, this higher MIC may not be detected by routine susceptibility testing, giving the appearance of a susceptible isolate with clinical failure when treated.

Heteroresistance may be difficult to diagnose and result in poor response to treatment. Examples include the following:

- *S. aureus* and vancomycin
- *C. neoformans* and azoles
- *M. tuberculosis* and rifampin
- *E. faecium* and vancomycin
- *A. baumanii* and carbapenems and colistin
- *H. pylori* and metronidazole and amoxicillin
- *S. pneumoniae* and penicillin.

Pharmacokinetics

This is what the body does to the drug; it comprises absorption, distribution, metabolism, and excretion (mnemonic: ADME)

Absorption

To be effective, a drug must reach the site of the infection. In some cases this is possible by topical application (e.g., nystatin suspension for oral candidiasis), but in many cases systemic absorption is required for drug delivery.

Some drugs are poorly absorbed when given by mouth (e.g., aminoglycosides and glycopeptides) and are therefore always given parenterally. Occasionally, oral drugs may be used to treat luminal infections when absorption is not needed, e.g., oral vancomycin for *C. difficile*.

If a drug is absorbed when given by mouth, the proportion absorbed into the systemic circulation is called the *bioavailability*. Drugs given intravenously have 100% bioavailability. Depending on the properties of the drug, the time profile of absorption versus elimination may be more important than the total amount of drug absorbed (see Pharmacodynamics, p. 14).

Absorption may be affected by interactions with other drugs or food that may bind the drug (e.g., quinolones should not be given with divalent cations such as calcium). Altered physiology (e.g., diarrhea) may reduce absorption. None of the commonly prescribed antibiotics are subject to significant first-pass metabolism in the liver.

Distribution

The *volume of distribution* is an estimate of the total distribution of the drug within the body. A drug with a small volume of distribution is largely confined to the plasma. A drug with a large volume of distribution is widely distributed, e.g., fat-soluble drugs.

Metabolism

Some antibiotics are metabolized in the liver by isoforms of cytochrome P450 (CYP), of which the CYP3A4 isoenzyme is the most abundant (Box 1.2). Rifampin induces the activity of CYP3A4, leading to increased metabolism (and reduced efficacy) of drugs that share this pathway, e.g., HIV protease inhibitors.

In contrast, the azole antifungals and some macrolides inhibit the activity of CYP3A4, which will reduce the metabolism (and may increase toxicity) of drugs also metabolized by this isoenzyme. Always check for interactions before starting or stopping antibiotics and seek expert advice if unsure.

Box 1.2 Examples of antimicrobials with interactions mediated by CYP3A4

- *Inducers:* rifampin
- *Inhibitors:* ketoconazole, itraconazole, erythromycin, clarithromycin
- *Substrates:* ritonavir, saquinavir, indinavir, nelfinavir

Excretion

This can be divided into *renal* (e.g., aminoglycosides, glycopeptides) and *nonrenal* (biliary tree, e.g., ceftriaxone; gastrointestinal tract [GI] tract, e.g., azithromycin). Together with metabolism, clearance determines the *half-life* of the drug (the time for the blood concentration to decrease by half).

Steady state occurs when a patient has taken the drug for a period of time equal to 5–7 half-lives. Calculating creatinine clearance (CrCl, see Antimicrobials in renal impairment, p 21) as a measure of renal function can be essential for safe dosing of some renally excreted drugs, such as aminoglycosides (see Aminoglycosides, p. 39).

Pharmacodynamics

Pharmacodynamics describes the dynamic interaction between drug, pathogen, and host. Together these components of pharmacodynamics describe how a particular anti-infective will work within a host to fight infection.

Bacteriostatic

These are antibiotics that inhibit growth and replication of bacteria but are nonlethal to the pathogen (e.g., drugs that inhibit folic acid synthesis, see pp. 7–8).

Bactericidal

These are antibiotics that cause bacterial cell death by inhibition of *(a)* cell wall synthesis, *(b)* nucleic acid synthesis, or *(c)* protein synthesis. Some antibiotics may be bacteriostatic at low concentrations but bactericidal at higher concentrations.

Minimum inhibitory concentration (MIC)

This is the concentration of antimicrobial required to inhibit the overnight growth of 90% (MIC_{90}) or 50% (MIC_{50}) of a particular bacterial or fungal isolate in vitro. Clinically, the MIC is used to assign an organism to a susceptibility category (sensitive, intermediate, resistant).

Minimum bactericidal concentration (MBC)

This is the concentration of antimicrobial required to kill 90% (MBC_{90}) or 50% (MBC_{50}) of a bacterial isolate in vitro. Typically, the MBC is 2 to 4 times the MIC for the same isolate.

Historically, the MBC was clinically used in the treatment of endocarditis but is now rarely determined or reported.

Synergism

This occurs when the activity of two drugs together is greater than the sum of their actions if each were given separately.

An example is the use of ampicillin and gentamicin for enterococcal infections (see Enterococci, p. 192). Ampicillin acts on the cell wall to enable gentamicin to gain entry to the cell and act on the ribosome.

Antagonism

Antagonism is present when one drug diminishes the activity of another. In this case, administering both antibiotics together may result in a worse clinical outcome than just giving one antibiotic.

For example, co-administration of a bacteriostatic agent (e.g., tetracycline) with a β-lactam may inhibit cell growth and prevent the bactericidal activity of the β-lactam.

Concentration-dependent killing

The antibiotic kills the organism when its concentration is well above the MIC of the organism. The greater the peak, the greater the killing, e.g., once-daily dosing of gentamicin (see Aminoglycosides, p. 39).

Time-dependent killing

The antibiotic *only* kills the bacteria when its concentration is above the MIC of the organism, but increasing the concentration does not lead to increased killing. Most recommended dosing schedules account for this (see Penicillins, p. 25; Cephalosporins, p. 27; Macrolides, p. 42).

On a practical level it is important when adjusting the dose of glycopeptides (see Glycopeptides, p. 36).

Post-antibiotic effect (PAE)

The *post-antibiotic effect* (PAE) is defined as the time during which bacterial growth is inhibited after antibiotic concentrations have fallen below the MIC. The mechanism for this is unclear, but it may be due to a delay in the bacteria re-entering a log-growth period.

Several factors influence the presence or duration of the PAE, including the type of organism, type of antimicrobial, concentration of antimicrobial, duration of antimicrobial exposure, and antimicrobial combinations.

In vitro, β-lactam antimicrobials demonstrate a PAE against Gram-positive cocci but not against Gram-negative bacilli. Antimicrobials that inhibit RNA or protein synthesis produce a PAE against Gram-positive cocci and Gram-negative bacilli.

The clinical relevance of the PAE is probably most important when designing dosage regimens. The presence of a long PAE allows aminoglycosides to be dosed infrequently; the lack of an in vivo PAE suggests that β-lactam antimicrobials require frequent or continuous dosing.

Eagle effect

This is a paradoxical effect, first described by Eagle in 1948, whereby higher concentrations of penicillin result in decreased killing of staphylococci and streptococci. Eagle also showed that this paradoxical effect seen in vitro correlated with an adverse outcome in vivo.

This effect has since been described with a number of other antimicrobials and organisms, e.g., ampicillin and *E. faecalis*, carbenicillin and *P. mirabilis*, cefotaxime and *S. aureus* and *P. aeruginosa*, and aminoglycosides and Gram-negative bacteria. Recently, a similar effect has been reported in vitro with *Candida* spp. and the echinocandins.

Preventing the development of resistance with pharmacodynamic targets

Studies are focusing on defining the breakpoints that predict the emergence of resistance. An ideal antibiotic should have a low rate of resistance mutation, high fitness cost of resistance, and low rate of fitness restoring complementary mutation.

Novel parameters that are being investigated include the following:

- *Mutant prevention concentration:* a target drug concentration that would restrict selection of resistant mutants
- *Mutant selection window:* the concentration range between the minimal concentration required to block growth of wild-type bacteria, up to the concentration needed to inhibit the growth of the least susceptible, single-step mutant. There are different concentration ranges for each organism–drug combination. In clinical practice, drug regimens would be designed to avoid this window and thus prevent resistance.

Choosing an antimicrobial

Before prescribing an antimicrobial, the following factors should be considered:

- *Host factors:* medical history (e.g., immune history of patient), severity of infection, allergies, renal and hepatic function, pregnancy, breast feeding, age, weight, ability to tolerate drugs by mouth, compliance
- *Organism factors:* known or likely organism(s) and known or likely antimicrobial susceptibility. Always consult your local antibiogram and institutional guidelines.
- *Drug factors:* pharmacokinetics (see Pharmacokinetics, p. 13), pharmacodynamics (see Pharmacodynamics, p. 14), side effects, interactions with other medications, previous therapy
- *Dose:* may depend not just on the severity of the infection but also on host factors (age, weight, renal function). An inadequate dose may result in a suboptimal clinical response and increase the likelihood of antibiotic resistance. Conversely, too large a dose may result in unnecessary toxicity and expense
- *Route of administration:* antimicrobials may be given by a variety of routes: orally (PO), intravenously (IV), intramuscularly (IM), per rectum (PR), per vagina (PV), aerosolized/nebulized (NEB), or topically (TOP)
- *Duration of treatment:* knowing the anticipated duration of treatment can help aid drug selection. For example, when a prolonged course of anti-infectives is needed, selecting a therapy with an oral formulation may be desirable. Ideally, duration of treatment should be adequate to cure infection but minimized to prevent collateral damage from the antimicrobial, such as *C. difficile* infection or other adverse effects.

Routes of administration

Oral administration (PO)

Many of the available antibacterial agents have an oral formulation available. If a drug is absorbed when given by mouth, the proportion that is absorbed into the systemic circulation is called the *bioavailability* (see Pharmacokinetics, p. 13). Often, the bioavailability of a drug is influenced by drug formulation and conditions at the time of administration.

For example, the quinolone antibacterials should not be administered with divalent cations such as calcium and magnesium, and oral itraconazole capsules are not absorbed in a high pH environment and must be avoided in patients on acid suppressive therapy. Some drugs are not absorbed at all when given orally.

Lack of absorption can be advantageous when treating luminal infections, e.g., oral vancomycin for *C. difficile* and neomycin in hepatic failure where systemic drug toxicity can be avoided while providing effective drug treatment at the site of infection.

Intravenous administration (IV)

The intravenous route of administration provides 100% bioavailability (see Box 1.3). This route guarantees systemic drug exposure in cases where gastrointestinal tract function is questionable.

Indications

Antimicrobials are given intravenously in the following situations:
- Life-threatening infections—e.g., meningitis, sepsis, and endocarditis require intravenous therapy. Antibiotics may be given as prolonged infusions or bolus doses, depending on the drug.
- Inability to take or absorb oral medications—e.g., NPO status, severe vomiting or diarrhea, esophageal or intestinal obstruction, postoperative ileus
- Poor oral bioavailability. Some drugs are not absorbed if given orally, e.g., aminoglycosides, glycopeptides, and colistin.

Disadvantages

Intravenous therapy may be associated with a number of problems:
- Side effects, which may be local (e.g., phlebitis) or systemic (e.g., rapid infusion may result in infusion-related reactions such as the "red man syndrome" with vancomycin)
- Line infections, which may be local (e.g., exit site, tunnel or pocket infections) or systemic (e.g., bacteremia, endocarditis)
- Inconvenience to patient
- Need to stay in the hospital. This may be overcome by the use of outpatient antimicrobial therapy (OPAT), which is now widely available but may be limited to certain agents and requires additional logistical considerations
- Intravenous antibiotics may be considerably more expensive than the oral formulation due to cost of the agent or additional healthcare personnel required for use.

IV-to-oral switch

As a result of the problems associated with IV therapy, many hospitals employ IV-to-oral switch protocols for certain conditions that encourage clinicians to change to oral antibiotics as soon as this is safe. Criteria include the following:
- Suitable oral agent available
- Signs and symptoms of infection resolving (including resolution of fever and normalization of white blood cell count [WBC])
- Patient can tolerate, swallow, and absorb oral antibiotics
- No symptoms or signs of ongoing sepsis
- Some conditions are specifically excluded (e.g., meningitis and endocarditis).

Box 1.3 Practical points regarding IV antibiotics

- Many people believe that IV antibiotics are somehow stronger than oral antibiotics. This is not necessarily the case (e.g., ciprofloxacin is as effective when given orally as when given IV).
- The oral and IV doses of the same antibiotic may be different (e.g., metronidazole, penicillin).

Intramuscular administration (IM)

This is an infrequent method of administration, largely because absorption is unpredictable and the injection may be painful. Local side effects include irritation and, more rarely, development of a sterile abscess. The advantages are that there is no question of compliance and the agent can easily be administered in the community.

Intramuscular administration is commonly used for vaccinations, in sexually transmitted disease clinics, and for tuberculosis (TB) treatment in the developing world. However, its use for outpatient management of certain infections has grown in recent years, particularly with IM ceftriaxone and the aminoglycosides.

Never give IM injections to patients with bleeding or clotting disorders, e.g., thrombocytopenia, hemophilia.

Examples of drugs given intramuscularly

- Procaine penicillin (procaine benzylpenicillin) is given as daily IM injections in early syphilis or late latent syphilis.
- Ceftriaxone IM may be given as secondary prophylaxis for contacts of meningococcal disease if the individual is unable to take rifampin or ciprofloxacin (although it is not licensed for this indication).
- Ceftriaxone IM is used for gonococcal infection (particularly pharyngeal or conjunctival infection).
- Streptomycin IM is commonly given for treatment of TB in the developing world.
- Gentamicin IM is sometimes given to manage resistant UTIs in patients in the community.

Topical administration (TOP)

Many antimicrobials are available as topical preparations. They are most commonly used to treat superficial infections, particularly in dermatology. However, they are not without risk and should be used with caution. Before prescribing a topical drug consider the following:

- Does the condition require treatment? Not all skin conditions that are oozing, crusted, or pustular are infected. Would improving hygiene resolve the situation? Even if an organism is cultured from a swab, it may represent colonization and not require treatment
- Would systemic antibiotics be more appropriate? Some skin infections (e.g., erysipelas, cellulitis) require systemic antibiotics, as the infection is too deep for topical antibiotics to penetrate adequately
- Development of resistance: topical antibacterials should be limited to those not used systemically, to prevent development of resistance.
- Duration of treatment: topical agents should only be used for short periods in defined infections.

Examples of drugs given topically

- Mupirocin may be used to treat impetigo (if MRSA positive) or given as part of MRSA decolonization regimens. It should not be used for more than 7–10 days.
- Neomycin is also used to treat skin infection but may cause localized sensitivity and, less commonly, ototoxicity if large areas of skin are treated, allowing absorption to occur.

- Ciprofloxacin may be given as eye drops or ear drops for conjunctivitis or otitis externa, respectively.
- Acyclovir cream may be used for the treatment of oral and genital herpes simplex infections.
- Nystatin suspension can be used for oral candidiasis.
- Clotrimazole cream is used for vulvovaginal candidiasis or athlete's foot.
- Lindane may be used for head lice.

Aerosolized administration (NEB)

Aerosolized antibiotics are usually given for treatment or prophylaxis of respiratory infections. They are administered directly to the site of infection and may have fewer systemic adverse effects. However, they are usually more difficult to give and there may be some systemic absorption.

Administration of agents via this method can be challenging. It is important that the specific recommendations regarding appropriate nebulizer and administration conditions be followed to ensure appropriate drug delivery.

One of the main groups to benefit from aerosolized antibiotics is patients with cystic fibrosis (CF), who may acquire multiresistant organisms (see Cystic fibrosis, p. 567).

Examples of antimicrobials given by inhalation

- *Tobramycin* (see Aminoglycosides, p. 39) is an aminoglycoside often given by nebulizer for chronic pulmonary infection with *P. aeruginosa* in CF patients. It can be given cyclically (twice daily for 28 days, followed by a 28-day tobramycin-free period). Not all patients respond to treatment, and some become less responsive as drug resistance develops.
- *Colistin* (see Polymyxins, p. 63) is a polymyxin antibiotic active against many Gram-negative organisms, including *P. aeruginosa* and *Acinetobacter* spp. It is not absorbed orally and is toxic when given systemically, so inhalation of a nebulized solution is the preferred route for treating respiratory infections. It is mainly used as an adjunct to standard antibiotics in CF patients. It has also been used for the prevention and treatment of ventilator-associated pneumonia due to *Acinetobacter* spp., although this practice is controversial. It should be noted that due to recent safety concerns, inhaled colistin should be used immediately after preparation to avoid serious adverse events.
- A new aerosolized anti-infective, *aztreonam*, is used in patients with CF colonized with *Pseudomonas aeruginosa*.
- *Pentamidine isetionate* (see Antiprotozoal drugs (2), p. 104) administered via nebulization is used as a third-line agent for the prevention of *Pneumocystis jiroveci* pneumonia (see *Pneumocystis jiroveci*, p. 429). In some cases of mild infection, inhaled pentamidine may be used in patients who are unable to tolerate co-trimoxazole, but in more severe cases it must be administered intravenously. Aerosolized pentamidine does not adequately penetrate the lung apices and has been associated with breakthrough infections at this site. Also, this

route of administration does not protect against extrapulmonary disease.

• Ribavirin (see Antivirals for respiratory syncytial virus, p. 84) is licensed for the treatment of severe respiratory synctial virus (RSV) bronchiolitis in infants and children, especially if they have other serious diseases. There is no evidence of mortality benefit. Side effects include worsening respiration, bacterial pneumonia, and pneumothorax.

CAUTION: Ribavirin is teratogenic, and exposure should be avoided in pregnant and breast-feeding women. Individuals wearing contact lenses should also avoid locations where ribavirin is being aerosolized.

Antimicrobials in renal impairment

General principles

• The use of drugs in patients with renal impairment can cause several problems:
  • Reduced excretion of a drug or its metabolites may cause toxicity.
  • Increased sensitivity to some drugs may occur.
  • Many side effects are poorly tolerated in patients with renal impairment.
  • Some drugs are not effective when renal function is impaired.
• Avoid nephrotoxic drugs in patients with potentially reversible renal impairment.
• Keep antibiotic prescriptions to a minimum for patients with severe renal disease.
• Some intravenous antibiotic preparations contain sodium (e.g., Zosyn®), which may cause difficulties in patients with renal impairment.
• Some of these problems may be avoided by reducing the dose (or using alternative drugs).

Assessment of renal function

Renal function can be assessed in a number of ways:
• *Serum creatinine* is the most commonly used parameter. It is affected by muscle mass, which may be reduced in elderly patients (resulting in underestimation of renal impairment) and immobile patients or increased in certain races (e.g., blacks). Serum creatinine does not rise until 60% of total kidney function is lost.
• *Creatinine clearance (CrCl)* is best measured using a 24-hour urine collection. Estimated CrCl is calculated using the Cockcroft and Gault formula (Box 1.4), which is based on age, weight, sex, and serum creatinine. Thus, estimated CrCl may be inaccurate in patients who are obese or have acute renal failure.

Box 1.4 Cockcroft and Gault formula for estimated creatinine clearance

CrCl (mL/min) = (140−age) × lean body weight (kg) (× 0.85 for females)
(The denominator is (72* serum creatinine (mg/dL)).

- *Glomerular filtration rate (GFR)* is the volume of fluid filtered from the renal glomerular capillaries into Bowman's capsule per unit time and can be measured by injecting inulin into the plasma. Estimated GFR (eGFR) can be calculated using the modification of diet in renal disease (MDRD) formula (Box 1.5), which is based on serum creatinine, age, sex, and race. Renal impairment was previously classified into three grades (mild, moderate, and severe). This has been superseded by the use of CrCl or GFR. Many automated laboratory systems that report an estimate of GFR use the MDRD equation. It is important to note that most drug dosing schema were prepared using the Cockcroft-Gault equation and not the MDRD, and caution should be used when applying drug dosing using results of the MDRD.

Box 1.5 MDRD formula for estimated glomerular filtration rate

$$\text{eGFR (mL/min/1.73m}^2) = 186 \times (\text{serum creatine/(mg/dL)})^{-1.154} \times (\text{Age})^{-0.203} \times (0.742 \text{ if female}) \text{ or} \times (1.212 \text{ if black})$$

Dose modification in renal impairment

The level of renal function below which the dose of a drug must be reduced depends on the proportion of the drug eliminated by renal excretion and its toxicity.

For drugs with only minor or no dose-related side effects, very precise modification of the dose regimen is unnecessary and a simple scheme for dose reduction is sufficient. For more toxic drugs with a small safety margin, dose regimens based on GFR should be used.

When both efficacy and toxicity are closely related to plasma-drug concentration, recommended regimens should be regarded only as a guide to initial treatment; subsequent doses must be adjusted according to clinical response and plasma-drug concentration (e.g., vancomycin, gentamicin).

The total daily maintenance dose of a drug can be reduced by either reducing the size of the individual doses or increasing the interval between doses, depending on the pharmacodynamic properties of the drug. For some drugs, a traditional loading dose may be required to achieve appropriate initial drug concentrations. These doses are often the same for patients with and without renal dysfunction.

Seek specialist advice from your hospital pharmacist for patients on hemodialysis, hemofiltration, or chronic ambulatory peritoneal dialysis.

Drugs to be used with caution

For up-to-date guidance, always consult your hospital pharmacist or on-line resources such as the renal book, which may be accessed at: http://kdp.louisville.edu/renalbook/.

A wide range of antimicrobials should be used with caution in patients with renal impairment, independent of whether or not they are eliminated renally. Some examples include the following:

- Antibacterials, e.g., aminoglycosides, aztreonam, cephalosporins, carbapenems, chloramphenicol, colistin, ethambutol, isoniazid, macrolides, ketolides, penicillins, quinolones, sulfonamides, tetracyclines, trimethoprim, vancomycin
- Antifungals, e.g., amphotericin B, flucytosine, fluconazole, itraconazole, voriconazole
- Antimalarials, e.g., atovaquone, chloroquine, proguanil, pyrimethamine, quinine, sulfadiazine
- Antivirals, e.g., acyclovir, adefovir, amantadine, antiretrovirals, famciclovir, foscarnet, ganciclovir, oseltamivir, pentamidine, ribavirin, valacyclovir, valganciclovir

Antimicrobials in liver disease

Metabolism by the liver is the main route of elimination for many drugs, but hepatic reserve is large and liver disease has to be severe before important changes in drug metabolism occur. Routine liver functions tests are a poor guide to metabolic capacity, and it is not possible to predict the extent to which the metabolism of a particular drug may be impaired in an individual patient.

Effect of liver disease on response to drugs

Liver disease may alter the response to drugs in several ways:
- Impaired drug metabolism may lead to increased toxicity.
- Hypoproteinemia results in reduced protein binding and increased toxicity of highly protein-bound drugs, e.g., phenytoin.
- Reduced synthesis of clotting factors increases the sensitivity to oral anticoagulants
- Hepatic encephalopathy may be precipitated by certain drugs, e.g., sedative drugs, opioid analgesics, diuretics, and drugs that cause constipation.
- Fluid overload (ascites, edema) may be exacerbated by drugs that give rise to fluid retention, e.g., non-steroidals and corticosteroids.
- Hepatotoxicity is either dose related or unpredictable (idiosyncratic) and is more common in patients with liver disease.

Drugs to be used with caution

For up-to-date guidance always consult your hospital pharmacist. The following antimicrobials should be used with caution in liver disease:
- Antibacterials, e.g., ceftriaxone, chloramphenicol, amoxicillin/clavulanate, co-trimoxazole, daptomycin, isoniazid, macrolides, ketolides, linezolid, meropenem, metronidazole, moxifloxacin, neomycin, quinupristin-dalfopristin, rifamycins, tetracyclines, tigecycline
- Antifungals, e.g., azoles, caspofungin, terbinafine
- Antimalarials, e.g., mefloquine, pyrimethamine
- Antivirals, e.g., antiretrovirals, interferons, ribavirin, valacyclovir, valganciclovir

Antimicrobial prophylaxis

Definitions
Prophylaxis is the administration of antibiotics to prevent infection. *Primary prophylaxis* aims to prevent initial infection or disease (e.g., to cover a surgical procedure), while *secondary prophylaxis* aims to prevent recurrent disease (e.g., giving trimethoprim-sulfamethoxazole to a patient with history of PCP). *Surgical prophylaxis* is usually primary and aims to target the operative period *when* the site may become contaminated.

Principles of antimicrobial prophylaxis
All hospitals should have a policy for prescribing antimicrobial prophylaxis for common procedures, which may be area, unit, or surgeon specific. The following factors should be considered:
- Before prescribing always consider:
  - Does the patient have any known drug allergies?
  - Has the patient received any recent antibiotics?
  - Is the patient known to be colonized with resistant organisms?
- Which drug? A bactericidal agent should be used that:
  - is active against the probable infecting organism(s).
  - penetrates the likely site of infection.
  - has a favorable safety profile.
- What dose? For surgical prophylaxis, the aim is to maintain the drug concentration above the target MIC throughout the operative period. The number of doses usually depends on the length of procedure and likely blood loss.
- Which route? This depends on the nature of the procedure or exposure, whether or not the patient is able to take oral medication, and the pharmacokinetics of the drug.
- Time of administration? Antimicrobial prophylaxis should be administered within 1 hour prior to surgical incision to ensure adequate tissue concentrations. This measure is publically reported for U.S. hospitals through the Surgical Care Improvement Project (SCIP) core measures initiative for certain surgical procedures.
- Duration? Prophylactic antibiotics should not usually be given for more than 24 hours following a surgical procedure. In many cases, a single, pre-operative dose of antimicrobial is sufficient.

If there is evidence of infection, the patient should be carefully assessed and appropriate cultures sent. The organisms responsible for postoperative infections are unlikely to be sensitive to the prophylactic antibiotics. Seek advice on antimicrobial therapy from an infection specialist in light of the clinical picture and likely infecting organisms.

In cases of prophylaxis for chronic infections, prophylaxis may be lifelong.

Risks of antimicrobial prophylaxis
While the benefit of prophylactic antibiotics is clear, there are also potential risks:
- Adverse effects associated with specific drug (e.g., penicillin anaphylaxis)

- Selection of antibiotic-resistant organisms
- Alteration of normal flora

Before prescribing antimicrobial prophylaxis for a procedure, consider whether it is actually needed. Consult national guidelines, your local antibiotic susceptibility data or an infectious diseases specialist to guide appropriate selection.

Other examples of antimicrobial prophylaxis

- *Selective decontamination of digestive tract* (SDD): administration of antibiotics that are poorly absorbed when given orally to eliminate normal GI flora. Some intensive care units use it to prevent ventilator-associated pneumonia. This practice is controversial.
- *Local infiltration into wound/incision line:* current data suggest this can lead to higher rates of infection, unless combined with systemic administration. There is no additional reduction in wound infections if antibiotics are given by both routes simultaneously, compared with systemic antibiotics alone.
- *Antibiotic-impregnated materials:* gentamicin cement is used routinely in joint replacement; this is also controversial. Antibiotic-soaked Dacron vascular grafts are used in vascular surgery.

In some institutions, antibiotic-impregnated catheters are used to prevent central line–associated bloodstream infections. In some cases, cations are used in lieu of antimicrobial agents to limit the development of resistance.

Penicillins

Penicillin was discovered by Alexander Fleming in 1928 but did not become widely available until the 1940s. The penicillins are closely related compounds comprising a β-lactam ring, a five-membered thiozolidine ring, and a side chain (Fig. 1.1). The ring structures are essential for antibacterial activity, and the side chain determines the spectrum and pharmacological properties.

Most penicillins in current use are semisynthetic derivatives of 6-aminopenicillic acid. They inhibit bacterial cell wall synthesis and are thus bactericidal.

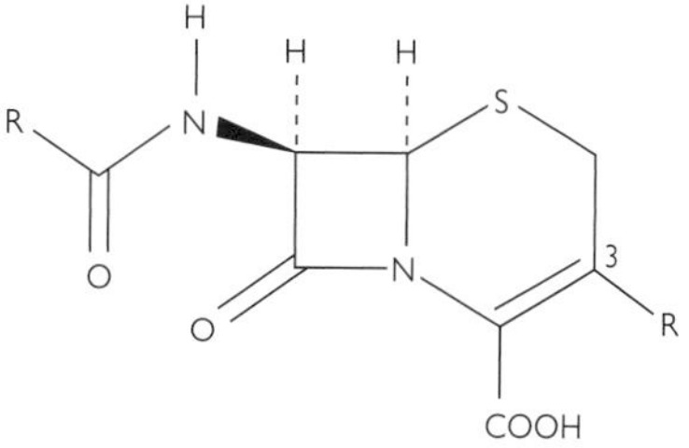

Fig. 1.1 Structure of penicillin.

Classification
- *Natural penicillins:* penicillin G, procaine penicillin, penicillin V, benzathine penicillin
- *Aminopenicillins:* ampicillin, amoxicillin
- *Antistaphylococcal penicillins:* methicillin, oxacillin, nafcillin, dicloxacillin
- *Extended-spectrum penicillins* (antipseudomonal penicillins): piperacillin, ticarcillin

Mechanism of action
The penicillins inhibit cell wall synthesis by binding to PBPs and inhibiting transpeptidation of peptidoglycan.

Resistance
Bacteria may become resistant to penicillins by a number of mechanisms:
- Destruction of the antibiotic by β-lactamases (β-lactamases, see p. 29). This is the most common mechanism.
- Failure to penetrate the outer membrane of Gram-negative bacteria
- Efflux across the outer membrane of Gram-negative bacteria
- Low-affinity binding of antibiotic to target PBPs

Some bacteria may display more than one resistance mechanism, e.g., in MRSA the *mecA* gene encodes for an additional PBP (i.e., altered target site), and most also produce a β-lactamase.

Clinical use
- Penicillin G is used in infections due to group A and group B streptococci; meningitis due to *S. pneumoniae* (if penicillin susceptible) and *N. meningitidis*; streptococcal endocarditis; and neurosyphilis.
- Aminopenicillins are used in respiratory tract infections, endocarditis, UTIs caused by susceptible organisms, and treatment of *H. pylori*.
- Extended-spectrum or antipseudomonal penicillins are used in infections due to resistant Gram-negative bacteria. These agents are also commonly employed as part of empiric antibiotic therapy.
- Penicillin V is also used prophylactically to prevent recurrent rheumatic fever, secondary cases in outbreaks of group A streptococcal disease, and pneumococcal and *H. influenzae* infections in asplenic patients.

Pharmacology
- Penicillins differ markedly in their oral absorption (penicillin V 60%, amoxicillin 75%, antipseudomonal penicillins 0%).
- They vary in degree of protein binding; metabolism is minimal.
- They are rapidly excreted by the renal tubular cells; excretion may be blocked by probenecid. Dose modification may be required in renal impairment.

Toxicity and side effects
- *Allergic* reactions (skin rashes, serum sickness, delayed hypersensitivity) occur in <10% of those exposed. Anaphylactic reactions are rare (0.004–0.4%).
- *Gastrointestinal:* diarrhea, enterocolitis (2–5%, usually ampicillin)
- *Hematological:* hemolytic anemia, neutropenia; thrombocytopenia (1–4%)

- *Laboratory:* elevated transaminases, electrolyte abnormalities (hypernatremia, hypo- or hyperkalemia)
- *Renal:* interstitial nephritis, hemorrhagic cystitis
- *Central nervous* system: encephalopathy or seizures are rare but may occur in renal failure or if high prolonged doses of penicillin are used.

Cephalosporins

Giuseppe Brotzu first demonstrated the antimicrobial activity of culture filtrates of the mold *Cephalosporium acremonium* in 1945. However, the cephalosporin class of antibiotics did not become widely used for another 20 years.

Cephalosporins consist of a β-lactam ring and a six-membered dihydro-thiazine ring, modified at certain positions to produce different compounds (Fig. 1.2). Most available cephalosporins are semi-synthetic derivatives of cephalosporin C.

Classification

Cephalosporins are classified into generations:

- *First generation:* primarily active against Gram-positive bacteria, e.g., cefazolin, cephalexin, cefadroxil
- *Second generation:* enhanced activity against Gram-negative bacteria, with varying degrees of activity against Gram-positive bacteria, e.g., cefuroxime, cefamandole, cefprozil, and cefaclor. The cephamycin group (e.g., cefotetan and cefoxitin) has additional anaerobic activity, e.g., *B. fragilis*. The cephem, loracarbef, is also traditionally considered a second generation cephalosporin.
- *Third generation:* markedly increased activity against Gram-negative bacteria, e.g., cefditoren, cefotaxime, ceftriaxone, ceftazidime, cefdinir, cefixime, cefpodoxime, ceftibuten, and ceftizoxime

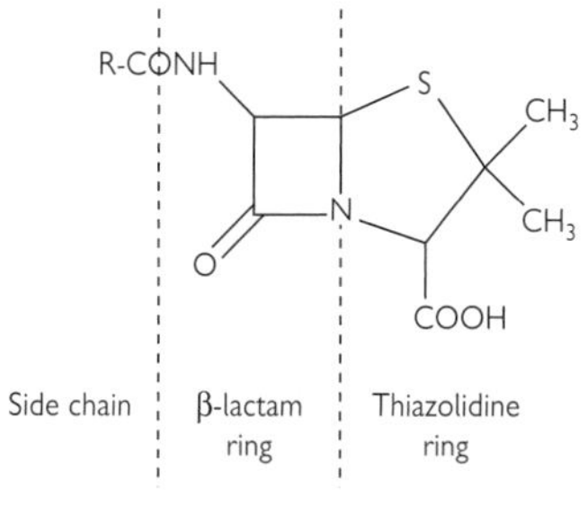

Fig. 1.2 Basic structure of cephalosporins.

- *Fourth generation:* broad spectrum of activity against Gram-positive cocci and Gram-negative bacteria, including *Pseudomonas* spp., e.g., cefepime
- *Advanced generation:* broad spectrum of activity against Gram-positive cocci, including MRSA and Gram-negative bacteria, e.g., ceftaroline, ceftobiprole.
- *NOTE:* No cephalosporin has appreciable activity against *Enterococcus* spp.

Mechanism of action

They inhibit cell wall synthesis by binding to PBPs and inhibiting transpeptidation of peptidoglycan. They are bactericidal and have significant post-antibiotic effect against Gram-positive (but not Gram-negative) bacteria.

Resistance

There are four common resistance mechanisms:
- Destruction of the antibiotic by β-lactamases (see β-Lactamases, p. 29, and Box 1.6)
- Reduced penetration through the outer membrane of Gram-negative bacteria
- Enhanced efflux
- Alteration in PBP target, resulting in reduced affinity binding.

Clinical use

- *First generation:* staphylococcal and streptococcal skin and soft tissue infections, UTIs, surgical prophylaxis
- *Second generation:* severe infections of the respiratory tract and uncomplicated UTIs
- *Cephamycins:* intra-abdominal, pelvic, and gynecological infections, infected decubitus ulcers, diabetic foot infections, mixed aerobic–anaerobic soft tissue infections
- *Third generation:* penicillin-resistant pneumococci, meningitis, upper and lower respiratory tract infections, sinusitis, otitis media, nosocomial infections caused by Gram-negative bacilli, *N. gonorrheae*, Lyme disease, severe *Shigella* spp., and nontyphoidal salmonella infection; outpatient antibiotic therapy for endocarditis and osteomyelitis
- *Fourth generation:* similar use to that of third-generation agents, traditionally reserved for cases of presumed or documented severe nosocomial Gram-negative infections
- *Advanced generation:* approved for treatment of skin and soft tissue infections as well as community-acquired pneumonia

---

Box 1.6 CAUTION: cephalosporins and ESCAPPM

The second and third generation cephalosporins are susceptible to inactivation by inducible β-lactamases (see β-Lactamases, p. 29). They should not be used as monotherapy to treat organisms that may have these enzymes, e.g., *Enterobacter* spp., *Serratia* spp., *Citrobacter freundii*, *Acinetobacter* spp., *Proteus vulgaris*, *Providencia* spp., *Morganella morganii* (mnemonic: ESCAPPM).

Pharmacology

Cephalosporins may be given orally (PO), intravenously (IV), or intramuscularly (IM). The fourth-generation agent (cefepime) and advanced generation agents only available parenterally. Oral preparations have 80–95% bioavailability.

Protein binding is variable (10–98%). Drugs are largely confined to the extracellular compartment. There is poor cerebrospinal fluid (CSF) penetration unless meningeal inflammation is present. They cross the placenta.

Most drugs are not metabolized, except cefotaxime and cephalothin, which are metabolized in the liver. Most drugs are excreted by the kidneys. Ceftriaxone is excreted by the biliary system.

Toxicity and side effects

- *Hypersensitivity:* rash (1–3%), urticaria and serum sickness (<1%), anaphylaxis (0.01%)
- *Gastrointestinal:* diarrhea (1–19%), nausea and vomiting (1–6%), transient hepatitis (1–7%), biliary sludging (ceftriaxone)
- *Hematological:* eosinophilia (1–10%), neutropenia, thrombocytopenia, clotting abnormalities (cefamandole and cefotetan), platelet dysfunction, hemolytic anemia
- *Renal:* interstitial nephritis
- *Central nervous system:* seizures
- *False-positive laboratory tests:* Coombs' test, glycosuria, elevated serum creatinine
- *Other:* drug fever, disulfiram-like reaction (cefamandole and cefotetan), phlebitis

β-Lactamases

β-Lactamases are enzymes that bind covalently to the β-lactam ring, hydrolyse it, and make the antibiotic ineffective. Emergence of resistance to β-lactam antibiotics began even before penicillin was widely available, with the first β-lactamase (penicillinase) being described in E. coli in 1940. This was followed by the emergence of resistance in S. aureus due to plasmid-encoded penicillinase.

Many genera of Gram-negative bacilli possess naturally occurring, chromosomally mediated β-lactamases (AmpC). These enzymes are thought to have evolved from PBPs, to which they are very similar.

The first plasmid-mediated β-lactamase in Gram-negative bacteria, TEM-1, was described in 1960. Within a few years it had spread worldwide and was found in many different species.

Over the past 20 years, many antibiotics have been developed in attempts to evade these resistance mechanisms. However, with each new class of drugs, new β-lactamases have emerged.

Classification

There are two classification systems for β-lactamases.

Ambler classification

This is a molecular classification with four classes (A to D) based on the nucleotide/amino acid sequences of the enzymes:

- *Classes A, C, and D* are PBPs, without cell wall synthetic activity (serine β-lactamases).
- *Class B* are zinc-dependent enzymes (metallo-β-lactamases) that hydrolyse the β-lactam ring through a different mechanism

Bush–Jacoby–Medeiros classification

This is a functional classification with four groups:

- *Group 1* β-lactamases are cephalosporinases that are not inhibited by clavulanic acid. They correspond to Ambler group C.
- *Group 2* β-lactamases are penicillinases and/or cephalosporinases that are inhibited by clavulanic acid. This group corresponds to Ambler groups A and D and includes the TEM and SHV enzymes.
- *Group 3* β-lactamases are zinc-dependent (metallo-β-lactamases) and are not inhibited by clavulanic acid. They correspond to Ambler group B.
- *Group 4* β-lactamases are penicillinases that are not inhibited by clavulanic acid. They do not yet have a molecular class.

AmpC β-lactamases

These are chromosomally mediated β-lactamases that are active against third generation cephalosporins and are not inhibited by clavulanic acid or other β-lactamase inhibitors. They fall into the molecular group C/functional group 1.

They are found in the ESCAPPM group of organisms: *E*nterobacter spp., *S*erratia spp., *C*itrobacter freundii, *A*cinetobacter spp., *P*roteus vulgaris, *P*rovidencia spp., *M*organella morganii.

Amp C β-lactamases are inducible in the Enterobacteriaceae but can also be plasmid mediated. The use of third generation cephalosporins to treat these infections results in the selection of stably derepressed mutants that hyperproduce AmpC and has been associated with clinical failure. These infections are thus usually treated with carbapenems.

Extended-spectrum β-lactamases (ESBLs)

These are β-lactamases capable of conferring bacterial resistance to the penicillins; first, second, and third generation cephalosporins; and aztreonam (but not the cephamycins or carbapenems) through hydrolysis of these antibiotics.

These enzymes are inhibited by β-lactamase inhibitors such as clavulanic acid. They fall into functional groups 2be and 2d.

ESBLs are most commonly found in *E. coli* and *K. pneumoniae* but have been described in many other Gram-negative bacilli. Most ESBLs are derivatives of the TEM, SHV, and CTX-M type enzymes.

TEM β-lactamases

TEM-1 is the most common β-lactamase in Gram-negative bacteria and is able to hydrolyse penicillins and early generation cephalosporins. TEM-2 has a similar spectrum. TEM-3 was the first ESBL, reported in 1989. Since then over 180 TEM enzymes have been described (see http://www.lahey.org/studies/temtable.htm).

Most of these are inhibited by clavulanic acid, but some inhibitor-resistant variants exist, particularly in Europe. TEM enzymes are most common in *E. coli* and *K. pneumoniae* but are increasingly found in other species of Gram-negative bacilli.

SHV β-lactamases

The SHV-1 β-lactamase is most commonly found in *K. pneumoniae* and accounts for up to 20% of ampicillin resistance in this species.

CTX-M β-lactamases

This family of plasmid-mediated β-lactamases was named for their preferential hydrolysis of cefotaxime. They have been found in *Salmonella enterica* serovar Typhimurium and in *E. coli* as well as other Enterobacteriaceae.

These enzymes are quite different from the TEM and SHV enzymes and show greater similarity to the chromosomal AmpC enzyme of *Kluyvera ascorbata*, which suggests that CTX-M may have originated from this species. CTX-M β-lactamases were previously associated with outbreaks in Europe, South America, and Japan, but now they are reported worldwide.

OXA β-lactamases

These are characterized by their high hydrolytic activity against oxacillin and cloxacillin and are poorly inhibited by clavulanic acid. They belong to molecular group D/functional group 2d.

OXA-type ESBLs are mainly found in *P. aeruginosa* but have been detected in other Gram-negative bacteria. More recently, non-ESBL OXA derivatives have been described.

Other ESBLs

A number of ESBLs that are unrelated to the established families of ESBLs have been described: PER-1, PER-2, VEB-1, GES, BES, TLA, SFO, and IBC. These are found primarily in *P aeruginosa* and are often limited to select geographic sites.

Although β-lactamases only inhibit β-lactam antibiotics, many ESBL-producing bacteria also display resistance to other commonly used anti-infectives, including trimethoprim-sulfamethoxazole, fluroquinolones, and the aminoglycosides. These resistance mechanisms can be carried by the genes responsible for ESBL production.

ESBL detection methods

There are several methods that can be used to detect ESBL production. The CLSI guidelines for detecting ESBL production include an initial screen with a cephalosporin (cefpodoxime, ceftazidime, cefotaxime, or ceftriaxone. Aztreonam may also be used.) followed by confirmatory testing with ceftazidime and cefotaxime disks combined alone and in combination with clavulanate.

An ESBL is confirmed if the clavulanate disk increases the zone of inhibition by ≥5 mm. In addition, many automated testing systems as well as E-test now offer the ability to screen for ESBL production and recent changes to CLSI breakpoints limit the need for this testing..

Carbapenemases

Carbapenemases are a diverse group of β-lactamases that confer resistance to the cephalosporins as well as carbapenems. The most clinically important carbapenemase is *Klebsiella pneumoniae* carbapenemase (KPC) or carbapenemase-producing Enterobacteriaceae (CPE). This is a class A β-lactamase that may be chromosomally or plasmid mediated.

The first CPE isolate was reported in North Carolina in the late 1990s. Testing for carbapenemase-producing isolates can be challenging, as traditional testing methods may report false susceptibility to imipenem or meropenem.

At present, ertapenem susceptibility appears to be the most sensitive predictor of carbapenemase production although recent changes by CLSI are designed to better discriminate susceptibility for the other carbapenems. Treating these pathogens is also a clinical challenge, as the production of carbapenemase confers resistance to all β-lactams, aztreonam, and the carbapenems.

β-lactamase inhibitors

β-Lactamase inhibitors are clavulanic acid and penicillanic acid sulfone derivatives. They have weak antibacterial activity but are potent inhibitors of many β-lactamases, e.g., penicillinases produced by *S. aureus*, *H. influenzae*, *M. catarrhalis*, and *Bacteroides* spp., and TEM and SHV β-lactamases produced by Enterobacteriaceae. They can restore the antibacterial activity of certain antibiotics, e.g., amoxicillin, ampicillin, piperacillin, and ticarcillin.

Three β-lactamase inhibitors are in clinical use: clavulanic acid, sulbactam, and tazobactam. All are only available in combination with a β-lactam antibiotic; the antibiotic spectrum is determined by the companion antibiotic.

Although there are minor differences in potency, activity, and pharmacology between the three compounds, they can be considered therapeutically equivalent (except for some *Klebsiella* spp., where clavulanate inhibits isolates resistant to sulbactam and tazobactam).

Amoxicillin/clavulanate (Augmentin®)

Clavulanate is a potent inhibitor of many plasmid-mediated β-lactamases and a weak inducer of some chromosomal β-lactamases.

It is available as a combination with amoxicillin and used for the treatment of a wide range of infections where β-lactamase-producing organisms may be present. Examples include otitis media, sinusitis, pneumonia, skin and soft tissue infections, diabetic foot infections, and human and animal bite infections.

It is only available as an oral formulation in both traditional and extended-release preparations.

Side effects are similar to those with ampicillin. Cholestatic jaundice may occur during or after therapy and is six times more common than with amoxicillin alone. A common adverse event with amoxicillin/clavulanate is diarrhea, which can occur in up to 30% of patients.

Ampicillin-sulbactam (Unasyn®)

Sulbactam is a 6-desaminopenicillin sulfone. It has a broader spectrum of activity but is less potent than clavulanic acid. It is available in a parenteral formulation only.

Ampicillin-sulbactam is used for the treatment of skin and soft tissue infections, intra-abdominal infections, and gynecological infections caused by β-lactamase–producing bacteria. It has also recently been used to treat carbapenem-resistant *Acinetobacter baumanii* infections.

Side effects are similar to those with ampicillin.

Ticarcillin-clavulanate (Timentin®)

This combination is useful against infections caused by *Pseudomonas* spp. and *Proteus* spp.

It has been used for the treatment of pneumonia, intra-abdominal infections, gynecological infections, skin and soft tissue infections, and osteomyelitis. It is only available in parenteral form and is given intravenously.

Side effects are similar to those of other β-lactams. Cholestatic jaundice may also occur because of the clavulanic acid component.

Piperacillin-tazobactam (Zosyn®)

Tazobactam is penicillanic acid sulfone β-lactamase inhibitor with a similar structure to sulbactam. Its spectrum of activity is similar to that of sulbactam but its potency is comparable to that of clavulanic acid.

It is available as a combination with piperacillin (an antipseudomonal penicillin) and is given parenterally.

It has a broad spectrum of activity and is used in the treatment of nosocomial pneumonia) skin and soft tissue infections, intra-abdominal infections, UTIs, polymicrobial infections, bacteremia, and febrile neutropenia.

Although commonly used as empiric therapy for presumed infections due to *Pseudomonas* spp., the β-lactamase inhibitor does not confer significant additional activity for this organism compared to piperacillin alone.

Side effects are similar to those of piperacillin.

Carbapenems

The carbapenems are β-lactam antibiotics derived from thienamycin, a compound produced by *Streptomyces cattleya*. Four carbapenems are licensed for use in the United States: doripenem, imipenem, meropenem, and ertapenem.

Mechanism of action

These agents show high affinity to most high-molecular-weight PBPs of Gram-positive and Gram-negative bacteria. Carbapenems, particularly imipenem, traverse the outer membrane of Gram-negative bacteria through different outer membrane proteins (OprD) than those used by penicillins and cephalosporins (OmpC and OmpF). They also have excellent stability to β-lactamases. Consequently, carbapenems have the broadest antibacterial spectrum of all the β-lactam antibiotics.

Imipenem is slightly more active against Gram-positive bacteria, whereas meropenem and ertapenem are slightly more active against Gram-negative species.

Meropenem is most active against *P. aeruginosa*. Ertapenem has poor activity against *P. aeruginosa*, *Enterococcus* spp., and *Acinetobacter* spp. and should not be used to reliably treat these pathogens.

Resistance

Resistance is due to one of four mechanisms:
• Production of a low-affinity PBP target
• Reduced outer membrane permeability due to absence of OprD in Gram-negative bacteria
• Efflux of the drug in Gram-negative bacteria
• Production of β-lactamases (see β-Lactamases, p. 29) that hydrolyse carbapenems (carbapenemases).

These enzymes fall into three groups. The molecular class A (functional group 2f) enzymes include SME, IMI, NMC, KPC, and GES. The molecular class B (functional group 3) enzymes include IMP, VIM, GIM, and SVM. The molecular group D (functional group 2d) includes OXA enzymes.

In Gram-negative bacteria, resistance is frequently due to a combination of impaired drug entry, drug efflux, and β-lactamase production.

Clinical use

Carbapenems may be used to treat a wide variety of severe infections, e.g., bacteremia, pneumonia, intra-abdominal infections, obstetric and gynecological infections, complicated UTIs, and soft tissue and bone infections.

Imipenem, meropenem, and doripenem are the most appropriate for treatment of infections caused by the cephalosporin-resistant AmpC-producing organisms, e.g., *Enterobacter* spp., *Serratia* spp., *Citrobacter freundii*, *Acinetobacter* spp., *Proteus vulgaris*, *Providencia* spp., and *Morganella morganii* (the ESCAPPM group).

Imipenem and meropenem are also used for the treatment of serious infections, e.g., patients with polymicrobial infections, febrile neutropenia, and nosocomial infections, such as those caused by *P. aeruginosa* and *Acinetobacter* spp.

Meropenem is also licensed for the treatment of bacterial meningitis. Imipenem should *not* be used because of its propensity to cause seizures.

Doripenem has a similar spectrum of activity to that of imipenem and meropenem. It currently is only licensed for treatment of complicated intra-abdominal and UTIs, although it has been studied for treatment of pneumonia with positive results.

Ertapenem has similar uses to those of imipenem and meropenem but cannot be used in infections caused by *P. aeruginosa* and *Acinetobacter* spp. Its long plasma half-life means that it can be administered once daily, making it useful for outpatient antibiotic therapy (OPAT). One of its most common uses is for surgical prophylaxis prior to intra-abdominal procedures.

Pharmacology

Imipenem, meropenem, doripenem, and ertapenem have poor oral absorption and are given parenterally.

Imipenem, doripenem, and meropenem are pharmacologically similar with a plasma half-life of 1 hour, whereas ertapenem has a plasma half-life of 4 hours, which permits once-daily dosing.

All carbapenems are widely distributed and penetrate inflamed meninges. All are renally excreted and require dose modification in renal failure.

Imipenem is a substrate for the renal dehydropeptidase-1 (DHP-1) enzyme and is therefore coadministered with cilastatin, a DHP-1 inhibitor.

Toxicity and side effects

Carbapenems are generally well tolerated.

β-lactam-related allergic reactions are the most common side effects, e.g., rash, urticaria, immediate hypersensitivity, and cross-reactivity with penicillin.

Imipenem causes nausea (if infused too quickly) and can cause seizures, particularly if not dosed appropriately for renal dysfunction.

Monobactams

The monobactams are monocyclic β-lactam antibiotics produced by some bacteria (e.g., *Chromobacterium violaceum*). They are only active against Gram-negative bacteria.

Aztreonam

Aztreonam is the only commercially available compound. It is active against most Enterobacteriaeceae, *H. influenzae*, and *Neisseria* spp. *S. maltophilia*, *B. cepacia*, and many *Acinetobacter* spp. are resistant. Some strains of *P. aeruginosa*, *E. cloacae*, and *C. freundii* are resistant.

Aztreonam passes through the outer membrane and binds to PBP3 of Gram-negative bacteria. It is resistant to hydrolysis by most β-lactamases, apart from the AmpC β-lactamases.

Aztreonam is not absorbed orally and is given intravenously or intramuscularly. It is widely distributed and penetrates inflamed meninges. It is mainly renally excreted and requires dose modification in renal failure.

It is used for the treatment of a variety of infections, e.g., UTIs, pneumonia, septicemia, skin and soft tissue infections, intra-abdominal infections, gynecological infections, wound and burn infections.

Aztreonam should never be used alone as empiric therapy as it has no activity against Gram-positive organisms.

Although it possesses a β-lactam ring structure, aztreonam has no immunological cross-reactivity with penicillin and can safely be administered to penicillin-allergic patients. Empiric Gram-negative therapy in patients with a documented penicillin allergy comprises the primary use for aztreonam.

Other cell wall agents

Bacitracin
Bacitracin binds to isoprenylphosphate and prevents dephosphorylation of the lipid carrier that transports the cell wall building block across the membrane. Without dephosphorylation, the native compound cannot be regenerated for another round of transfer.

Similar reactions in eukaryotic cells may be why this agent is so toxic and is therefore used topically. It is also used to identify group A streptococci (bacitracin resistant) in the diagnostic laboratory.

Fosfomycin
Fosfomycin inhibits pyruvyl transferase and thus formation of N-acetylglucosamine from N-acetylmuramic acid. It is a naturally occurring antibiotic with a fairly broad spectrum, particularly against Gram-negative rods.

It is mainly used to treat urinary tract infections. It offers convenient single-dose therapy, and its activity against multi-drug-resistant urinary tract pathogens has made its use more common in recent years.

Cycloserine
This drug is often part of the second-line regimen for drug-resistant tuberculosis. It is a structural analog of D-alanine and acts on alanine racemase and synthetase to inhibit the synthesis of the terminal D-alanyl-D-alanine. It thus prevents formation of the pentapeptide chain of muramic acid. See Antituberculous agents—second line (p. 68).

Isoniazid and ethambutol
These are first-line drugs used in the treatment of tuberculosis. They interfere with mycolic acid synthesis in mycobacterial cell walls. See Antituberculous agents—first line (p. 65).

Glycopeptides

The glycopeptide antibiotics, vancomycin and teicoplanin, are bactericidal against most Gram-positive bacteria. Vancomycin was first isolated from Nocardia orientalis and introduced into clinical practice in 1958. Teicoplanin was obtained from Actinoplanes teichomyceticus in 1978 and is available in Europe and Asia but not in the United States.

Mechanism of action
Glycopeptides inhibit cell synthesis by binding to D-alanyl-D-alanine tail of the muramylpentapeptide and inhibiting production peptidoglycan matrix.

Antimicrobial activity

Glycopeptides have broad activity against Gram-positive organisms, e.g., staphylococci, *E. faecalis*, *S. pneumoniae*, groups A, B, C, and G streptococci, *S. bovis*, *S. mutans*, viridans group streptococci, *Bacillus* spp., *Corynebacterium* spp., *Peptostreptococcus* spp., *Actinomyces* spp., *Propionibacterium* spp., and most *Clostridium* spp.

Glycopeptides show no activity against Gram-negative species (except nongonococcal *Neisseria* spp.).

Resistance

Vancomycin resistance may be intrinsic or acquired. Intrinsic vancomycin resistance occurs in *Leuconostoc, Pediococcus, Lactobacillus*, and *Erysipelothrix rhusiopathiae*.

- *Enterococci*: six types of glycopeptide resistance have been described (VanA, VanB, VanC, VanD, VanE, and VanG), named on the basis of their ligase genes (*vanA, vanB*, etc, see Table 1.3). These result in the formation of a peptidoglycan precursor with decreased affinity for glycopeptides. Resistance may be intrinsic (e.g., in *E. gallinarum*, *E. casseliflavus*) or acquired (e.g., in *E. faecium* and *E. faecalis*).
- *Staphylococcus aureus*: the first clinical isolate of *S. aureus* with diminished susceptibility to vancomycin was reported in Japan in 1997. This is referred to as a vancomycin-intermediate *S. aureus* (VISA) or glycopeptide intermediate *S. aureus* (GISA). VISA isolates have a thickened cell wall that may prevent glycopeptides from reaching their target sites. In 2002, two isolates of truly vancomycin-resistant *S. aureus* (VRSA) were reported, both of which carried the *vanA* gene, suggesting horizontal transfer of this gene from enterococci.
- *S. pneumoniae*: vancomycin tolerance has recently been reported.

Clinical use

Glycopeptides are used to treat the following conditions:
- Severe infections caused by MRSA

Table 1.3 Vancomycin resistance in enterococci and staphylococci

	Van A	Van B	Van C	Van D	Van E	Van G
Vanc MIC	64->500	4->500	2-32	64-128	16	12-16
Expression	Inducible	Inducible	Constitutive, inducible	Constitutive	Inducible	
Location	P, C	P, C	C	C	C	C
Species	E. faecalis, E. faecium, S. aureus	E. faecalis, E. faecium	E. gallinarum, E. casseliflavus, E. flavescens	E. faecium	E. faecalis	E. faecalis

C, chromosome; MIC, minimum inhibitory concentration (mcg/mL); P, plasmid; Vanc, vancomycin

- Meningitis due to penicillin-resistant S. *pneumoniae*
- *C. difficile*–associated diarrhea (oral vancomycin only)
- Febrile neutropenia
- Continuous ambulatory peritoneal dialysis (CAPD) peritonitis
- Endophthalmitis
- Empiric treatment of intravascular catheter-related infections and CSF shunt infections

Pharmacology

Vancomycin is usually given intravenously but may also be given orally (for treatment of *C. difficile* only), intraperitoneally, intrathecally, or intraocularly.

It is widely distributed but has poor CSF penetration in the absence of meningeal inflammation. Vancomcyin is excreted unchanged in the kidneys, and dose reduction is required in renal impairment.

Therapeutic drug monitoring of trough concentrations is performed after the third dose (in patients with normal renal function) and should be 10–20 mcg/mL, based on clinical indication. Vancomycin shows time-dependent killing. Therefore, monitoring of peak serum concentrations is not recommended.

Vancomycin is not orally bioavailable.

Toxicity and side effects

Toxicity is more common with vancomycin than with teicoplanin.

Ototoxicity is rare unless there is renal impairment. Nephrotoxicity has been reported with high doses and is often associated with concomitant nephrotoxin, such as aminoglycoside or piperacillin/tazobactam usage.

Infusion-related reactions can occur, e.g., "red man syndrome" with rapid infusion of vancomycin.

Others, e.g., neutropenia, thrombocytopenia, rashes, and drug fever, occur more rarely.

Lipoglycopeptides

The lipoglycopeptides are considered second-generation glycopeptide anti-infectives. Currently, there is only one agent available, televancin; however, two additional agents, oritavancin and dalbavancin, are both in various stages of development.

These agents are semisynthetic derivatives of vancomycin and demonstrate rapid, bactericidal activity against Gram-positive pathogens, including MRSA, vancomycin-resistant enterococci (VRE), and resistant streptococci.

Mechanism of action

The lipoglycopeptides inhibit bacterial cell wall synthesis by blocking the transglycosylation of peptidoglycan synthesis in a manner similar to vancomycin. These agents also possess a second mechanism of activity and at clinically achievable concentrations can also disrupt integrity and function of the bacterial cell membrane.

Resistance

VRE strains with high vancomycin MICs will also be resistant to televancin, but the drug does retain activity to VAN-B strains (vancomycin resistant but teicoplanin susceptible). To date, all glycopeptides resistant strains of MRSA have retained activity to televancin, although resistance can evolve with time.

Clinical use

Televancin has been approved for the treatment of complicated skin and soft tissue infections and nosocomial pneumonia as well as other resistant Gram-positive infections not responding to other therapies.

Pharmacology

Televancin must be administered intravenously. It demonstrates linear and predictable pharmacokinetics. With a half-life of 6 to 9 hours and a post-antibiotic effect of up to 4 hours for S. aureus, it can easily be administered once daily.

The drug is highly protein bound, making CNS penetration unlikely. Televancin is renally eliminated with more than 60% excreted unchanged in the urine. Dose reductions are necessary for renal impairment.

Toxicity and side effects

Commonly reported side effects include the following:

- Mild taste disturbance
- Nausea and vomiting
- Renal dysfunction; in addition, efficacy may decrease with estimated creatinine clearance of <50 mL/min
- Infusion related reactions: "red-man" syndrome similar to that with vancomycin
- QTc prolongation
- Teratogenicity: pregnancy category C, due to significant risks to the fetus. In the United States, patient education materials are required prior to administration.
- Interference with laboratory testing for prothrombin time (PT), International Normalized Ratio (INR) < activated partial thromboplastin time (PTT), clotting time, and factor Xa based testing for anticoagulation. To avoid interference, obtain samples for testing 23 hours after televancin administration.

Aminoglycosides

Streptomycin, produced by Streptomyces griseus, was the first aminogly-coside used in the initial treatment trials of tuberculosis in the 1940s. Today aminoglycosides remain an important part of the antibiotic arse-nal. All aminoglycosides have an essential six-member ring with amino group constituents (aminocyclitol). The term aminoglycoside results from glycosidic bonds between the aminocyclitol and two or more sugars.

They are active against many Gram-negative and some Gram-positive organisms. In the United States, the currently available aminoglycosides are: streptomycin, neomycin, kanamycin, paromomycin, gentamicin, tobramycin, amikacin, and netilmicin.

Despite eight different agents being approved, gentamicin, tobramycin, and amikacin are the most frequently prescribed.

Mechanism of action

Aminoglycosides bind to the A site of 30S ribosomal subunit, resulting in a conformational change that interferes with mRNA translation and translocation, and hence inhibit protein synthesis. Avidity of binding varies among aminoglycosides.

The transport of aminoglycosides into the cell by energy-dependent mechanisms (EDP-I and EDP-II) results in accumulation of high concentrations of drug in the cell. The onset of cell death is coincident with the transition from EDP-I to EDP-II.

The activity of aminoglycosides is pH dependent and is significantly reduced in acidic environments.

Resistance

Resistance to aminoglycosides may be intrinsic or acquired.
Intrinsic resistance may be non-enzymatic or enzymatic:
- Anaerobes are unable to generate a sufficient electrical potential difference across the membrane and are intrinsically resistant.
- Mutations in the 16S ribosomal subunit can result in resistance to streptomycin in *M. tuberculosis*.
- Methylating enzymes that modify the 16S rRNA may cause intrinsic resistance; this has not yet been seen in clinical isolates.

Acquired resistance may occur through a variety of mechanisms:
- Reduced drug uptake
- Efflux pumps, e.g., activation of the Mex XY pump in *P. aeruginosa*
- Enzymatic modification of the drug may occur as a result of aminoglycoside-modifying enzymes (AMEs) that phosphorylate, acetylate, or adenylate exposed amino or hydroxyl groups. The enzymatically modified drugs bind poorly to ribosomes, resulting in high levels of resistance.

Clinical use

- *Empiric therapy*: aminoglycosides may be given as empiric therapy for serious infections suspected to be due to Gram-negative bacteria. Depending on the clinical indication, they are usually combined with a β-lactam, vancomycin, and/or an anaerobic agent.
- *Specific therapy*: once culture results are available, aminoglycosides may be useful for the specific treatment, e.g., infections due to *Pseudomonas* spp. or resistant Gram-negative species, or for synergy in Gram-positive endocarditis.
- *Prophylaxis*: aminoglycosides are sometimes used prophylactically, e.g., to prevent enterococcal endocarditis in at-risk patients undergoing genitourinary or gastrointestinal procedures.

- Gentamicin and tobramycin are the most commonly used aminoglycosides. Their main use is in the empirical treatment of serious infections (e.g., bacteremia, febrile neutropenia, biliary sepsis, acute pyelonephritis, endocarditis). Gentamicin is often incorporated into cement in orthopedic procedures. Gentamicin drops are used in superficial eye infections and bacterial otitis externa.
- Amikacin is used in gentamicin- and tobramycin-resistant infections, mycobacterial infections, or nocardiosis.
- Tobramycin is slightly better for *P. aeruginosa* than gentamicin and may be inhaled in patients with cystic fibrosis.
- Neomycin is given orally for bowel sterilization pre-surgery or for selective decontamination of the digestive tract.
- Netilmicin is used in Gram-negative infections resistant to gentamicin. Although rarely used, it is considered to demonstrate comparable efficacy for certain indications.
- Streptomycin is used to treat tuberculosis, particularly in the developing world. It is sometimes used synergistically in enterococcal endocarditis (if there is gentamicin resistance).
- Paromomycin is used to treat cryptosporidiosis.

Pharmacology

The aminoglycosides share a number of important characteristics (see Pharmacodynamics, p. 14):
- Concentration-dependent bactericidal activity
- Significant post-antibiotic effect
- Synergism, particularly with cell wall–active agents

Aminoglycosides have poor oral absorption and are usually administered intravenously or intramuscularly for systemic administration. They may also be administered orally (e.g., neomycin, paromomycin), topically, intra-pleurally, intraperitoneally, or intrathecally.

Aminoglycosides are highly soluble with low protein binding, resulting in distribution in the vascular and interstitial compartments. CSF penetration is poor, apart from in neonates. Aminoglycosides are excreted unchanged in the urine (99%).

Aminoglycosides may be given once daily or in multiple daily doses. Once-daily dosing is simpler, as efficacious as multiple dosing in certain indications, and may lower the risk of drug-induced toxicity. The usual suggested dose of gentamicin is 5–7 mg/kg/day. The dose is reduced in renal failure to 3 mg/kg/day. Exceptions include children, pregnancy, burns, endocarditis, and monotherapy of pseudomonal infections outside of the urinary tract.

If patients need to continue therapy beyond 48 hours, a random concentration obtained 6–14 hours following the dose should be obtained and the dosing interval adjusted according to the Hartford nomogram (Fig. 1.3).

Toxicity and side effects

Nephrotoxicity is the most common adverse effect (5–25%).

Ototoxicity (cochlear and vestibular) may be irreversible.

Neuromuscular blockade is rare. It typically occurs in patients with other disease states that interfere with neuromuscular transmission. Aminoglycosides are contraindicated in patients with myasthenia gravis.

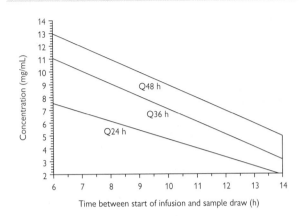

Fig. 1.3 Hartford nomogram for once-daily aminoglyco-sides. Reproduced with permission from Nicolau et al. (1995). Experience with a once daily aminoglycoside program administered to 2,184 patients. Antimicrob Agents Chemother 39:650–655.

Macrolides

The macrolides (erythromycin, clarithromycin, azithromycin) and the lincosamides (lincomycin and clindamycin), although chemically unrelated, have some similar properties such as antimicrobial activity, mechanisms of action, resistance, and pharmacology. The ketolides are a new class of antibiotics, derived from erythromycin, with activity against macrolide-resistant strains.

Erythromycin
Erythromycin was derived from *Saccharopolyspora erythraea* in 1952. Erythromycin A is the active component. It consists of a 14-member macrocyclic lactone ring attached to two sugars.
   Mechanism of action: inhibits RNA-dependent protein synthesis at the step of chain elongation by interacting with the peptidyl transferase site. It also inhibits the formation of the 50S ribosomal subunit.
   Resistance: there are four resistance mechanisms:
- Decreased outer membrane permeability, e.g., Enterobacteriaceae, *Pseudomonas* spp. *Acinetobacter* spp. are intrinsically resistant.
- Efflux pumps, e.g., *msr(A)* gene of *S. aureus* and *mef(A)* gene of *S. pneumoniae* and Group A. streptococci
- Alterations of 23S rRNA by methylation of adenine. This confers resistance to macrolides, lincosamides, and streptogramins type B and is referred to as the MLS$_B$ phenotype. It is encoded by *erm* (erythromycin ribosomal methylase) genes.

- Enzymatic inactivation by phosphotransferases, mediated by *mph* genes. Hydrolysis of the macrocyclic lactone is encoded by esterase genes, *ere(A)* and *ere(B)*, on plasmids.

Clinical use includes community-acquired pneumonia, atypical pneumonia (e.g., *M. pneumoniae, C. pneumoniae, L. pneumophila*), *B. pertussis*, and *Campylobacter* gastroenteritis. It is used topically to treat acne vulgaris and ophthalmically to treat and prevent superficial infections.

Pharmacology: given orally (stimulates GI motility) or intravenously. It is widely distributed in the tissues and excreted in the bile and urine. Some is inactivated in the liver. It is a substrate for (CYP2D6 and CYP3A4) as well as inhibitor of (CYP1A2 and CYP3A4) CYP enzymes.

Toxicity and side effects: gastrointestinal symptoms (nausea, vomiting, abdominal cramps, diarrhea) are common. Skin rash, fever, eosinophilia, cholestatic jaundice, transient hearing loss, QT prolongation, torsades de pointes, candidiasis, pseudomembranous colitis, and infantile pyloric stenosis can also occur.

Clarithromycin

- *Structure:* 14-member ring with methoxy group at position 6
- *Mechanism of action:* same as for erythromycin. More active than erythromycin against *S. pneumoniae,* Group A. streptococci, MRSA, *M. catarrhalis,* and *L. pneumophila.* Also active against *M. leprae, M. avium* complex (MAC), and *T. gondii*
- *Resistance:* similar to erythromycin
- *Clinical use:* similar to erythromycin. Treatment of MAC and other nontuberculous mycobacterial infections, *H. pylori* eradication
- *Pharmacology:* given orally or intravenously. Metabolized in the liver to active metabolites by CYP3A4. It is also a potent inhibitor of this enzyme, making it responsible for many drug–drug interactions.

Azithromycin

- *Structure:* 15-member lactone ring (azalide)
- *Mechanism of action:* same as for erythromycin. Greater activity against Gram-negative species than that of erythromycin and clarithromcyin. Also active against MAC and *T. gondii*
- *Resistance:* similar to erythromycin
- *Clinical use:* similar to erythromycin. Also use for treatment of *B. microti, B. burgdorferi,* cryptosporidiosis
- *Pharmacology:* given orally but should be taken 1 hour before or 2 hours after food. Widely distributed in tissues with half-life of 2–4 days. Mostly not metabolized, and excreted in the bile. Also available in IV form. An extended release formulation is available but associated with significant gastrointestinal toxicity.
- *Toxicity and side effects:* similar to those of erythromycin

Ketolides

Ketolides are a new class of antibiotics derived from erythromycin A that have increased potency against bacteria that have become resistant to macrolides, e.g., *S. pneumoniae* and *S. pyogenes*. Telithromycin is currently the only available drug.

Telithromycin

- *Structure:* 14-member ring with ketone instead of L-cladinose at position 3. This prevents induction of macrolide-lincosamide-streptogramin B (MLS$_B$) resistance (see Lincosamides, Box 1.7, p. 45).
- *Mechanism of action:* similar to that of erythromycin
- *Resistance:* this is uncommon, as ketolides are poor inducers of efflux pumps and MLS$_B$ methylase genes. *S. aureus* strains with constitutive *erm* genes are resistant, whereas *S. pneumoniae* strains with constitutive *erm* genes remain sensitive
- *Toxicity and side effects:* similar to those of clarithromycin and azithromycin. Reports of exacerbation of myasthenia gravis, prolonged QTc, and acute hepatic failure. Carries a black box warning cautioning use in patients with myasthenia gravis and requires a medication guide be given to patients with each prescription.
- *Pharmacology:* good oral absorption and bioavailability. Metabolized in the liver by CYP3A4
- *Clinical use:* community-acquired pneumonia, acute exacerbation of chronic obstructive pulmonary disease (COPD), tonsillitis, pharyngitis, and sinusitis

---

Box 1.7 MLS$_B$ resistance (also known as inducible resistance)

Macrolides, lincosamides, and streptogramin type B (MLS$_B$) antibiotics bind to closely related sites on the 50S ribosome of bacteria. One consequence is that some bacteria (e.g., staphylococci, streptococci, and enterococci) with inducible resistance to erythromycin also become resistant to the other MLS$_B$ agents, in the presence of erythromycin. The methylase enzyme involved is not induced by lincosamides or streptogramins, which therefore remain active in the absence of macrolides.

Over 20 *erm* genes encode the MLS$_B$ resistance, and it is becoming more common in group A streptococci and pneumococci.

When using clindamycin to treat staphylococcal infections, it is important to screen for the presence of inducible resistance to clindamycin by performing a D test in the microbiology laboratory.

Lincosamides

This group of antibiotics includes lincomycin (not available in the United States) and clindamycin. Lincomycin was isolated from *Streptomyces lincolnensis* in 1962. Clindamycin, which was produced by the chemical modification of lincomycin, has better oral bioavailability and increased bacterial potency compared with that of lincomycin.

Although chemically unrelated to erythromycin, many of the biological properties of lincosamides are similar to those of the macrolides.

Mechanism of action

Lincosamides inhibit protein synthesis by interacting with the peptidyl transferase site of the 50S ribosomal subunit. They also inhibit the formation of the 50S ribosomal subunit.

Clindamycin is highly active against anaerobes (e.g., *B. fragilis*), pneumococci, group A streptococci, methicillin-sensitive *S. aureus* (MSSA), *T. gondii*, and *P. falciparum*.

Resistance

There are several resistance mechanisms:

- Alteration of 50S ribosomal proteins of the receptor site confers resistance to macrolides and lincosamides.
- Alteration in the 23S subunit by methylation of adenine results in the MLS_B phenotype (see Box 1.7) and confers resistance to macrolides, lincosamides, and type B streptogramins. This MLS_B phenotype is encoded by *erm* (erythromycin ribosomal methylase) genes.
- Inactivation by 3-lincomycin, 4-clindamycin 0-nucleotide transferase. This is plasmid mediated and encoded by *linA*   .
- Decreased membrane permeability in Gram-negative species, e.g., Enterobacteriaceae, *Pseudomonas* spp., *Acinetobacter* spp.

Clinical use

- Alternative to β-lactams in penicillin-allergic patients with skin and soft tissue infections
- Treatment of skin and soft tissue infections due to MRSA. Clindamycin is useful as it can also inhibit bacterial toxins, including Panton-Valentine leukocidin (PVL)
- Staphylococcal bone and joint infections
- Severe group A streptococcal infections, e.g., necrotizing fasciitis, toxic shock syndrome
- Anaerobic infections, e.g., intra-abdominal sepsis, anaerobic bronchopulmonary infections
- *Pneumocystis jirovecii* pneumonia (in combination with primaquine)
- *P. falciparum* malaria (in combination with quinine)

Pharmacology

- Clindamycin is given orally, intravenously, or by deep intramuscular injection.
- The drug is well absorbed orally and widely distributed with good tissue penetration, especially bone. CSF penetration is negligible.

- Most of the drug is metabolized to products with variable antibacterial activity.
- It is excreted in the bile and urine.
- Dose reduction is required for severe hepatic disease.

Toxicity and side effects
- *C. difficile* colitis: discontinue clindamycin
- *Allergic reactions:* rashes, fever, erythema multiforme, anaphylaxis
- *Laboratory abnormalities:* transient hepatitis, neutropenia, thrombocytopenia

Streptogramins

Streptogramins are a group of antibiotics derived from various *Streptomyces* spp. They consist of two macrocyclic lactone peptolide components referred to as streptogramin A and streptogramin B. A number of compounds exist:
- Quinupristin-dalfopristin (Synercid®) is the only drug available in the United States and is used for the treatment of resistant Gram-positive infections.
- Other examples of streptogramins include virginiamycin, which is mainly used as an animal growth promoter.

Mechanism of action

Streptogramins exert their action on the second, or elongation, stage of protein synthesis. The two components act synergistically as follows:
- Streptogramin A molecules (e.g., dalfopristin) bind to the 50S ribosomal subunit and prevent aminoacyl-tRNA from attaching to the catalytic site of the peptidyl transferase, thus inhibiting transfer of the growing peptide chain.
- Streptogramin B molecules (e.g., quinupristin) prevent the peptide bond forming, which leads to the premature release of incomplete polypeptides.

Quinupristin-dalfopristin is active against most Gram-positive organisms (except *E. faecalis*, which is intrinsically resistant).

Resistance

There are three mechanism of resistance:
- Modification of the ribosomal target site (quinupristin). This results in resistance to macrolides, lincosamides, and streptogramin B (MLS_B phenotype) and is encoded by various *erm* genes (see Lincosamides, p. 45, Box 1.7).
- Enzymatic inactivation by acetyltransferases, encoded by *vat(A)*, *vat(B)*, and *vat(C)* in staphylococci, and *vat(D)* in *E. faecium* (quinupristin and dalfopristin)
- Active transport out of the cells by efflux pumps, encoded by *vga(A)* and *vga(B)* genes in staphylococci (quinupristin and dalfopristin)

Clinical use

- Vancomycin-resistant *E. faecium* (not active against *E. faecalis*)
- Skin and soft tissue infection caused by MSSA or group A streptococci
- Serious Gram-positive infections for which there is no alternative antibiotic available

Pharmacology

- Quinupristin-dalfopristin is given intravenously, preferably into a central vein.
- The drug exhibits significant post-antibiotic effect: 2.8 hours for pneumococci, 4.7 hours for staphylococci, and 2.6–8.5 hours for enterococci
- There is a wide volume of distribution but poor CSF penetration. Case reports exist citing intrathecal injection.
- The drug is metabolized in the liver and excreted in the feces.

Toxicity and side effects

- Injection site reactions occur in >30% of patients, so the drug should be given via a central vein.
- Arthralgia and myalgia are common and may be dose related.
- Nausea, vomiting, diarrhea, skin rash, and pruritis can occur.
- Laboratory abnormalities include hepatitis and hyperbilirubinemia.
- Inhibition of hepatic CYP3A4 results in increased concentrations of drugs metabolized by this enzyme.

Lipopeptides

Daptomycin (Cubicin®), a fermentation product of *Streptomyces roseosporus*, was discovered in the 1980s. It is a 13-member cyclic amino acid lipopeptide antibiotic with a lipophilic tail.

It was approved in the United States in 2003 for the treatment of complicated skin and soft tissue infections.

Mechanism of action

The exact mechanism of action is unknown, although it appears to bind to the cell membrane of Gram-positive bacteria in a calcium-dependent manner, disrupting the cell membrane potential. Daptomycin is active against Gram-positive organisms, e.g., staphylococci, streptococci, and enterococci, including those that are glycopeptide resistant.

Resistance

Resistance to daptomycin is rare; strains with reduced susceptibility have been obtained after serial passage in vitro.

Clinical use

Daptomycin is used for complicated infections caused by Gram-positive bacteria including skin and soft tissue infections, bacteremia, and right-sided endocarditis. The drug is inactivated by surfactant and thus cannot be used to treat pneumonia.

Pharmacology

Daptomycin is given by intravenous infusion. The AUC/MIC profile and prolonged PAE enable once-daily dosing. Daptomycin is highly protein bound and is eliminated largely unchanged by the kidneys.

Toxicity and side effects

- *Common side effects:* nausea, vomiting diarrhea, headache, rash, and injection site reactions
- *Muscle toxicity:* myalgia, muscle weakness, and myositis are uncommon; rhabdomyolysis is rare. Serum creatinine kinase (CK) should be checked before starting treatment and weekly during treatment. Stop treatment if symptoms develop.
- *Interference with PT/INR assay:* clotting sample should be taken just prior to administration of daptomycin. This reaction can be reagent dependent and should be investigated with the laboratory if suspected.

Oxazolidinones

The oxazolidinones are a new, purely synthetic class of antimicrobials with activity against staphylococcal and streptococcal species. Linezolid (Zyvox®) is the only oxazolidinone available. It was introduced in 2001.

It is active against Gram-positive bacteria and is used for infections resistant to other antibiotics (e.g., MRSA and VRE). The oxazolidinones also possess activity against atypical mycobacteria, including *M. tuberculosis.*

Mechanism of action

Oxazolidinones are protein synthesis inhibitors that are bacteriostatic against Gram-positive organisms. They bind to the 50S ribosomal subunit at its interface with the 30S ribosomal subunit, preventing formation of the 70S initiation complex.

Resistance

Despite its recent introduction, resistance to linezolid among strains of MRSA and VRE has already been reported. The mechanism appears to be mutation in the 23S RNA domain V region. It is usually associated with long durations of therapy or prior exposure to linezolid.

Clinical use

Linezolid is approved for use in Gram-positive infections:
- Pneumonia and complicated skin or soft tissue infections caused by Gram-positive bacteria
- Serious infections due to resistant Gram-positive bacteria (e.g., MRSA, VRE, and penicillin-resistant pneumococci)

Because of higher mortality rates in patients receiving linezolid for empiric treatment of bacteremia, use for this indication should be limited to situations where the risk–benefit ratio has been carefully considered.

Pharmacology

Linezolid may be given orally (100% bioavailability) or intravenously. Linezolid is widely distributed with good tissue and CSF penetration. It is metabolized by oxidation in the liver and excreted in the urine (85%) or feces. No dose adjustment is required for renal or hepatic disease.

Toxicity and side effects

Linezolid is generally well tolerated.

- GI symptoms, e.g., nausea, vomiting, and diarrhea, are common.
- Myelosuppression such as thrombocytopenia, neutropenia, and pancytopenia has been reported. This is more common with prolonged therapy (>10 days) and usually reversible. Complete blood count (CBC) should be monitored weekly in patients taking linezolid.
- Monoamine oxidase inhibition: linezolid is a monoamine oxidase inhibitor. Patients should be told to avoid tyramine-rich foods. Linezolid has been associated with serotonin syndrome in patients taking concomitant selective serotonin reuptake inhibitors (SSRIs).
- Optic neuropathy has been reported in patients taking >28 days' treatment. Patients should be told to report visual symptoms and referred to an ophthalmologist, if necessary.
- Lactic acidosis has been associated with prolonged treatment.

Chloramphenicol

Chloramphenicol, initially called *chloromycetin*, was first isolated from *Streptomyces venezuelae* in 1947. It has a broad spectrum of activity against a wide range of bacteria, spirochaetes, rickettsiae, chlamydiae, and mycoplasmas.

Soon after its introduction in 1949, reports of aplastic anemia emerged, limiting its use. Furthermore, widespread use in the developing world has resulted in resistance, particularly in *S. typhi*. Despite this, chloramphenicol remains useful for the treatment of serious infections that are resistant to other antibiotics.

Mechanism of action

Chloramphenicol inhibits protein synthesis by binding to the 50S subunit of the 70S ribosome at a site that prevents the attachment of tRNA. This prevents association of the amino acid with peptidyltransferase and peptide band formation. This is a bacteriostatic effect in most organisms but is bactericidal in some meningeal pathogens, e.g., *H. influenzae, S. pneumoniae*, and *N. meningitis*.

Resistance

There are several resistance mechanisms:

- Reduced permeability or uptake
- Ribosomal mutation
- Production of acetyl transferase, an enzyme that acetylates the antibiotic into an inactive form. This mechanism also confers resistance to tetracyclines (see Tetracyclines, p. 51) and is responsible for

widespread epidemics of chloramphenicol resistance to *S. typhi* and *S. dysenteriae* seen in the developing world.

Clinical use

In the developed world chloramphenicol is rarely used (because of toxicity), but it remains a commonly used antibiotic in the developing world.

- Enteric fever due to *S. typhi* and *S. paratyphi*: high rates of drug resistance have been reported in India, Vietnam, and Central and South America
- Severe infections such as meningitis, septicemia, epiglottitis due to *Haemophilus influenzae*
- Sometimes used in infective exacerbations of COPD
- An alternative agent for infections in pregnancy, young children, or patients with immediate penicillin hypersensitivity
- Eye drops and ointment are widely used for superficial eye infections.
- Ear drops are used for bacterial otitis externa.

Pharmacology

Chloramphenicol may be administered orally, intravenously, intramuscularly, or topically. It has high lipid solubility and low protein binding, resulting in a wide volume of distribution in body fluids and tissues.

CSF and ocular penetration is good. Chloramphenicol is metabolized in the liver by glucuronidation and excreted in the bile. Only 5–10% is excreted in the urine.

Toxicity and side effects

- Bone marrow suppression is common, dose related, and reversible. It is a direct pharmacological effect of the antibiotic, resulting from inhibition of mitochondrial protein synthesis. Manifestations include anemia, reticulocytosis, leukopenia, and thrombocytopenia. Monitor CBC twice a week during treatment.
- Aplastic anemia is a rare, idiosyncratic, and often fatal complication, which may occur during or after the completion of therapy. It occurs in 1 in 40,000 patients. The pathogenesis of this condition is incompletely understood. Monitor CBC twice a week during treatment and discontinue the drug if the WBC falls below 2.5×10^9/L.
- There are also reports of hemolytic anemia in patients with glucose-6-phosphate dehydrogenase (G6PD) deficiency and childhood leukemia after chloramphenicol therapy.
- Gray baby syndrome may occur with high doses in neonates (abdominal distension, vomiting, cyanosis, circulatory collapse) because of the inability to metabolize and excrete the drug. If the drug is required in neonates, the dose should be reduced and drug concentrations monitored.
- Other side effects include rash, fevers, Jarisch–Herxheimer reactions, gastrointestinal symptoms, glossitis, stomatitis, optic neuritis, bleeding disorders, acute intermittent porphyria, and interference with development of immunity after immunization.

Tetracyclines

Tetracyclines are a group of broad-spectrum bacteriostatic antibiotics active against Gram-positive, Gram-negative, and intracellular organisms, e.g., *Chlamydia*, mycoplasmas, rickettsiae, and protozoan parasites.

The first tetracycline, aureomycin (chlortetracycline), was isolated from *Streptomyces aureofaciens*, a soil organism. Since then, a number of other tetracyclines have been developed.

Tetracyclines differ in their pharmacological properties rather than spectrum of activity, although minocycline has slightly broader spectrum.

Classification
- *First generation:* tetracycline, chlortetracycline, oxytetracycline, demeclocycline, lymecycline, and methacycline
- *Second generation:* doxycycline and minocycline
- *Third generation* (glycylcyclines): tigecycline

Mechanism of action
Tetracyclines inhibit bacterial protein synthesis by reversibly binding to the 30S ribosomal subunit. This blocks binding of aminoacyl–tRNA to the ribosomal A site, preventing the addition of new amino acids. As their binding is reversible, these agents are mainly bacteriostatic.

Tetracyclines also inhibit mitochondrial protein synthesis by binding to 70S ribosomal subunits in mitochondria in eukaryotic parasites. The mechanism of their antiprotozoal activity is unknown.

Resistance
The widespread use of tetracyclines has been accompanied by increasing drug resistance. This is mediated by acquisition of genes on mobile genetic elements (MGEs; see Molecular genetics of resistance, p. 9). Many tetracycline-resistance genes have been identified, most belonging to the *tet* family and some to the *otr* family. These genes confer resistance through the following mechanisms:
- *Efflux pumps:* these membrane-associated proteins pump tetracyclines out of the cell. They confer resistance to first-generation tetracyclines.
- *Ribosomal protection proteins* are cytoplasmic proteins that release tetracyclines from their binding site by guanosine diphosphate (GDP)-dependent mechanisms. They protect the ribosome from first- and second-generation tetracyclines.
- *Enzymatic inactivation* is seen in *B. fragilis*, where the *tet(X)* gene codes for a protein that modifies tetracyclines in the presence of nicotinamide adenine dinucleotide phosphate-oxidase (NADPH) and oxygen.

Clinical use
- Chlamydial infections
- Rickettsial infections
- Q-fever
- Brucellosis (doxycycline with either streptomycin or rifampicin)
- Lyme disease (*Borrelia burgdorferi*)
- *Mycoplasma* spp. infections

- Infective exacerbations of COPD (due to their activity against *H. influenzae*)
- They are also used in treatment of acne, destructive (refractory) periodontal diseases, sinusitis, chronic prostatitis, pelvic inflammatory disease, and melioidosis.

Pharmacology

- Tetracyclines are usually given orally. Absorption of tetracycline and oxytetracycline is reduced by milk, antacids, and some salts. Doxycycline and minocycline are highly bioavailable.
- To maximize bioavailability, tetracycline administration should be separated from food and milk
- They are sometimes divided into three groups on the basis of their half-lives: short acting (tetracycline, oxytetracycline), intermediate acting (demeclocycline) and long acting (doxycycline, minocycline).
- Tetracyclines are widely distributed and show good tissue penetration.
- Tetracycline is eliminated in the urine. Minocycline is metabolized in the liver. Doxycycline is mainly eliminated in the feces.

Toxicity and side effects

- Nausea, vomiting, diarrhea, dysphagia, and esophageal irritation are common.
- Photosensitivity reactions are common and appear to be toxic rather than allergic.
- Prolonged minocycline administration can cause skin, nail, and scleral pigmentation.
- Deposition occurs in growing bones and teeth, so tetracyclines should not be given to children <12 years of age or to pregnant or breast-feeding women.
- Hepatotoxicity due to fatty change may be fatal.
- Tetracyclines exacerbate renal impairment. All tetracyclines (except minocycline and doxycycline) should be avoided in renal failure. Demeclocycline causes nephrogenic diabetes insipidus and is used as a treatment for inappropriate antidiuretic hormone (ADH) secretion.
- Vertigo is unique to minocycline.
- Benign intracranial hypertension has been described with all tetracyclines.
- Superinfection: mucocutanous candidiasis is common. *C. difficile* colitis may occur.
- Allergic reactions (rashes, urticaria, anaphylaxis) are uncommon.

Tigecycline (Tygacil®)

- A glycylcycline antibiotic, structurally related to the tetracyclines
- Active against Gram-positive and Gram-negative bacteria, including tetracycline-resistant organisms, and some anaerobes. It is also active against MRSA and VRE but not against *P. aeruginosa* and

Proteus spp. Tigecycline also retains activity against some isolates of *Stenotrophomonas maltophilia*.
- Reserved for the treatment of complicated skin and soft tissue infections and complicated abdominal infections caused by multi-drug-resistant organisms. Data have also emerged supporting use of this agent for community-acquired pneumonia.
- Because of low serum drug concentrations, this agent should not be used to treat bacteremia.
- Side effects are similar to those of the tetracyclines.
- Nausea and vomiting are reported in up to 30% of patients.

Sulfonamides

The era of antimicrobial chemotherapy began in 1932 when Domagk reported the antimicrobial effects of Prontosil (a sulfachrysoidine dye) against murine streptococcal infections. This compound was found to exert its antibacterial effect through the release of sulfanilamide, which acted as a competitive inhibitor of dihydropteroate synthetase in the folate synthesis pathway (Fig. 1.4).

Although many sulfonamide drugs were developed, relatively few are in clinical use today, mainly because of their toxicity and increasing drug resistance. Those currently available in the United States include sulfamethoxazole, sulfadiazine, sulfadoxine, sulfasalazine, mafenide acetate, and sulfacetamide sodium.

Classification

The sulfonamides can be classified as follows:
- Short- or medium-acting sulfonamides, e.g., sulfisazoxole, sulfamethoxazole, sulfadiazine
- Long-acting sulfonamides, e.g., sulfadoxinetopical sulfonamides, e.g., silver sulfadiazine, mafenide acetate, sulfanilamide, sulfacetamide.

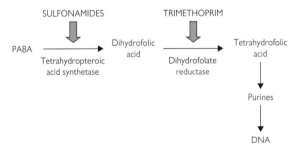

Fig. 1.4 Action of sulfonamides and trimethoprim on the bacterial folate synthesis pathway.

Mechanism of action

The sulfonamides are bacteriostatic and inhibit bacterial growth by interfering with folic acid synthesis. They are analogs of PABA and competitively inhibit the incorporation of PABA into tetrahydropteroic acid by means of the enzyme tetrahydropteroic acid synthetase.

They are active against a broad spectrum of Gram-positive and Gram-negative bacteria as well as *Actinomyces, Chlamydia, Plasmodium,* and *Toxoplasma* spp.

Resistance

Resistance to sulfonamides is widespread and increasingly common; cross-resistance between different sulfonamides occurs.

Resistance may be due to the following:
- Chromosomal mutations that result in
  - Overproduction of PABA, e.g., *S. aureus, N. gonorrheae.*
  - Alterations in dihydropteroate synthetase that in turn lead to reduced affinity for sulfonamides, e.g., *E. coli.*
- Plasmids that carry genes coding for
  - Production of drug-resistant enzymes.
  - Decreased bacterial permeability.

Plasmid-mediated sulfonamide resistance is common in Enterobacteriaceae and has increased greatly in recent years, often in conjunction with trimethoprim resistance.

Clinical use

- Sulfadiazine may be used for the treatment of UTIs, nocardiosis, toxoplasmosis, and prevention of rheumatic fever.
- Sulfadiazine is used in combination with pyrimethamine (see Antiprotozoal drugs 2, p. 104) for treating toxoplasmosis.
- Sulfadoxine is used in combination with pyrimethamine for treatment of falciparum malaria (see Miscellaneous antimalarials, p. 101).
- Silver sulfadiazine (Silvadene®) and mafenide acetate are used topically to prevent or treat infections in patients with burns.

Pharmacology

- Sulfonamides are usually administered orally. Sulfacetamide is used topically in eye drops. Silver sulfadiazine, sulfacetamide, and mafenide acetate are available in topical formulations.
- Oral sulfonamides are rapidly absorbed. Topical sulfonamides are also absorbed and may be detectable in the blood, particularly when applied to broken skin as in burn patients.
- The drug class is widely distributed with high concentrations in body fluids, including CSF.
- These agents are metabolized in the liver and excreted in the urine. Dose modification is required in renal impairment.

Toxicity and side effects

- *General:* nausea, vomiting, diarrhea, rash, fever, headache, depression, jaundice, hepatic necrosis, drug-induced lupus, serum sickness-like syndrome

- *Hematological:* acute hemolytic anemia, aplastic anemia, agranulocytosis, leukopenia, thrombocytopenia
- *Hypersensitivity reactions:* drug eruption, vasculitis, erythema nodosum, erythema multiforme, Stevens–Johnson syndrome, anaphylaxis
- Neonatal kernicterus can occur if given in the last month of pregnancy.

Trimethoprim

Trimethoprim is a diaminopyrimidine that was synthesized by Bushby and Hitchings in 1968. The other members of this class are pyrimethamine (an antiprotozoal), cycloguanil (a product of proguanil; see Miscellaneous antimalarials, p. 101), and flucytosine (an antifungal).

Trimethoprim has a fairly broad spectrum of activity against many Gram-positive bacteria and most Gram-negative rods except *P. aeruginosa* and *Bacteroides* spp.

Mechanism of action
Trimethoprim inhibits the bacterial enzyme dihydrofolate reductase (DHFR), preventing the conversion of dihydrofolate to tetrahydrofolate in the folate synthesis pathway (see Fig. 1.4). It works on the same pathway as the sulfonamides but at a later point, resulting in synergistic activity. It is bactericidal or bacteriostatic, depending on the organism and drug concentration.

Resistance
Resistance is common in Enterobacteriaceae, particularly in developing countries. It may be chromosomal or plasmid mediated and caused by the following:
- Chromosomal mutations in the gene for DHFR (or its promoter), resulting in overproduction or modification of the target enzyme
- Plasmid-encoded resistance (*dfr* genes in Enterobacteriaceae), which may result in synthesis of an additional trimethoprim-resistant DHFR enzyme
- Change in cell permeability/efflux pumps
- Alterations in metabolic pathway

More than one mechanism can occur in the same cell, resulting in higher resistance levels.

Clinical use
- UTIs
- Prophylaxis of recurrent UTIs
- Treatment of prostatitis and epididymo-orchitis
- An option for oral treatment of MRSA (community-associated isolates of MRSA retain susceptibility to MRSA in most instances)

Pharmacology
- Trimethoprim is given orally and is rapidly absorbed from the gut.
- It is widely distributed in tissues and body fluids, including CSF. High concentrations are achieved in the kidney, lung, sputum, and prostatic fluid; 60–80% is excreted in the urine within 24 hours; the remainder is excreted as urinary metabolites or in the bile.
- Synergism with sulfamethoxazole, polymixins, and aminoglycosides

Toxicity and side effects
- Avoid use in pregnancy, especially the first trimester (antifolate).
- Contraindicated in blood dyscrasias
- Side effects are similar to those of co-trimoxazole, but less severe and less frequent with trimethoprim alone.
- Other side effects include GI disturbance, pruritis, rashes, and hyperkalemia.

Co-trimoxazole

Co-trimoxazole (Bactrim® or Septra®) is a synergistic combination of trimethoprim and sulfamethoxazole, in the ratio of 1:5.

Mechanism of action
Sequential inhibition of two enzymes (tetrahydropteroic acid synthetase and dihydrofolate reductase) occurs in the bacterial folate synthesis pathway (see Sulfonamides, p. 53).

Resistance
Resistance may be due to a variety of mechanisms (see Sulfonamides, p. 53 and Trimethoprim, p. 55 for details). Increasing drug resistance rates have been seen in *S. aureus*, many Enterobacteriaceae, and *Pneumocystis jirovecii*.

Clinical use
- *Pneumocystis jiroveciii* pneumonia (treatment and prophylaxis)
- Toxoplasmosis (prophylaxis and second-line therapy)
- Nocardiosis (second-line therapy)
- Multi-drug-resistant organisms, e.g., *Acinetobacter* spp., *B. cepacia*, *S. maltophilia*, *M. marinum*, *M. kansasii*. Seek advice from an infection diseases specialist for treatment of these difficult infections.
- UTIs
- Acute otitis media in children (if the organism is sensitive and there are no other options)
- Skin and soft tissue infections due to community-associated MRSA infections

Pharmacology
Co-trimoxazole may be given orally or intravenously. Components have different volumes of distribution, so seek advice if treating complicated cases (e.g., at an unusual site).

Toxicity and side effects
- Avoid use in blood disorders, infants <6 weeks old, hepatic impairment, renal impairment, and women who are pregnant or breast-feeding.
- Side effects are mainly due to the sulfonamide component and may be more severe in the elderly.
- Nausea, vomiting, diarrhea, anorexia, and hypersensitivity are most common.

- Rashes, including erythema multiforme, Stevens–Johnson syndrome, and toxic epidermal necrolysis, are rare.
- Hematological toxicity
- Renal dysfunction, interstitial nephritis, hyperkalemia
- Drug-induced hepatitis, pancreatitis, hepatic failure
- Hyperkalemia due to trimethoprim component

Quinolones

Nalidixic acid, the first quinolone antibiotic, was identified in 1962. Development of the fluoroquinolones in the 1980s led to an expanded spectrum of activity and greater potency.

Currently available quinolones include ciprofloxacin, gemifloxacin, levo-floxacin, moxifloxacin, and ofloxacin. Several quinolones, e.g., gatifloxacin, grepafloxacin, and trovafloaxin, have been withdrawn from use because of their toxicity.

Classification

- *First generation:* active against Enterobacteriaceae, e.g., nalidixic acid
- *Second generation:* increased Gram-negative activity, including against *Pseudomonas* spp., and some Gram-positive cocci, e.g., ciprofloxacin, norfloxacin, ofloxacin
- *Third generation:* improved spectrum against *S. pneumoniae* and other Gram-positive cocci, e.g., levofloxacin, moxifloxacin, gemifloxacin
- *Group 4:* enhanced activity against Gram-positive cocci, *S. pneumoniae*, and anaerobes, e.g., trovafloxacin (not available in the United States)

Mechanism of action

The quinolones prevent bacterial nucleic acid synthesis by inhibiting two enzymes, DNA gyrase and topoisomerase IV. DNA gyrase consists of α- and β-subunits, which are encoded by the *gyrA* and *gyrB* genes, respectively. Quinolones inhibit DNA supercoiling, mainly through action on the A-subunit of DNA gyrase.

Topoisomerase IV also consists of two subunits, encoded by the *parC* and *parE* genes. Topoisomerase IV is involved in DNA relaxation and chromosomal segregation. DNA gyrase is the primary target for quinolones in Gram-negative bacteria, whereas topoisomerase IV is the main target in Gram-positive bacteria.

Resistance

Resistance is mainly due to spontaneous chromosomal mutations that:
- Alter the target enzymes. Exposure to quinolones results in the selection of drug-resistant mutants. Stepwise increasing resistance occurs through sequential mutations in *gyrA* (or *gyrB*) and *parC* (or *parE*).
- Alter cell membrane permeability. This may be due to mutations that reduce entry through porin channels or increase efflux. In *P. aeruginosa*, resistance has been shown to be due to over-expression of genes that encode the MexAB–OprM efflux pump, comprising a membrane-fusion protein (MexA), inner-membrane efflux pumps (MexB), and an outer-membrane protein (OprM).

Box 1.8 Indications for consideration of higher dose ciprofloxacin

- Infections in which antibiotic penetration is likely to be suboptimal, e.g., septic arthritis, osteomyelitis, VAP, infections in patients with CF, meningitis, intraocular infections
- Serious pseudomonal infections

Recently, plasmid-mediated quinolone resistance encoded by the *qnr* gene has been identified in *K. pneumoniae, E. coli,* and others.

Clinical use

- *Ciprofloxacin:* UTIs, prostatitis, gonorrhea, pseudomonal infections, prophylaxis of meningococcal meningitis, anthrax. An extended-release preparation is available to facilitate easy dosing. See also Box 1.8.
- *Levofloxacin:* sinusitis, COPD exacerbation, community-acquired pneumonia, UTI, chronic prostatitis, skin and soft tissue infections. It is also active against *M. tuberculosis.*
- *Moxifloxacin:* COPD exacerbation and community-acquired pneumonia. It is also active against *M. tuberculosis.* Because of the lack of urinary penetration, moxifloxacin cannot be used to treat UTIs.
- *Ofloxacin:* primarily used as for ophthalmic and otic administration, although oral tablets remain commercially available. An ophthalmic preparation of moxifloxacin is also available.
- *Gemifloxacin:* treatment of multi-drug resistant *S. pneumoniae* infection.
- Given the development of resistance, as of 2007, the CDC no longer recommends quinolones for the treatment of gonococcal infections.

Pharmacology

- The drug is well absorbed, with bioavailability ranging from 50% to 100%. Oral bioavailability is reduced by co-administration of antacids and divalent cations.
- Gemifloxacin may only be given orally; the other available quinolones are also available in IV formulations. Protein binding is low and volumes of distribution are high. Concentrations in prostate, lung, bile, and stool may exceed plasma concentrations.
- Ciprofloxacin, levofloxacin, ofloxacin, and gemifloxacin are eliminated renally, and dose reductions should be considered in patients with renal insufficiency. Moxifloxacin undergoes extensive metabolism and is eliminated as inactive drug in the urine and feces.

Toxicity and side effects

- Gastrointestinal side effects are common (3–17%), e.g., nausea, vomiting, abdominal discomfort, diarrhea (risk factor for *C. difficile* disease).
- CNS symptoms occur in 0.9–11% of patients, e.g., headache, dizziness, insomnia, and altered mood. Hallucinations, delirium, and seizures are

rare. Quinolones may induce seizures and should be used with caution in patients with a seizure history.

- Allergic reactions include rash, photosensitivity, drug fever, urticaria, angioedema, vasculitis, serum sickness, and interstitial nephritis.
  - Gemifloxacin is associated with a higher risk of rash, particularly in women who receive greater than 7 to 10 days of therapy. This is controlled by using the drug primarily for community-acquired infections for a duration of 5 days or less.
- Arthropathy has been observed in animals and tendon rupture in adults. Quinolones are not recommended in young children (but may be used for specific indications under expert guidance) or in adults with a history of tendon disorders. The entire class now carries a boxed warning regarding risk of tendon rupture in the United States.
- QT prolongation may predispose to ventricular arrhythmias.
- Laboratory abnormalities include leukopenia, eosinophilia, hepatitis (moxifloxacin), and dysglycemia.

Nitroimidazoles

Metronidazole (Flagyl®)

Metronidazole is a nitroimidazole drug that was introduced for the treatment of *T. vaginalis* infections in 1959. It was subsequently found to be bactericidal for most anaerobic and facultatively anaerobic bacteria and protozoa.

Mechanism of action

Metronidazole is a prodrug that needs to be activated in susceptible organisms. It has a low molecular weight and enters the bacterial cell by passive diffusion.

It is activated by reduction of its nitro group by a nitroreductase, resulting in the formation of metronidazole radicals. These highly reactive compounds interact with nucleic acids and proteins, causing breakage, destabilization, and cell death.

Resistance

Resistance to metronidazole is rare and a combination of mechanisms is required. Both chromosomally mediated and plasmid-mediated forms of resistance have been described. Reports of resistance in *Bacteroides* spp. have been attributed to the transferable genes *nimA* and *nimD*.

Metronidazole resistance in *H. pylori* is associated with mutational inactivation of the *rdxA*, *frxA*, and *fdxB* genes. Metronidazole resistance in *T. vaginalis* and *Giardia* is probably multifactorial, with reduced activation of metronidazole and/or reduced transcription of the ferrodoxin gene.

Clinical use

- Parasitic infections, e.g., bacterial vaginosis, intestinal amoebiasis, giardiasis, amoebic liver abscess

---

Box 1.9 Antibiotics with anaerobic coverage

Commonly, metronidazole is added to regimens to provide anaerobic coverage. The following agents offer anti-anaerobic activity and therefore may not require the addition of metronidazole:

- Amoxicillin/clavulanate
- Imipenen or meropenem
- Clindamycin
- Piperacillin–tazobactam
- Moxifloxacin

- Anaerobic infections (see Box 1.9)
- *C. difficile* colitis
- *H. pylori* eradication therapy
- Small-bowel bacterial overgrowth
- Infected leg ulcers and pressure sores
- Pelvic inflammatory disease
- Acute ulcerative gingivitis
- Surgical prophylaxis when anaerobic coverage is needed

Pharmacology

- Metronidazole may be given orally, intravenously, per vagina, or topically. *It should never be taken with alcohol because of the risk of a disulfiram-like reaction* (see Toxicity and side effects).
- When given orally, it is absorbed rapidly and almost completely.
- Protein binding is low and the drug is widely distributed in fluids and tissues. Metronidazole shows excellent penetration into abscesses.
- It is metabolized in the liver via the cytochrome P450 enzyme system.
- Metronidazole and its metabolites are primarily eliminated by the kidneys.

Toxicity and side effects

Metronidazole is generally well tolerated.

- Abnormal metallic taste is commonly reported.
- Gastrointestinal effects include nausea, anorexia, epigastric discomfort, vomiting, diarrhea, and constipation.
- Peripheral neuropathy occurs with prolonged treatment.
- A disulfiram-like reaction occurs with alcohol, e.g., nausea, vomiting, flushing, tachycardia, hypotension, acute confusion or psychosis, and sudden death.
- Genitourinary symptoms include transient darkening of the urine, dysuria, cystitis, and incontinence.
- Allergic reactions include rash, urticaria, flushing, bronchospasm, and serum sickness.
- CNS symptoms include headache, dizziness, syncope, vertigo, sleep disturbance, confusion, excitation, and depression. Cerebellar toxicity has been seen with high doses and/or prolonged therapy.
- Other side effects include fever, mucocutaneous candidiasis, neutropenia, and thrombophlebitis with IV infusion.

Nitrofurans

The nitrofuran group of antibiotics comprises the single agent nitrofuran-toin (Furadantin®, Macrobid®, Macrodantin®).

Mechanism of action

The mechanism of action is poorly understood but requires enzymatic reduction within the bacterial cell (like metronidazole). The reduced derivatives bind to ribosomal proteins and block translation. They also appear to directly damage bacterial DNA (like quinolones) and inhibit DNA repair.

Nitrofurans are bactericidal against urinary pathogens such as *E. coli, Citrobacter*, group B streptococci, *S. saprophyticus, E. faecalis*, and *E. faecium*. However, only a minority of *Enterobacter* spp. are sensitive, and most members of *Proteus, Providencia, Morganella, Serratia, Acinetobacter*, and *Pseudomonas* spp. are resistant.

Resistance

Resistance is rare. In *E. coli*, resistance may be chromosomal or plasmid mediated and is associated with inhibition of nitrofuran reductase activity.

Clinical use

- Acute uncomplicated cystitis (not pyelonephritis)
- Treatment of recurrent UTIs
- Prophylaxis of recurrent UTIs

Pharmacokinetics

- Nitrofurantoin has good oral absorption, which is enhanced by food.
- Serum concentrations are low but urine concentrations are high.
- Renal elimination: dose reduction is required in renal impairment.
- There is limited efficacy in patients with renal impairment and an estimated creatinine clearance of <30 mL/min.

Toxicity and side effects

- *Gastrointestinal:* nausea, vomiting
- *Pulmonary:* acute hypersensitivity (fever, cough, dyspnea, pulmonary infiltrates, myalgia, eosinophilia), chronic (pulmonary fibrosis, bronchiolitis obliterans organizing pneumonia)

Rifamycins

These are semisynthetic derivatives of rifamycin B, a natural product origi-nally isolated from *Streptomyces mediterranei*. Rifamycin B is poorly active but readily converted into rifamycin S, from which most active compounds are derived.

The rifamycins have a number of features in common:
- They inhibit bacterial DNA-dependent RNA polymerase.
- They have bactericidal effect against a variety of bacteria.

- They have rapid emergence of resistance due to mutation in *rpoB* gene (encodes ß-subunit of DNA-dependent RNA polymerase).
- They are used in combination with unrelated antibiotics to suppress emergence of resistance.
- They stimulate hepatic metabolism by CYP450 enzyme system.
- Excretion is predominantly biliary.

Rifampin

This is the most important rifamycin and is widely used for the treatment of tuberculosis and other bacterial infections.

- *Mechanism of action:* inhibits DNA-dependent RNA polymerase. Bactericidal against *S. aureus* (including MRSA), group A streptococcus, *S. pneumoniae*, *N. gonorrheae*, *N. meningitidis*, *H. influenzae*, *M. tuberculosis*, *M. kansasii*, *M. marinum*, *M. leprae*, *Legionella* spp.,
- *L. monocytogenes*, *Brucella* spp.
- *Resistance:* mutations in *rpoB* gene
- *Clinical use:* TB, leprosy, serious or device-related infections with antibiotic-resistant staphylococci, pneumococci, *Legionella*, elimination of nasopharyngeal carriage of *N. meningitidis* and *H. influenzae*
- *Pharmacology:* >90% oral absorption, widely distributed, low CSF penetration unless meningeal inflammation, metabolized in liver, predominantly excreted in bile, available as oral and IV formulations
- *Interactions:* enhances its own metabolism and that of other drugs, e.g., warfarin, oral contraceptives, corticosteroids, protease inhibitors
- *Toxicity and side effects:* orange discoloration of body fluids, skin rashes, GI upset, hepatitis, thrombocytopenia (stop drug), "rifampicin flu" (intermittent therapy)

Rifabutin

Rifabutin is mainly used to treat atypical mycobacterial infections.

- *Mechanism of action:* similar to that of rifampin but more active against *M. avium* complex (MAC)
- *Resistance:* mutations in *rpoB* gene. Lower frequency of spontaneously resistant strains than for rifampin
- *Clinical use:* prophylaxis against MAC in patient with AIDS, treatment of nontuberculous mycobacterial disease, treatment of TB in those who cannot have rifampin (unacceptable interactions, intolerance)
- *Pharmacology:* 12–20% oral absorption; widely distributed, with concentrations in organs being higher than that of plasma
- *Interactions:* CYP3A4 inhibitors can increase rifabutin concentrations. Rifabutin also induces CYP3A4, although to a lesser extent than rifampin.
- *Toxicity and side effects:* skin rashes, GI upset, hepatitis, neutropenia, uveitis, and arthralgia (with higher doses)

Rifapentine

- *Mechanism of action:* similar to that of rifampin but more active against MAC. Also active against *L. monocytogenes* and *Brucella* spp.

- *Clinical use:* used once weekly in continuation phase of TB treatment in noncavitatory, drug-susceptible, smear-negative (at 2 months) TB. It should not be given in HIV-infected patients as it has high treatment failure rates.
- *Pharmacology:* 70% oral absorption; well distributed with tissue concentrations exceeding plasma concentrations except CSF and bone
- *Interactions:* potent inducer of cytochrome P450, resulting in reduced concentrations of coadministered drugs, e.g., protease inhibitors
- *Toxicity and side effects:* neutropenia, hepatitis; animal evidence of teratogenicity and fetal toxicity (avoid use in pregnancy)

Other rifamycins

Rifaximin is used in traveler's diarrhea and hepatic encephalopathy. It may have a role in preventing recurrence of *C. difficile*–associated disease.

Polymyxins

The polymyxins (polymyxin B and polymyxin E/colistin) were discovered in 1947 and were used parenterally until the 1960s, when aminoglycosides entered common usage. In the 1980s, polymyxins fell into disuse mainly because of nephrotoxicity. With the emergence of multi-drug-resistant Gram-negative organisms, e.g., *Pseudomonas* spp. and *Acinetobacter* spp., injectable polymyxins are playing an increasing clinical role.

Mechanism of action

Polymyxins are cyclic cationic polypeptide detergents. They penetrate cell membranes and interact with phospholipids to disrupt the membranes. They are rapidly bactericidal.

Clinical use

Polymyxin B is used for the treatment of severe infections caused by multi-drug-resistant Gram-negative organisms. Colistin sulfate has been used for intestinal decontamination.

Aerosolized colistimethate has been used to treat CF patients with pulmonary colonization or infection with multi-drug-resistant *Pseudomonas* spp. IV colistimethate has been used to treat severe multi-drug-resistant Gram-negative infections, e.g., ventilator-associated pneumonia.

Pharmacology

The drug is not absorbed orally. Good serum concentrations occur after IV administration but with poor penetration of CSF, biliary tract, pleural fluid, and joint fluid. The drug is renally excreted, so reduce dosage in patients with renal impairment.

Polymyxin B is available topically and as a parenteral preparation that can be given intravenously or intramuscularly.

Colistin is available as colistin sulfate for topical use, and colistimethate sodium for intramuscular or intravenous use.

Toxicity and side effects

Dose-related nephrotoxicity and neurotoxicity (paraesthesia, peripheral neuropathy, and neuromuscular blockade) can occur. Caution should be used with preparations for aerosolized administration. These should not be used more than 24 hours after preparation due to the development of a toxic breakdown product that has been associated with patient deaths.

Fusidic acid

Fusidic acid is a member of the fusidane class of antibiotics, derived from *Fusidium coccineum* and chemically related to cephalosporin P. The sodium salt of fusidic acid (fucidin) was introduced into clinical practice in 1962. This agent has recently been the focus of renewed clinical interest given its ability to treat otherwise resistant staphylococcal infections. However, it is not available in the United States at this time.

Mechanism of action

Fusidic acid inhibits protein synthesis by blocking elongation factor G. Fusidic acid also has in vitro and in vivo immunosuppressive effects.

Resistance

Resistance occurs via chromosomal mutations in the *fusA* gene, which codes for elongation factor. There is also plasmid-mediated resistance, resulting in reduced permeability of the drug. It is a particular concern with long-term monotherapy, so fusidic acid is often combined with another agent.

Clinical use

Fusidic acid is mainly used for the treatment of staphylococcal infections, e.g., skin and soft tissue infections, bacteremia, septic arthritis, osteomyelitis, and lower respiratory tract infections in patients with CF.

It has also been used to treat erythrasma due to *Corynebacterium minutissium* and lepromatous leprosy.

Pharmacology

Fusidic acid may be given orally, topically, or intravenously. Oral absorption is rapid and almost complete. It is highly protein bound and widely distributed in most tissues. It is metabolized in the liver by cytochrome P450 and eliminated in the bile.

Toxicity and side effects

Fusidic acid is generally well tolerated, but the oral form may cause nausea, vomiting, and reversible jaundice (6%). The IV form is associated with thrombophlebitis and jaundice (17%).

Ophthalmic preparations may cause itching or stinging. A drug-induced immune-mediated thrombocytopenia has been described.

Mupirocin

Mupirocin is a pseudomonic acid, produced by *Pseudomonas fluorescens*, that is not related to any other antibiotic in clinical use.

Mechanism of action

Its mechanism of action is bacteriostatic: it inhibits bacterial RNA and protein synthesis by binding to bacterial isoleucyl tRNA synthetase, preventing the incorporation of isoleucine into protein chains in the bacterial cell wall.

Resistance

Low-level resistance is due to spontaneous mutation resulting in altered access to binding sites in isoleucyl tRNA synthetase. High-level resistance is mediated on transferable plasmids by the *mupA* gene, which codes for a modified enzyme. Mupirocin resistance in MRSA has been associated with widespread use, thus prolonged use (>7 days) is discouraged.

Clinical use

Mupirocin is primarily used for skin infections, e.g., impetigo and folliculitis, and for nasal decolonization of *S. aureus* or MRSA carriage. Mupirocin has also been used for treatment of secondarily infected eczema, burns, lacerations, and ulcers.

Pharmacology

The drug is given topically as a cream (Bactroban®) or nasal ointment (Bactroban nasal®).

Toxicity and side effects

Local reactions such as pruritis, burning sensation, rash, and urticaria may occur, particularly if used on broken skin.

Antituberculous agents – first line

Streptomycin was the first drug used in a randomized clinical trial in 1948 and was shown to reduce mortality from pulmonary tuberculosis. Since then, a number of antituberculous agents have been developed. For treatment guidelines, see *M. tuberculosis* (p. 309).

Classification

First-line drugs have superior efficacy and more acceptable toxicity and include isoniazid, rifampin, pyrazinamide, and ethambutol. In select clinical scenarios, rifabutin or rifapentene may be preferable to rifampin as a first-line option.

　　Second-line drugs are reserved for cases of resistant or refractory disease or drug intolerance. The agents are often more toxic or perhaps lack efficacy data as a primary therapy. Second-line agents include fluoroquinolones (levofloxacin and moxifloxacin), aminoglycosides (streptomycin, kanamycin, and amikacin), para-aminosalicyclic acid, cycloserine, ethionamide, and capreomycin.

Mechanisms of action

- Bactericidal drugs are active against replicating tubercle bacilli in cavities, e.g., isoniazid, rifampicin, ethambutol, and streptomycin.
- Sterilizing drugs are active against slowly replicating organisms (persisters) or intracellular organisms, e.g., pyrazinamide, and isoniazid.

Isoniazid (INH)

INH, or isonicotinic acid hydrazide, is a synthetic agent.

- *Mechanism of action:* inhibits mycolic acid synthesis. Rapidly bactericidal against actively replicating M. tuberculosis (MIC 0.01–2 mg/L). Most other mycobacteria are resistant.
- *Resistance:* isoniazid resistance is one of the two most frequent forms of resistance. It is associated with mutations in *inhA* (mycolic acid synthesis), *katG* (catalase peroxidase), and *oryR-ahpC* genes.
- *Clinical use:* treatment of all forms of TB infection, including latent TB; chemoprophylaxis in contacts and highly susceptible patients
- *Pharmacology:* >95% oral absorption, widely distributed, good CSF penetration, metabolized in liver (N-acteyl transferase), excreted in urine. Patients may be fast or slow acetylators, depending on genetic polymorphism (no clinical significance). Dose reduction in renal failure is required.
- *Adverse effects:* neurotoxicity and peripheral neuropathy (reduced with pyridoxine), hepatitis that can be severe and is age-dependent and is increased with alcohol use, arthralgias, hypersensitivity, antinuclear antibody (ANA)-positive lupus-like syndrome
- *Drug interactions:* increases plasma concentration of antiepileptic drugs

Rifampin (RIF)

(see Rifamycins, p. 61)
RIF is a semisynthetic derivative of rifamycin B.

- *Mechanism of action:* inhibits mycobacterial DNA-dependent RNA polymerase, thereby inhibiting RNA synthesis. It is bactericidal against actively replicating M. tuberculosis and other mycobacteria (M. kansasii, M. marinum, M. leprae). It is also active against a variety of other bacteria (see Rifamycins, p. 61).
- *Resistance* emerges rapidly during monotherapy. It is caused by a point mutation in the *rpoB* gene (encodes ß-subunit of RNA polymerase).
- *Clinical use:* treatment of all forms of TB infection; chemoprophylaxis of contacts and susceptible individuals (second line)
- *Pharmacology:* >90% oral absorption, widely distributed, low concentrations in CSF unless meningeal inflammation. It is metabolized in the liver (cytochrome P450 enzyme system). It is excreted in bile and undergoes enterohepatic circulation; some is

excreted in the urine. Dose reduction in patients with liver failure is required.
- *Adverse effects:* orange discoloration of body fluids, skin rash, GI upset, hepatitis, hypersensitivity, "rifampicin flu" (intermittent therapy), "red man syndrome" (overdose)
- *Drug interactions:* induces its own metabolism (autoinduction) and that of corticosteroids as well as many other drugs metabolized via the cytochrome P450 enzyme system. Drug interactions often limit use in select patient populations (such as HIV).

Other rifamycins

(see Rifamycins, p. 61)
- Rifabutin induces cytochrome P450 less than rifampin. It is used to treat tuberculosis in HIV-infected patients on protease inhibitors or with atypical mycobacterial infections (see Rifamycins, p. 61).
- Rifapentene has a significantly longer half-life than that of rifampin and can be administered once weekly in the continuation phase of TB treatment.
- Rifapentine is a greater inducer of cytochrome P450 than rifampin.
- Rifapentene has been used to treat TB in HIV-infected patients but is not recommended for intermittent therapy in this patient population because of a high rate of resistance developing on therapy.

Pyrazinamide (PZA)

PZA, or pyrazinoic acid amide, is a synthetic nicotinamide analog.
- *Mechanism of action:* unknown. Activity requires conversion to pyrazinoic acid by mycobacterial pyrazinamidase. It is active against replicating intracellular organisms and those in an acid pH environment, e.g., within necrotic inflammatory foci.
- *Resistance* is uncommon and is due to mutations in the *pncA* (pyrazinamidase) gene.
- *Clinical use:* essential component of short-course therapy. There are high relapse rates if not given in the first 2 months of treatment.
- *Pharmacology:* >90% oral absorption, widely distributed, good CSF penetration. It is metabolized in the liver and excreted by the kidneys. Dose reduction in patients with renal failure is required. Increase dosage in patients on dialysis.
- *Adverse effects:* GI upset is fairly common; hepatotoxicity, gout (inhibits excretion of uric acid), arthralgia

Ethambutol (EMB)

EMB, or hydroxymethyl propyl ethylenediamine, is a synthetic compound.
- *Mechanism of action:* inhibits arabinosyl transferase enzymes (synthesis of arabinogalactan and lipoarabinomannan). Bacteriostatic. It is active against mycobacteria (*M. tuberculosis, M. kansasii, M. xenopi, M. malmoense*) and *Nocardia*.
- *Resistance* is uncommon. It is caused by point mutations in the genes encoding arabinosyl transferase enzyme (*embA, embB,* and *embC*).
- *Clinical use:* first 2 months of TB treatment (if suspected or known drug resistance); other mycobacterial infections

- *Pharmacology:* 75–80% oral absorption, widely distributed, 25–40% CSF penetration. It is metabolized in the liver, with renal excretion. Dose modification in renal failure is required.
- *Adverse effects:* optic neuritis (reversible), peripheral neuropathy, arthralgia, hyperuricemia, rashes

Antituberculous agents – second line

These drugs may be used to treat tuberculosis if there is the following:
- Intolerance to first-line drugs
- Resistance to one or more first-line drugs
- Multi-drug resistance (resistance to isoniazid and rifampicin, MDR-TB)
- Extensively drug-resistant TB (MDR plus resistance to a quinolone and an injectable agent)
- Co-infection with HIV

Treatment in these situations may be complicated, and advice should be sought from a specialist experienced in treating such patients.

Para-aminosalicyclic acid (PAS)

- *Mechanism of action:* interferes with the salicylate-dependent biosynthesis of iron-chelating compounds called mycobactins. PAS is bacteriostatic against *M. tuberculosis*.
- *Clinical use:* this inexpensive oral agent has limited use in developing countries because of poor compliance and primary resistance. It is used for multi-drug-resistant TB in developed countries.
- *Pharmacology:* incomplete oral absorption, hepatic metabolism, renal excretion. In the United States it is only available as delayed-release granules.
- *Adverse effects:* GI upset, hepatotoxicity. It interferes with iodine metabolism and is associated with significant sodium load.
- *Drug interactions:* it may enhance toxicity of salicylates and corticosteroids and diminish antihypertensive effects of some medications.

Capreomycin

This cyclic polypeptide antibiotic is produced by *Streptomyces capreolus*.
- *Mechanism of action:* unknown
- *Resistance:* mechanism is unknown; partial cross-resistance with other aminoglycosides (amikacin and kanamycin)
- *Clinical use:* first-line injectable agent in multi-drug-resistant TB, particularly if streptomycin resistant
- *Pharmacology:* administered IM or IV, has renal excretion
- *Adverse effects:* injection site reactions; ototoxic, nephrotoxic, neuromuscular blockade. An audiogram and vestibular testing are recommended at baseline.

Streptomycin (SM) (see Aminoglycosides, p. 39)

This aminoglycoside antibiotic is derived from *Streptomyces griseus*.
- *Mechanism of action:* binds to 16S rRNA, inhibits protein synthesis. It is bactericidal against *M. tuberculosis* and various other bacteria.
- *Resistance:* mutation in *rpsL* gene (encodes ribosomal protein S12)
- *Clinical usage:* treatment of tuberculosis, *M. kansasii* infections, plague, enterococcal endocarditis
- *Pharmacology:* not absorbed from GI tract, administered intravenously or intramuscularly. The drug is widely distributed but has poor penetration of CSF and abscesses, with 99% renal excretion.
- *Adverse effects:* injection site reactions, ototoxicity, hypersensitivity, neuromuscular blockade, peripheral neuritis, optic neuritis

Other aminoglycosides

- Amikacin and kanamycin are used third line after streptomycin and capreomycin for treatment of multi-drug-resistant TB.
- Amikacin is ototoxic and nephrotoxic; monitor serum concentrations.
- Kanamycin offers no advantage over amikacin apart from cost.

Cycloserine

This naturally occurring amino acid is derived from *Streptomyces orchidaceus*. It has a broad spectrum of antibiotic activity: *S aureus*, streptococci, enterococci, Enterobacteriaceae, *Nocardia* spp., *Chlamydia* spp., and mycobacteria.
- *Mechanism of action:* inhibits cell wall synthesis
- *Primary resistance* is rare; secondary resistance develops slowly.
- *Clinical use:* primary treatment of drug-resistant TB with documented susceptibility to cycloserine, non-tuberculous mycobacteria
- *Pharmacology:* well absorbed, widely distributed including CSF, 50% metabolized, 50% excreted unchanged in urine
- *Adverse effects:* dose-related CNS events including psychosis, worsens underlying disease in patients with seizure disorders. Pyridoxine may decrease neurotoxicity. Consider monitoring serum drug concentrations

Ethionamide

Ethylthiosonicotinamide, an isonicotinic acid derivative, was introduced in 1956.
- *Mechanism of action:* inhibits mycolic acid synthesis. Bacteriostatic
- *Resistance:* mechanism is unknown, but some INH- and ETH-resistant isolates harbor mutations in the *inhA* gene involved in mycolic acid synthesis.
- *Clinical use:* drug-resistant and multi-drug-resistant TB; sometimes used in leprosy
- *Pharmacology:* well absorbed, widely distributed, including in CSF; metabolized in liver, 99% excreted as metabolites in urine
- *Adverse effects:* GI upset, metallic taste, hypersensitivity, hepatitis
- *Drug interactions:* PAS increases ethionomide toxicity, and seizures may occur with concomitant cycloserine administration.

Fluoroquinolones (see Quinolones, p. 57)

Ciprofloxacin, ofloxacin, levofloxacin, and moxifloxacin can be used to treat multi-drug-resistant TB or atypical mycobacterial infections (see Nontuberculous mycobacteria, p. 70).

Drug concentration monitoring for antituberculous agents

Therapeutic drug monitoring for agents used to treat tuberculosis is available for most agents with activity against tuberculosis. One laboratory conducting such monitoring is the Advanced Diagnostic Laboratories (ADL) at National Jewish Health in Denver, Colorado.[1]

Nontuberculous mycobacteria

These organisms may be called atypical mycobacteria, environmental mycobacteria, opportunist mycobacteria, nontuberculous mycobacteria (NTM), or mycobacteria other than tuberculosis (MOTT). They can cause a variety of diseases (pulmonary, skin, soft tissue, bone and joint infections, disseminated disease), particularly in immune-deficient individuals.

Treatment depends on the causative organism and often requires a prolonged course of a combination of antibiotics. Surgical excision of lesions may also be required.

The most commonly used drugs are as follows:
- Clarithromycin, azithromycin (see Macrolides, p. 42)
- Ethambutol (see Antituberculous agents—first line, p. 65)
- Rifampin, rifabutin (see Rifamycins, p. 61)
- Clofazimine (see Antileprotics, p. 70)
- Ciprofloxacin, moxifloxacin (see Quinolones, p. 57)
- Amikacin (see Aminoglycosides, p. 39)
- Minocycline, doxycycline (see Tetracyclines, p. 51)
- Co-trimoxazole (see Co-trimoxazole, p. 56).

Antileprotics

Introduced by the WHO in 1982, multi-drug therapy (MDT) with a combination of dapsone, clofazimine, and rifampin is the current treatment for infections with *M. leprae* (see Table 1.4). It has been very successful with a high cure rate, few side effects, and low relapse rate.

Dapsone

Since first used to treat leprosy by Cochrane in 1947, dapsone has remained the cornerstone of treatment. The emergence of drug resistance in the 1960s has necessitated the addition of other drugs.

---

[1] For more information visit: www.nationaljewish.org/research/diagnostics/adx/labs/pharmacokinetics/aspx

Dapsone is a diaminodipheny salphane that is active against many bacteria and some protozoa.

- *Mechanism of action:* inhibition of dihydropterate synthetase, inhibiting synthesis of dihydrofolic acid. Bacteriostatic and weakly bactericidal against *M. leprae*
- *Resistance:* resistance acquired by sequential mutations
- *Clinical use:* leprosy, malaria (treatment and prophylaxis), toxoplasmosis (prophylaxis), pneumocystis pneumonia (treatment and prophylaxis), dermatitis herpetiformis
- *Pharmacology:* >90% oral absorption; widely distributed but selectively retained in skin, kidneys, and liver; metabolized by oxidation and acetylation; mostly renally excreted
- *Adverse effects:* GI upset, anorexia, headaches, dizziness, insomnia, "dapsone syndrome" (fever, skin rash ± lymphadenopathy, jaundice, hepatomegaly), hemolystic anemia(especially in G6PD deficiency), methemoglobinemia, sulfhemoglobinemia

Clofazimine

Clofazimine is an iminophenazine dye active against mycobacteria (*M. tuberculosis, M. scrofulaceum, M. leprae, M. avium intracellulare, M. fortuitum, M. chelonae*), *Actinomyces* spp., and *Nocardia* spp.

- *Mechanism of action:* unknown; has anti-inflammatory properties and is weakly bactericidal against *M. leprae*
- *Resistance* is rare (one case report)
- *Clinical use:* leprosy
- *Pharmacology:* well absorbed orally, taken up by adipose tissue and monocytes/macrophages, long half-life (10–70 days), excreted in urine and feces
- *Adverse effects:* GI upset, skin discoloration (dose related, reversible), small-bowel edema/subacute obstruction (prolonged use)

NOTE: Clofazimine is no longer commercially available in the United States but may be obtained through the National Hansen's Disease Program (part of the division of the Department of Health and Human Services) by calling 1-800-642-2477. More information is available on the Web site: www.hrsa.gov/hansens/clinical/regimens.htm.

Rifampin

This is the most effective antileprotic, rendering the patient non-infectious within days of starting therapy. It is also used for treatment of TB and other bacterial infections (see Rifamycins, p. 61).

Second-line therapies

One problem with MDT is the prolonged duration of treatment (up to 2 years in multibacillary leprosy). Recent research has focused on determining alternative regimens of shorter duration. Antibiotics that have been shown to have potent bactericidal activity against *M. leprae* are as follows:

- Minocycline is the only tetracycline with activity against *M. leprae*. It demonstrates potent bactericidal activity (see Tetracyclines, p. 51)

Table 1.4 MDT regimens for treatment of M. leprae infections

Regimen	Drug	Duration
Paucibacillary leprosy	Dapsone 100 mg daily	6–12 months
	Rifampin 600 mg monthly	
Multibacillary leprosy	Dapsone 100 mg daily	2 years
	Clofazimine 50 mg daily	
	Rifampin 600 mg monthly	

- Ofloxacin, levofloxacin (which may have increased activity over that of ofloxacin) and moxifloxacin have demonstrated bactericidal activity (see Quinolones, p. 72).
- Clarithromycin is the only macrolide with activity against M. leprae and demonstrates bactericidal activity(see Macrolides, p. 42).

Single dose therapy

Although slightly less efficacious than conventional MDT, a single-dose regimen (rifampin, ofloxacin and minocycline) is available for single-lesion paucibacillary leprosy.

Adjunctive treatments

- Neuritis or silent neuropathy is a common reaction that can occur while on treatment for leprosy.
- Corticosteroids have been shown to be efficacious in the treatment of nerve damage.
- Reversal reactions (type 1 reactions) can be treated with aspirin (if mild) or prednisone (if moderate to severe).
- Erythema nodosum leprosum (type 2 reactions) can be treated with aspirin (if mild), prednisolone, clofazimine at high doses (300 mg daily followed by a taper), or thalidomide (if severe).

Antifungals

A number of antifungal agents are currently available:

- Alkylamines inhibit ergosterol biosynthesis by inhibiting squalene epoxidase, e.g., terbinafine.
- Antimetabolites that interfere with DNA synthesis, e.g., flucytosine
- Azoles, e.g., imidazoles and triazoles, inhibit ergosterol synthesis by blocking 14-α-demethylase
- Glucan synthesis inhibitors, e.g., echinocandins
- Polyenes, e.g., nystatiin, amphotericin, bind to the fungal cell membrane and cause it to leak electrolytes.
- Miscellaneous agents, e.g., griseofulvin

Polyenes

The polyene antifungal agents are the most broad-spectrum antifungal drugs available today. This group includes amphotericin and nystatin. Both drugs have the same mechanism of action but have very different clinical uses. Neither drug is absorbed when given orally.

Nystatin is too toxic to be given parenterally so is limited to topical treatment of mucosal *Candida* infections of the oropharynx, esophagus, intestinal tract, and vagina.

Amphotericin can be given topically, including administration via the oral route, but is usually used IV for the systemic treatment of invasive fungal infections.

Mechanism of action

Polyenes bind to ergosterol in the fungal cell membrane, resulting in increased membrane permeability, leakage of cell content, and cell death.

Resistance

- *Intrinsic resistance:* the following organisms are intrinsically resistant to amphotericin: *Aspergillus terreus, Fusarium* spp., *Pseudallescheria boydii, Scedosporium prolificans, Trichosporon beigelii*, and some *Candida lusitaniae*.
- *Acquired resistance* is rare but has been reported in AIDS patients with relapsing cryptococcal disease.

Clinical use

Conventional amphotericin B deoxycholate, given by IV infusion, is used to treat systemic fungal infections (including dimorphic fungi). Because of its significant toxicity, its use is often limited to patients with irreversible renal failure or, in some cases, as primary therapy for cryptococcal meningitis, either alone or with flucytosine (see Other antifungals, p. 78).

Lipid formulations of amphotericin B are recommended if toxicity or renal impairment precludes use of conventional amphotericin. The lipid formulations are very costly, so many institutions have guidelines for use.

Currently, there are three lipid formulations of amphotericin B available for use in the United States (Table 1.5). Although slight differences exist in FDA-approved indications for these agents, there are few clinical differences between the drugs. Amphotericin B colloidal dispersion (ABCD) is associated with a higher rate of infusion-related reactions than that of the other agents and is therefore rarely used.

Nystatin suspension is used for mucosal candidiasis. Oral formulations of amphotericin B are no longer commercially available but can be compounded extemporaneously if needed.

Amphotericin solution can be used for continuous bladder irrigation in funguria, but the clinical advantages of this approach are unclear.

Nystatin cream is used to treat vaginal candidiasis. It stains clothes yellow and damages latex condoms and diaphragms.

Table 1.5 Lipid formulations of amphotericin

Name	Formulation
Liposomal amphotericin (AmBisome®)	Drug is encapsulated in phospholipid-containing liposomes
Amphotericin B colloidal dispersion (ABCD; Amphotec®)	Drug is complexed with cholesterol sulfate to form small lipid discs
Amphotericin B lipid complex (ABLC; Abelcet®)	Drug is complexed with phospholipids to form ribbon-like structures

Pharmacology

Amphotericin is usually given IV with a carrier (e.g., deoxycholate). It is highly protein bound and penetrates CSF and other body fluids poorly. Liver or renal impairment and dialysis have little effect on serum concentrations. The lipid formulations have widely diverse pharmacokinetics.

Toxicity and side effects

Despite the selective toxicity to fungal cell membranes compared with that to human cell membranes, conventional (micellar) amphotericin B is associated with infusion-related reactions (chills, fever, headache, nausea, vomiting) and nephrotoxicity. Premedication with acetaminophen and diphenhydramine is advised to minimize these reactions.

Routine monitoring of patients receiving an amphotericin B product should include CBC, liver function tests (LFTs), renal function, and electrolytes. The new lipid formulations minimize but do not completely eliminate these toxicities. One proposed strategy for minimizing nephrotoxicity is to administer the drug via continuous infusion. However, this should be avoided in patients with confirmed fungal infection, as the drug exhibits concentration-dependent activity and this approach may lead to suboptimal treatment.

Additional side effects of IV amphotericin include GI symptoms (anorexia, nausea and vomiting, diarrhea, epigastric pain), muscle and joint pain, anemia and other blood disorders, cardiovascular toxicity (including arrhythmias, especially if infused too quickly), neurological disorders, abnormal LFTS, and rash and pain at the infusion site.

The liposomal preparation (AmBisome®) is associated with a unique triad of symptoms that presents as an acute infusion reaction including chest pain in some cases. This appears to be associated with the lipid carrier, and patients can safely receive an alternate lipid formulation.

Triazoles

The triazoles include fluconazole, itraconazole, voriconazole, and posaconazole.

Mechanism of action

Triazoles inhibit the synthesis of ergosterol (the main sterol in fungal cell membranes) by inhibiting cytochrome P450 14-α-demethylase. They are all essentially fungistatic, but some may be fungicidal at high concentrations.

Fluconazole (Diflucan®)

- *Activity:* against *Candida* spp. and *Cryptococcus* spp. Fluconazole is also active against *Coccidioides immitis* and has limited activity against *Histoplasma capsulatum* and *Blastomyces dermatitidis*. It has no meaningful activity against *Aspergillus* spp. or most other molds.
- *Resistance:* C. krusei is intrinsically resistant to fluconazole. *C. glabrata* is associated with high fluconazole MICs; 10–15% are resistant. Acquired resistance to fluconazole has been reported in *C. albicans* in HIV patients.
- *Clinical use:* treatment of oropharyngeal, vulvovaginal, and invasive candidiasis; also for prophylaxis in oncology and transplant patients
- *Pharmacology:* available as PO and IV preparations. Well absorbed orally. Renal excretion; dose reduction required in renal impairment
- *Side effects:* generally well tolerated. It may cause abnormal LFTs.
- *Drug interactions:* At doses >200 mg daily, fluconazole is a potent inhibitor of CYP3A4.

Itraconazole (Sporanox®)

- *Activity:* against yeasts, molds, and dimorphic fungi, e.g., *Candida* spp., *Cryptococcus* spp., *Aspergillus* spp., *Pseudallescheria boydii, Sporothrix schenkii, Histoplasma capsulatum, Blastomyces dermatitidis, Coccidiodes immitis, Paracoccidioides braziliensis, Pencillium marneffei,* and dermatophytes. It may retain activity against fluconazole-resistant *C. krusei* and *C. glabrata*. It has limited activity against *Fusarium* spp. and Zygomycetes.
- *Clinical use:* used in treatment of yeast and mold infections, especially fluconazole-resistant *Candida* spp. and *Aspergillus* spp.
- *Resistance:* detectable in most of the species above as well as others.
- *Pharmacology:* available as oral capsule or oral suspension (in cyclodextrin). An IV formulation was withdrawn from the market due to lack of use. Absorption of capsules is highly variable, dependent on acid and unpredictable. The capsules should not be administered with acid-suppressive therapy. Absorption and bioavailability of solution is better but is still <50%. Gastric acidity and food affect absorption of capsules but not solution. The drug is highly lipophilic; it achieves high concentrations in fatty tissues and purulent exudates.
- *Adverse effects:* Hypertension, hypokalemia, edema, headache, and altered mental state have been reported. Seek advice before giving itraconazole to patients at risk of heart failure. Given the cyclodextran excipient, significant diarrhea can be associated with the oral solution formulation.

Voriconazole (Vfend®)

Voriconazole is structurally similar to fluconazole, with a higher affinity for 14-α-demethylase conferring a broader spectrum of activity that includes *Aspergillus* spp.

- *Activity:* against a wide variety of fungi: *Candida* spp. (fungistatic), *Cryptococcus* spp. (fungistatic), *Aspergillus* spp. (fungicidal), *Blastomyces dermatitidis, Coccidioides immitis, Histoplasma capsulatum, Fusarium* spp., and *Penicillium marneffei.* Active against fluconazole-resistant *C. krusei, C. glabrata,* and *C. guilliermondii.* Zygomycetes, e.g., *Mucor* spp. and *Rhizomucor* spp., have high MICs, and breakthrough infections with these pathogens can occur while on voriconazole.
- *Clinical use:* first-line treatment of choice for invasive aspergillosis. It is also effective against invasive candidiasis, but benefit over other azole therapies is uncertain. It can be used in salvage therapy of *Scedosporium apiospermum* and *Fusarium* spp. Voriconazole is frequently used for fungal prophylaxis in the oncology setting.
- *Pharmacology:* available as PO or IV formulations, metabolized in the liver by cytochrome P450 enzymes. The drug exhibits nonlinear pharmacokinetics, thus dose escalation should be done with caution. The IV formulation should be used with caution in patients with renal dysfunction. The oral formulation should be taken on an empty stomach.
- *Side effects:* dose-related, transient visual disturbance, skin rash, and abnormal LFTs are common and should be routinely monitored. Hepatic failure has been reported.
- *Drug interactions:* voriconazole is a potent inhibitor of CYP 3A4 and 2C19, resulting in major drug interactions with immunosuppressant agents and other medications relying on CYP450 for elimination.

Posaconazole (Noxafil®)

- *Activity:* Excellent activity against *Candida* spp., including those that have reduced fluconazole susceptibility. Also active against *Aspergillus* spp., *Sporothrix schenkii, Histoplasma capsulatum, Blastomyces dermatitidis, Coccidiodes immitis, Paracoccidioides braziliensis, Pencillium marneffei,* and agents causing chromoblastomycosis, mycetoma, and phaeohyphomycosis, including *Scedosporium apiospermum* and species of *Exophiala, Alternaria,* and *Bipolaris.* It is the only azole with consistent activity against Zygomycetes.
- *Clinical use:* used in prevention of invasive fungal infections in high-risk patients with neutropenia or graft-versus-host disease. It is also used as salvage therapy in patients with invasive fungal infections that failed primary therapy (usually amphotericin B). Preliminary data suggest that posaconazole may be effective for zygomycosis unresponsive to amphotericin B.
- *Pharmacology:* oral suspension available and must be taken with a high-fat meal. IV formulation under development. Nonrenal elimination
- *Adverse effects:* nausea, headache, rash, dry skin, taste disturbance, abdominal pain, dizziness, and flushing may occur.
- *Drug interactions:* posaconazole is an inhibitor of CYP3A4.

Echinocandins

This relatively new class of drugs inhibits glucan synthesis and is rapidly fungicidal for yeasts; their activity against molds is more complex. Three drugs are currently licensed: caspofungin, micafungin, and anidulafungin.

Mechanism of action

The echinocandins block the synthesis of 1–3-β-glucan (a fungal cell wall component) by inhibiting the enzyme 1–3-β-glucan synthase. This selective action results in fewer side effects (as there is no mammalian target) and lack of cross-resistance with other antifungals.

Spectrum of activity

All echinocandins are active against *Candida* spp. and *Aspergillus* spp. They have no activity against *Cryptococcus neoformans, Fusarium* spp., *Pseudallescheria* spp., or the Zygomycetes. Acquired resistance has not yet been described.

Caspofungin (Cancidas®)

- *Clinical use:* used for invasive *Aspergillus* infections unresponsive to traditional therapies. It is also used for the treatment of invasive candidiasis and as empirical therapy in neutropenic patients. Caspofungin is active against *Pneumocystis jiroveciii* but has not been studied for this indication in humans.
- *Pharmacology:* available as an IV formulation. Protein binding is >90%. It is widely distributed with high concentrations in the lungs, liver, spleen, and kidneys and lower concentrations in CSF. It is metabolized by the liver (not by cytochrome P450). Reduce dosage in patients with moderate hepatic impairment are recommended. Metabolites are eliminated in the urine and feces. No dose adjustment is required in renal impairment.
- *Adverse effects:* nausea, vomiting, and injection site reactions. Transient LFT abnormalities occur in 11–24% of patients, as well as infusion-related histamine release.

Anidulafungin (Eraxis®)

- *Clinical use:* similar to that of capsofungin, primarily used for treating invasive candidal infections
- *Pharmacology:* available as an IV formulation only. Elimination is non-renal and non-hepatic, so no dose adjustments are required.
- *Adverse effects:* abnormal LFTs, infusion-related histamine release

Micafungin (Mycamine®)

- *Clinical use:* similar to that of other echinocandins, including prevention of *Candida* infections after bone marrow transplantation
- *Pharmacology:* available as an IV formulation only, hepatic elimination
- *Adverse effects:* abnormal LFTs, infusion-related histamine release

Other antifungals

Flucytosine (Ancobon®)

Flucyosine is a fluorine analog of cytosine (pyrimidine) that inhibits DNA synthesis.

- *Mechanism of action:* converted to metabolites that either inhibit thymidylate synthetase (interfering with DNA synthesis) or cause aberrant transcription of RNA
- *Resistance:* may be due to loss of cytosine permease (which permits entry of the drug) or loss of enzymes that convert it into its active metabolites. Resistance emerges rapidly with monotherapy.
- *Clinical use:* cryptococcosis, candidiasis, and chromoblastomycosis; usually used as combination therapy, e.g., with amphotericin, because of rapid development of resistance
- *Pharmacology:* available orally only. Rapidly and almost completely absorbed. Low protein binding. CSF concentrations are 74% of plasma concentrations; 90% is excreted unchanged in the urine. Dose reduction is required in patients with renal impairment.
- *Adverse effects:* rash, diarrhea, and abnormal LFTs. Leukopenia, thrombocytopenia, and enterocolitis may occur in patients with renal impairment; monitor CBC, renal function, LFTs, and serum flucytosine concentrations during treatment if prolonged treatment is needed (target peak concentration <100 mcg/mL to minimize toxicity). Flucytosine is teratogenic in rats and contraindicated in pregnancy.

Griseofulvin

Griseofulvin was previously used for fungal nail infections, but poor response rates and significant relapse rates have limited its use. It is used in children for tinea capitis.

- *Mechanism of action:* disruption of fungal cellular microtubules
- *Clinical use:* tinea capitis in children. Dermatophyte infections of skin, scalp, nails, and hair where topical therapy has failed or is inappropriate
- *Pharmacology:* given orally; two different preparations are available. The microsize (tablet and alcohol-containing suspension) is subject to variable absorption and is best administered with a high-fat meal. The ultramicrosize (tablet) is nearly completely absorbed.
- *Adverse effects:* mental confusion, headache, nausea, vomiting, and rashes. Avoid use in pregnancy, breast-feeding, systemic lupus erythematosus (risk of exacerbation), and liver disease
- *Drug interactions* may diminish the anticoagulant effect of warfarin and enhance the effects of alcohol.

Terbinafine (Lamisil®)

- *Mechanism of action:* acts on the enzyme squalene epoxidase, blocking the transformation of squalene to lanosterol and thus inhibiting ergosterol synthesis. The intracellular accumulation of squalene also results in disruption of fungal cell membranes.
- *Resistance:* not yet reported

- *Clinical use:* dermatophyte and ringworm infections (including tinea pedis, cruris, and corporis) for which oral therapy is appropriate. Fingernail infections need a 6-week course, toenails usually require 12 weeks. It is also available topically to treat fungal skin infections.
- *Pharmacology:* given PO or topically. Metabolized by cytochrome P450 enzymes and eliminated renally. Dose reduction is required in patients with renal disease.
- *Adverse effects:* abdominal discomfort, anorexia, nausea, diarrhea, headache, rash, and urticaria. Rare events include liver toxicity and serious skin reactions (e.g., Stevens–Johnson syndrome).
- *Drug interactions:* inhibitor of CYP2D6

Antivirals for HSV and VZV: acyclovir and valacyclovir

Acyclovir was the first agent with demonstrated effectiveness against herpes simplex virus (HSV) infection. Valacyclovir is the L-valyl ester prodrug of acyclovir and is preferred because of its better oral bioavailability. It is rapidly and nearly completely converted to acyclovir in first-pass enzymatic hydrolysis in the liver.

Penciclovir and its prodrug, famciclovir, are similar to acyclovir.

Mechanism of action
- An acyclic nucleoside analog, substrate for HSV-specific thymidine kinase (TK)
- Phosphorylated in HSV-infected cells to form acyclovir-triphosphate, a competitive inhibitor of viral DNA polymerase
- Incorporated into viral DNA chain. Causes chain termination. Chain-enzyme complex formation may irreversibly inactivate the polymerase.

Resistance
- Most commonly associated with reduced TK activity
- Cross-resistance to other agents activated by TK (e.g., ganciclovir)
- Acyclovir-resistant HSV is in <1% immunocompetent patients, 6–8% immunocompromised, and up to 17% in patients with AIDS and transplant patients receiving over 2 weeks of acyclovir therapy.
- Acyclovir-resistant varicella zoster virus (VZV) is less common; increased risk in chronic suppressive therapy with subtherapeutic doses

Pharmacology
- Oral bioavailability: acyclovir 15–20%, valacyclovir up to 54%
- Oral valacyclovir achieves similar total acyclovir exposure to that of IV acyclovir but with lower peak plasma concentrations.
- 60–90% is renally excreted, the remainder is metabolized. It is removed by hemodialysis. Reduce dosage in renal impairment.
- Topical absorption is low.
- Crosses placenta, high concentrations in breast milk. It is not known to be harmful in pregnancy but manufacturers still advise caution.

Adverse effects
- Topical agents may cause skin irritation.
- Nausea, rash, headache
- Neurotoxicity in 1–4% of those receiving IV acyclovir, increased in renal impairment
- Reversible crystalluria and resulting renal impairment in up to 5% receiving IV acyclovir
- High-dose valacyclovir may cause GI disturbance, confusion, and hallucinations.
- Valacyclovir has been associated with hemolytic uremic syndrome (HUS) in neutropenic and other immunosuppressed patients. Use in these populations should be avoided.

Drug interactions
- Zidovudine: lethargy
- Cyclosporine and other nephrotoxic agents: renal impairment
- Probenecid: decreased clearance and prolonged half-life
- These antivirals may decrease the clearance of other drugs eliminated by active renal secretion (e.g., methotrexate).

Antivirals for HSV and VZV

Table 1.6 Antiviral therapy for HSV and VZV

Drug	Preparations	Use
Acyclovir	Oral	Treatment and prophylaxis for HSV, treatment of VZV
	Intravenous	Treatment of HSV in immunocompromised patients, treatment of severe genital herpes, VZV, and HSV encephalitis
	Topical	Skin and eye infections (e.g., dendritic corneal ulcer)
Valacyclovir	Oral	Treatment of herpes zoster and HSV infections of skin and mucous membranes
Penciclovir (acyclic guanosine analog)	Topical	Similar to acyclovir in potency and spectrum of activity. Cross-resistance common. Labial HSV treatment
Famciclovir (penciclovir prodrug)	Oral	Treatment of herpes zoster, acute and recurrent genital HSV
Cidofovir (see Antivirals for CMV, p. 81)	Intravenous	Acyclovir-resistant HSV strains, as activation is not dependent on virus-specified enzymes

Antivirals for cytomegalovirus

Ganciclovir, foscarnet, and cidofovir all act by inhibiting viral DNA polymerase and are effective in treating cytomegalovirus (CMV) end-organ disease. Valganciclovir is an ester of ganciclovir, which may be given orally; it has an identical toxicity profile.

Ganciclovir and valganciclovir

These agents have inhibitory activity against herpesviruses, with particularly potent inhibition of CMV replication; 33% of patients receiving IV therapy interrupt or prematurely stop therapy because of marrow or CNS toxicity. Given side effects associated with ganciclovir, it is restricted to life-threatening or sight-threatening CMV infections in immunocompromised patients or for prevention of CMV disease during immunosuppressive therapy after organ transplantation.

Valganciclovir is used for induction and maintenance of CMV retinitis in AIDS and for prevention of transplant-associated CMV disease.

- *Mechanism of action:* nucleoside analog of guanosine—phosphorylated by a CMV viral protein kinase (not TK as in HSV). It inhibits viral DNA chain elongation but does not necessarily cause chain termination (unlike acyclovir), leading to accumulation of short noninfectious viral DNA fragments
- *Resistance:* due to mutations in the protein kinase or DNA polymerase. High-level resistance is seen in prolonged therapy for those with AIDS or transplantation-related disease. The most common mechanism of resistance is defects in UL97, which is involved with phosphorylation of ganciclovir.
- *Pharmacology:* oral bioavailability is 5–10%. Aqueous, vitreous, and subretinal concentrations are similar to that of serum. Most of the drug is eliminated unaltered by the kidney and removed by hemodialysis. It is available as intravitreal implant. It is usually administered IV given poor oral bioavailability.
- *Adverse effects:* myelosuppression, e.g., neutropenia and thrombocytopenia, occurs in 15–20% of AIDS patients receiving IV therapy (less in transplantation patients). This is usually seen in the second week of therapy and is reversible within 1 week of cessation in most cases. Recombinant granulocyte colony-stimulating factor (G-CSF) may be useful; 5–15% have CNS effects—headache to confusion and convulsions. Other effects include renal impairment, LFT abnormalities, rash, fever, and phlebitis at the IV site.
- *Drug interactions:* increases didanosine concentrations and may increase cyclosporine. With zidovudine and other cytotoxic agents myelosuppression is significantly increased; they should not be given together. Probenecid has decreased clearance and prolonged half-life. Renal dysfunction occurs with concurrent cyclosporine or amphotericin B.

Foscarnet

- *Mechanism of action:* inorganic pyrophosphate analog inhibitory for herpesviruses and HIV. No intracellular metabolism. Directly inhibits viral DNA polymerase or reverse transcriptase (100-fold greater effect than with cellular DNA polymerase). It is active against most ganciclovir-resistant CMV strains (and acyclovir-resistant HSV/VZV).
- *Resistance:* due to point mutations in DNA polymerase of HSV/CMV or reverse transcriptase of HIV. It occurs in <5% of patients.
- *Clinical use:* for refractory CMV treatment and acyclovir-resistant mucocutaneous HSV, with 90% of CMV retinitis patients experiencing clinical stabilization. In those with persistent or relapsed retinitis, combined foscarnet/ganciclovir delays progression longer than use of high doses of the individual agents. Foscarnet is used in AIDS-related CMV GI and pulmonary infections.
- *Pharmacology:* oral bioavailability is 8%. Vitreous concentrations are 1.4 times higher than in plasma. The drug has renal elimination, most of it unaltered. It is removed by hemodialysis. Its prolonged terminal half-life is due to bone deposition.
- *Interactions:* hypocalcemia with concomitant IV pentamidine. Renal dysfunction occurs with concurrent cyclosporine, amphotericin B, and other nephrotoxic agents.
- *Adverse effects:* nephrotoxicity, proteinuria, sometimes acute tubular necrosis (one-third develop significant renal impairment, which is reversible within 3–4 weeks of cessation of therapy). Saline loading may reduce incidence. Metabolic effects include hypo- and hypercalcemia, hypo- and hyperphosphatemia, hypomagnesemia, and hypokalemia. CNS symptoms are secondary to hypocalcemia; direct effects are seizures and hallucinations. Nausea, rash, abnormal LFTs, and heart block can occur.

Cidofovir

Cidofovir is used in CMV in patients with AIDS, particularly when ganciclovir or foscarnet therapy is not tolerated or has failed. Topical gel is used in mucocutaneous lesions. It has been used intravitreally for CMV retinitis but is very toxic. There is anecdotal (and conflicting) evidence for its use in treatment of progressive multifocal leukoencephalopathy (caused by reactivation of JC virus).

- *Mechanism of action:* acyclic phosphonate nucleotide analog of deoxycytidine monophosphate active against herpesviruses and other DNA viruses. Activation doesn't require virus-specific enzymes, thus it is inhibitory for certain acyclovir- and ganciclovir-resistant HSV and CMV strains. Cellular enzymes metabolize it to the active form, which competitively inhibits viral DNA polymerase.
- *Resistance:* some ganciclovir and foscarnet cross-resistance. Development of resistance secondary to cidofovir therapy is uncommon.
- *Pharmacology:* oral bioavailability is <5%. There is renal elimination with most of the drug unaltered. Cidofovir has a very long half-life as reflected by doses given every 2 weeks.

- *Interactions:* nephrotoxic drugs can enhance renal toxic effects.
- *Adverse effects:* dose-related nephrotoxicity. It should not be used if CrCl is <55 mL/min; concomitant probenecid and saline prehydration reduce incidence. Neutropenia occurs in 20%. Dose-related topical reactions and intravitreal dosing can cause iritis, vitreitis, and visual loss. Cidofovir should not be used in pregnant women, and men should avoid fathering children for at least 3 months after discontinuation.

Antivirals for influenza

Vaccination is the most effective way of preventing influenza. Antiviral agents are not a substitute (see Influenza—treatment and prevention, p. 325). Osetalmavir and zanamivir are licensed for the treatment and prophylaxis of influenza A and B in at-risk groups.

Amantadine and rimantadine are licensed but no longer recommended for the treatment and prophylaxis of influenza A because of resistance in recent seasonal influenza strains.

Zanamavir

This is effective against both influenza A and B.

- *Mechanism of action:* selective inhibitor of the viral neuraminidase and administered by inhalation
- *Resistance:* some reported but the impact is not yet clear
- *Clinical use:* treatment of influenza A and B in those over 12 years if given within 48 hours of symptom onset. It can also be used for post-exposure prophylaxis.
- *Pharmacology:* poor oral bioavailability, thus given by inhalation. Concentrations far above those required for viral inhibition are achieved at respiratory mucosa after inhaling.
- *Adverse effects:* GI disturbance. Rarely, angioedema, rash, and bronchospasm occur (use with care in those with asthma and COPD; bronchodilators should be available).

Osetalmavir

- *Mechanism of action:* A neuraminidase inhibitor effective against both influenza A and B
- *Resistance* has developed rapidly in the H1 strain, the vast majority of H1N1 now being resistant. H3 strains are mostly susceptible. Resistance is described in human cases of H5N1 virus infection in Vietnam. There are reports of in vitro cross-resistance with zanamivir.
- *Pharmacology:* prodrug that is hydrolyzed in the liver to produce the active agent. The drug is excreted in the urine. Dose adjustments are required in the setting of renal dysfunction.
- *Side effects and toxicity:* nausea, vomiting, abdominal pain, headache, fatigue, and insomnia. Rarely, rashes, hypersensitivity, and Stevens–Johnson syndrome occur.

Amantadine and rimantadine

Amantadine and rimantadine, comprising the adamantine class, are symmetric tricyclic amines that specifically inhibit replication of influenza A at low concentrations. Initiation of therapy within 2 days of symptoms reduces the duration of illness by 1–2 days. Use of these agents is limited by their side-effect profile, limited antiviral spectrum, and rapid development of resistance.

- *Mechanism of action:* at low concentrations they interact with the M2 protein of susceptible viruses, preventing viral uncoating in endosomes. Higher concentrations increase lysosomal pH and inhibit virus-induced membrane fusion.
- *Resistance:* common; over 90% of influenza isolates were inherently resistant to the adamantines. These agents are no longer recommended for treatment or prevention of seasonal influenza.
- *Pharmacology:* well absorbed orally. Amantadine is excreted unchanged by the kidney (decrease dose in elderly and renally impaired). Rimantadine is extensively metabolized by the liver before renal excretion (reduce doses in those with severe liver or renal dysfunction).
- *Adverse effects:* diarrhea, nausea, difficulty concentrating. Neurotoxicity occurs at high doses or in those with renal impairment, e.g., tremor, seizures, coma. Anticholinergic symptoms accompany high doses of amantadine, e.g., dry mouth, papillary dilation, toxic psychosis, and cardiac arrhythmias. Psychiatric symptoms in those with Parkinson's disease or schizophrenia have been associated with amantadine.
- *Drug interactions:* increased CNS side effects with concomitant antihistamines or anticholinergics

Antivirals for respiratory syncytial virus

Ribavirin

This broad-spectrum antiviral is used in the treatment of respiratory syncytial virus (RSV), hepatitis C, influenza, and Lassa fever. Studies assessing its role in the treatment of RSV infection in children have been small, and although they show no reduction in hospital stay, there is a beneficial effect on pulmonary function at 1 year. It is currently used in the treatment of RSV bronchiolitis and pneumonia in hospitalized children, especially those with complicated or severe disease.

- *Mechanism of action:* guanosine analog, which interferes with nucleic acid synthesis and may also block production of viral mRNA
- *Resistance* is not demonstrated in RSV.
- *Pharmacology:* excreted renally (around 40%) and in feces (15%) and is metabolized by the liver. Some drug is retained in tissues and red blood cells. It is given by nebulizer in bronchiolitis, orally or IV in other conditions (IV ribavirin is no longer available in the United States but can be obtained for compassionate-use purposes).
- *Adverse effects:* dose-related anemia (extravascular hemolysis) and marrow suppression at high doses. Itch, nausea, depression, and cough.

With aerosolized preparations, conjunctivits, rash, and bronchospasm can occur. Because of the teratogenic risk, pregnant women and people wearing contact lenses should not be present when ribavirin inhalation is being administered. The drug should also not be used in pregnant patients via any route of administration.

Other therapies for RSV

These are discussed in more detail later (see Bronchiolitis, p. 550). Some authorities advocate the use of ribavirin in combination with RSV immunoglobulin, particularly in immunosuppressed individuals.

Antivirals for chronic viral hepatitis

A number of drugs are licensed for the treatment of viral hepatitis. These are generally used for the treatment of chronic hepatitis B (HBV, see Hepatitis B virus, p. 361) and hepatitis C (HCV, see Hepatitis C virus, p. 364) virus infections. They have rarely been used in fulminant acute viral hepatitis but this approach is experimental and referral to a transplant center is recommended.

Indications for therapy

- Chronic HBV infection with ongoing viral replication for at least 6 months: HbsAg, HbeAg and HBV DNA-positive (wild-type infection) or HbsAg, anti-Hbe and HBV DNA-positive (anti-HBe variant)
- Chronic HCV infection with moderate to severe disease, defined as significant and/or bridging fibrosis and/or significant necrotic inflammation

Interferon-α

This is a synthetic analog of a natural compound with a number of antiviral and immunomodulatory effects.

- *Indications:* treatment of chronic HBV and HCV infections
- *Pharmacology:* given by IM or SC injection. The usual dose is 5–10 MU 3 times weekly for 3–6 months. Pegylated interferon-A has a longer half-life and can be given weekly.
- *Duration of treatment:* 24 weeks for HCV genotype 2 or 3 infections; 12 weeks initially for genotypes 1, 4, 5, and 6; continued to 48 weeks if viral load is suppressed to <1% of baseline level (2 log reduction)
- *Side effects:* fever, chills, fatigue, myalgia, myelotoxicity (monitor CBC), impaired concentration, altered mood, exacerbation or development of autoimmune thyroid diseases, alopecia, arthralgia, hypersensitivity (rare), pulmonary infiltrates (rare)

Ribavirin

Ribavirin is a guanosine analog with broad-spectrum antiviral activity.

- *Indications:* used orally in combination with interferon-α or pegylated interferon-α for treatment of chronic HCV infection
- *Mechanism:* inhibits inosine monophosphate dehydrogenase

- *Resistance* is not reported.
- *Pharmacology:* rapidly absorbed orally, rapidly metabolized in liver; excreted in urine (50%), feces (15%), or retained in tissues, principally in red blood cells
- *Side effects:* hemolytic anemia (monitor CBC), pruritis, rash, hypersensitivity (rare), teratogenicity (avoid conception)

Lamivudine

This nucleoside analog is widely used for the treatment of HIV and HBV infection.

- *Indications:* end-stage HBV disease pre-, peri- and post-transplant; patients who have failed interferon therapy; patients for whom interferon is contraindicated
- *Mechanism:* inhibits viral reverse transcriptase enzyme, inhibiting viral replication
- *Resistance* emerges with monotherapy, e.g., the YMDD variant. Resistance rates are 50% at 2 years, 90% at 4 years.
- *Pharmacology:* given orally, usual dose is 100 mg once daily, well absorbed, renal excretion (reduce dose in renal impairment)
- *Side effects* are minimal.
- *Outcome:* response rate increases with time: 17% at 1 year, 27% at 2 years. One study showed 66% response rate at 4 years.

Adefovir dipivoxil

This is a prodrug of the nucleotide analog adefovir, with activity against herpes viruses and HBV.

- Lamivudine-resistant strains have been shown to be sensitive to adefovir.
- Treatment with 10 mg daily decreases HBV DNA levels, improves hepatic histology scores, and induces loss of HbeAg.
- Concerns about renal toxicity when used as HIV therapy

Entecavir

Entecavir is a nucleoside analog that inhibits HBV DNA polymerase.

- *Indications:* treatment of chronic HBV, active against lamivudine-resistant strains
- *Resistance* is rare in nucleoside-naive patients.
- *Pharmacology:* given orally
- *Side effects:* GI symptoms, elevated amylase, and CNS symptoms

Tenofovir disoproxil fumarate

This synthetic nucleotide analog has activity against HIV and HBV. It may be used in treatment-naive patients or as additional therapy in patients with lamivudine, telbivudine, or entecavir resistance.

- *Pharmacology:* 25% oral absorption, not metabolized, renal excretion
- *Side effects:* GI symptoms, renal impairment, lactic acidosis, and hepatic steatosis (rare)

Telbivudine

Telbivudine is a nucleoside reverse transcriptase inhibitor that appears to have more potent activity than lamivudine or adefovir.

- It selects for the same resistant mutants as lamivudine.
- High cost has limited its use a first-line agent.

Telaprevir and beceprevir

Recently, these two protease inhibitors have shown promising results in treating HCV infection in combination with traditional therapies (interferon + ribavirin). FDA approval for use of both agents in the United States was recently granted.

Immunomodulatory agents

A number of strategies have been tried in HBV, but these have generally shown no benefit, e.g., corticosteroids ± interferon, thymic hormones, levimasole, and inosine pranobex. Trials are currently under way with lamivudine + corticosteroids.

Future therapies

Combination therapy with interferon and nucleotide analogs is likely to become standard for HBV. HCV has serine protease and helicase activity to which specific inhibitors may be developed in the future.

Principles of HIV treatment

Before 1988, the treatment of HIV and AIDS was primarily the treatment and prevention of opportunistic infections. Early studies of zidovudine monotherapy showed short-term benefits in delaying disease progression in symptomatic patients, but this finding was later refuted by the Concorde trial.

In 1995, several studies proved that dual nucleoside analog regimens were superior to monotherapy. In 1996, introduction of the protease inhibitors allowed the development of potent triple-drug combinations, and the era of highly active antiretroviral therapy (HAART) began.

Although HAART (now referred to as ART) has dramatically decreased HIV-related morbidity and mortality in the developed world, a number of problems remain: ongoing viral replication, emergence of drug resistance, high treatment failure rates, and concerns about the long-term metabolic complications of antiretroviral therapy.

Antiretroviral drugs

There are five main classes of antiretroviral drugs:
- Nucleoside/nucleotide reverse transcriptase inhibitors = NRTIs (see Nucleoside/nucleotide analog reverse transcriptase inhibitors (NRTIs), p. 89)
- Protease inhibitors = PIs (see Protease inhibitors, p. 93)
- Non-nucleoside reverse transcriptase inhibitors = NNRTIs (see Non-nucleoside reverse transcriptase inhibitors (NNRTIs), p. 91)
- Entry inhibitors (see Other HIV therapies, p. 95)
- Integrase inhibitors = INSTI (see Other HIV therapies, p. 95).

Considerations when starting antiretroviral therapy (Table 1.7)

The aim of antiretroviral therapy is to prolong and improve quality of life by maintaining viral load suppression for as long as possible. Factors determining when to start and choice of therapy are as follows:

- Risk of disease progression (CD4 count, HIV viral load)
- Compelling indications to initiate therapy (pregnancy, HIV-associated nephropathy, and HBV coinfection requiring treatment)
- Willingness of the patient to start therapy
- Clinical effectiveness of combination regimen
- Ability of patient to adhere to therapy
- Comorbidities, e.g., tuberculosis, liver disease, cardiovascular disease, psychiatric conditions
- Pill burden, dosing schedule, food considerations
- Adverse effects
- Drug–drug interactions
- Pregnancy potential
- Gender and CD4 count (if considering nevirapine)
- Coreceptor tropism assay (if considering CCR5 antagonist)
- HLA-B*5701 testing (if considering abacavir)
- Drug resistance potential/results of genotypic testing
- Future therapeutic options.

Primary HIV infection

The rationale for starting treatment during or shortly after infection is to attempt to maintain specific and robust CD4 T-cell responses, which are generally lost in chronic HIV infection. This should be balanced against the risks of toxicity, development of drug resistance, and difficulties of long-term adherence. This remains an area of active research.

Table 1.7 Recommendations for starting antiretroviral therapy in adults

Disease stage	UK guidelines*	US guidelines†
Primary HIV infection	Only in clinical trial	Consider treatment
Established infection, CD4 <200 cells/mm³	Treat	Treat
Established infection, CD4 201–350 cells/mm³	Treat	Treat
Established infection, CD4 >350 cells/mm³	Defer	May be considered
Symptomatic disease or AIDS	Treat	Treat
Special situations		Pregnant women, HIV nephropathy, HBV infection requiring treatment

CD4, CD4 T-cell count;.

* British HIV Association guidelines (2008): http://www.bhiva.org
† U.S. DHHS guidelines (2011): http://www.aidsinfo.nih.gov

Established HIV infection

According to the 2011 Department of Health and Human Service Guidelines,[1] antiretroviral therapy is recommended for patients with CD4 counts <500 cells/mm^3 and can be considered for >500 cells/mm^3. This reflects a change from previous recommendations where therapy was not recommended until the CD4 cell count fell below 350 cells/mm^3.

It should be noted the recent change was controversial and the strongest data remain for patients with a CD4 count <200 cells/mm^3 or an AIDS-defining condition.

Special circumstances

Antiretroviral therapy should also be started in the following patients, regardless of CD4 cell count:
• Pregnant women
• HIV-associated nephropathy
• HBV infection requiring treatment

Initial regimen in treatment naive patients

Any HAART regimen should be individualized to achieve the best potency, adherence, and tolerability and to minimize drug interactions and toxicity. Although baseline drug resistance testing is recommended before starting antiretroviral therapy, this is unavailable in developing countries.

Recommended initial combinations are as follows:
• NNRTI based: NNRTI plus two NRTIs
• PI based: PI (preferably boosted with ritonavir) plus two NRTIs
• Integrase inhibitor based: INSTI plus two NRTIs

Regimens that are not recommended are as follows:
• Monotherapy (rapid development of resistance, inferior efficacy)
• Dual therapy (inferior efficacy)
• Triple NRTI combinations (inferior efficacy).
• Quadruple (abacavir plus lamivudine plus zidovudine plus tenofovir) NRTI combinations (inferior efficacy)

Nucleoside/nucleotide analog reverse transcriptase inhibitors

HIV reverse transcriptase is an RNA-dependent DNA polymerase that is essential for virus replication. It enables transcription of virus RNA into a DNA copy, which is then integrated into the host genome. This enzyme can be inhibited by the following:
• Nucleoside or nucleotide reverse transcriptase inhibitors (NRTIs)
• Non-nucleoside reverse transcriptase inhibitors (NNRTIs, (see Non-nucleoside reverse transcriptase inhibitors, p. 91).

NRTIs (Table 1.8) are commonly used as the backbone of therapy for chronic HIV infection, in combination with protease inhibitors (PIs, see Protease inhibitors, p. 93) or NNRTIs. For treatment guidelines, see http://AIDSinfo.nih.gov.

Table 1.8 Characteristics of NRTIs

Drug	Pharmacology	Adverse effects
Abacavir	83% oral bioavailability; metabolized in liver, metabolites excreted in urine	Hypersensitivity reaction (can be fatal)
Didanosine	Take 1 hour before or 2 hours after meals; 30–40% oral bioavailability; renal excretion 50%—adjust dose in renal impairment	Pancreatitis, peripheral neuropathy. Coadministration with tenofovir increases didanosine concentrations
Emtricitabine	93% oral bioavailability; renal excretion—adjust dose in renal impairment	Minimal toxicity
Lamivudine	86% oral bioavailability; renal excretion—adjust dose in renal impairment	Minimal toxicity
Stavudine	86% oral bioavailability; renal excretion 50%—adjust dose in renal impairment	Peripheral neuropathy, pancreatitis, lipodystrophy, rapidly progressive ascending neuro-muscular weakness (rare)
Tenofovir	Bioavailability: 25% if fasting, 39% with high-fat meal; renal excretion—adjust dose in renal impairment	Rare reports of renal insufficiency. Coadministration with didanosine increases didanosine concentrations
Zidovudine	60% oral bioavailability; metabolized to glucuronide, renal excretion of metabolite	Bone marrow suppression

Specific drugs
- Abacavir (ABC, Ziagen®)
- Didanosine (ddl, Videx®, Videx EC®)
- Emtricitabine (FTC, Emtriva®)
- Lamivudine (3TC, Epivir®)
- Stavudine (d4T, Zerit®)
- Tenofovir disoproxil fumarate (TDF, Viread®)
- Zidovudine (AZT, ZDV, Retrovir®)

Combination drugs
- Combivir® (zidovudine + lamivudine)
- Trizivir® (abacavir + zidovudine + lamivudine)
- Epzicom® (abacavir + lamivudine)
- Truvada® (emtricitabine + tenofovir)
- Atripla® (emtricitabine + tenofovir + efavirenz; see NNRTIs below)

Structure
- Nucleoside or nucleotide analogs

Mechanism of action
- Inhibit HIV reverse transcriptase enzyme
- Also inhibit mitochondrial DNA polymerases, resulting in toxicity

Resistance
- Caused by one or more mutations in reverse transcriptase gene
- Some specific mutations confer cross-resistance to other NRTIs.

Pharmacology
- Variable oral absorption (25–93%), reduced by food
- Widely distributed
- Variable CSF penetration (12–50%)
- Cross the placenta, secreted in breast milk
- Some metabolized in liver
- Renal excretion: most need dose adjustment in renal impairment

Adverse effects
- All may cause GI symptoms, lipodystrophy, neurological symptoms, and lactic acidosis with hepatic steatosis (rare but may be fatal).
- Some also cause myelosuppression (AZT), peripheral neuropathy (d4T, ddI, ddC), pancreatitis (d4T, ddI, ddC), hyperlipidemia (d4T), renal insufficiency or Fanconi syndrome (TDF), osteomalacia or decrease in bone mineral density (TDF), and hypersensitivity (ABC).
- Severe acute exacerbation of hepatitis may occur in patients with hepatitis B who abruptly discontinue lamivudine, emtricitabine, and/or tenofovir.
- Didanosine has been associated with noncirrhotic portal hypertension and possible risk of myocardial infarction (MI) with recent or current abacavir studies, although the data remain controversial.

Non-nucleoside reverse transcriptase inhibitors

This is the third class of commonly used antiretrovirals. Based on clinical trial data, efavirenz-based regimens are considered superior to other regimens in terms of antiviral potency, durability, and safety. However, because of teratogenicity in primates, efavirenz is not recommended in pregnancy and in women of childbearing potential.

Nevirapine-containing regimens are also potent, but the data for antiviral activity compared to that of other regimens are less consistent. Nevirapine also has a higher incidence of serious adverse toxicities (hepatitis, Stevens–Johnson syndrome), making it more appropriate as an alternative to efavirenz in treatment-naive patients.

Delaviridine is the least potent NNRTI and is not recommended as part of an initial antiretroviral regimen.

For treatment guidelines, see http://www.bhiva.org and http://AIDSinfo.nih.gov.

Specific drugs

Four NNRTIs (Table 1.9) are currently marketed for use:
- Delaviridine (Rescriptor®)
- Efavirenz (EFV, Sustiva®)
- Nevirapine (NVP, Viramune®]
- Etravirine (TMC-125, INTELENCE™).

Mechanism of action

- Inhibit HIV reverse transcriptase

Resistance

- Associated with mutation in reverse transcriptase gene
- Single mutation confers resistance to most of the drugs available in this class.

Pharmacology

- Well absorbed orally
- Metabolized by cytochrome P450 enzyme system
- Excretion of metabolites in urine
- Unchanged drug excreted in feces
- Long half-life. This is a particular problem when used in pregnancy as monotherapy, as it results in development of resistance, which may affect future treatment options. The long half-life is also an issue when stopping drug regimens because of the mismatch in half-life of nevirapine and that of NRTIs and PIs

Table 1.9 Characteristics of NNRTIs

Drug	Pharmacology	Adverse effects
Delaviridine	85% oral bioavailability; CYP3A4 inhibitor; excretion: 51% in urine, 44% in feces	Rash, increased transaminases, headaches
Efavirenz	Take on an empty stomach; oral bioavailability not known; mixed CYP3A4 inducer and inhibitor; excretion: 14–34% in urine, 16–61% in feces	Rash, CNS symptoms (52%), increased transaminases, false-positive cannabinoid test, teratogenic in monkeys
Nevirapine	>90% oral bioavailability; CYP3A4 inducer; excretion: 80% in urine, 10% in feces	Rash, hepatitis, Stevens–Johnson syndrome, toxic epidermal necrolysis, DRESS syndrome (drug rash with eosinophilia and systemic symptoms)
Etravirine	Take with food; oral bioavailability not known; 99% protein bound; metabolized by CYP3A4; eliminated in feces and urine	Rash, GI symptoms, fatigue, peripheral neuropathy, headache, hypertension

Adverse effects
- Rash common
- Elevated transaminases
- CNS symptoms are common with efavirenz (dizziness, insomnia, somnolence, abnormal dreams, confusion, impaired concentration, amnesia, agitation, hallucinations, euphoria). Take tablets at night on an empty stomach to minimize these adverse effects. Symptoms usually resolve in 2–4 weeks.
- Hepatitis (most common with nevirapine, especially in women with high CD4 counts)
- Stevens–Johnson syndrome (rare, most common with nevirapine)
- Teratogenicity in monkeys (efavirenz, no data on other NNRTIs)

Protease inhibitors

HIV protease inhibitors (PIs, Table 1.10) are a group of structurally related molecules that represent synthetic analogs of one of the HIV *gag-pol* cleavage sites. The introduction of PIs in 1996 heralded the era of ART, enabling the combination of drugs with two different enzymatic sites of action in the virus life cycle. They are used in combination with NRTIs for treatment and post-exposure prophylaxis of HIV infection. For treatment guidelines see http://www.bhiva.org and http://AIDSinfo.nih.gov

Specific drugs
- Atazanavir (ATV, Reyataz®)
- Darunavir (DRV, Prezista®)
- Fosamprenavir (FPV, Lexiva®)
- Indinavir (IDV, Crixivan®)—no longer recommended
- Lopinavir + ritonavir (LPV/r, Kaletra®)
- Nelfinavir (NFV, Viracept®)—no longer recommended
- Ritonavir (RTV, Norvir®)
- Saquinavir (SQV) hard gel capsule (Invirase®): due to QTc prolongation issues, boosted regimens only recommended with caution
- Tipranavir (TPV, Aptivus®)

Mechanisms of action and resistance
- Inhibit HIV protease, so inhibiting cleavage of viral polypeptides to form structural proteins and viral enzymes
- Mutations in HIV protease gene; many mutations confer cross-resistance to other PIs.

Pharmacology
- Oral absorption is variable (13–78%), not known for some drugs
- Metabolized by cytochrome P450 enzyme system
- Distribution unknown for some drugs, CNS penetration variable
- Eliminated primarily in feces
- Low-dose ritonavir is used in combination with other PIs to decrease metabolism and increase plasma concentrations of the other PI. This is known as "ritonavir-boosted therapy."

Table 1.10 Characteristics of PIs

Drug	Pharmacology	Adverse effects
Amprenavir	Avoid high-fat meal; oral bioavailability not determined; CYP3A4 inhibitor	GI symptoms, rash, oral paraesthesia, raised transaminases, hyperglycemia, hyperlipidemia, fat redistribution
Atazanavir	Take with food; oral bioavailability not determined; CYP3A4 inhibitor and substrate	Hyperbilirubinemia, prolonged PR interval, hyperglycemia, fat redistribution
Darunavir	Administer with food; oral bioavailability 37%; CYP3A4 inhibitor and substrate	Skin rash, diarrhea, nausea, hyperglycemia, transaminitis, hyperglycemia, fat redistribution, possible increased bleeding in hemophiliacs
Fosamprenavir	No food restrictions; oral bioavailability not determined; CYP3A4 inhibitor, inducer and substrate	Skin rash, GI symptoms, headache, raised transaminases, hyperglycemia, hyperlipidemia, fat redistribution
Indinavir	Take 1 hour before or 2 hours after meals; 65% oral bioavailability; CYP3A4 inhibitor	Nephrolithiasis, GI symptoms, headache, asthenia, blurred vision, dizziness, rash, metallic taste, hyperglycemia, hyperlipidemia, fat redistribution
Lopinavir + ritonavir	Take with food; oral bioavailability not determined; CYP3A4 inhibitor; refrigerate (liquid only)	GI symptoms, asthenia, raised transaminases, hyperglycemia, hyperlipidemia, fat redistribution
Nelfinavir	Take with food; oral bioavailability 20–80%; CYP3A4 inhibitor	Diarrhea, hyperglycemia, hyperlipidemia, fat redistribution
Ritonavir	Take with food; oral bioavailability not determined; inhibits CYP2D6 > CYP2D6; refrigerate (capsules, not tablets)	GI symptoms, parasthesias, hepatitis, pancreatitis, asthenia, taste disturbance, hyperglycemia, hyperlipidemia, raised transaminases, uric acid, CK
Saquinavir	No food effect; bioavailability: 4% (hard gel). CYP3A4 inhibitor	GI symptoms, headache, raised transaminases, hyperglycemia, hyperlipidemia, fat redistribution, QTc prolongation with boosted regimens
Tipranavir	Take with food; CYP3A4 inhibitor and substrate; refrigerate capsules	Hepatotoxicity, skin rash, hyperlipidemia, hyperglycemia, fat redistribution, intracranial hemorrhage (rare)

Adverse effects and toxicity
- Gastrointestinal symptoms (nausea, vomiting, diarrhea)
- Neurological symptoms (headache, paraesthesias)
- Skin rash
- Fat redistribution
- Abnormal liver function tests, hyperglycemia, hyperlipidemia
- Indirect hyperbilirubenemia (ATV and IDV)
- Nephrolithiasis (ATV, IDV, and FPV)
- PR interval prolongation (ATV, LPV/r)
- Fatal and nonfatal cases of intracranial hemorrhages (rare) (TPV)
- QTc prolongation, all protease inhibitors, particularly Kaletra (LPV/r)

Interactions

Drugs that should *not* be administered with PIs include the following:
- Antiarrhythmics: amiodarone, IV lidocaine, quinidine
- Antihistamines: astemizole, terfenadine
- Ergot derivatives: ergotamine, dihydroergotamine, ergonovine, methylergonovine
- Inhaled steroids: fluticasone
- Motility agents: cisapride
- Neuroleptics: pimozide
- Sedatives: midazolam, triazolam
- Antimycobacterials: rifampin, rifapentine
- Statins: simvastatin, lovastatin
- Herbal products: St John's wort

Other HIV therapies

These include the following:
- Fusion entry inhibitors, e.g., T20
- Chemokine receptor antagonists, e.g., maraviroc, vicriviroc
- Integrase inhibitors, e.g., raltegravir
- Immunotherapies, e.g., interleukin-2 (IL-2), therapeutic vaccines.

Enfuvirtide (T20, Fuzeon®)
- The first of a new class of drugs called the *entry inhibitors*
- Binds to the HIV surface protein gp41, preventing binding of gp41 to CD4 cells
- Reserved for use in treatment-experienced patients
- Given twice daily by subcutaneous (SC) infection
- Adverse effects include injection site reactions, increased risk of bacterial pneumonia, and hypersensitivity reactions (<1%).

Maraviroc (MVC, Selzentry")
- A chemokine receptor antagonist that prevents the binding of HIV to the CCR5 receptor on CD4 T cells
- Used in treatment-naive and treatment-experienced patients
- Requires a tropism assay prior to initiating treatment to determine if the virus is CCR5 (susceptible) or CXCR4 (not susceptible)

- Given orally (no food effect)
- Metabolized in the liver by CYP3A
- Adverse effects include abdominal pain, cough, dizziness, musculoskeletal symptoms, pyrexia, rash, upper respiratory tract infections, hepatotoxicity, and orthostatic hypotension.

Vicriviroc (SCH-D)

- A chemokine receptor antagonist that prevents the binding of HIV to the CCR5 receptor on CD4 T cells
- Investigational drug still undergoing clinical trials; it is not yet Food and Drug Administration (FDA) approved
- Adverse effects include headache, fatigue, nausea, dizziness, and abdominal pain.

Raltegravir (RAL, Isentress®)

- Novel agent that inhibits integration of viral genetic material into the human chromosome (strand transfer inhibitor)
- Used in treatment-naive and treatment-experienced patients
- Given orally (no food restrictions)
- Metabolized by glucuronidation
- Side effects include nausea, diarrhea, pyrexia, and CK elevation.

Interleukin-2 (IL-2)

- Aldesleukin is a synthetic IL-2 derivative with antineoplastic and immunomodulating activities.
- Previous studies have shown that IL-2 in combination with antiretroviral therapy significantly increases CD4 counts.
- Studies are now under way to see if IL-2 in combination with approved and investigational HIV treatments can improve the immune system and delay disease progression.

Therapeutic HIV vaccines

- Therapeutic HIV vaccines are designed to boost the host immune response to HIV in order to control the infection.
- There are currently no licensed HIV therapeutic vaccines, although clinical trials are ongoing.

Antimalarials

Historical aspects

Quinolines have been the mainstay of antimalarial therapy since the 17th century when Peruvian Indians used the bark of the cinchona tree. Despite its longevity, quinine remains an important drug in the treatment of malaria, although resistance to it is gradually increasing. Another quinoline, chloroquine, was widely used but has succumbed to global resistance in *P. falciparum* and increasing resistance in *P. vivax*. A newer quinoline, mefloquine, is also used to treat malaria.

The antimalarial activity of the biguanides (proguanil) was discovered during the Second World War. These, along with the diaminopyrimidines (pyrimethamine), are referred to as the *antifolate drugs*. They are used in combination with other drugs for prophylaxis (e.g., chloroquine + proguanil or atovaquone + proguanil) or treatment (e.g., sulfadoxine-pyrimethamine).

Qinghao, derived from *Artemisia annua*, has been used by the Chinese to treat fever for over 2000 years. Artemisin in and its derivatives (dihydroartemisin, artemether, and artesunate) have been found to have potent antimalarial activity and are widely used for the treatment of malaria in Southeast Asia. In uncomplicated malaria, these drugs are used in combination with other drugs, e.g., mefloquine-artesunate.

Resistance mechanisms

Antimalarial drug resistance arises through the selection of rare naturally arising mutants with reduced drug susceptibility. Unlike bacteria, plasmodia do not have transferable resistance mechanisms but are eukaryotes and can acquire or lose polygenic resistance mechanisms during meiosis. Resistance arises readily to drugs such as the antifolates or atovaquone because a single point mutation confers resistance, and per-parasite mutation frequencies are relatively high.

- Resistance to antifolates is associated with progressive acquisition of mutations in the dihydrofolate reductase (DHFR) gene or dihydropterate synthetase (DHPS) gene, respectively.
- The mechanism of resistance in quinoline antimalarials remains controversial but has been associated with mutations in *pfmdr1* (an efflux mechanism similar to that found in multi-drug-resistant mammalian tumor cells) and *pfCRT* (a food vacuolar membrane protein with transporter function).
- Atovaquone resistance arises from point mutations in the gene encoding cytochrome bc_1 mitochondrial complex.
- Although resistance to artemisinin and its derivatives occurs in vitro, clinical resistance has yet to be reported.

Rationale for combination therapy

The simplest reason to combine antimalarials is to increase efficacy. Drug combinations can also shorten duration of treatment, hence increasing compliance and decreasing the risk of resistant parasites arising by mutation during therapy.

As with other infectious diseases such as TB and HIV, the emergence of resistance can be prevented by the use of drugs with different mechanisms of action. If two drugs with different mechanisms of action are combined, then the per-parasite probability of developing resistance is the product of their individual per-parasite probabilities. There are some limitations, however:

- If some patients receive only one component of the combination or there is already high resistance to one of the components, resistance can arise to the other.
- Combinations are more expensive than single drugs (but the increased cost is outweighed by longer-term benefits).
- Although artemisinin combinations appear to be the most promising, the best combinations have yet to be determined.

Guidelines for the prevention and treatment of malaria are given in Box 1.10.

> **Box 1.10 Guidelines for prevention and treatment of malaria**
>
> *Prophylaxis*
> - U.S. guidelines: National Center for Infectious Diseases Travelers' Health. *The Yellow Book – Health Information for International Travel 2010.* Atlanta: Centers for Disease Control and Prevention. http://wwwn.cdc.gov/travel/ybToc.aspx
> - WHO guidelines: World Health Organization. *International Travel and Health: Vaccination Requirements and Health Advice.* Geneva: WHO, 2011. http://www.who.int/ith/en/index.html
>
> *Treatment*
> - U.S. guidelines: CDC. *Treatment of Malaria (Guidelines for Clinicians).* http://www.cdc.gov/malaria/diagnosis_treatment/tx_clinicians.htm
> - WHO Treatment of Malaria (2nd ed.) Geneva: WHO, 2010. http://www.who.int/malaria/publications/atoz/9789241547925/en/index.html

Quinine and related compounds

Quinine/Quinidine

4-methanolquinoline is derived from the bark of the cinchona tree. It inhibits erythrocytic stages of human malaria parasites but not all liver stages. It is also active against gametocytes of *P. vivax, P. ovale,* and *P. malariae*

Quinidine is a stereoisomer of quinine that is only administered parenterally.

- *Resistance* is widespread in Southeast Asia where some strains are also resistant to chloroquine, mefloquine, and sulfadoxine-pyrimethamine. There is cross-resistance with mefloquine in Central Africa.
- *Clinical use:* treatment of *P. falciparum* malaria. Quinidine, an antiarrhythmic drug with greater toxicity, is used more commonly in the United States. IV quinidine is not commercially available in the United States but can be obtained through the CDC at 770-488-7788 or from Eli Lilly at 800-821-0538.
- *Pharmacology:* well absorbed orally; IM administration more predictable than IV administration. Extensive hepatic metabolism. Urinary clearance is <20%.
- *Adverse effects:* cinchonism (tinnitus, vomiting, diarrhea, headache), hypoglycemia (monitor blood glucose), hypotension, cardiac arrhythmias, hemolytic anemia (blackwater fever)

Mefloquine (Lariam®)

Mefloquine is a synthetic 4-methanolquinoline, formulated as hydrochloride. It is active against erythrocytic stages of *Plasmodium* spp. It is effective against strains of *P. falciparum* that are resistant to chloroquine, sulfonamides, and pyrimethamine. It is also active against bacteria (e.g., MRSA) and some fungi.

- *Resistance* is increasing; there is 15% high-grade resistance and 50% low-grade resistance in Southeast Asia. There is cross-resistance with quinine and halofantrine and an inverse relationship with chloroquine resistance.
- *Clinical use:* prophylaxis in areas of chloroquine resistance. Treatment of uncomplicated multi-drug-resistant malaria
- *Pharmacology:* well absorbed orally, concentrated in erythrocytes, metabolites not active, predominantly excreted in bile
- *Adverse effects:* nausea, dizziness, fatigue, confusion, and sleep disturbance. Psychosis, encephalopathy, and convulsions occur in 1/1200–1700 patients; 1/10,000 patients have risk of serious toxicity in prophylaxis. Rarely, mefloquine-induced pneumonitis has been reported. Mefloquine is contraindicated in patients with a history of psychiatric or seizure disorders.

Chloroquine (Aralen®)/ hydroxychloroquine (Plaquenil®)

These are synthetic 4-aminoquinolines, active against erythrocytic stages of all four human malaria species and gametocytes of *P. vivax*, *P. ovale*, and *P. malariae*.

- *Mechanism of action:* inhibits parasite heme detoxification
- *Resistance* of *P. falciparum* to chloroquine is widespread and is due to increased drug efflux (mutation in *pfmdr1* gene) and/or decreased drug uptake (mutation in *pfCRT* gene).
- *Clinical use:* prophylaxis and treatment of chloroquine-sensitive malaria. Hydroxychloroquine is also used to treat lupus and rheumatoid arthritis.
- *Pharmacology:* 80–90% oral absorption. Widely distributed. Extensive tissue binding with high affinity for melanin-containing tissues. Extensive metabolism to active metabolite; 50% renal excretion.
- *Adverse effects:* dizziness, headache, rashes, nausea, diarrhea, and pruritis. Long-term treatment may cause cardiovascular CNS effects and retinopathy. Rarely, aplastic anemia, photosensitivity, tinnitus, and deafness may occur. Use with caution in patients with G6PD deficiency or pre-existing liver disease. In some patients with chloroquine intolerance, hydroxychloroquine may be better tolerated.

Primaquine

Primaquine is a synthetic 8-aminoquinoline, formulated as diphosphate. It is active against hepatic stages of *Plasmodia* spp., including the hypnozoite stage of *P. vivax*. It has poor activity against erythrocytic stages but is active against gametocytes. It is also active against *Pneumocystis* spp., *Babesia* spp., *Leishmania* spp., and *Trypanosoma cruzi*.

- *Mechanism of action* is not known
- *Resistance:* failure rates of up to 35% are reported in Southeast Asia in patients treated for *P. vivax*.
- *Clinical use:* treatment and prevention of relapse of *P. vivax* and *P. ovale*. Second-line treatment of *Pneumocystis jirovecii* (in combination with clindamycin)

- *Pharmacology:* well absorbed orally, extensive tissue distribution, metabolized to carboxyprimaquine, methoxy and hydroxy metabolites, <4% excreted unchanged in urine
- *Adverse effects* are generally mild: abdominal cramps, anemia, leukocytosis, and methemoglobinemia. Hemolytic anemia occurs in G6PD deficiency (patients should be screened prior to therapy).
- *Drug interactions:* avoid concomitant use with other marrow-suppressing medications.

Artemisinin and its derivatives

Artemisinin (quinghao) is derived from *Artemisia annua* (sweet worm-wood). Artemisinin and its derivatives act by inhibiting *P. falciparum*–encoded sarcoplasmic-endoplasmic reticulum calcium ATPase.

Most clinically important artemisinins are metabolized to dihydroartem-isinin, in which form they have comparable antimalarial activity. They are highly effective alternatives to quinine for the treatment of chloroquine-resistant falciparum malaria. In both uncomplicated and severe infections they have shown faster fever and parasite clearance times and have proved effective in treating cerebral malaria.

They are widely used in the developing world to treat malaria. Their use in the developed world is hampered by a lack of availability of GMP (good manufacturing practice) products.

Artemether

Artemether is methyl and ester of dihydroartemisin. It is sold commer-cially in combination with lumefantrine (Coartem™).
- *Resistance:* there have been clinically documented cases of atermisinin resistance.
- *Pharmacology:* absorbed slowly and erratically; not suitable for severely ill patients, available orally only in the United States.
- *Adverse effects:* generally well tolerated. Type I hypersensitivity has been reported.

Artesunate

- Water-soluble hemisuccinate of dihydroartemisinin
- Can be given PO, PR, or IV
- Widely used in treatment of malaria in the developing world but not licensed in the United States.
- Shown to be superior to quinine in efficacy (mortality 15% vs. 24%) and tolerability for the treatment of severe malaria
- IV artesunate is available through the CDC under investigational protocols (CDC malaria hotline: 770-488-7788).

Artemisin in combination therapies

These are generally accepted as the best treatments for uncomplicated falciparum malaria. Recently, the WHO called for only combination products of atermisinin derivatives to be produced in order to prevent resistance.

These combinations are rapidly and reliably effective; their efficacy is determined by the drug partnering the artemisinin derivative and is usually >95%. The use of certain combinations is limited by resistance in the partner drug.

They are safe and well tolerated, although hypersensitivity may occasionally occur. The adverse-effect profiles are determined by the partner drug. They should not be used in the first trimester of pregnancy (safety not established) unless there is no alternative.

Artemether-lumefantrine (Coartem®) is the only available combination product in the United States. It has been associated with irreversible hearing loss.

Miscellaneous antimalarials

Proguanil (Paludrine®)

Proguanil is a synthetic arylbiguanide. Its metabolite cycloguanil inhibits the erythrocytic stages of all four *Plasmodium* species and the hepatic stage of *P. falciparum*. It acts synergistically with atovaquone.

- Worldwide resistance of *P. falciparum* is associated with point mutations in *DHFR* gene. Resistance of *P. vivax* and *P. malariae* is reported in Southeast Asia.
- *Clinical use:* antimalarial prophylaxis (with chloroquine); treatment and prophylaxis of drug-resistant falciparum malaria (with atovaquone)
- *Pharmacology:* >90% oral absorption; 75% protein bound; concentrated in erythrocytes; 20% metabolized by cytochrome P450 enzyme system to cycloguanil (active metabolite). Nonmetabolizers occur in Japan and Kenya, leading to resistance; 60% is excreted in urine
- *Adverse effects:* GI and renal effects at high doses (>600 mg/day)

Atovaquone-proguanil (Malarone®)

Atovaquone is a hydroxynaphthoquinone that is more active than standard antimalarials against all stages of *P. falciparum*. It is also active against *Babesia* spp., *Toxoplasma gondii*, and *Pneumocystis jirovecii*.

- *Resistance* is due to point mutations in the parasite's cytochrome *bc*1 gene. Resistance emerges rapidly. It is therefore used in combination with proguanil, with which it appears to have synergistic activity.
- *Clinical use:* prophylaxis and treatment of malaria; treatment of *Pneumocystis* pneumonia (atovaquone alone)
- *Pharmacology:* poor oral absorption, improved when given with meals; 99% protein bound; poor CSF penetration (<1%). Not metabolized. Elimination half-life is 73 hours.
- *Adverse effects:* fever, nausea, diarrhea, and rash

Tetracycline and doxycycline

Tetracycline and doxycycline (see Tetracyclines, p. 51) are both protein synthesis inhibitors. They are well absorbed orally with elimination half-lives of 8 hours (tetracycline) and 20 hours (doxycycline).

Quinine + tetracycline has been used for treatment of multi-drug-resistant falciparum malaria in Thailand for years.

Quinine + doxycycline is recommended for treatment of falciparum malaria in the United States. Doxycycline also used in prophylaxis of malaria (in regions with chloroquine or mefloquine resistance).
- *Main limitations:* contraindicated in children and pregnant women; photosensitivity with doxycycline. There is emergence of parasite resistance to tetracycline in areas where it has been extensively used.

Clindamycin
Clindamycin (see Lincosamides, p. 45) is a lincosamide antibiotic that also acts on the malaria parasite's apicoplast.

Although studies of quinine + clindamycin have shown good efficacy and safety profiles in various populations, it has not been widely used.

Antiprotozoal drugs (1)

Albendazole
This is a benzimidazole derivative, active against a variety of parasites.
- *Clinical use:* giardiasis, microsporidiosis, intestinal worm infections, trichinosis, cutaneous larva migrans, hydatid disease, neurocysticercosis, lymphatic filiariasis

Amphotericin B (see Polyenes, p. 73)
This polyene antifungal is active against a variety of fungi and some protozoa, e.g., *Leishmania* spp., *Naegleria*, and *Hartmanella*.
- *Clinical use:* treatment of leishmaniasis

Antimony compounds
Sodium stibogluconate (Pentostam®) is a pentavalent antimony compound that is not approved in the United States but can be obtained through the CDC by calling 404-639-3670.
- Active against amastigotes of *Leishmania* spp. within macrophages, with variation in sensitivity of different species
- Acquired resistance results in poor response and high resistance rates. Relapse is also common in immunosuppressed or HIV patients.
- *Clinical use:* treatment of leishmaniasis
- *Pharmacology:* given IM or IV with peak concentrations occurring after 1 hour. Slow accumulation in CNS and tissues. Excreted in urine
- *Adverse effects:* cough/vomiting (if infused too quickly), arthralgia, myalgia, bradycardia, abdominal cramps, diarrhea, rash, pruritis, increased LFTs, increased creatinine, increased amylase

Atovaquone (see Miscellaneous antimalarials p. 101)
This antimalarial has activity against other protozoa, e.g., *Babesia* spp., *Toxoplasma gondii*, and *Pneumocystis jirovecii*.
- *Clinical use:* treatment of *Pneumocystis jirovecii* pneumonia. It has also been used in cerebral toxoplasmosis and babesiosis, but further studies required.

Ciprofloxacin (see Quinolones, p. 57)

A fluoroquinolone antibiotic, ciprofloxacin is active against a wide variety of bacteria, *Legionella*, *Mycoplasma*, *Chlamydia*, mycobacteria, *Cyclospora cayetanensis*, and *Isospora belli*.

- *Clinical use*: second-line treatment of cyclospora and isospora

Clarithromycin (see Macrolides, p. 42)

This macrolide antibiotic is active against a variety of bacteria, *Legionella* spp., *Mycoplasma pneumoniae*, *Chlamydia* spp., atypical mycobacteria, and *Toxoplasma gondii*.

- *Clinical use*: second-line treatment of toxoplasmosis

Clindamycin (see Lincosamides, p. 45)

Clindamycin is a lincosamide antibiotic that is active against Gram-positive and anaerobic bacteria and some protozoa, e.g., *P. falciparum*, *Babesia* spp., *Toxoplasma gondii*, and *Pneumocystis jirovecii*.

- *Clinical use*: second-line treatment of *Pneumocystis jirovecii* pneumonia; second-line treatment and prophylaxis of cerebral toxoplasmosis

Co-trimoxazole (see Co-trimoxazole, p. 56)

This diaminopyrimidine-sulfonamide antibiotic is active against a wide variety of bacteria, atypical mycobacteria, *Nocardia* spp., *Pneumocystis jirovecii*, *Toxoplasma gondii*, *Cyclospora cayetanensis*, and *Isospora belli*.

- *Clinical use*: treatment and prophylaxis of *Pneumocystis jirovecii* pneumonia and cerebral toxoplasmosis

Dapsone (see Antileprotics, p. 70)

This sulfonamide derivative is active against *Mycobacterium leprae*, *Plasmodium* spp., *Toxoplasma gondii*, and *Pneumocystis jirovecii*.

- *Clinical use*: treatment and prophylaxis of *Pneumocystis jirovecii* pneumonia and cerebral toxoplasmosis

Fluconazole (see Triazoles, p. 75)

This triazole antifungal is active against a wide variety of fungi and *Leishmania* spp. It is used to treat cutaneous leishmaniasis.

Melarsoprol

This is an arsenical compound active against *Trypanosoma brucei* spp.

- *Resistance*: due to reduced uptake by trypanosomes
- *Pharmacology*: given IV, rapidly metabolized to melarsen oxide, which crosses the blood–brain barrier; biphasic elimination
- *Clinical use*: late-stage African sleeping sickness (available only from the CDC: 404-639-3670)
- *Adverse effects*: fever, abdominal pain, vomiting, peripheral neuropathy; 10% risk of post-treatment encephalopathy (may be reduced by prednisolone), 2–4% risk of death secondary to treatment

Metronidazole (see Nitroimidazoles, p. 59)

This nitroimidazole antibiotic is active against anaerobic bacteria and protozoa, e.g., *Trichomonas vaginalis*, *Giardia lamblia*, *Entamoeba histolytica*, *Balantidium coli*, and *Blastocystis hominis*.

- *Clinical use:* anaerobic bacterial infections, bacterial vaginosis, giardiasis, intestinal and amoebiasis, amoebic liver abscess

Miltefosine

This hexadecylphosphocholine is active against *Leishmania* spp., *Trypanosoma* spp., and *Entamoeba histolytica*. It is not currently available in the United States unless through compassionate-use protocols with the FDA. It is approved and widely used in South America and India.

- *Pharmacology:* well absorbed and widely distributed
- *Clinical use:* treatment of leishmaniasis
- *Adverse effects:* vomiting, diarrhea, teratogenic (avoid in pregnancy); rarely, QTc prolongation, leukocytosis, and thrombocytopenia

Antiprotozoal drugs (2)

Nifurtimox

This nitrofuran antibiotic is active against a variety of bacteria and *Trypanosoma cruzi*. It is available only through the CDC (404-639-3670).

- *Clinical use:* treatment of Chagas disease
- *Adverse effects:* GI symptoms (40–70%), CNS symptoms (33%), skin rash, hemolysis (G6PD deficiency)

Nitazoxanide

This broad-spectrum antiparasitic heterocycle is active against *Cryptosporidium parvum* and *Enterocytozoon bieneusi*.

- *Clinical use:* HIV-associated cryptosporidiosis (if ART fails), refractory *C. difficile*

Paromomycin (see Aminoglycosides, p. 39)

Paromomycin is an aminoglycoside antibiotic that is similar to neomycin.

- *Clinical use:* intestinal amoebiasis (oral), cutaneous leishmaniasis (topical), nitroimidazole-resistant trichomiasis (topical)

Pentamidine isethionate

This synthetic diamidine is active against *Plasmodium falciparum*, *Toxoplasma gondii*, *Leishmania* spp., *Trypanosoma* spp., *Babesia* spp., and *Pneumocystis jirovecii*.

- *Resistance:* relapse rates of 7–16% reported in the treatment of *Trypanosoma brucei gambiense*
- *Clinical use:* treatment of African trypanosomiasis (early stage), prophylaxis and treatment of *Pneumocystis* pneumonia (IV and inhaled), treatment of leishmaniasis (antimony-resistant)
- *Pharmacology:* negligible oral absorption, given IV or by nebulizer, hepatic metabolism, 15–20% excreted in urine. Poor CSF penetration (<1%). It is retained in tissues, e.g., liver, kidneys, adrenals, spleen, and lungs, resulting in a long terminal half-life (>12 days).
- *Adverse effects:* phlebitis, injection site abscess, GI symptoms, hypotension, hypoglycemia/hyperglycemia, hypocalcemia, neutropenia, increased creatinine and increased LFTs, pancreatitis, rash

Primaquine (see Quinine and related compounds, p. 98)

This is a synthetic 8-aminoquinoline that is active against hepatic stages of *Plasmodium vivax* and *ovale*, *Pneumocystis jirovecii*, *Babesia* spp., *Leishmania* spp., and *Trypanosoma cruzi.*
* *Clinical use:* treatment of *P vivax* or *P ovale* malaria, treatment of pneumocystis pneumonia (with clindamycin)

Pyrimethamine (see Miscellaneous antimalarials, p. 101)

This synthetic diaminopyrimidine is active against *Plasmodium* spp., *Toxoplasma gondii*, and *Pneumocystis jirovecii.*
* *Clinical use:* treatment of malaria (in combination with sulfadoxine or dapsone), toxoplasmosis (with sulfadiazine), and pneumocystis pneumonia (with dapsone)

Spiramycin

This macrolide antibiotic is active against a variety of bacteria and *Toxoplasma gondii.* Currently it is investigational in the United States; one needs to contact the FDA (1-888-463-6332) for IND.
* *Clinical use:* toxoplasmosis (especially in pregnancy)
* *Adverse effects:* dizziness, dry mouth, rarely, cholestatic hepatitis, and QTc prolongation

Sulfadiazine (see Sulfonamides, p. 53)

This sulfonamide antibiotic is active against a variety of bacteria and *Toxoplasma gondii.*
* *Clinical use:* toxoplasmosis (in combination with pyrimethamine)

Suramin

Suramin is a sulfated naphthylamine that is active against *Trypanosoma brucei* spp. It is not available in the United States except through the CDC (404-639-3670).
* *Mechanism of action:* binds to plasma proteins and is taken up into trypanomes by endocytosis. Acts synergistically with nitroimidazoles and enflornithine
* *Resistance:* clinical relapse rates of 30–50% reported in East Africa
* *Clinical use:* African sleeping sickness (early stage), onchocerciasis
* *Pharmacology:* poor oral absorption, given by slow IV infusion, >99% protein bound, poor CSF penetration, plasma half-life >40 days, not metabolized, high tissue distribution (liver, kidney, adrenal glands), renal excretion
* *Adverse effects:* highly toxic especially in malnourished patients. Immediate reactions (nausea, vomiting, cardiovascular collapse) can be avoided by use of slow IV injection. It may be followed by fever and urticaria. Anaphylaxis is rare (<1 in 2000). Delayed reactions include exfoliative dermatitis, anemia, leukopenia, jaundice, and diarrhea.

Tetracycline (see Tetracyclines, p. 51)

This tetracycline antibiotic is active against a variety of bacteria, *Chlamydia*, rickettsia, spirochetes, *Plasmodium falciparum, Balantidium coli,* and *Dientamoeba fragilis.*

- *Clinical use:* treatment and prophylaxis of drug-resistant falciparum malaria, treatment of *Balantidium coli* and *Dientamoeba fragilis*

Tinidazole (see Nitroimidazoles, p. 59)

This nitroimidazole antibiotic has similar activity to that of metronidazole.
- *Clinical use:* amoebiasis, giardiasis, trichomoniasis, *C. difficile* colitis

Anthelmintic drugs

Most anthelmintics were discovered and developed for use in veterinary medicine. Although no new antihelmintics have come to the market in recent years, satisfactory results can be achieved with current drugs. The exceptions to this are the treatment of larval cestodes, disseminated strongyloidiasis, and guinea worm.

Generic properties

- *Mechanism of action:* cause degenerative alterations in the tegument and intestinal cells of the worm by inhibiting its polymerization into microtubules. This results in an inability of the larva and adult stage to uptake glucose.
- *Drug resistance:* clinical drug resistance is rare.
- *Adverse effects:* the main side effects are GI and neurological symptoms, although allergic/anaphylactic reactions may rarely occur as a result of the death of large numbers of worms.

Albendazole

This benzimidazole carbamate is active against *Enterobius vermicularis, Ascaris lumbricoides, Ancylostoma duodenale, Necator americanus, Strongyloides stercoralis, Trichuris trichura, Trichinella spiralis*, animal hookworms, microfilaria, and *Echinococcus* spp. It is also active against *Giardia lamblia*, microsporidia.
- *Clinical use:* intestinal worm infections, trichinosis, cutaneous larva migrans, hydatid disease (± surgery), neurocysticercosis, lymphatic filiariasis (± ivermectin), giardiasis, microsporidiosis
- *Pharmacology:* well absorbed orally, metabolized to albendazole sulfoxide (active metabolite), half-life of 8 hours, renal excretion. Topical albendazole is also available and can be used for some helminths (e.g., cutaneous larva migrans)
- *Adverse effects:* GI symptoms common, leukopenia and increased LFTs with prolonged use. Rarely, neutropenia, pancytopenia, agranulocytosis, or thrombocytopenia can occur. Avoid use in pregnancy (teratogenic).

Diethylcarbamazine

This carbamyl derivative of piperazine is active against filarial worms: *Loa loa, Brugia malayi, Wuchereria bancrofti,* and *Onchocerca volvulus.* It is not approved in the United States but available through the CDC (404-639-3670).
- *Clinical use:* filiariasis
- *Pharmacology:* >90% oral absorption, 50% metabolized and excreted by feces, 50% excreted unchanged in urine

- *Adverse effects:* drug-induced death of microfilariae may trigger Mazotti reactions, e.g., skin rash, fever, headache, malaise, nausea, myalgia, arthralgia, vertigo, tachycardia, hypotension, cough, respiratory distress, ocular signs, neurological problems

Ivermectin

This is a mixture of two semisynthetic derivatives of avermectins, a complex of macrocyclic lactone antibiotics produced by *Streptomyces avertimilis*. It is active against *Ascaris lumbricoides*, *Strongyloides stercoralis*, *Onchocerca volvulus*, *Loa loa*, and *Sarcoptes scabiei*.

- *Clinical use:* onchocerciasis, nondisseminated strongyloidiasis, lymphatic filiariasis (with albendazole), scabies
- *Pharmacology:* 60% oral absorption, rapidly metabolized by liver, highest concentrations in liver and fat, excreted in feces
- *Adverse effects:* Mazotti reactions, GI symptoms, neurological symptoms

Mebendazole

This benzimidazole carbamate is active against *Enterobius vermicularis*, *Ascaris lumbricoides*, *Ancylostoma duodenale*, *Necator americanus*, *Strongyloides stercoralis*, and *Trichuris trichura*.

- *Clinical use:* intestinal worm infections, trichinosis
- *Pharmacology:* poor oral absorption, most of the drug and its metabolites (inactive) are retained in GI tract and excreted in feces, <2% excreted by kidneys
- *Adverse effects:* GI symptoms. Avoid use in pregnancy.

Praziquantel

This synthetic pyrazinoquinolone is active against schistosomes, larval tapeworms, *Fasciolopsis buski*, *Metagonimus yokogawi*, *Heterophyes heterophyes*, *Nanophytes salmincola*, *Clorchis* spp., *Opisthorcis* spp., *Paragonimus* spp., and *Fasciola hepatica* (variable activity).

- Resistance is emerging in schistosomes.
- *Clinical use:* schistosomiasis, tapeworm infections, trematode infections (except *Fasciola hepatica*)
- *Pharmacology:* >80% oral absorption, undergoes rapid first-pass metabolism to inactive metabolites, low plasma concentrations, 90% excreted in urine by 24 hours
- *Adverse effects:* GI symptoms, mild neurological effects during treatment of schistosomiasis; cerebral inflammation and edema during treatment of neurocysticercosis; risk of visual impairment with ocular cysticercosis

Pyrantel

This tetrahydropyrimidine is active against *Enterobius vermicularis*, *Ascaris lumbricoides*, *Ancylostoma duodenale*, and *Necator americanus*.

- *Clinical use:* pinworm, ascariasis, hookworm (especially *Ancylostoma duodenale*), trichostrongyliasis
- *Pharmacology:* <5% absorbed orally, metabolized, and excreted in urine; the rest passes unchanged in the feces
- *Adverse effects:* GI symptoms and neurological effects (rare).

Thiabendazole

This thiazoloyl benzimidazole is active against most common intestinal nematodes. It is also effective against strongyloidiasis, trichinosis, and cutaneous and visceral larva migrans.

- *Clinical use:* intestinal worms, strongyloidiasis, trichinosis, cutaneous larva migrans
- *Pharmacology:* well absorbed orally, peak plasma concentrations after 1–2 hours, metabolized to 5-hydroxyderivative (inactive), 90% excreted in urine within 24 hours, remainder excreted in feces
- *Adverse effects:* GI symptoms, fever, rare neurological symptoms (vertigo, disorientation, hallucinations)

Infection control

Introduction to infection control

At any one time in the United States, it is estimated that 5–10% of hospital inpatients are suffering from a health care–associated infection (HAI).[1] The top four most common HAIs are as follows:
- Urinary tract infection (UTI)
- Central line–associated bloodstream infection
- Surgical site infection
- Lower respiratory tract infection (LRTI)

The socioeconomic impact in terms of increased length of stay and financial cost is immense, as is the personal cost to each individual who acquires an essentially preventable infection. HAIs have triggered considerable political interest over recent years, resulting in reorganization of hospital and community infection control services and the publication of numerous related documents (see Table 2.1).

In many ways, infection control is the epitome of patient safety (see Box 2.1 for important definitions in infection control and Box 2.2 for common abbreviations used). As such, at no time has as much attention

---

Box 2.1 Important definitions in infection control

- *Infection:* the deposition and multiplication of organisms in tissues or on body surfaces, which usually causes adverse effects.
- *Colonization:* organisms are present but cause no host response.
- *Carrier:* organisms remain in the individual (e.g., tissues or body cavity) after a clinical infection but cause no symptoms. An immunological response may remain. Typhoid Mary was one of the most famous carriers of all time (see Enteric fever, p. 587).
- *Hospital-onset, health care–associated infection:* Formerly described as "nosocomial," the infection was not present or incubating at the time of admission. Instead, symptom onset began more than 48–72 hours following hospital admission.
- *Community-onset, health care–associated infection:* infection with symptom onset that occurs outside of the hospital but following exposure to health care. *Health care exposure* is defined as the presence of an indwelling device at admission or hospitalization, with hemodialysis, or during residence in a long-term care facility in the 12 months prior to symptom onset.
- *Community-associated infection:* infection in the community that occurs in the absence of health care exposure.
- *Decontamination:* a process or treatment that renders a medical device, instrument, or environmental surface safe to handle.
- *Disinfection:* the destruction of pathogenic and other microorganisms by physical or chemical means. Disinfection is less lethal than sterilization, because it destroys most recognized pathogenic microorganisms but not necessarily all microbial forms, such as bacterial spores (see p. 144).
- *Sterilization:* a physical or chemical procedure that destroys all organisms, including large numbers of resistant bacterial spores (see p. 146).

Table 2.1 Important infection control documents published since 2005

Year	Organization	Title
2005	ATS/IDSA	Guidelines for the management of adults with hospital-acquired, ventilator-associated, and healthcare-associated pneumonia. *Am J Respir Crit Care Med* 2005;171:388–416.
2007	IDSA/SHEA	Infectious Diseases Society of America and the Society for Healthcare Epidemiology of America guidelines for developing an institutional program to enhance antimicrobial stewardship. Dellit et al. (2007). *Clin Infect Dis* 44:159–177.
2006	HICPAC	Management of Multidrug-Resistant Organisms in Healthcare Settings, 2006. http://www.cdc.gov/ncidod/dhqp/pdf/ar/MDROGuideline2006.pdf
2007	HICPAC	2007 Guideline for Isolation Precautions: Preventing Transmission of Infectious Agents in Healthcare Settings. http://www.cdc.gov/hicpac/2007IP/2007isolationPrecautions.html
2008	SHEA/IDSA	Compendium of Strategies for the Prevention of Healthcare-associated Infections in Acute Care Hospitals. http://www.shea-online.org/about/compendium.cfm
2008	SHEA/APIC	SHEA/APIC guideline: infection prevention and control in the long-term care facility. Smith et al. (2008). *Infect Control Hosp Epidemiol* 29:785–814.
2008	HICPAC	Guideline for Disinfection and Sterilization in Healthcare Facilities, 2008. http://www.cdc.gov/hicpac/Disinfection_Sterilization/acknowledg.html
2009	IDSA	Guidelines for the management of intravascular catheter–related Infections. Mermel et al. (2009). *Clin Infect Dis* 49:1–45.
2009	HICPAC	Guideline for Prevention of Catheter-Associated Urinary Tract Infections, 2009. http://www.cdc.gov/hicpac/cauti/001_cauti.html
2010	IDSA	Diagnosis, prevention, and treatment of catheter-associated urinary tract infection in adults: 2009 International Clinical Practice Guidelines from the Infectious Diseases Society of America. Hooten et al. (2010). *Clin Infect Dis* 50:625–663.
2010	SHEA/IDSA	Clinical practice guidelines for *Clostridium difficile* infection in adults: 2010 update by the Society for Healthcare Epidemiology of America (SHEA) and the Infectious Diseases Society of America (IDSA). Cohen et al. (2010). *Infect Control Hosp Epidemiol* 31:431–455.

Box 2.2 Infection control abbreviations used in the U.S.

- **APIC:** Association of Professionals in Infection Control
- **BSI:** bloodstream infection
- **CAUTI:** catheter-associated urinary tract infection
- **CDC:** Centers for Disease Control and Prevention (Atlanta, GA)
- **CDI:** *Clostridium difficile* infection
- **CLABSI:** central line–associated bloodstream infection
- **DHHS:** Department of Health and Human Services
- **ECDC:** European Centre for Disease Prevention and Control (Stockholm, Sweden)
- **EPA:** Environmental Protection Agency
- **HICPAC:** Healthcare Infection Control Practices Advisory Committee Program
- **ICC:** infection control committee
- **IDSA:** Infectious Diseases Society of America
- **IHI:** Institute for Healthcare Improvement
- **IOM:** Institute of Medicine
- **IP:** infection preventionist
- **OSHA:** Occupational Safety and Health Administration
- **SHEA:** Society for Healthcare Epidemiology of America
- **SSI:** surgical site infection
- **VAP:** ventilator-associated pneumonia

Box 2.3 Clinical trials in infection control and hospital epidemiology

Historically, there have been few controlled trials in infection control, and the evidence base for many procedures is sparse. There have been several initiatives to rectify this in recent years, including formation of ORION (Outbreak Reports and Intervention Studies of Nosocomial Infection). They have published a CONSORT (Consolidated Standards of Reporting Trials) equivalent statement, in order to raise the standards of research and publication. It consists of a 22-item checklist and a summary table. The emphasis is on transparency to improve the quality of reporting and on the use of appropriate statistical techniques, so that the work is robust enough to influence policy and practice.[2]

been paid to infection control as now. Infection control has emerged as a key consideration for health care workers, administrators, public interest groups, and politicians (see Box 2.3 for discussion of clinical trials). It is likely that infection control will maintain its high political profile.

References to relevant topics in other chapters
- Management of rash contact in pregnancy, p. 711
- Bioterrorism, p. 753
- Glycopeptide resistance in S. aureus, p. 186

Useful infection control Web sites

- CDC Hospital Infection Program: www.cdc.gov/ncidod/dhqp/index.html
- National Healthcare Safety Network: www.cdc.gov/nhsn
- World Health Organization: www.who.int/csr/resources
- Association of Professionals in Infection Control: www.apic.org
- Society for Healthcare Epidemiology of America: www.shea-online.org
- CDC Vaccines and Immunizations: www.cdc.gov/vaccines/
- National Institute for Occupational Safety and Health (NIOSH): www. cdc.gov/niosh/
- Occupational Safety and Health Administration (OSHA): www.osha.gov
- Association of PeriOperative Registered Nurses (AORN): www.aorn.org
- Institute of Medicine: www.iom.edu
- Institute for Healthcare Improvement: www.ihi.org
- World Alliance for Patient Safety: www.who.int/patientsafety/worldalliance

References

1. Plowman R, Graves N, Griffin MA, et al. (2001). The rate and cost of hospital acquired infections occurring in patients admitted to selected specialties of a district general hospital in England and the national burden imposed. *JHI* 47:198–209.

2. Stane S, Cooper B, Kibbler C, et al. (2007). The ORION statement: guidelines for transparent reporting of outbreak reports and intervention studies of nosocomical infection. *Lancet Infect Dis* 7(4):282–288.

Basic epidemiology of infection (1)

In order to introduce effective infection control measures, the basic epidemiology of an infection (route of transmission, host risk factors, etc.) must be considered. The incidence and nature of a HAI (as with any infection) depend on the following:

- The organism
- The host (patients and staff)
- The environment

The organism

The organisms responsible for common HAIs are listed in Table 2.2. These may be acquired endogenously or exogenously.

Endogenous infection

Endogenous infection, also called *autoinfection* or *self-infection*, occurs when the infection is caused by organisms from the patient's own body. These may be part of their normal flora or acquired in the hospital.

Antibiotics change the normal flora of the host and may select for resistant organisms. Risk of infection may be reduced by protecting any potential sites of entry, e.g., intravascular lines.

Exogenous infection

Exogenous infection refers to infection in which the causal organism originates outside the patient. It is usually from the environment. Organisms are generally acquired by airborne, contact, or percutaneous routes.

Table 2.2 Organisms commonly involved in hospital-acquired infections

Infection	Organism(s) involved
Urinary tract infections	Gram-negative bacteria, e.g., *E. coli*, *Proteus* spp., *Klebsiella* spp., *Serratia* spp., *P. aeruginosa*
	Other than *Staphylococcus saphrophyticus*, Gram-positive bacteria are less common, e.g., *Enterococcus* spp.; and fungi are less common, e.g., *C. albicans*
Respiratory infections	Bacteria, e.g., *H. influenzae*, *S. pneumoniae*, *S. aureus*, Enterobacteriaceae, *P. aeruginosa*
	Viruses: respiratory viruses
	Fungi, e.g., *Candida* spp., *Aspergillus* spp.
Wounds and skin sepsis	Bacteria, e.g., *S. aureus*; *S. pyogenes*; *E. coli*; *Proteus* spp.; anaerobes; *Enterococcus* spp.;
Bloodstream infection (BSI)	Gram-positive bacteria, e.g., *S. aureus*, methicillin-resistant *S. aureus* (MRSA), *Enterococcus* spp., coagulase-negative staphylococci
	Gram-negative bacteria, e.g., *E. coli*, *Proteus* spp., *Klebsiella* spp., *Serratia* spp., *P. aeruginosa*
	Fungi, e.g., *Candida* spp.
Gastrointestinal infections	Bacteria, e.g., *C. difficile*
	Viruses, e.g., norovirus

Within the hospital setting, environmental infection is usually due to a contaminated item of equipment and can be minimized by implementing the correct decontamination, sterilization, and infection control procedures. *Cross-infection* refers to infection acquired in the hospital from another person, either patients or staff.

Risks can be reduced by focusing on measures to interrupt transmission, e.g., handwashing.

The host

Patient risk factors that result in increased likelihood of acquiring an infection in hospital include the following:
- Degree of underlying illness – more-severely ill patients are more vulnerable to acquiring an infection and more likely to become sicker
- Use of medical devices – these breach host defenses and provide possible portals of entry for organisms
- Extremes of age – the elderly and very young are at higher risk of infection
- Duration of hospitalization
- Immunosuppression, e.g., diabetes mellitus, transplantation

Staff risk factors include the following:
- Immunosuppression, e.g., HIV; pregnancy

- Staff who perform exposure-prone procedures are more likely to be exposed to blood-borne viral infections
- Skin conditions (e.g., eczema) increase prolonged carriage of organisms such as MRSA.

Basic epidemiology of infection (2)

The environment

The hospital environment includes all of the physical surroundings of the hospital, patients, and staff, i.e., the building, fittings, fixtures, furnishings, equipment, and supplies. The following are important environmental issues in the control of infection:

- Environmental cleaning—see Box 2.4
- Environmental disinfection
- Decontamination of equipment
- Building and refurbishment, including air-handling systems
- Clinical waste management
- Pest control
- Food services and food hygiene
- Isolation facilities and ability to cohort patients

Routes of transmission

The isolation precautions required depend on the likely route of transmission of the organism. The main routes are as follows:

- *Airborne:* when the infection usually occurs by the respiratory route and the agent is carried in aerosols (<5 micrometer diameter)
- *Droplet:* large droplets carry the infectious agent (>5 micrometer diameter)
- *Direct contact:* infection is directly transmitted between the source of infection and the recipient, i.e., person-to-person spread
- *Indirect contact:* infection occurs through contact with a secondarily contaminated object, i.e., via equipment contaminated with body fluids such as urine, feces, and wound exudates. This route also

---

Box 2.4 Hospital cleaning

"Dirty hospitals" are frequently reported by the media, with attention drawn to the lack of investment and poor support for hospital cleaning. Although there is no known correlation between the cleanliness of wards and infection rates, spread of some organisms has been clearly linked to environmental contamination (e.g., MRSA, VRE, and *C. difficile*).

As such, resources should be directed toward education and training of medical and nursing staff, and employment of adequate cleaning services. The physical removal of dirt, fomites, dust, and human body fluids is most important.

New approaches and adjunctive technologies look promising, including objective assessment of cleaning, water-based cleaning using ultra-microfibers (UMF), ultraviolet (UV) light, and dry H_2O_2 steam vapor.

includes contact via an environmental source, e.g., an outbreak of gastroenteritis transmitted by food

- *Inoculation:* infection occurs through direct inoculation, e.g., needlestick injury. Other routes are via blood products (hepatitis A, hepatitis B, hepatitis C, HIV), total parenteral nutrition (TPN), and other fluids (*Enterobacter*; *B. cepacia*). Multi-dose vials should be avoided.

Overview of surveillance

Definitions

Surveillance comes from the French "to watch over" and means "vigilant supervision" or "ongoing scrutiny." Langmuir, the founder of the CDC, described surveillance as "the continued watchfulness over the distribution and trends of diseases through systematic collection, consolidation, and evaluation of data."

Often, in the real world, total accuracy of the data must be sacrificed in favor of the practicability, cost-effectiveness, uniformity, and timeliness in which the information can be collected. An important point to remember is that there is no value in just collecting interesting data; you need to do something with it, as emphasized by an alternative definition of *surveillance:* "information for action."

Surveillance may be active or passive. *Direct* surveillance is when a special effort is made to collect the data, e.g., daily rounds with patient evaluation for signs of a specific infection. *Indirect* surveillance uses routine data that have already been collected, e.g., review of microbiological records.

Aims of surveillance

The main aims of surveillance of hospital infection are to provide valid data on the number and rates of infections occurring, to feed back these data in order to change behavior when necessary, and to recognize, prevent, and control outbreaks.

The infection control team typically performs this surveillance and provides data to administration, unit directors, and health care workers. Every member of medical and nursing staff and every department has a responsibility to perform best practices and respond to relevant data on infection rates. In addition, routine surveillance from the laboratory can identify new antibiotic resistant or "alert" organisms.

Methods of surveillance

Those employed in HAI control usually involve a combination of active and passive surveillance systems. Though direct surveillance is believed to lead to the most accurate data, it is typically impractical and inefficient. Thus, practice varies within and between hospitals and is largely dependent on availability of staff and resources.

In practice, a number of surveillance methods are used, as each provides different information:

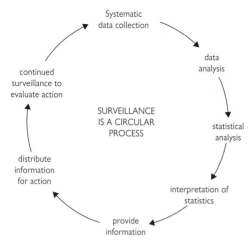

Fig. 2.1 Principles of surveillance. Surveillance is a circular process.

- The Infection Preventionist reviews patients with significant microbiology cultures and also visits each ward to discuss all patients with the ward staff.
- The infection control team performs regular analysis of outcome data to detect changes from baseline rates.
- Each unit collects data on specific process measures (e.g., compliance with "bundles"). This is particularly relevant in areas such as the intensive care unit (ICU) and surgical wards.
- Electronic database surveillance: many hospitals are expanding surveillance by using various hospital databases, e.g., administrative and pharmacy databases.
- Other methods include review of patients on antibiotics or those with known risk factors or indwelling devices (see principles of surveillance in Fig 2.1).

Evaluation of a surveillance system

- Define the event to be measured (case definition)
- Define the population under surveillance
- List the objectives of system
- Define the public health importance of the health event (e.g., number of deaths, case fatality ratio, morbidity, economics, preventability)

Some characteristics of a surveillance system are listed in Box 2.5.

Does surveillance work?

There is good evidence that surveillance in hospitals actually reduces infection rates. The SENIC study (Study on Efficacy of Nosocomial Infection

---

Box 2.5 What makes a good surveillance system?

For surveillance to succeed, it should have the following attributes:
- Simple (well-designed reporting forms make all the difference!)
- Flexible
- Acceptable to the population studied
- Sensitive
- Representative
- Timely
- Reasonable cost

Control) was carried out over two decades ago in the United States.[1] One of the main objectives was to determine whether surveillance and infection control programs lowered the rate of HAIs.

An important finding of the SENIC study was the need to close the loop and present data back to the clinicians. This study demonstrated that hospitals with direct surveillance and infection-control programs could reduce the incidence of infection by 32%. Clinical audit was also found to be important.

Reference

1. Haley RW, Morgan WM, Culver DH (1985). Study on efficacy of nosocomial infection control. *An J Infect Control* 13(3);97–108.

Surveillance of alert organisms

In most U.S. hospitals, the infection control team performs surveillance for patients suffering from the following infections, to ensure that all staff are aware of infection control precautions:
- Infectious diarrhea (*Campylobacter, Salmonella, Shigella, C. difficile,* rotavirus, norovirus, etc.)
- Group A streptococcus
- Meningococcal disease
- Influenza-like illness (e.g., influenza or respiratory syncytial virus [RSV])
- HIV
- Hepatitis A–E
- Severe herpes simplex
- Legionnaire's disease
- Varicella zoster virus (VZV; shingles or chickenpox)
- Lice or scabies
- Tuberculosis (TB)

Many of the above infections don't require specific isolation in the hospital setting but must be reported to local health departments.

Multi-drug-resistant organisms (MDROs)

Practice varies between hospitals, but in general, infection control staff perform surveillance for the following MDROs:
- MRSA
- Vancomycin-resistant enterococci (VRE)

- *Clostridium difficile* infection (CDI)
- Multi-drug-resistant Gram-negative organisms—the definition of this varies between hospitals

Originally, aminoglycoside-resistant organisms were usually flagged; however, these have become so widespread that in many hospitals this would not be practical. Some hospitals flag isolates producing extended-spectrum β-lactamases (ESBLs).

Often the patient's notes and electronic records are flagged if an MDRO has been isolated in the past.

The quality of the data provided can be evaluated in terms of
- Sensitivity and specificity
- Predictive value (positive and negative)
- Usefulness, in relation to the goals of the surveillance (quality indicators)

It is sometimes more valuable to focus on the outcome (e.g., the number of cases of polio) rather than the process (e.g., the number of polio vaccinations).

Ownership is important; feeding the data back to key stakeholders will make them more willing to help again in the future!

Surveillance of hospital-onset, health care—associated infection

Definition
Hospital-onset, health care–associated infection (formerly known as "nosocomial") is an infection that was neither present nor incubating at the time of hospital admission. Symptoms typically manifest more than 48 hours later.

The term *health care–associated infection* (HAI) encompasses any infection by any infectious agent acquired as a consequence of a person's exposure to health care.

Criteria for HAI surveillance schemes
In order to obtain accurate results with both inter- and intrahospital validity, the following criteria are important:
- Agreed-upon definitions of infection
- Accurate denominator data
- Correction of infection rates for risk factors, e.g., risk stratification for pre-existing diseases
- Identification of HAI post-discharge.

The nature of risk and its assessment

Risk management is something we do every day in our personal lives, such as when crossing the road, but has recently evolved as an important science in health care settings. In combination with total quality management (TQM), its aim is to integrate and coordinate all quality-assessment activities and focus on the identification and correction of any problems, with the ultimate goal of protecting patients.

Key definitions
- *Risk management* is a systematic process of risk identification, analysis, treatment, and evaluation of potential and actual risks.
- *Hazard versus risk:* a *hazard* is the potential to cause harm, while a *risk* is the likelihood of harm (in defined circumstances and usually qualified by some statement of the severity of the harm).
- *Total quality management* is a management strategy aimed at embedding awareness of quality in all organizational processes.
- *Controls assurance:* the need to be seen to be doing our "reasonable best" to reduce risk by using resources effectively.
- *Clinical governance and quality improvement:* a framework through which health care organizations are accountable for continually improving the quality of their services and safeguarding high standards of care, by creating an environment in which excellence in clinical care will flourish.

Risk management and economics
Health economics and cost-effectiveness play a big part in risk management. It is particularly important today because of rising health care costs, governmental cost containment, and medical malpractice claims.

Goals of risk management
- Survival of the organization
- Enhanced quality and standard of care
- Minimization of risk of medical or accidental injuries and losses
- Improvement of program effectiveness and efficiency through administrative direction and control
- Coordination and integration of current policies, functions, programs, committees, and other aspects relative to the risk management process

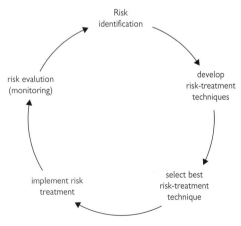

Fig. 2.2 The risk-management cycle.

- Avoidance of adverse publicity
- Minimization of cost of risk transfer (insurance)

The risk-management cycle is outlined in Fig. 2.2.

Management of outbreaks

Definition
There are various definitions of the word *outbreak*. Essentially, an outbreak is an incident in which the observed number of cases exceeds the expected number of cases. In certain circumstances, the emergence of one new infection may constitute an outbreak.

Here are some examples to illustrate these definitions:
- 2 cases of MRSA bacteremia on the neonatal unit
- 1 case of human avian flu or 1 case of vancomycin-resistant *S. aureus*
- 2 new hepatitis C–positive hemodialysis patients, identified by regular screening tests
- An unusual number of cases of diarrhea on a medical ward
- Increased numbers of *Campylobacter* isolates sent to the state reference laboratory, compared to the same period in previous years

Steps in outbreak management
1. Identification of an outbreak
2. Investigation of an outbreak
3. Case definition
4. Describing the outbreak
5. Proposing and testing the hypothesis
6. Control measures and follow-up
7. Communication

Management of hospital outbreaks
Outbreaks of health care–associated infections must be identified and thoroughly investigated. Because of their importance in terms of morbidity and mortality, outbreak investigations are necessary to identify any breakdown in a process and to prevent spread or future recurrences.

The transfer of patients between clinical areas and different wards (and different hospitals) can make contacts difficult to identify, and outbreak investigation is often time consuming. In addition to short-term benefits, effective outbreak investigations often lead to sustained improvement in patient care.

Management of risks to health care workers from patients

Numerous practices are in place to reduce the risk of health care workers (HCWs) acquiring infections from their patients. However, HCWs (including laboratory staff) do become infected at work with organisms ranging from the relatively benign norovirus to life-threatening conditions.

Infection control procedures for patients infected with HIV, hepatitis B, or hepatitis C may be considered together because routes of acquisition are similar. The main risk of transmission is from the accidental inoculation of blood (see Management of risk from sharps, p. 123).

Clearly, it is impossible to identify all carriers of blood-borne viruses, so universal infection control precautions (see p. 131) are required for all patients.

Infectivity of body fluids from patients with HIV or hepatitis B or C

The following fluids are potentially infectious:
- Blood and any fluid visibly contaminated with blood
- Cerebrospinal fluid (CSF), peritoneal fluid, pleural fluid, pericardial fluid, synovial fluid, amniotic fluid, semen, vaginal secretions, saliva in the context of dentistry.

The following are *not* regarded as infectious, unless visibly contaminated with blood: feces, nasal secretions, saliva (except in dentistry), sputum, sweat, tears, urine, and vomit.

Care of patients with HIV or hepatitis B or C

Patients known to be positive for these viruses (or likely to be positive as a result of certain risk factors) should have a risk assessment performed. The risk assessment should fully respect patient confidentiality. The likelihood of exposure of staff or other patients to the patient's blood or body fluids should be considered.

Medical and nursing care of infected patients depends on local hospital policy, but here are a few practical suggestions:
- *Single-room isolation:* this is only usually required if uncontrolled bleeding or loss of other body fluids is likely or if the patient has another condition requiring isolation (e.g., diarrhea; pulmonary TB; salmonellosis; herpes zoster).
- *Disposal of sharps:* sharps must be disposed of in a sharps bin inside the room per hospital policy.
- *Spills:* any spills of blood or body fluids should be covered and disinfected with an EPA-registered agent; a hypochlorite (bleach) containing solution is preferred.
- *Equipment disinfection and sterilization:* use single-use or disposable items whenever possible.
- *Protective clothing:* depends on the likelihood and degree of exposure to the patient's blood and body fluids. Gloves, mask, and protective eyewear are required wherever there is a possibility of blood contact or aerosolization.
- *Linen* from patients in isolation or contaminated with blood or body fluids should be regarded as infected linen.
- *Toilet and bathroom facilities:* patients may use the ward facilities except if there is bleeding (or risk of bleeding). In this scenario, toilet and bathroom facilities must be reserved for this patient only (or use a commode).
- *Waste:* clinical waste and disposable items must be placed in red OSHA bags, with double-bagging if leakage of body fluids is possible.
- *Specimen transport:* label specimens and accompanying forms with "Biohazard" stickers.

Other infections acquired by HCWs from patients

While many infections may be transmitted to hospital staff, the following are recognized more frequently or have more significant consequences:

- Viral gastroenteritis
- *Neisseria meningitidis* in HCWs who intubate the patient or perform mouth-to-mouth resuscitation.
- *Mycobacterium tuberculosis* (MTB)
- Varicella zoster
- Influenza
- Others: pertussis, diphtheria, rabies, viral hemorrhagic fevers (Box 2.6)

Further information

- NHSN Healthcare Personnel Safety module: www.cdc.gov/nhsn/hps.html
- NHSN Blood and Body Fluid Exposure module: www.cdc.gov/nhsn/hps_bbf.html
- OSHA bloodborne pathogens and needlestick prevention: www.osha.gov/SLTC/bloodbornepathogens/
- U.S. Public Health Service Guidelines for Management of Healthcare Exposures, including recommendations for post-exposure prophylaxis:
  HIV: www.cdc.gov/mmwr/preview/mmwrhtml/rr5409a1.htm
  Hepatitis B or C: www.cdc.gov/mmwr/preview/mmwrhtml/rr5011a1.htm
- Joint working party of Hospital Infection Society and Surgical Infection Study Group. Risks to surgeons and patients from HIV and hepatitis. *BMJ* 1992;305:1337–1343.

Box 2.6 Education in infection control procedures works!

During the SARS epidemic (2004), the proportion of infected HCWs varied from 20 to 60% of cases worldwide, with notable differences between hospitals. The better the education in infection control, the lower the risk of acquiring the infection.[1]

Reference

1. McDonald L, Simor AE, Sn IJ, et al. (2004). SARS in healthcare facilities, Toronto and Taiwan. *Emerg Infect Dis* 10(5)777–781.

Management of risk from sharps

By following universal infection control precautions, all health care workers can minimize risks of infection associated with blood and body fluids. The main risk associated with needlestick and other sharps injuries is transmission of blood-borne viruses.

The rate of transmission with a significant inoculation of blood through a hollow bore needle is as follows:

- Approximately 30% if the donor is hepatitis B surface antigen positive (the risk is as high as 30% if the patient is hepatitis B e antigen positive, while it decreases to 3% if hepatitis B e antibody positive)
- Approximately 3% if the donor is hepatitis C antibody positive

- Approximately 0.3% if the donor is HIV positive
- There is also the risk of emerging or unknown agents.

Prevention of sharps injuries

Sharps are often disposed of improperly. Good clinical practice is important in preventing needlestick injuries, e.g.:

- Handle needles and other sharps carefully.
- Never re-cap needles.
- Staff using needles or other sharps are responsible for safe disposal.
- Use sharps bins as indicated.

Action in event of sharps injury

- *Immediate first aid:* encourage bleeding of the area, wash with soap under running water, and cover with waterproof dressing. For an eye splash irrigate well with running water. If splash is into the mouth, do not swallow and rinse out the mouth several times with cold water.
- *Contact an occupational health or other expert* about hospital guidelines immediately (e.g., microbiology or infectious diseases physician). Most hospitals have an exposure "hotline."
- *Risk assessment:* consider the hazard (potential to cause harm) and risk (likelihood that harm will occur) based on the injury, the source, and the recipient (see Box 2.7).

Management of a needlestick injury

(see Box 2.9)

- Always seek expert advice, usually from occupational health, microbiology, or infectious diseases staff.
- Refer the recipient to occupational health, microbiology, or infectious diseases staff immediately. They will make a risk assessment of the severity of the injury.
- Consult your hospital policy. Most hospitals have a needlestick hotline to receive immediate attention and assessment following an exposure.

Box 2.7 Risk assessment

Consider the injury, the source, and the recipient.

Injury
- Extent and depth of injury (see Box 2.8)
- Size and type of needle
- Visible contamination with blood
- Site

Source
Usually the source is the patient undergoing the procedure, but it may be unknown.
- Hepatitis B and C, HIV status (if known)
- Viral load and stage of illness if HIV positive

Recipient
- Hepatitis B vaccine status and antibody level
- Any conditions that may affect treatment, e.g., pregnancy

- If this was a significant injury, a member of the team looking after the donor (but not the recipient of the injury) should counsel the donor. Blood should be requested for HIV, HBs Ag, and HCV antibody. See Table 2.3 for management of sharps injury from an infected donor.

Table 2.3 Management of sharps injury from infected donor

Donor known positive or likely positive	Action
HIV	*URGENT.* Discuss with an infection expert who will consider PEP. In general, PEP is not mandatory when HIV status is unknown, but the decision must be made on a case-by-case basis. The risks associated with PEP vs. the risk of acquiring HIV will be explained to the recipient. PEP usually consists of a 3-day starter pack of antiviral therapy, with plans for ongoing counseling and treatment depending on results. Specific guidelines for PEP have been published by the CDC.
Hepatitis B (HBV)	*URGENT.* Discuss with an infection expert who will consider hepatitis B immune globulin (HBIG) and accelerated vaccination or booster(s) as in Table 3.6.
Hepatitis C (HCV)	No immediate intervention. If donor is anti-HCV positive, HCV RNA will be tested in the recipient by PCR at 6 and 12 weeks, and anti-HCV will be tested at 12 and 24 weeks. If signs of infection occur in the recipient, the test will be confirmed and the patient may be referred to further experts to consider HCV chemotherapy.

Box 2.8 Grading of exposure

Risk associated with type of exposure is graded as follows:

Negligible risk
- Intact skin visibly contaminated with blood or body fluids, i.e., no actual injury occurred

Low risk
- Mucous membranes or conjunctival contact with blood or body fluids
- Intradermal injury associated with a needle or instrument contaminated by blood or body fluids (possible parenteral exposure)

Medium risk
- Skin-penetrating needle contaminated with blood or body fluids or wound that causes bleeding and is produced by an instrument that is visibly contaminated (definite parenteral exposure)

High risk
- Significant exposure to blood or body fluids from source known to be hepatitis B (see Table 2.4), hepatitis C, or HIV positive.

Table 2.4 Management of significant exposure to hepatitis B virus (HBV)*

HBV status of person exposed	Significant exposure	
	HBsAg-positive source	**Unknown source**
1 dose or less of HBV vaccine pre-exposure	Accelerated course of HBV vaccine (doses at 0, 1, and 2 months. May need booster dose at 12 months if there is continuing risk of exposure)	Accelerated course of HBV vaccine (doses at 0, 1, and 2 months. May need booster dose at 12 months if continuing risk of exposure)
	Also give HBIG x1	
2 doses or more of HBV vaccine pre-exposure (anti-HBS not known)	1 dose of HBV vaccine followed by second dose 1 month later	1 dose of HBV vaccine
Known responder to HBV vaccine (anti-HBS >10 microunits/mL)	Consider booster dose of HBV vaccine	Consider booster dose of HBV vaccine
Known nonresponder to HBV vaccine (anti-HBS <10 microunits/mL) 2–4 months post immunization	HBIG x1	HBIG x1
	Consider booster dose of HBV vaccine	Consider booster dose of HBV vaccine

*In addition to percutaneous inoculation (needlestick, scratch, bite, etc), exposure may result from contamination of mucous membranes (e.g., spillage into eyes or mouth) or contamination of non-intact skin (open wounds, dermatitis, eczema).

- If pre-test counseling is required, involve trained personnel.
- Provide patient information leaflets as appropriate.
- If the injury was negligible (see Box 2.8), blood will be taken for storage and to check anti-hepatitis B surface antigen (HBsAg) if unknown. This is an opportunity for hepatitis B vaccination.
- If the injury was significant (see Box 2.8), blood will be taken for HBsAg and long-term storage. Hepatitis B vaccination (booster) will be considered. With a high-risk donor, post-exposure prophylaxis (PEP) and/or hepatitis B immunoglobulin may be considered.

Box 2.9 Summary flowchart for needlestick injury

Check that basic first aid has been performed
Discuss with occupational health, infectious diseases, and/or microbiology
Risk assessment – significant injury?

No	Yes
• Occupational health referral for routine assessment • Obtain anti-HBsAg if unknown • Encourage HBV vaccination if not done	• Obtain anti-HBsAg if unknown • Request source sample for HbsAg; anti-HCV; anti-HIV testing • Unknown source: gather as much information as possible to make a risk assessment. HIV PEP only in specific scenarios

Further risk assessment:
• Known or highly likely to be HIV positive – URGENT: infection expert will consider PEP
• Known or highly likely to be HBV positive – URGENT: infection expert will consider HBIG and accelerated vaccine/booster
• Known or highly likely to be HCV positive – no immediate intervention. Infection expert will check HCV RNA on source if known anti-HCV positive donor. Follow up recipient at 6 and 12 weeks (PCR), and at 12 and 24 weeks (anti-HCV)

Reporting

All injuries should be reported to occupational health, typically via the needlestick hotline. A review of equipment and procedures should occur, led by a senior member of the department.

Additional notes regarding management of significant exposure to HIV

Factors known to increase the risk of transmission of HIV
• Deep and penetrating injury
• Visibly blood-stained device
• Needle involved has been in the source patient's artery or vein
• Source has terminal HIV disease or high viral load

Further information

US Public Health Service Guidelines for Management of Healthcare Exposures, including recommendations for post-exposure prophylaxis:
• HIV: www.cdc.gov/mmwr/preview/mmwrhtml/rr5409a1.htm
• Hepatitis B or C: www.cdc.gov/mmwr/preview/mmwrhtml/rr5011a1.htm

Risk from tissues for transplantation

The number of organs and tissues that can be successfully transplanted is increasing. The current list of organ transplants includes heart, kidneys, liver, lungs, pancreas, and intestine. Tissues include bones, tendons, cornea, heart valves, veins, and skin.

Rejection and infection arising from anti-rejection therapy are the main risks. Hematology and oncology patients who have received bone marrow transplants are at particularly high risk of infection.

Infection in a transplant recipient may either be transmitted from the donor with the organ or arise due to the immunosuppressed state of the recipient. Certain infectious agents are particularly recognized as causing infections post-transplant. Depending on which organ has been transplanted, different infectious agents are commonly implicated at different time periods. Box 2.10 describes typical problems after a renal transplant.

Box 2.10 Example – infections post–renal transplant

Minor infections are common after a kidney transplant. Urine infections affect ~50% of transplant recipients, especially if the patient has reflux nephropathy or diabetes. More serious infections in the first 6 months post-transplant include pneumonia (e.g., *Pneumocystis* pneumonia [PCP], pneumococcus), cytomegalovirus (CMV), chickenpox, BK virus, and disseminated fungal infection.

Each transplant unit will have guidelines for prophylaxis, which may include the following:
- Co-trimoxazole (PCP)
- Amphotericin (oral candida)
- Isoniazid for those at risk of TB
- Antibiotics (if urinary tract infections are common)
- Valganciclovir or valacyclovir if CMV-positive donor into CMV-negative recipient
- Vaccination, e.g., influenza, Pneumovax®

Surveillance of infections among tissue donors

A tissue donation and banking program is operated by the United Network for Organ Sharing (UNOS). Donations may come from living and/or cadaveric donors, and include surgical bone (mainly femoral heads), tendons, skin, and heart valves. The National Marrow Donor Program operates a bone marrow registry and a cord blood bank.

All tissue donors (including stem cell and cord blood donors) are routinely tested for HIV, HCV, HBV, human T-cell lymphotropic virus (HTLV), and syphilis infections.

Management of risk from virally infected health care workers

Virally infected staff are usually managed by the occupational health department. The following is a guide to current recommendations at the time of this publication.

The Society for Healthcare Epidemiology of America (SHEA) recently published a guideline for management of health care workers (HCWs) with hepatitis B, hepatitis C, and/or HIV.* This document provides recommendations based on the type of infection, amount of viremia, and type of procedures that the HCW might perform (see Box 2.11).

Furthermore, these guidelines recommend that each HCW with a potentially transmissible viral infection be reviewed by an independent board at each hospital and submit to routine testing and evaluation.

Finally, HCWs with infection from a potentially transmissible infection should double-glove for all procedures for which gloving is required.

Box 2.11 Common procedures according to risk for bloodborne pathogen exposure

For a full list of procedures, see http://www.shea-online.org/Assets/files/guidelines/BBPathogen_GL.pdf.

Category 1: Minimal risk of transmission
- Regular history-taking or examination
- Routine rectal or vaginal examination
- Elective peripheral phlebotomy
- Sigmoidoscopy and colonoscopy

Category 2: Transmission is theoretically possible but unlikely
- Minor local procedure with local anesthesia (e.g., skin excision, abscess drainage, biopsy)
- Bronchoscopy
- Angiography and cardiac catheterization
- Minor gynecological procedures
- Vaginal delivery

Category 3: "Exposure-prone" or definite risk of transmission
- General, cardiothoracic, neurosurgical, obstetrical or gynecological, orthopedic, transplantation, or trauma surgery
- Extensive plastic surgery
- Interaction with a patient who has a high risk of biting the HCW
- Any open surgical procedure lasting longer than 3 hours

---

* http://www.shea-online.org/Assets/files/guidelines/BBPathogen_GL.pdf

Hepatitis B-infected and/or hepatitis C-infected HCWs

- HCWs with a viral load <10,000 copies/mL have no restrictions but must undergo testing twice each year.
- HCWs with viral load ≥10,000 copies/mL should not perform Category 3 procedures.

HIV-infected HCWs

- HCWs with a viral load <50 copies/mL have no restrictions but must undergo testing at least twice each year.
- HCWs with a viral load ≥50 copies/mL should not perform Category 3 procedures.

Containment levels

The *containment level* (CL) refers to the physical requirements necessary for working with organisms of different pathogenicity and includes guidance about the facilities, working environment, safety equipment, and procedures (e.g., staff training).

There are four different levels (CL1–CL4), and the CL of an organism usually corresponds to its categorization, e.g., all group 3 organisms must be handled at CL3.

Summary of requirements

Containment level 1 (CL1), i.e., low individual and community risk

- No special facilities, equipment, or procedures are required. Standard well-designed laboratory facilities and basic safe laboratory practices suffice.
- Handwashing facilities must be provided.
- Disinfectants must be properly used.

Containment level 2 (CL2), i.e., moderate individual risk, limited community risk

- Laboratory should be separated from other activities and have a biohazard sign. Room surfaces are impervious and readily cleanable.
- Equipment should include an autoclave, certified high-efficiency particulate air (HEPA)-filtered class I or II biological safety cabinet for organism manipulations, and personal protective equipment, including laboratory coats worn only in the laboratory.
- All contaminated material should be properly decontaminated.

Containment level 3 (CL3), i.e., high individual risk, low community risk

- Specialized design and construction of laboratories, with controlled-access double-door entry and body shower. All wall penetrations must be sealed. Ventilation system design must ensure that air pressure is negative to surrounding areas at all times, with no recirculation of air; air should be exhausted through a dedicated exhaust or HEPA filtration system. There are minimum furnishings, all readily cleanable and sterilizable (fumigation). Laboratory windows are sealed and unbreakable. Backup power is available.
- Equipment must include an autoclave, certified HEPA-filtered class II biological safety cabinet for organism manipulations, and a dedicated

handwashing sink with foot, knee, or automatic controls, located near the exit. Personal protective equipment should include solid front laboratory clothing worn only in the laboratory, head covers and dedicated footwear, gloves, and appropriate respiratory protection, depending on the infectious agents in use.

- All activities involving infectious materials are conducted in biological safety cabinets or other appropriate combinations of personal protective and physical containment devices.
- Laboratory staff must be fully trained in the handling of pathogenic and other hazardous material, in the use of safety equipment, disposal techniques, handling of contaminated waste, and emergency response. Standard operating procedures must be provided and posted within the laboratory, outlining operational protocols, waste disposal, disinfection procedures, and emergency response. The facility must have a medical surveillance program appropriate to the agents used.

Containment level 4 (CL4), i.e., high individual risk, high community risk

- CL4 is the highest level of containment and represents an isolated unit that is completely self-contained to function independently. Facilities are highly specialized and secure, with an air lock for entry and exit, class III biological safety cabinets, or positive pressure-ventilated suits, and a separate ventilation system with full controls to contain contamination.
- Only fully trained and authorized personnel may enter the CL4 containment laboratory. On exit from the area, personnel will shower and redress in street clothing. All manipulations with agents must be performed in class III biological safety cabinets or in conjunction with one-piece, positive-pressure-ventilated suits.

Universal infection control precautions and barrier nursing

Universal infection control precautions (UICP) involve following simple infection control precautions for *all* patients. It is difficult to tell which patients are infected and which ones are not, so all patients should be regarded as potentially infected.

Adherence to UICP for all patients should minimize the transmission of HIV, hepatitis B and C, and other infectious agents. It also eliminates confusion among staff as to which patients are to be treated as infected and should also prevent any breach of confidentiality.

The main components of UICP

- Handwashing (p. 135)
- Protective clothing
- Gloves should be worn if the patient contact involves blood or body fluid, but the risk of splashing is low. If the risk of splashing is high, a waterproof gown, mask, and eye protection should also be worn.
- Disposal of linen and waste
- Broken skin
  - Clinical staff should cover all skin lesions with a waterproof dressing.

> **Box 2.12 Preventing risk of microbial contamination during a procedure**
>
> The elements of the care process listed below form the basis of reducing the risk of bacterial contamination during any procedure. The three elements are as follows:
>
> *Hand hygiene*
> - Decontaminate hands before and after each patient contact.
> - Use correct hand hygiene procedure.
> - Use personal protective equipment (PPE).
> - Wear examination gloves if there is risk of exposure to body fluids.
> - Gloves are single-use items.
> - Gowns, aprons, eye and face protection may be indicated if there is a risk of splashing with blood or body fluids.
>
> *Aseptic technique*
> - Gown, gloves, and drapes as indicated should be used for the insertion of invasive devices.
>
> *Sharps*
> - Safe disposal of sharps
> - Sharps container available at point of use
> - No disassembling of needle and syringe
> - Sharps should not be passed from hand to hand.
> - The container should not be overfilled.

- Sharps (Box 2.12)
  - Never re-cap, bend, or break a needle or any other sharp.
  - Dispose of all sharps as a single unit, in a suitable sharps bin.
  - Never attempt to retrieve anything from a sharps bin.
  - Only fill a sharps bin to full, and secure the lid before disposing of it according to local policy,
- Spills
  - Any spill of blood or other body fluid that contains blood should be treated with an EPA-registered hypochlorite-containing agent and left in place for 2 minutes. Afterwards, this should be cleared up with paper towels, wearing gloves and aprons. The area should then be washed with hot water and detergent.

Patient isolation

The use of universal infection control precautions (UICP, p. 131) should minimize the need for isolation of most patients. In practice, isolation depends on a risk assessment for each patient and the facilities available in each hospital. Always act on the patient's clinical presentation, and do not wait for laboratory results to be available, as it may be too late. Involve the infection control team early for further advice (Box 2.13).

Box 2.13 Isolating patients with HAI

Guidance and a summary of best practice on isolating patients with health care-acquired infection have been published by the CDC and HICPAC (http://www.cdc.gov/hicpac/pdf/isolation/Isolation2007.pdf)

Recommendations cover the following:

1. Single-room nursing
2. Cohort nursing
3. Management of the patient once isolated
   • Hand hygiene and personal protective equipment (PPE)
   • Cleaning and decontamination
   • Movement of the patient

Effective isolation relies on all staff following the necessary procedures to make sure that none of the transmission barriers are breached. The simplest solution is to use single-rooms, but in an outbreak multi-bed rooms or even whole wards may be used.

Patients are isolated for two reasons:

• *Source isolation* to minimize the chance of infecting other patients, e.g., patient with active TB. The air inside the isolation room should be at negative pressure (exhaust-ventilated) compared to that of the corridor. Patients with highly contagious infections such as the viral hemorrhagic fevers must be nursed in a high-security isolation unit.

• *Protective isolation* to minimize that patient becoming infected, e.g., to protect susceptible or immunosuppressed patients. The air inside the isolation room should be at positive pressure (pressure-ventilated) compared to that of the corridor. In some critical situations such as bone marrow transplant units, where airborne contamination with fungal spores is a problem, the efficiency of air filtration may be increased and laminar flow maintained as a barrier around the patient.

Source isolation

The following measures apply to all patients in source isolation:

• Limit transport to other departments (e.g., X-ray) to essential investigations only.

• If a patient does need to go to another department, brief the porters and other staff on what precautions are necessary.

• Do not transfer the patient to another ward or health care institution without discussion with the infection control team.

• If the patient is well enough, consider sending them home.

• Keep staff caring for infected patients to a minimum. Try not to let these staff work elsewhere in the hospital.

• After death of an infected patient, maintain infection control precautions and consult hospital policy for dealing with the body.

In addition to standard or universal precautions, three specific types of source isolation exist: airborne, contact, and droplet.

• *Airborne isolation* is used to stop transmission of organisms that can be spread on airborne droplets (<5 micrometers in diameter, e.g., TB). Airborne isolation involves the use of gowns, gloves, and fit-tested

N95 masks (or a powered air-purifying respiratory [PAPR] system if not fit-tested).
- *Contact isolation* is used to stop transmission of organisms by direct contact with the patient when performing care activities or indirect contact (touching) with environmental surfaces or patient care items (e.g., MRSA). Contact isolation involves the use of gown and gloves.
- *Droplet isolation* is used to stop transmission of organisms by respiratory droplets created when a patient coughs or sneezes or during cough-producing procedures (e.g., influenza). Droplet isolation involves wearing a surgical mask when interacting with the patient.

Antibiotic policies

An antibiotic policy consists of written guidance that recommends antibiotics and their dose for treating and preventing specific infections. In general, a hospital antibiotic policy covers empirical treatment (when the initial diagnosis is made and before a causative organism is isolated), directed treatment (when causative organism is known), and agents for prophylaxis. See Box 2.14 for an example. Antibiotic policies are typically governed by the Antibiotic Stewardship committee of the hospital.

Box 2.14 Antimicrobial prescribing – summary of best practice

This strategy aims to reduce the risk of infections from MRSA, other resistant bacteria, and *Clostridium difficile* infection (CDI), and maintain the effectiveness of antibiotics by reducing antibiotic resistance.
- Every hospital should have an antimicrobial stewardship program and policies with a strategy for implementation.
- Every hospital should have an antimicrobial formulary and guidelines for antimicrobial treatment and prophylaxis.
- The decision to prescribe should always be clinically justified.
- IV therapy should only be used for severe infections and/or those who cannot take oral medications.
- Antimicrobial treatment should be reviewed at least daily.
- Broad-spectrum antimicrobials should be minimized.
- A single dose should be used for surgical prophylaxis.

Key objectives of an antibiotic policy
- Best possible treatment for individual
- Tailored to local units with their specific microbiological issues
- Reduce antibiotic resistance
- It is clear and easy to follow. Information on practical aspects, e.g., dose, duration, should be included.
- Minimal side effects and toxicity (but should include information about monitoring levels)
- Low cost

Advantages
- Ensure patients receive effective treatment
- Minimal side effects and complications, e.g., *C. difficile*
- Reduce the overuse of broad-spectrum agents
- Reduce emergence of resistance
- Limit unnecessary treatment
- Education

Disadvantages
- Poor compliance among clinicians
- May lead to overuse of antibiotics if clinical decision making is poor
- No control for quality of diagnosis

Handwashing

The importance of handwashing has been recognized since the 19th century when Semmelweiss encouraged medical students in Vienna to wash their hands in chlorinated lime solution on the delivery unit. The maternal mortality rate from puerperal fever in patients attended to by medical students was far lower than that of those attended to by midwives who did not wash their hands.

Handwashing practices are not always ideal.
- Average compliance of health care workers with handwashing is typically <50% and technique is often poor and rushed.
- Research has begun to focus on how to change the culture and behavior on the ward and improve adherence to policies.
- There is no doubt that good handwashing practice reduces transmission of infections, but to be effective, all HCWs must always comply.

Skin flora can be divided into two types:
- *Transient organisms* are not normally part of the normal flora and can be picked up from the patient or their environment. Examples include *E. coli, S. aureus, Klebsiella* spp., and *Pseudmomonas* spp. They are usually removed by a "social" hand wash (Box 2.15), with soap and water. The aim of hygienic hand disinfection (Box 2.15), e.g., with alcohol gel, is to remove or destroy all transient flora, and there may be a prolonged effect.
- *Resident organisms* are usually found deep in the dermis. They do not usually cause infection, except if introduced during invasive procedures, e.g., line insertion or surgical procedures. Examples include coagulase-negative staphylococci and aerobic and anaerobic diphtheroids. They are not usually removed by a single handwashing procedure.

How to wash?
Use of a good handwashing technique (Fig. 2.3) will clean areas that are often missed (e.g., between the fingers, thumbs, fingertips, areas of palms, and backs of the hands). This should only take 15–30 seconds. Make sure hands are wet before applying soap, and rinse thoroughly before drying.

If using a gel, effective decontamination only occurs when the alcohol is rubbed in until the skin is dry.

Box 2.15 Common handwashing terms[1]

Social hand wash
- Cleaning of hands with plain nonmedicated bar or liquid soap and water, for the removal of dirt, soil, and various organic substances

Hygienic hand wash
- Cleaning of hands with antimicrobial or medicated soap and water. Most antimicrobial soaps contain a single active agent and are usually available as liquid preparations.

Hygienic hand disinfection
- Normally consists of the application of an alcohol-based hand rub onto dry hands without water

Surgical scrub
- The aim of this procedure is to remove or destroy all transient flora and reduce resident flora. There must also be a prolonged effect. Chlorhexidine, povidone-iodine, alcohol, or a mixture thereof is usually used.

When to wash?

Wash hands after any process that contaminates the skin and before food preparation, patient contact, or any clinical procedure. Examples include after leaving a source isolation room, or before entering a protective isolation room.

What to use?

In most clinical situations, soap and water or an alcohol rub is adequate. The length of time and handwashing technique are more important than which soap is used. There are specifications for sinks in clinical areas. Hand lotions and creams may be used after handwashing to prevent soreness.

Measuring compliance with handwashing

The gold standard for measuring compliance with handwashing is direct observation. This may, however, be subject to the Hawthorne effect, in that behavior tends to improve when an individual is being watched. Newer methods include devices to electronically monitor use of soap and hand wash dispensers.

Hand care in general

- Nail care: keep nails short and clean. Artificial nails should not be worn because they have been the source of HAI, including endocarditis and outbreaks due to *Serratia*.
- Jewelry and watches may harbor bacteria and hinder handwashing. Some hospitals often limit the wearing of certain types of jewelry.
- If hands get dry and sore, as often occurs after repeated handwashing, transient flora may become resident in skin cracks. HCWs should consult occupational health staff if they are concerned.

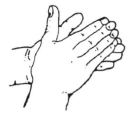

1. Palm to palm

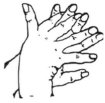

2. Right palm over left dorsum and left palm over right dorsum

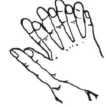

3. Palm to palm fingers interlaced

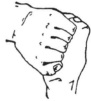

4. Backs of fingers to opposing palms with fingers interlocked

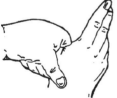

5. Rotational rubbing of right thumb clasped in left palm and vice versa

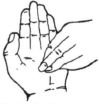

6. Rotational rubbing, backwards and forwards with clasped fingers of right hand in left palm and vice versa

Fig. 2.3 Hand decontamination. Technique based on the procedure described by Aycliffe et al. in *J Clin Pathol* 1978;31:923. Reproduced with permission from BMJ Publishing Group Ltd.

Changing the culture

The main factors preventing compliance with hand hygiene are time and system constraints. Many feel that full compliance with complete guidance is unrealistic. Washing with soap and water can take 60–90 seconds; therefore, many institutions have moved to alcohol-based hand rub at the point of care (i.e., at the bedside rather than at the entrance to the ward). This is easier, takes only 15–20 seconds, is microbiologically efficacious for all but a few organisms (e.g., C. difficile and norovirus).

Multifaceted approach

Evidence suggests a multipronged approach is the only way to bring about change. For example, key parameters in compliance with alcohol-based hand rubs include education of HCWs, monitoring and feedback to HCWs, good administrative support, and introducing a system change (i.e., putting alcohol gel by each patient).

References for best-practice guidelines are listed in Table 2.5.

Table 2.5 Best practice guidelines for handwashing

	Body	Reference
HICPAC	Healthcare Infection Control Practices Advisory Committee	http://www.cdc.gov/mmwr/pdf/rr/rr5303.pdf Also in *Morbidity and Mortality Weekly Report* 2002;51:1–44.
WHO Patient Safety	WHO	www.who.int/patientsafety. These hand hygiene guidelines on the WHO site should be applicable to all healthcare settings.
CDC	Centers for Disease Control and Prevention	http://www.cdc.gov/handhygiene/index.html
Clean Your Hands	National Patient Safety Agency	Implementation of guidelines and results of pilot campaign available at http://www.npsa.nhs.uk/cleanyourhands

Reference

1. Kampf G, Kramer E (2004). Epidemiological background of hand hygiene and evaluation of the most important agents for scrubs and rubs. *Clin Microbial Rev* 17(4):863–893.

Management of antibiotic-resistant organisms

In the following section, management of antibiotic-resistant organisms will be discussed at the population level. For treatment of individuals see sections MRSA (p. 184), vancomycin-intermediate *S. aureus* (VISA) (p. 186), and Gram-negative bacteria (p. 241).

Control of outbreaks of antibiotic-resistant organisms

The main steps in controlling most outbreaks of antibiotic-resistant organisms are as follows.

Identify reservoirs of resistant organisms
- Colonized and infected patients
- Environmental contamination

Halt transmission
- Improve handwashing and asepsis
- Isolate colonized and infected patients
- Eliminate any common source and disinfect environment
- Separate susceptible from infected and colonized patients
- Consider closing unit to new admission

Modify host risk
- Discontinue compromising factors, if possible
- Control antibiotic use (consider restriction or discontinuing antibiotics)

Control of endemic antibiotic resistance
- *Appropriate use of antibiotics:* this should include optimal choice of agent, the dose, and its duration, based on defined antibiotic policies for both treatment and prophylaxis. The use of topical antibiotics should be limited.
- *Infection control:* institute guidelines for intensive infection control procedures and provide adequate facilities and resources, especially for handwashing, barrier precautions (isolation), and environmental control measures.
- Improve antimicrobial prescribing practices through educational and administrative methods.
- Monitor local antibiotic resistance rates and ensure that antimicrobial guidelines are up to date.

MRSA prevention guidelines

In recent years, various guidelines covering management of MRSA have been published (Table 2.6)..

The evidence for treatment of MRSA nasal and extranasal colonization has been evaluated (www.clinicalevidence.com) and is controversial (see Box 2.16).

Antibiotics that have activity against MRSA are listed in Box 2.17.

Table 2.6 Guidelines for management of MRSA

Publication title	Reference	Notes
Management of Patients with Infections Caused by Methicillin-Resistant *Staphylococcus aureus*: Clinical Practice Guidelines by the Infectious Disease Society of America (IDSA)	Liu C et al. (2010) *Clin Infect Dis*; 52: 1–38	First guidelines for the treatment of specific infections due to MRSA
Strategies to Prevent Transmission of MRSA in Acute Care Hospitals	Calfee DP et al. (2008). *Infect Control Hosp Epidemiol* 29 (Suppl. 1): S62–S80	Strategies to detect and prevent MRSA transmission
Guidelines for the Control and Prevention of MRSA in Healthcare Facilities (UK)	Coia JE (2006). *J Hosp Infect* 63S:S1–S44	Infection control guidance and strategies for preventing spread of MRSA or infection with MRSA
Guidelines for the Prophylaxis and Treatment of MRSA Infections (UK)	Gemmel CG (2006). *J Antimicrob Chemother* 57:589–608	Prevention and treatment with antibiotics
Strategies for Clinical Management of MRSA in the Community	Gorwitz RJ et al. (2006). http://www.cdc.gov/ncidod/dhqp/ar_mrsa_ca.html	Summary of expert opinion for management of community-associated MRSA

Box 2.16 MRSA treatment of nasal and extranasal colonization (www.clinicalevidence.com)

Likely to be beneficial
- Mupirocin nasal ointment in select populations

Unknown effectiveness
- Antiseptic body washes
- Chlorhexidine-neomycin nasal cream (not available in the United States)
- Systemic antimicrobials

Unlikely to be beneficial
- Tea tree preparations

Box 2.17 Antibiotics with activity against MRSA

Almost always susceptible
- Vancomycin
- Daptomycin
- Linezolid (compared with glycopeptides)
- Quinupristin-dalfopristin

Typically effective against certain strains (community-associated MRSA)
- Trimethoprim-sulfamethoxazole
- Clindamycin
- Doxycycline, minocycline, tetracycline
- Rifampin

Screening for MRSA colonization

The aim of this strategy is to reduce MRSA infection by screening patients for MRSA colonization. Once colonization has been detected, patients are placed in contact isolation to prevent subsequent spread to other patients. This practice remains controversial but is likely effective in high-risk patients and units.

Individual hospitals must determine if this practice is appropriate and practical for their patients and, if performed, must have a specific policy in place to ensure that the protocol is performed correctly.

Screening should be considered in the following groups:
- Preoperative patients in certain surgical specialties when the rate of surgical site infection due to MRSA is high
- Critical care (including intensive care units (ICU) and high-dependency units)
- Other specific patient groups (depending on local risk assessment and practicalities) include all patients previously known to be MRSA positive, all elective surgical patients, oncology and chemotherapy inpatients, patients admitted from high-risk settings, and all emergency admissions.

Control of TB in hospitals

While most TB infections are acquired in the community, the risk of health care–associated TB remains for patients and HCWs. Most health care–acquired TB cases result from delayed diagnosis of TB, inadequate treatment of latent TB, and lack of isolation facilities. The successful control and prevention of TB in hospitals may be achieved through three approaches:
- *Administrative:* i.e., early investigation and diagnosis of those suspected to have TB
- *Environment/engineering:* patients undergoing evaluation for possible TB should be placed in negative pressure rooms.
- *Personal respiratory protection:* patients undergoing evaluation for possible TB should be placed on airborne isolation (see p. 133).

Transmission of TB from patients

The CDC has published guidelines for preventing the spread of TB in health care settings.[*] In general, transmission of TB from patients can be prevented by ensuring that staff are aware of the appropriate isolation facilities and infection control precautions to be taken for patients with infectious or potentially infectious TB or who have drug-resistant TB.

Transmission of TB from HCWs

When an HCW develops TB, this may lead to expensive, time-consuming, large-scale contact investigations to determine the extent of transmission and to prevent further spread. The incidence of acute and latent TB is higher among foreign-born HCWs.

Difficulties arise in interpretation of tuberculin skin tests in this group, although standard practice is to interpret any positive tuberculin skin test as indicative of latent TB (and thus requiring therapy) regardless of whether the HCW has received bacillus Calmette–Guérin (BCG) before or not.

Management of HCWs with TB is usually shared by occupational health and infection control departments.

Control of CJD and transmissible spongiform encephalopathies

The transmissible spongiform encephalopathies (TSEs) include Creutzfeld–Jakob disease (CJD) (which may be sporadic, familial, iatrogenic, or variant CJD [vCJD]) and Gerstmann–Sträussler–Scheinker syndrome (GSS) (p. 411 and 414). These conditions are characterized by neurodegeneration, with spongiform changes in the brain and central nervous system (CNS).

The prion proteins associated with TSEs are unusually resistant to inactivation by heat and chemicals, so special decontamination procedures are required. Cases of iatrogenic CJD have been transmitted by contaminated pituitary-derived hormones, dura mater grafts, neurosurgical instruments, corneal transplantation, organ transplantation, and blood transfusion.

Current challenges faced are in the early detection and diagnosis of vCJD, therapy and support for those affected, and improved understanding of transmission risks.

Variant CJD/new-variant CJD (vCJD)

This disease emerged in the late 1990s. Only 3 cases have been identified in the United States, although more than 160 cases have been documented in the UK. It has a distinct clinical presentation (p. 411) and tends to infect a younger age group than that with classical CJD. The number of new cases of vCJD is falling, but the total number of predicted cases is still a topic of debate.

In vCJD, prion proteins are detected in systemic lymphoid tissue before the patient is symptomatic, and the infectious agents are more resistant to inactivation than previously observed. These issues have had widespread consequences

[*] Available at: http://www.cdc.gov/mmwr/preview/mmwrhtml/rr5417a1.htm?s_cid=rr5417a1_e

in infection control procedures, such as increased use of single-use devices, traceability of endoscopes, and quarantining of surgical instruments.

Risk assessments

All patients admitted for surgery should have a risk assessment performed. The potential for transmission depends on the following factors:
- Prevalence of disease in the population
- Type and frequency of invasive procedures involving potentially infectious tissues
- Effectiveness of strategies for instrument decontamination and management
- Donor screening and selection (e.g., in transplantation)

Classification of risk

Risk for each individual patient should be classified as follows:
- Low risk i.e., no identified risk
- Asymptomatic but potentially at risk of CJD (e.g., recipients of pituitary hormones or dura mater grafts, or relatives with familial CJD)
- Symptomatic (definite, probable, or possible CJD or vCJD, or diagnosis actively under consideration)

Prevention of transmission of CJD

Always consult Hospital policy and involve the infection control team. Some general principles are advised for the processing of instruments

---

Box 2.18 Precautions regarding processing of instruments to minimize transmission of CJD

- Staff should practice universal precautions.
- Clean all surgical instruments to remove organic matter before sterilization.
- Consider using single-use instruments whenever possible. Never reprocess single-use kits; throw them away immediately. Use single-use kits for all lumbar punctures.
- The following methods are effective for prions: high-vacuum porous-load autoclaving at 134–137°C for 18 minutes or 132°C for 60 minutes. The following methods are ineffective for prions: autoclaving at 134°C for 3 minutes; alcohol; ethylene oxide; glutaraldehyde; formalin.
- Record the unique identification number of all flexible endoscopes every time they are used, and ensure that all instruments are traceable through the audit trail.
- Recent research in mice has suggested that dental tissue may be infective, thus instruments used for root canal work should be single-use.

Further information is available from the following Web sites:
- CDC—information on classic CJD: http://www.cdc.gov/ncidod/dvrd/cjd/
- CDC—information on vCJD: http://www.cdc.gov/ncidod/dvrd/vcjd/index.htm
- National Prior Disease Pathology Surveillance Center: http://www.cjdsurveillance.com/
- Spongiform Encephalopathy Advisory Committee (SEAC): www.seac.gov.uk/

Box 2.19 Care of symptomatic or at-risk patients with possible CJD

All patients should be subject to universal precautions. Patients known to have CJD do not require special nursing precautions or special precautions for management of sharp injuries, exposure to blood and body fluids, used and infected linen, and the disposal of clinical waste.

However, particular care must be taken to adhere to hospital policy for the following:

- *Collection, labeling, and transport of clinical specimens:* use biohazard stickers and provide adequate clinical information for laboratory staff to undertake a risk assessment.
- *CNS and lymphoid tissue biopsies:* these procedures should be performed by experienced staff, using disposable equipment. Gloves, goggles, and aprons should be worn, and any contaminated objects should be incinerated.
- *Surgical procedures on symptomatic or at-risk patients:* perform a risk assessment considering the likelihood that the patient is carrying the infectious agent and the chance that the agent could be transmitted by the specific procedure. Consult hospital policy for details about single-use protective clothing, single-use instruments, incineration, cleaning of operating rooms, and other precautions.

(Box 2.18) and in blood transfusion (Box 2.19) in order to minimize transmission of CJD.

All clinical specimens from known, suspected, or at-risk patients should be handled at CL3 in the microbiology laboratory, as the agent of CJD is in hazard group 3.

Disinfection

Disinfection is the process of killing microorganisms by physical or chemical means to render the object safe. It does not imply complete inactivation of all viruses or removal of bacterial spores (as occurs in sterilization).

A *disinfectant* is defined as a chemical used to destroy microorganisms. These agents only act on surfaces (environmental surfaces, equipment, or body surfaces) and do not penetrate layers of dirt or grease. Thus disinfection is not a substitute for cleaning. Disinfectants do not usually have a persistent effect.

Use of disinfectants

The environmental use of disinfectants should be restricted to accidental spills or build-up of infected material in areas where this may be a hazard to patients or HCWs.

Different disinfectants have different properties: many are corrosive and toxic, and the speed of action is highly variable. Some, if used correctly

Table 2.7 Environmental and skin disinfectants

Class	Use	Notes
Environmental disinfectants		
Hypochlorite (bleach)	Best general-purpose disinfectant available. However, not suitable for particularly dirty situations. Generally, use a solution of 1000 ppm (parts per million) available chlorine, but increase concentration to 1 ppm if need to destroy hepatitis viruses (e.g., dialysis units). Use hypochlorite granules for spillage of body fluids, except urine.	Sodium hypochlorite acts by the release of chlorine on contact with organic matter, so rapidly destroys all bacteria and viruses. However, some agents are unstable, and disinfecting properties may be lost through the rapid release of chlorine on contact with blood, feces, or textiles. Strong solutions are corrosive to aluminum and other metals.
Quaternary ammonium compounds (QAC)	Hospital-grade QACs are the most commonly used agents for environmental disinfection in the US. They are cheap and quickly and effectively kill most hospital pathogens	QACs are not sporicidal (e.g., C. difficile) and are not virucidal against hydrophilic (non-enveloped) viruses (e.g., Norovirus).
Phenolics	Not for routine environmental cleansing or disinfection; used in laboratory and postmortem rooms	Derived from coal-tar and in common use in hospitals for over a century. Reasonable in visibly dirty situations. However, many bacteria and viruses are resistant and prolonged exposure is needed for effective action. It is also toxic, so handle with special precautions.
Chlorxylenols	Household disinfectant	Said to combine some of the properties of the phenolics with hypochlorites. Less effective at killing Gram-negatives than the phenolics, and expensive
Skin disinfectants		
Alcohol	Often used as a base for other skin disinfectants, e.g., iodine or chlorhexidine	Ethyl alcohol (70%) effectively kills organisms on the skin, but this effect ceases after evaporation. Isopropyl alcohol evaporates less rapidly, but is thought to be less effective against some viruses.
Iodine	Surgical scrubs, shampoos, etc.	Iodine dissolved in 70% alcohol is less popular now, as it is messy and may be an irritant.
Chlorhexidine	Surgical scrubs, popular disinfectant in hospitals and laboratories	Often marketed with other disinfecting agents and in alcoholic or aqueous solution. Some hospital organisms show resistance to it, but this is not a problem when using the alcoholic solution.

can kill all germs (i.e., sterilize), but most are highly selective and only kill a limited range of organisms. They fall into two main groups:

- *Environmental disinfectants* are often too toxic for use on skin and may require protective clothing. Quaternary ammonium compounds (QACs) are the most commonly used but, notably, do not kill C. *difficile* spores.
- *Skin disinfectants* (also called *antiseptics*) often have limited range of action so are inappropriate for environmental disinfection and usually are relatively expensive. Chlorhexidine is the preferred agent. Alternatives are alcohol and iodine.

Other disinfectants may be used to sterilize instruments, but heat treatment is usually preferred.

Selection of a disinfectant

Considerations include the following:

- Which organisms do you want to destroy?
- What is the construction of the object to be disinfected?
- Does the object need cleaning first?
- When an agent has been chosen, what concentration of disinfectant is required?

Sterilization

Sterilization is the process by which transmissible agents are killed or eliminated. Standard sterilization works against fungi, bacteria, viruses, and spores, but not prions. There are two main types of sterilization:

- *Physical sterilization:* this includes heat sterilization and radiation (e.g., electron beams, X-rays, gamma rays)
- *Chemical sterilization:* this includes ethylene oxide, ozone, chlorine bleach, glutaraldehyde, formaldehyde, hydrogen peroxide, and peracetic acid.

Cleaning of instruments

Regardless of the type of sterilization process deemed most appropriate, thorough cleaning is required. Otherwise, any dirt or biological matter may shield any organisms present.

Physical scrubbing with detergent and water is recommended. Cool water is needed to clean organic matter from instruments, as warm or hot water may cause coagulation of organic debris.

Alternative cleaning methods include ultrasound or pulsed air.

Physical sterilization: heat

This can be either dry-heat or moist-heat sterilization.

Dry-heat sterilization uses hot air, which is free (or almost free) from water vapor, so any moisture plays no role in the process of sterilization. Methods include the hot-air oven, radiation, and microwave. The dry heat coagulates the proteins in any organism and causes oxidative free-radical damage and drying of cells.

Moist-heat sterilization uses hot air heavily laden with water vapor. Moist heat coagulates the proteins in any organism, which is helped by the water vapor that has a very high penetrating property, and also causes oxidative free-radical damage. Methods include autoclaving, pressure cooking, pasteurization of milk, boiling, and steam sterilizing (steam at atmospheric pressure for 90 minutes).

Autoclaves

Steam sterilization with autoclaves is commonly used in hospitals and provides an inexpensive means of sterilizing large numbers of surgical instruments. To achieve sterility, a holding time of >15 minutes at 121°C or 3 minutes at 134°C is required. Liquids and instruments packed in cloth may take longer to reach the specified temperature, so they usually need more time.

Autoclave treatment inactivates all bacteria, fungi, viruses, and spores. Certain prions may be eradicated by autoclaving at 121–132°C for 60 minutes or 134°C for >18 minutes, but this process is not 100% reliable for CJD. Monitoring of an autoclave cycle is important and involves recording of temperature and pressure over time.

To ensure that adequate conditions have been met, most hospitals use indicator tape that changes color. Bioindicators (e.g., based on the spores of *B. sterothermophilus*) are also used to independently confirm autoclave performance. These indicators should be positioned to ensure that steam penetrates the most difficult places. Note that autoclaving is often used to sterilize medical waste prior to disposal.

Chemical sterilization

Chemical sterilization is generally used when heat methods are inappropriate, e.g., for sterilizing heat-sensitive materials such as plastics, paper, biological materials, fiber optics, and electronics. Options include the following:

- *Ethylene oxide (EO)* sterilization is very common, particularly for disposable medical devices. Sterilization is usually carried out between 30°C and 60°C, for objects that are sensitive to higher temperatures e.g., plastics and optics. EO gas penetrates well and is highly effective, killing all viruses, bacteria, fungi, and spores. However it is highly flammable, takes longer than any heat treatment, and produces toxic residues. *B. subtilis* spores are used as a rapid biological indicator for EO sterilizers.
- *Ozone* is used to sterilize water and air in industrial settings and as a surface disinfectant. It can oxidize most organic matter but may be impractical because it is toxic and unstable and must be produced on site.
- *Chlorine bleach* will kill bacteria, fungi and viruses, and most spores (including *C. difficile*). Household bleach (5.25% sodium hypochlorite) is usually diluted to 1/10 before use. To kill MTB, it should only be diluted 1/5, and to inactivate prions it should be 1/2.5 (1 part bleach and 1.5 parts water). For full sterilization, bleach should be allowed to react for 20 minutes. It is highly corrosive (including of some stainless steel surgical instruments).
- *Glutaraldehyde and formaldehyde* are volatile liquids that are only effective if the immersion time is long enough. It can take up to 12

hours to kill all spores in a clear liquid with glutaraldehyde and even longer with formaldehyde. Both liquids are toxic if inhaled or if they come into contact with skin. Glutaraldehyde is expensive and has a shelf life of <2 weeks. Formaldehyde is cheaper but much more volatile (it may be used as a gaseous sterilizing agent).

- *Orthophthalaldehyde* has many advantages over glutaraldehyde: it shows better mycobactericidal activity, kills glutaraldehyde-resistant spores, is more stable, less volatile, and less irritating, and acts faster. However it is more expensive, and stains skin and proteins gray.
- *Hydrogen peroxide* is a nontoxic chemical at low concentrations and leaves no residue. It can be used to sterilize endoscopes, either in low-temperature plasma sterilization chambers or mixed with formic acid. It can also be used at a concentration of 30–35% under low-pressure conditions in the dry sterilization process (DSP). This process achieves bacterial reduction of 10–6 to 10–8 in approximately 6 seconds, and the surface temperature is increased only 10–15°C.

Ventilation in health care premises

Definitions of different ventilation systems

Positive-pressure ventilation

Positive-pressure isolation rooms are used to prevent the entry of microorganisms if patients are susceptible to infections (e.g., stem cell transplant recipients). The air is filtered before entering a sealed room, with a HEPA filter, and air is pumped into the room at a greater rate than it is expelled. This forces air out of the isolation room, keeping the room free of microorganisms.

There is usually an anteroom to facilitate the donning of protective clothing and airflows of at least 12 air changes per hour.

Negative-pressure ventilation

Negative-pressure isolation rooms are used to prevent pathogens (e.g., TB) from an infected patient infecting other patients or HCWs in the hospital. It is usually a sealed room except for a small gap under the door, through which air enters.

Direction of airflow can be confirmed by a smoke test (hold a smoke tube ~5 cm in front of the bottom of the door, and if the room is at negative pressure, the smoke will travel under the door and into the room).

HEPA filter

HEPA filters can remove almost all airborne particles 0.3 micrometers in diameter, e.g., *Aspergillus* spores.

Plenum ventilation

This is the most frequently used system in general-purpose operating rooms. Atmospheric air is filtered in two stages:

- Coarse filter to remove dust and debris
- Bacterial filter of ~2 micrometers pore size with 95% efficiency is used inside the inlet grill.

Some air may be recirculated within the suite. An exhaust system removes the air to the outside. There are ~15 air changes per hour.

Laminar flow

Laminar flow is used in some orthopedic operating rooms to reduce the number of microorganisms present. This may be of most value in preventing prosthetic joint infections, but definitive data are lacking.

A continuous flow of filtered air is recirculated under positive pressure into the operating field, and any air contaminants generated under surgery are removed from the site. There are approximately 300 air changes per hour, which should result in <10 cfu/m^3 (colony-forming units).

Different systems include introduction of air horizontally or vertically, in an enclosed, semi-enclosed, or open manner.

Box 2.20 Rituals and behaviors in operating rooms

All operating rooms (ORs) should have their own up-to-date infection control policy. This should include standard precautions for every invasive procedure, and outline the need for an additional risk assessment for each patient to see if other specific precautions are required.

There are many rituals and behaviors that have crept into standard practice in many ORs, some of which are beneficial, some being harmful. The standard of evidence varies, but a few practical pointers are listed below.

- Patients' clothes: it may not be necessary for them to change, e.g., for cataract surgery. Jewelry only needs to be removed (for infection control purposes) if near the site of operation.
- Shaving should be avoided. Ideally, no hair removal is performed. If hair removal is required, however, depilatory cream the day before surgery is preferable, or clippers in the anesthetic room immediately preoperatively.
- Hand hygiene: scrubbing brushes should not be used on the skin.
- Drapes: there is no evidence for adhesives around the edge of wounds.
- Gloves: needle puncture is not an indication to change gloves; if necessary, a second pair should be worn on top.
- Masks: there is no good evidence that masks reduce infection rates; however, they are recommended to protect the surgeon. The scrub team should wear masks and hats for implants, and the mask should be changed for each procedure. Ideally, hair is completed covered.
- Linen should be waterproof and disposable

References

1. Walker JT, Hoffman P, Bennett AM, et al. (2007). Hospital and community acquired infection and the built environment—design and testing of infection control rooms. *J Hosp Infect* 65 (Suppl 2):43–49.

2. Woodhead K, Taylor EW, Bannister G (2002). Behaviors and rituals in the operating theatre. A report from the HIS Working Party. *J Hosp Infect* 51(4):241–255.

Introduction to prevention of HAI

As many as 5–10% of hospital inpatients have an HAI during their stay. Patients in intensive care units (ICUs) are at increased risk, and estimates suggest that 15–40% of patients in the ICU will have at least one HAI. Given the shift of health care outside of the ICU, however, the majority of HAIs occur outside of the ICU.

In 2009, the CDC estimated that 1.6 million HAIs and 99,000 attributable deaths occur each year in the United States. In addition, HAIs lead to significant morbidity, leading to increased hospital costs, increased lengths of hospitalization, and disability. The estimated cost to the U.S. health care system is $36–45 billion annually.[*]

It is estimated that around 25–50% of HAIs are preventable through better application of good practice.[†] It is difficult to calculate the costs of introducing prevention methods on a hospital basis, but all research so far suggests that it is cheaper to focus on prevention than to pay for costs of treating HAI. A recent CDC report noted that a reduction in HAI by 20–50% could save $9–25 billion.[*]

Prevention is everyone's business— not just infection control!

There is clearly a need to change hospital culture and staff behavior. This has been highlighted as one of biggest obstacles. Evidence suggests that a variety of approaches are required so that the individual HCW accepts personal responsibility for infection control.

Training and education must be continual, and constant reminders, e.g., poster campaigns, handwashing publicity, and infection awareness days, are effective. Named individuals acting as liaison representatives and role models or "champions" in each specialty are beneficial.

Feedback of infection rates at ward and team level is vital to engage staff, encourage a sense of ownership, and encourage continual review of good practice.

Focus points regarding prevention
- Education and training for health care staff, especially doctors
- Better compliance with hand hygiene, care of indwelling lines, catheter care, and aseptic technique
- Good antibiotic prescribing
- Hospital cleanliness
- Consultation with infection control staff on wider issues, e.g., new-build projects

Infections in intensive care

Health care–associated infections complicate 25–40% of all ICU admissions. Although ICUs represent <5% of hospital beds, health care–associated infections in the ICU consume a significant amount of hospital resources.

---

[*] http://www.cdc.gov/ncidod/dhqp/pdf/Scott_CostPaper.pdf

[†] http://www.shea-online.org/Assets/files/0408_Penn_Study.pdf

Patients in the ICU are exposed to more broad-spectrum antibiotics, more invasive medical devices, and more procedures than those on normal hospital wards. Hand hygiene, barrier precautions, and antibiotic policies are particularly important in controlling infection.

Organisms

- The causal organism(s) isolated often depend on length of ICU stay (Table 2.8).
- Gram-positive infections are typically more common than Gram-negative ones, probably because of increased line- and device-associated infections (see Box 2.21). Recent preventative efforts have led to a decline in Gram-positive infections in many ICUs.

Table 2.8 Organisms isolated depend on the length of ICU stay

Early infection (≤4 days)	Late infection (>4 days)
S. aureus: MRSA > MSSA	S. aureus: MRSA > MSSA
H. influenzae	Enterococcus spp.
Enterobacteriaceae spp.	Enterobacteriaciaea spp.
S. pneumoniae	P. aeruginosa
Streptococcus spp.	Fungi
Anaerobes	Serratia spp.
	Acinetobacter spp.

MRSA, methicillin-resistant S. aureus; MSSA, methicillin-sensitive S. aureus.

Box 2.21 Studies of HAIs on the ICU

The National Healthcare Safety Network (NSHN) regularly reports rates of device-related HAIs from hospitals that participate in the network. Although rates typically vary according to the type of ICU, in 2008, the most common ICU-related infections were urinary catheter–associated urinary tract infection (3.1–7.4 CAUTI/1000 catheter days), central line–associated bloodstream infection (1.3–5.0 CLABSI/1000 central-line days), and ventilator-associated pneumonia (0.5–10.7 VAP/1000 ventilator days).[1]

The European Prevalence of Infection in Intensive Care (EPIC) study was a 1-day point prevalence study looking at >10,000 patients from 17 countries on all ICUs except pediatrics and coronary care units.[2] The infection data were linked to the patients' APACHE score and 6-week outcome, presence of lines, specific interventions, and demographics. Overall, 45% of patients had some sort of an infection, and 20% had at least one infection acquired in the ICU. The most common were pneumonia (47%), lower respiratory tract infection (18%), UTI (18%), bacteremia (12%), and wound infection (7%). Organisms were split 50/50 between Gram-positive and Gram-negative, the most common being S. aureus, P. aeruginosa, coagulase-negative staphylococci and enterococcus.

The Study on the Efficacy of Nosocomial Infection Control (SENIC) looked at the relative change in nosocomial infection over a 5-year period.[3] Overall, when infection control measures were introduced, "nosocomial" infections were reduced by 32%.

- There is increasing prevalence of *Candida* infections including non-*albicans*, which may be more drug resistant.
- There are more infections with antibiotic-resistant organisms: MRSA, VRE, and multi-drug-resistant Gram-negative species, such as *E. coli*, *Klebsiella* spp., *Serratia* spp., *Acinetobacter* spp., *S. maltophilia*, and *Enterobacter* spp.

Patients

- Increasing population of immunosuppressed patients, e.g., HIV, bone marrow transplant (BMT), solid organ transplant patients
- Increasing use of devices, e.g., lines, balloon pumps, pacing wires, endotracheal tubes
- Increasingly invasive procedures, e.g., use of ventilator, drains

ICU environment

Isolation of patients with resistant organisms is the aim. There should also be sufficient space around each bed, wash hand basins between every other bed, adequate ventilation, and adequate storage and utility space.

How to minimize infections on the ICU

- Follow evidence-based guidelines and policies.
- Use good infection control measures, e.g., handwashing.
- Practice close adherence to isolation policies.
- Practice good antibiotic control, e.g., a specific policy based on local knowledge.
- Have close liaison with infection services, pharmacy, engineers, estates.
- Feed back results of surveillance of resistant organisms.

Selective decontamination of the digestive tract (SDD)

This is a prophylactic technique that remains controversial. The aim is to eradicate aerobic Gram-negative rods (GNR) from the oropharynx. SDD consists of four components:

- Oral antimicrobial applied topically to the mouth four times daily
- A liquid suspension containing the same antimicrobials given via nasogastric tube
- IV antimicrobials for 3 days
- Stringent infection control measures

A systematic review and meta-analysis of >50 randomized controlled trials showed that SDD resulted in a significant decrease in levels of overall bloodstream infections (BSIs), Gram-negative BSIs, and overall mortality, but had no effect on Gram-positive BSIs.[4] Despite these results, this practice has not become widespread in the United States because of concerns about emergence of resistance.

Infection prevention and control in adult critical care

Best practices for prevention of HAIs are similar regardless of whether the patient is in the ICU or not.

- Sustainable reductions in HAIs require the engagement and active involvement of all staff working in the ICU, supported by the infection control and clinical champions.

- No single action will produce effective infection prevention and control practice. This is achieved by sustained and close adherence to best practice by every member of the ICU team.
- All individuals who come into contact with ICU patients have a responsibility to ensure effective infection prevention and control afforded to them.

References

1. Edwards JR, Peterson KD, Banerjee S, et al. (2009). National Healthcare Safety Network (NHSN) report: data summary for 2006 through 2008, issued December 2009. *Am J Infect Control* 37:783–805.

2. Vincent JL, Bihari DJ, Suter PM (1995). EPIC study (1992). *JAMA* 274: 639–44.

3. Haley RW, Morgan WM, Culver DH (1985). Study on efficiency of nosocomial infection control. *Am J Infect Control* 13(3):97–108.

4. Silvestri L, van Saene HK, Milanese M, Gregori D, Gulls A (2007). Selective decontamination of the digestive tract reduces bacterial bloodstream infection and mortality in critically ill patients. Systematic review of randomized, controlled trials. *J Hosp Infect* 65(3):187–203.

Surgical site infection

Introduction

Surgical site infections (SSIs) are seen in 2–5% of patients undergoing a surgical procedure. SSIs can lead to minor, superficial infections that require no antibiotic therapy or to severe, life-threatening invasive infections. SSIs make up almost 20% of all HAIs and cause significant morbidity, increased length of stay, and increased costs.

Most infections are endogenous (i.e., result from contamination of the incision by the patient's own microbes during surgery). The other route of acquisition is exogenous from the environment or other people.

Factors associated with SSI are generally separated into patient-related factors and procedure-related or perioperative factors (Table 2.9).

Table 2.9 Factors associated with SSI[3]

Patient related	Procedure related
Colonization with *S. aureus*	Antimicrobial prophylaxis
Diabetes mellitus	Duration of procedure
Extremes of age	Foreign material
Immunosuppression	Sterilization of instruments
Longer hospital stay	Operating room ventilation
Malnutrition	Preoperative shaving
Obesity	Preoperative skin preparation
Remote infection	Skin antisepsis
Smoking	

Multiple guidelines and recommendations have been published with the aim of preventing SSIs from occurring.

National surveillance of surgical site infection

The NHSN provides regular reports on SSI data from hospitals that participate in the network.[1] Procedures are listed as specific codes and are risk stratified by the NHSN Risk Index, a validated score to determine preoperative risk of infection. Approximately 50% of reported cases are "superficial-incisional," although the diagnosis of superficial infections (which typically do not require hospitalization) is poorly sensitive. *S. aureus* is the most common cause of SSIs.

MRSA is at least as common as MSSA, although recent data suggest that MRSA is now more common than MSSA in both tertiary and community hospitals. Patients with MRSA SSI have increased mortality and higher hospital costs compared with patients with MSSA SSI.[2]

Nonpharmacological measures for reducing SSI[3]

- Appropriate hair removal
- Appropriate operating room air exchanges
- Appropriate surgical attire
- Glycemic control
- Maintenance of good oxygenation
- Limit in-and-out traffic
- Maintain normothermia during the surgical procedure
- Proper preparation of the surgical field

Other useful resources

- American Healthcare Infection Control Practices Advisory Committee (HICPAC) guidelines for prevention of SSI (1999)[4]
- SHEA/IDSA Compendium of Strategies for Prevention of SSIs in Acute Care Hospitals[3]
- Institute for Healthcare Improvement Bundle to Prevent SSI (see Box 2.22)[5]

Box 2.22 Care bundle for preventing SSI

Preoperative
- *Hair removal:* no hair removal, if possible. If necessary, use a clipper with a disposable head. Shaving with a razor is not recommended.

Perioperative
- *Prophylactic antimicrobial:* provide an appropriate antimicrobial within 1 hour prior to incision (within 2 hours for fluoroquinolones and vancomycin, when indicated). Remember to repeat dosing in longer procedures.
- *Glucose control:* maintaining a blood glucose <200 mmol/L following the surgical procedure has been shown to reduce wound infection.
- *Normothermia:* maintaining a body temperature above 36°C in the perioperative period has been shown to reduce infection rates following colorectal procedures, but this recommendation remains controversial.

References

1. Edwards JR, Peterson KD, Banerjee S, et al. (2009). National Healthcare Safety Network (NHSN) report: data summary for 2006 through 2008, issued December 2009. *Am J Infect Control* 37:783–805.

2. Engemann JJ, Carmeli Y, Cosgrove SE, et al. (2003). Adverse clinical and economic outcomes attributable to meticillin resistance among patients with *Staphylococcus aureus* surgical site infection. *Clin Infect Dis* 36:592–598.

3. Anderson DJ, Kaye KS, Classen D, et al. (2008). Strategies to prevent surgical site infections in acute care hospitals. *Infect Control Hosp Epidemiol* 29 (Suppl 1):S51–561.

4. Mangram AJ, Horan TC, Pearson ML, et al. (1999). Guideline for prevention of surgical site infection. Centers for Disease Control and Prevention (CDC) Hospital Infection Control Practices Advisory Committee. *Am J Infect Control* 27(2):97–132.

5. http://www.ihi.org/IHI/Programs/Campaign/SSI.htm

Bloodstream infection (BSI)

Definitions

Primary bacteremia is commonly defined as organisms cultured from the blood when signs and symptoms are not attributed to infection at another location. Over 95% of BSIs on ICUs are primary bacteremias, most of which are line related.[1]

Secondary bacteremia is when organisms are cultured from the blood and are related to a documented focus of infection, e.g., infected leg ulcer.

Approximately 250,000 primary BSIs occur each year in the United States.

Central line–associated bloodstream infections (CLABSI)

Peripheral venous catheters are more commonly used for vascular access, but the risk of BSI is low. BSIs are more commonly associated with central venous catheter (CVC) insertion, which are a significant cause of mortality and morbidity. The estimated additional cost of a CLABSI is between $7,000 and $29,000.[2]

Prevention of CLABSI

The combination of a CVC insertion guideline (Box 2.23) and monitoring tool has been shown to significantly reduce the incidence of CLABSI in an ICU.[3,4] Coated catheters and antibiotic-containing locks may be helpful in certain scenarios and, in particular, when rates of CLABSI remain high despite adherence to standard recommendations (p. 156).[2]

Taking blood cultures: a summary of best practice

The aim of these recommendations is to ensure that blood cultures are taken for the correct indication at the correct time using the correct technique.

- Only take blood for culture when there is a clinical need to do so and not as routine.
- Members of staff taking blood cultures should be trained and competent in the procedure.
- Always make a fresh stab.

Box 2.23 Central venous catheter care

On insertion
- *Catheter type:* single lumen unless indicated otherwise for patient care; Consider antimicrobial impregnated line if 1–3 wks duration likely and high risk BSI, and rates of CLABSI are high despite adherence to standard recommendations
- *Insertion site:* subclavian or internal jugular
- Use chlorhexidine gluconate for skin preparation and allow to dry.
- Prevent microbial contamination—use hand hygiene, aseptic technique, and full barrier precautions
- Sterile, transparent, semipermeable dressing

Continuing care
- Full documentation
- Regular observation of line insertion site, at least daily
- Catheter site care—intact, clean dressing
- Catheter access
- Aseptic techniques when accessing catheter ports
- No routine catheter replacement

For further discussion of line-related sepsis, including the care of peripheral lines, see Line-related sepsis, p. 162 and 571.

- Thoroughly disinfect the skin before inserting the needle. Chlorhexidine gluconate–containing disinfectants are superior to povidone-iodine.
- Once disinfected, don't touch the skin again (no-touch technique).
- Disinfect the culture bottle cap before transferring the sample.

Other useful resources
- American Healthcare Infection Control Practices Advisory Committee (HICPAC) guidelines (2002)
- SHEA/IDSA Compendium of Strategies to Prevent CLABSI in Acute Care Hospitals (2008)[2]
- IDSA Guidelines for Detection and Management of Intravascular Catheter-Related Infection (2009)[5]

References

1. Richards MJ, Edwards JR, Culver DH, Gaynes RP (1999). Nosocomial infections in medical intensive care units in the United States. National Nosocomial Infections Surveillance System. *Crit Care Med* 25(5):887–92..

2. Marschall J, Mermel LA, Classen DK, et al. (2008). Strategies to prevent CLABSI in acute care hospitals. *Infect Control Hosp Epidemiol* 29;S22–30.

3. Berenholtz SM, Pronovost PJ, Lipsett PA, et al. (2004). Eliminating catheter-related bloodstream infections in the intensive care unit. *Crit Care Med* 32:2014–2020.

4. Pronovost PJ, Needham D, Berenholtz SM, et al. (2006). An intervention to decrease catheter-related bloodstream infection in the ICU. *N Engl J Med* 355:2725–2732.

5. Mermel LA, Allon M, Bouza E, et al. (2009). Clinical practice guidelines for the diagnosis and management of intravascular catheter-related infection: 2009 update by the Infectious Disease Society of America. *Clin Infect Dis* 49:1–45.

Catheter-associated urinary tract infection (CAUTI)

Urinary tract infections are the largest single group of HAIs, accounting for 32%.[1] The presence of a urinary catheter and the length of time it is in place are the two biggest contributing factors.[2] In total, 80% of health care–associated UTIs are attributable to an indwelling urinary catheter.

Though not believed to be as severe as other HAIs, CAUTIs still lead to increased morbidity, including increased length of hospitalization and increased cost. Each CAUTI leads to additional cost of approximately $1000. Recently published guidelines include specific recommendations to reduce the risk of CAUTI (Box 2.24).[3]

Box 2.24 Urinary catheter care bundle

At insertion

- Assess need for catheterization—avoid if possible.
- Clean the urethral meatus prior to catheter insertion.
- Sterile, closed drainage systems are recommended.
- Use correct hand hygiene, aseptic technique, and personal protective equipment.

Continuing care

- Sterile sampling of urine: perform aseptically via designated catheter port
- Drainage bag position: above the floor but below bladder level to prevent reflux or contamination
- Examination gloves should be worn to manipulate a catheter, preceded and followed by hand decontamination.
- Use correct hand hygiene.
- Clean catheter site regularly.
- Remove catheter as soon as possible.

Risk factors

- Presence of urinary catheter
- Duration of catheter
- Advanced age, diabetes, or immunosuppression
- Not maintaining a closed drainage system

Prevention

Before inserting a urinary catheter

Is it really necessary? Review the indication for inserting a catheter in this particular patient at this particular time. Only use an indwelling urethral catheter after considering alternative options (e.g., condom catheter, incontinence pads).

Choose the correct catheter type, catheter size, and drainage system. By selecting the optimum equipment, the risk of infection from re-catheterization can be reduced. Use the smallest catheter possible that allows adequate drainage, and make sure the length is appropriate for male and female patients. In general, a catheter with a 10 mL balloon capacity should be used, except for specific urology cases.

Document the date of insertion and the type and size of catheter.

Insertion of the catheter

Use aseptic technique for insertion, including hand hygiene, sterile equipment, gloves, and drape. Clean the urethral meatus prior to insertion, using soap and water (antiseptic preparations are not necessary). Use of a sterile lubricant in both male and female patients should reduce urethral trauma, thus decreasing the risk of infection.

Antibiotic prophylaxis is *NOT* indicated in most patients.

Ongoing management of a catheterized patient

- Review the need for the catheter daily. Remove it as soon as possible.
- If possible, set up automatic reminders for review of catheter necessity.
- Empty the urinary drainage system frequently to ensure adequate flow and to prevent reflux. Use a separate container for each patient and avoid contact between the drainage tap and container. The drainage bag should only be changed when necessary, according to the manufacturer's instructions.
- Management of the drainage bag requires universal precautions. Wash your hands and wear a new pair of gloves before manipulating the catheter. Always position the drainage bag below the level of the bladder (to prevent backflow). If this is not possible, e.g., when the patient is being moved, clamp the drainage tube, and ensure that the clamp is removed as soon as dependent drainage can be resumed.
- Clean the catheter urethral meatus junction daily with soap and water. Do not use antiseptic creams as these may increase infection. Advise the patient to have a shower rather than a bath.
- Maintain the connection between the urinary catheter and the drainage system, and only break it for good clinical reasons.
- Only flush a drainage bag if there is a clear indication (e.g., after some surgical procedures or to manage obstructive problems).
- Do not change a catheter routinely; assess each patient's needs.
- Record ongoing management in the care plan and nursing notes.
- Do not routinely use antiseptic- or antibacterial-impregnated catheters.

Obtaining a urine sample from a catheterized patient

Clean the sampling port with an alcohol swab, then use sterile equipment and an aseptic no-touch technique. If there is no sampling port available, send a sample from the drainage bag (and label it as such). Do not screen for asymptomatic bacteriuria (i.e., only send urine cultures when clinically indicated).

Other useful resources
- SHEA/IDSA Compendium of Strategies for Prevention of CAUTI[*]
- IDSA Guidelines—Diagnosis, Prevention, and Treatment of CAUTI in Adults: 2009 International Clinical Practice Guidelines[*]
- HICPAC Guideline for Prevention of CAUTI 2009[†]

References

1. http://www.cdc.gov/ncidod/dhqp/hai.html

2. Lo E, Nicolle L, Classen D, et al. (2008). Strategies to prevent catheter-associated urinary tract infections in acute care hospitals. *Infect Control Hosp Epidemiol* 29:S41–S50.

3. http://www.cdc.gov/ncidod/dhqp/pdf/Scott_CostPaper.pdf

Ventilator-associated pneumonia

Hospital-acquired pneumonia

Respiratory infections are the third largest contributor to HAI in the United States, leading to 15% of HAIs each year.[1] Approximately 1% of hospitalized patients will be diagnosed with hospital-acquired pneumonia.

These infections cause significant morbidity, leading to increased length of stay (7–9 days), increased cost (>$40,000 per infection), and increased health complications. Attributable mortality is estimated to be 30–50%.

Epidemiologically, these pneumonias can be separated into three categories: hospital-acquired pneumonia (HAP), health care–associated pneumonia (HCAP), and ventilator-associated pneumonia (VAP) (Box 2.25).

When considering treatment for these infections, it is important to consider the time of onset of symptoms and the likely microbiology (Table 2.10). The American Thoracic Society and IDSA have published joint

---

Box 2.25 Epidemiologic definitions of pneumonias

- *Hospital-acquired pneumonia:* pneumonia with symptom onset more than 48 hours after admission to the hospital.
- *Health care–associated pneumonia:* pneumonia that occurs in any patient who was hospitalized in an acute care hospital for 2 or more days within 90 days of the infection; resided in a nursing home or long-term care facility; received recent IV antibiotic therapy, chemotherapy, or wound care within the past 30 days of the current infection; or attended a hospital or hemodialysis clinic.
- *Ventilator-associated pneumonia:* pneumonia that occurs more than 48–72 hours following intubation. The NHSN definition for VAP includes pneumonias diagnosed any time following intubation and for 48 hours after a patient is extubated.

---

* http://www.journals.uchicago.edu/doi/pdf/10.1086/650482

† http://www.cdc.gov/hicpac/pdf/CAUTI/CAUTIguideline2009final.pdf

Table 2.10 Microbiology of hospital-acquired pneumonia

Early onset <5 days	Late onset >5 days	Others based on specific risks
S. pneumoniae	P. aeruginosa	Anaerobic bacteria
H. influenzae	Enterobacter spp.	Legionella pneumophila
S. aureus	Acinetobacter spp.	Viruses: influenza A and B; RSV
Enterobacter spp.	Klebsiella spp.	Fungi
	S. marcescens	
	E. coli	
	Other GNRs	
	S. aureus/MRSA	

guidelines that discuss prevention, diagnosis, and treatment of these pneumonias in detail.[2] See also Hospital-acquired pneumonia, p. 561.

Ventilator-associated pneumonia (VAP)

Pneumonia occurring during mechanical ventilation is the most common infection in ICUs, leading to 45% of all ICU infections. As many as 10–20% of patients undergoing ventilation will develop VAP, but more recent estimates are lower. Estimates vary, however, based on type of unit and patient risk factors.

VAP may be due to microaspiration of oropharyngeal secretions, aspiration of gastric contents, colonization of the aerodigestive tract, use of contaminated equipment or medications, or direct inoculation from staff (cross-infection).[2]

Predisposing factors include duration of intubation, impaired conscious level, presence of endotracheal or nasogastric tubes, extremities of age, replacement of normal flora due to prior antibiotic treatment, underlying illness, and immunocompromised patients.

About 50% is defined as early VAP, i.e., within the first 5 days. VAP has significant consequences at the individual and population level:
• Increased duration of ventilation
• Increased length of ICU stay and hospital stay
• Increased cost (estimated at almost $25,000 per patient)
• Increased mortality

Emphasis here is on the prevention of VAP. For further discussion of pathogenesis, clinical features, diagnosis, and treatment of VAP, see Ventilator-associated pneumonia in Chapter 4 (p. 561).

Prevention of VAP

Recommendations to prevent VAP in the ICU include the following:
• Use noninvasive ventilation when appropriate
• Appropriate disinfection and care of tubing, ventilators and humidifiers to limit contamination
• No routine changes of ventilator tubing
• Avoid antacids and H_2 blockers

- Sterile tracheal suctioning
- Place patient in semi-recumbent position with head of bed elevated 30–45 degrees
- Subglottic suctioning
- Regular oral care with an antiseptic solution
- Only replace tubing when visibly soiled or mechanically malfunctioning
- Hang hygiene before care of patient or manipulation of ventilator or tubing
- Use of selective decontamination of digestive tract (p. 152) is controversial.

The ventilator care bundle was initially introduced as part of the 100,000 Lives Campaign.[3] Its success in preventing VAP depends on all five individual steps of the bundle being performed:
- Elevation of head of bed to 30–45 degrees
- Daily "sedation vacations" or gradually lightening the use of sedatives
- Daily assessment of readiness to extubate or wean from the ventilator
- Peptic ulcer prophylaxis
- Deep venous thrombosis prophylaxis

Impact of ventilator care bundle

A study from Alabama reported no cases of VAP for 255 days after implementing the ventilator bundle.[4] Similarly, introduction of ventilator bundles in 35 ICUs in the United States resulted in an average 44.5% reduction of VAP.[5]

Other benefits associated with reduced VAP include better patient outcome, shorter hospital stay, lower costs, and improved staff morale.

Other useful resources

- CDC and Healthcare Infection Control Practices Advisory Committee (HICPAC) Guidelines (2003)[6]
- IDSA/SHEA Compendium of Strategies for Prevention of VAP[7]

References

1. http://www.cdc.gov/ncidod/dhqp/hai.html

2. Guidelines for the management of adults with hospital-acquired, ventilator-associated, and healthcare-associated pneumonia *Am J Respir Crit Care Med* 2005;171:388–416.

3. http://www.ihi.org/IHI/Programs/Campaign/ (ref = 100k lives)

4. Vincent JL, Bihari DJ, Suter PM (1995). EPIC study (1992). *JAMA* 274:639–644.

5. Resar R, Pronovost P, Haraden C, et al. (2005). Using a bundle approach to improve ventilation care process and reduce ventilator-associated pneumonia. *Jt Comm J Qual Patient Saf* 31(5):243–238.

6. http://www.cdc.gov/mmwr/preview/mmwrhtml/rr5303a1.htm

7. Coffin SE, Klompas M, Classen D, et al. (2008). Strategies to prevent ventilator-associated pneumonia in acute care hospitals. *Infect Control Hosp Epidemiol* 29:S31–S40.

Line-related sepsis

Intravascular devices may be complicated by local infections (e.g., phlebitis) or systemic infections (e.g., BSI, endocarditis, osteomyelitis). The most common organisms that cause line-related sepsis are coagulase-negative staphylococci, S. aureus (including MRSA), enterococci, Enterobacteriaceae, Pseudomonas spp., and Candida spp.

Infection may arise in numerous ways. Usually lines become contaminated by the patient's skin flora at the insertion site or by the introduction of other organisms via the cannula hub or injection port.

Always consider whether a line is absolutely necessary or whether an alternative route of administration may suffice (e.g., nasogastric, rectal, subcutaneous). Review the continued need for a line daily.

Peripheral intravenous catheters (PIVs)

PIVs are used most frequently for vascular access. Although they have a low risk of systemic complications, the overall total morbidity is high because they are so widely used.

Almost all systemic infections are preceded by a visible phlebitis, which should act as a trigger for their removal (see Table 2.11). The approach for minimizing peripheral line infections is summarized in Box 2.26.

Box 2.26 Peripheral line care

On insertion
- Asepsis: prevent microbial contamination by correct hand hygiene and personal protective equipment
- Skin preparation: use (2%) alcoholic chlorhexidine gluconate, allow to dry for maximal effect
- Dressing: a sterile, semi-permeable, transparent dressing to allow observation of insertion site
- Documentation: date and site of insertion recorded in notes

Continuing care
- Continuing clinical indication: ensure all lines and associated devices are still indicated. If there is no indication then the lines or devices should be removed
- Line insertion site: regular observation for signs of infection, at least daily
- Dressing: an intact, dry, adherent transparent dressing is present
- Line access: use aseptic techniques and swab ports or hub with alcohol prior to accessing the line or administering fluids or injections
- Administration set replacement: immediately after administration of blood, blood products or lipid feeds. Replace all other fluid sets after 72 hours
- Routine line replacement: replace in a new site after 72 hours, or earlier if indicated clinically
- See Bloodstream infection (p. 156; Box 2.23).

Table 2.11 Visual infusion phlebitis (VIP) score[3]

Score	Description
0	Site looks healthy
1	Mild pain or redness near site
2	Two of the following evident at site: redness, pain, swelling
3	All of the following evident: redness, pain along cannula site, swelling
4	All of the following evident and extensive: redness, pain along path of cannula, swelling, palpable venous cord
5	All of the following evident and extensive: redness, pain along path of cannula, swelling, palpable venous cord and pyrexia

Central vascular catheters (CVCs)

CVCs (nontunneled), or central lines, lead to higher rates of BSI. A *central line* is defined as any IV catheter that terminates in the central vasculature. These infections are less easy to prevent than PIC infections.

Many ICUs use more peripherally inserted central catheters (PICC) in place of traditional CVCs. While this approach may be advantageous for some reasons (e.g., risk of trauma), the rate of central line–associated BSI (CLABSI) is approximately the same for CVCs and PICCs in hospitalized patients.

For a full discussion of advances in diagnosis, prevention and management see publications by Raad et al[1] and Mermel et al.[2]

Risk factors

Risk factors associated with line infection include the following:
- *Patient characteristics:* age, underlying illness, immunosuppression
- *Catheter characteristics:* material, type, size, coating/impregnation
- Infusate and dressing type
- Experience of person inserting the line, site preparation, anatomical insertion site, and duration of insertion
- Standard of daily line care

Minimizing line infections

- *Hand decontamination:* wash hands thoroughly first (see Handwashing, p. 135).
- *Aseptic technique:* maintain a strict no-touch aseptic technique when manipulating any part of the line or cannula.
- *Cannula selection:* chose the smallest possible lumen for the fluid to be infused; use a single-lumen CVC unless multiple ports are required; consider antimicrobial-impregnated or coated CVCs if a line is needed for >3 days. PICC lines may be considered for patients anticipated to need vascular access for a longer time period.
- *Perform "scrub the hub":* properly disinfect the catheter port or hub prior to accessing.
- *Insertion site:* for PIVs, look on the distal arm, away from previous sites and joint areas. For nontunneled CVCs, consider each case carefully as

choice of site is important in minimizing infection. Avoid the femoral vein if possible.

- *Skin preparation:* preferentially use chlorhexidine gluconate plus alcohol prior to insertion of any intravenous catheter.
- *Dressing:* a transparent film or sterile gauze is ideal. Write the date of insertion on the dressing. Always replace the dressing after inspecting the insertion site or if it becomes damp, loosened, or soiled.
- *Observation:* at least daily or whenever the line is manipulated. The visual infusion phlebitis (VIP) score may be useful (Table 2.11).[3]
- *Catheter removal:* replace any lines inserted as emergency within 24 hours. Remove any catheter after 72 hours (PIC) or if there are signs of infection e.g., VIP score ≥2. Do not routinely replace or remove CVCs unless they are no longer indicated, are malfunctioning, or appear infected.
- Training and audit play an integral part.

Antimicrobial-coated or impregnated catheters

There is increased interest in using antimicrobial-coated or impregnated catheters. Agents include antiseptics (e.g., chlorhexidine and silver sulfadiazine, silver, quaternary ammonium compounds) or antibiotics (e.g., minocycline and rifampin). Ideally, compounds should be active on internal and external surfaces and mainly target Gram-positive organisms.

Current evidence supports their use, particularly in patients who will require a CVC for 5 or more days or in settings where the rate of CLABSI is unacceptably high despite adherence to standard recommendations. Some trials were poorly designed and cost-effectiveness has been questioned. Follow your hospital guidelines.

Antibiotic-containing locks

Antibiotic-containing locks remain controversial. They may be useful as an adjunctive treatment of a CLABSI when the central line can not be removed.[2] This strategy should not be employed, however, if the CLABSI is caused by specific organisms, such as MRSA. In addition, there may be concerns about increasing resistance, e.g., VRE.

Other strategies, including tetrasodium EDTA and alcohol, have also been used to decrease the risk of CLABSI but remain controversial. In contrast, heparin locks may actually promote the growth of biofilm and, thus, might increase the risk of infection.

Other useful resources

- American Healthcare Infection Control Practices Advisory Committee (HICPAC) Guidelines (2002)
- SHEA/IDSA Compendium of Strategies for Prevention of CLABSI in Acute Care Hospitals
- Canadian Intravascular Access Devices Infection Control Guidelines
- IDSA Clinical Practice Guidelines for Diagnosis and Management of Intravascular Catheter–Related Infection (2009)[2]

References

1. Raad I, Hanneit, Maki D (2007). Intravascular catheters-related infections: advances in diagnosis, prevention and management. *Lancet Inf Dis* 7:645–657.

2. Mermel LA, Allon M, Bouza E, et al. (2009). Clinical practice guidelines for the diagnosis and management of intravascular catheter-related infection: 2009 update by the Infectious Disease Society of America. *Clin Infect Dis* 49:1–45.

3. Jackson A (1998). Infection control—a battle in vein: infusion phlebitis. *Nurs Times* 94;68, 71.

Hospital epidemics of diarrhea and vomiting

Most outbreaks of diarrhea and vomiting in hospitals are caused by viruses (e.g., norovirus). However, remember to exclude other important causes, such as *C. difficile*, *Salmonella* spp. and *Shigella* spp., although these bacteria predominantly cause diarrhea, rather than vomiting.

Precautions for patients with gastroenteritis

In general, continent patients diagnosed with gastroenteritis do not require additional isolation, though some variation from this recommendation is required on the basis of type of pathogen identified (see Box 2.27).

The CDC recommends using contact precautions (see p. 134) for any diapered or incontinent patient with gastroenteritis. Furthermore, contact precautions should be implemented for all patients with gastroenteritis in the setting of an institutional outbreak.

In cases of viral diarrhea, these precautions should be applied from the time when diarrhea first starts until complete resolution of symptoms, at

---

Box 2.27 Recommended isolation for patients with gastroenteritis based on patient- and pathogen-specific factors

All patients with gastroenteritis and bowel incontinence should be placed on contact precaution.

Standard precautions (e.g., good hand hygiene)
- Adenovirus
- *Campylobacter* spp.
- Cholera
- *Cryptosporidium*
- *E. coli* (including enteropathogenic O157:H7 strains)
- *Giardia lamblia*
- *Salmonella* spp.
- *Shigella* spp.
- *Yersinia enterocolitica*

Contact precautions
- *Clostridium difficile*
- Rotavirus
- Norovirus

Note: Hospitals may have different policies for some of these pathogens. For example, some hospitals require contact precautions for patients diagnosed with some of these pathogens if the patient is incontinent. Check with infection control.

a minimum. Many hospitals, however, elect to continue precautions for longer (e.g., 48 hours after symptom resolution or even until discharge), so check your hospital policy. If an alternative cause for the diarrhea is found (e.g., C. difficile, see p. 167), contact precautions may be required for different lengths of time, so seek advice from infection control staff.

The following can be considered reasonable guidance for preventing the spread of viral gastroenteritis within a hospital:

- As soon as the diarrhea starts, move patients to single rooms, if available. Do not wait for the stool culture result to come back. Ideally, each patient with diarrhea or vomiting should have their own toilet, commode, or bedpan. If isolation is not feasible, clean equipment after use with a hypochlorite-containing solution (1000ppm).
- Clean the bed space the patient has moved from with a hypochlorite-containing solution (1000ppm).
- Careful handwashing is vital, after each contact with the patient.
- Use soap and water for patients diagnosed with C. difficile or norovirus (instead of alcohol foam).
- Clean up diarrhea or vomit immediately and clean the area with a hypochlorite-containing solution (1000 ppm). Aerosols from vomiting are an important route of transmission in viral gastroenteritis.
- During an outbreak, clean all toilets on the ward with a hypochlorite-containing solution (1000 ppm) at least twice a day. Pay particular attention to toilet flush handles, toilet seats, and door handles.
- Dispose of used linen as contaminated laundry.

Hospital outbreaks of diarrhea and vomiting

Patients
- Involve infection control, and consider holding an outbreak meeting. Notify infection control of any new cases immediately.
- Patients may need to be cohorted together in a specific unit or a specific part of a unit.
- Consider sending one sample of vomit for virology and one stool sample for virology, culture, and C. difficile toxin. Once an outbreak has been confirmed, further testing may not be necessary, as a clinical definition can be applied.
- In most states, microbiology or infection control is responsible for notifying both county and state health departments. In others, however, treating clinicians are also responsible for reporting to the health department.
- Patients may be sent home at any time, even if they still have symptoms.

Staff
- Staff should pay particular attention to handwashing.
- No food or drink should be consumed in clinical areas.
- If symptoms develop, staff should report to occupational health immediately. A sample of stool or vomit can be submitted and the member of staff should stop work immediately. They can return to work 24–48 hours after symptoms have settled. Check hospital policy to determine the time frame for return to work.

- Nursing staff must not work in any other clinical area without consulting infection control.
- Key areas of the ward should be cleaned regularly with a hypochlorite-containing solution at 1000 ppm. This includes the environment around symptomatic patients, the toilets, commodes, bedpans, bathrooms, and showers.
- Terminal cleaning or environmental decontamination is important.

Clostridium difficile infection

C. difficile was originally defined as the cause of antibiotic-associated colitis in 1978 and continues to have a significant impact on patient morbidity and mortality. C. difficile leads to 20–30% of all cases of antibiotic-associated diarrhea and is the most common type of health care–associated diarrhea.

On average, patients with C. difficile infection (CDI) have an increased length of stay of 21 days. CDI also leads to higher risk of death and excess cost. In total, excess annual costs for CDI likely exceed $3 billion.[1]

The epidemiology of CDI has changed in the last decade. Formerly believed to be a "nuisance" infection, CDI is associated with increasing rates of incidence, colectomy, and mortality and is being diagnosed in patients in the community. The change in epidemiology is most likely due to the emergence of a new, virulent strain, the ribotype 027/NAP-1 strain.

To better describe CDI in the setting of this changing epidemiology, the CDC has released new surveillance definitions (see Box 2.28).[2]

See Antibiotic-associated colitis in Chapter 4 (p. 591) for epidemiology, clinical features, pathogenesis, diagnosis and management of CDAD.

Box 2.28 New surveillance definitions for CDI[2]

Health care facility associated
- *Hospital onset:* symptom onset after day 3 of admission
- *Community onset:* symptom onset upon admission or within first 3 days of admission AND discharged from a hospital in the past 4 weeks

Community associated
- Symptom onset upon admission or within first 3 days of admission AND no prior hospitalization OR hospitalization >12 weeks prior to admission

Indeterminate
- Symptom onset upon admission or within first 3 days of admission AND discharged from a hospital between 4 and 12 weeks prior to admission

Each type of CDI is subsequently labeled as follows:
- *New:* no prior CDI OR more than 8 weeks since prior CDI
- *Recurrent:* CDI between 2 and 8 weeks prior to onset of current CDI
- *Continuation:* CDI within the past 2 weeks

Diagnosis

Current tests for diagnosis of CDI include enzyme-linked immunosorbent assays (ELISAs) for toxins A and/or B, vero-cell culture for cytopathic effect, and examination under fluorescent light after culture on specific agar (CCFA: cefoxitin cycloserine fructose agar, or CCEY: cefoxitin cycloserine egg yolk). Real-time polymerase chain reaction (PCR)-based testing has been approved and is being used more commonly. This strategy leads to higher test sensitivity and specificity as well as higher cost.

Policies for testing samples vary. In some hospitals, tests for *C. difficile* must be specifically requested, while elsewhere all unformed stools are tested. Given the changing epidemiology, it is important for clinicians to consider CDI even in "nontraditional" patients. It is usual practice not to repeat the test once a patient has a positive result.

The practice of sending three stool samples to increase the sensitivity of ELISA-based tests is not evidence based. In fact, no diagnostic advantage is gained by sending more than one specimen.[3]

Typing

Various typing techniques have been placed in order of decreasing discriminatory ability. These are (most discriminatory first): multiple loci variable-number tandem-repeat analysis (MLVA), restriction endonuclease analysis (REA), pulsed-field gel electrophoresis (PFGE), surface layer protein A gene sequence typing (slpAST), PCR-ribotyping, multi-locus sequence typing (MLST), and amplified fragment length polymorphism (AFLP).[4]

In practice, these techniques are not employed in most hospitals but are reserved for research or outbreak investigations.

Control of infection

CDI is transmitted by clostridial spores, which are shed in large numbers by infected patients and are capable of surviving for long periods in the environment. Contact precautions should be followed, as outlined in Hospital epidemics of diarrhea and vomiting. See also Box 2.29.

Box 2.29 Reducing risk of infection from *C. difficile*

- Prudent antibiotic prescribing, as per local policy. Minimize use of broad-spectrum agents, review prescription daily, and include stop dates.
- *Hand hygiene:* wash hands with soap and water before and after each patient contact; alcohol foam is ineffective against *C. difficile* spores
- *Enhanced environmental cleaning:* use chlorine-based disinfectants to reduce environmental contamination with *C. difficile* spores as per local policy. Deep clean and decontaminate a room after a CDI patient has been discharged.
- *Isolation:* always use a single room if available; cohort patient care if a single room is not available.
- *Personal protective equipment:* always use disposable gloves and gown when handling body fluids and when caring for CDI-infected patients.

Specific issues relating to the management of patients with CDI include the following.

Management of the patient

- Review the individual's antibiotic prescription. Consider stopping antimicrobial agents. Seek advice from an infection expert if in doubt.
- Recently published guidelines recommend treating mild to moderate cases of CDI with metronidazole (500 mg by mouth three times a day for 10–14 days).[1] Metrodnidazole is cheaper than oral vancomycin and results in less VRE than using oral vancomycin. Some data suggest that metronidazole may be less efficacious for ribotype 027.
- Oral vancomycin is recommended for treatment of severe CDI (125 mg by mouth [or by rectum] four times a day for 10–14 days).[1] Consult your local hospital policy.
- Contact precautions must continue until the diarrhea settles. If in doubt, seek advice from infection control. Stool may remain positive for *C. difficile* toxin for considerable time afterward, so microbiological clearance and repeat specimens are not required or recommended.
- The management of recurrence (which can be as high as 25%) is not well known. Typically, patients are treated with the same regimen used for the first infection. The preferred strategy for a second recurrence and beyond is vancomycin with tapering doses or pulse doses. Other strategies may include anion-exchange resins to absorb toxins, intravenous immunoglobulin, stool transplantation, or rifampin "chasers."
- Probiotics are not recommended for either prevention or treatment of CDI and may lead to harm.[1]
- Areas of research and development include tolevamer (a polymer that binds toxin and reduces the recurrence rate), rifaximin, monoclonal antibody, nitazoxanide (antiparasitic agent), and fidaxomicin.

Prevention of infection

- *C. difficile* spores survive in the environment for long periods of time. Disinfect all furniture and surfaces with a hypochlorite-containing solution (1000 ppm).
- When contact precautions are discontinued, the patient's room should undergo "terminal cleaning."
- *Handwashing:* By washing with soap and water, the dilutional effect of the water and friction through rubbing the hands may help to remove some of the spores. Alcohol foam is not effective for hand hygiene for patients with CDI.
- *C. difficile* vaccines and anti-toxin immunoglobulins are still in research and development stages.
- There is no evidence that giving pre-emptive metronidazole or vancomycin when a patient starts broad-spectrum antibiotics is beneficial.

Other useful resources

- SHEA-IDSA Guidelines for *Clostridium difficile* Infection in Adults[1]
- SHEA/IDSA Compendium of Strategies for Prevention of *Clostridium difficile* in Acute Care Hospitals

C. difficile *ribotype 027/NAP1*

This new epidemic strain causes disease that is more frequent, more severe, and more refractory to normal treatment than previous types. Ribotype 027 produces more toxin A and B in vitro (due to an 18 base pair deletion in the *tcdC* gene) and also more binary toxin (significance is uncertain).

Ribotype 027 is resistant to fluoroquinolones and has higher MICs to metronidazole (but is still sensitive to this agent). This new strain is spreading rapidly throughout the world.

References

1. Cohen SH, Gerding SN, Johnson S, et al. (2010). Clinical practice guidelines for *Clostridium difficile* infection in adults: 2010 update by the Society for Healthcare Epidemiology of America (SHEA) and the Infectious Diseases Society of America (IDSA). *Infect Control Hosp Epidemiol* 31:431–455.

2. http://www.cdc.gov/nhsn/PDFs/pscManual/12pscMDRO_CDADcurrent.pdf

3. Peterson LR, Robicsek A (2009). Does my patients have *Clostridium difficile* infection? *Ann Intern Med* 151:176–179.

4. Killgore G, Thompson A, Johnson S, et al. (2008). Comparison of seven techniques for typing international epidemic strains of *Clostridium difficile*: restriction endonuclease analysis, pulsed-field gel electrophoresis, PCR-ribotyping, multilocus sequence typing, multilocus variable-number tandem-repeat analysis, amplified fragment polymorphism, and surface layer protein. A gene sequence typing. *J Clin Microbiol* 46(2):431–437.

Infection control in the community

The burden of HAI outside hospitals is unknown. As more patients continually move between hospitals and the community, particularly older and more dependent patients, in the future, HAI in hospitals and the community will be managed as one.

At the present time, infection control in the community is defined as the infection control service provided outside acute and major hospitals to those in another care setting. This covers a wide group, including nursing home residents, renal patients on home dialysis, and outbreaks of diseases in school and places of work. The nurses responsible for infection control in the community have many other responsibilities, which may include contact tracing for TB.

Until recently, infection control in the community has been an underdeveloped area with considerable uncertainty about local arrangements and no single pattern of service provision.

Community *C. difficile*

CDI is being increasingly recognized in the community. It is generally defined as diagnosis of CDI in patients in the community or in those within 48 hours of hospital admission, in the absence of recent hospitalization. Research suggests that most patients have received antibiotics.

Community-acquired MRSA.

This is genetically distinct from hospital-acquired MRSA and is becoming more common (p. 184).

Control of antimicrobial resistance in the community

Some countries have launched campaigns to educate doctors and patients about antibiotic misuse and the threat of drug resistance.

In the United States, the "Get Smart" campaign has been driven by the Centers for Disease Control and Prevention (http://www.cdc.gov/drugresistance/community), and Health Canada is behind the "Do Bugs Need Drugs" initiative (http://www.dobugsneeddrugs.org).

Systematic microbiology

Identification of bacteria

Identification of bacteria in the diagnostic laboratory is based on phenotypic characteristics such as the following:

- Microscopic appearance
- Growth requirements
- Colonial morphology
- Hemolysis pattern
- Biochemical tests
- Antimicrobial susceptibility patterns

Many laboratory technicians are able to make a preliminary identification to genus level on the basis of clinical data, morphological characteristics, and a limited range of rapid tests. Commercial identification systems such as the Analytical Profile Index (API) system (bioMérieux) contain a battery of biochemical tests that can identify the organism to species level.

Microscopy

Staining and microscopic examination of samples or cultures reveals the size, shape, and arrangement of bacteria and the presence of inclusions, e.g., spores. The following stains are commonly used.

Gram stain

A fixed slide is flooded with 0.5% methyl/crystal violet (30 seconds), followed by Lugol's iodine (30 seconds), followed by rinsing with 95–100% ethanol or acetone, followed by counterstaining with 0.1% neutral red, safranin, or carbolfuchsin (2 minutes). Gram-positive organisms stain deep blue to purple and Gram-negative organisms stain pink to red.

Acridine orange (AO) stain

AO is a fluorochrome that intercalates into nucleic acid. The slide is stained with AO (5–10 seconds), decolorized with alcoholic saline (5–10 seconds), and rinsed with normal saline. Once dry, a drop of saline or distilled water and a coverslip are added, and the slide is examined under fluorescence microscopy.

AO is more sensitive than Gram stain and is often used to evaluate Gram stain–negative blood culture broths, CSF, or buffy coat. Bacterial and fungal DNA fluoresce orange, while mammalian DNA stains green.

Auramine Rhodamine (AR) stain

AR binds to mycolic acids. Used to identify mycobacteria in clinical specimens, auramine is considered more sensitive than the Ziehl Neelsen or Kinyoun stains (discussed later).

A heat-fixed slide is flooded with auramine solution for 15 minutes. It is rinsed with water and then decolorized with 1% acid–alcohol for 3–5 minutes (until no further stain seeps from film). It is rinsed and stained with 0.5% potassium permanganate for 2–4 minutes. It is rinsed and allowed to air dry before examination under fluorescence microscopy.

Acid-fast bacilli (AFB) appear bright yellow to green against a dark background.

Ziehl–Neelsen (ZN) stain

ZN provides better morphological detail than an auramine stain.

A heat-fixed slide is flooded with strong carbolfuchsin and heated gently until it is just steaming. It is left to cool (3–5 minutes), rinsed with water, and decolorized with a 3% acid–alcohol solution (5–7 minutes, until the slide is faintly pink). The slide is rinsed with water and counterstained with 1% methylene blue or malachite green (30 seconds). It is allowed to air dry before examination under oil immersion light microscopy. AFB appear red on a blue or green background.

Kinyoun stain

The only difference between the ZN and Kinyoun stain is the substitution of phenol for steam. Kinyoun (cold) staining is less time consuming and easier to perform than ZN, with an equivalent sensitivity and specificity for AFB.

Modified acid-fast stain

This is a modified ZN stain (1% sulfuric acid is used as the decolorizer) for the identification of *Nocardia* spp. and cryptosporidia.

Nigrosin (India ink) stain

This stain is used to identify *Cryptococcus neoformans* in clinical specimens. A drop of India ink is put on the slide, followed by a drop of the specimen, and mixed together. A coverslip is applied and the slide is examined under light microscopy. *Cryptococcus neoformans* is identified by a clear zone (capsule) around the organism.

Growth requirements

These can vary considerably and include the following.

Atmosphere

Organisms can be divided into categories according to their atmospheric requirements:

- *Strict aerobes* grow only in the presence of oxygen.
- *Strict anaerobes* grow only in the absence of oxygen.
- *Facultative organisms* grow aerobically or anaerobically.
- *Microaerophilic organisms* grow best in atmospheres with reduced oxygen concentration (e.g., 5–10% CO_2).
- *Capnophilic organisms* require additional CO_2 for growth.

Temperature

Organisms can also be differentiated by their temperature requirements:

- *Psychrophilic organisms* grow at temperatures of 10–30°C.
- *Mesophilic organisms* grow at temperatures of 30–40°C.
- *Thermophilic organisms* grow at temperatures of 50–60°C.

Most clinically encountered organisms are mesophilic.

Nutrition

Some organisms grow readily on ordinary nutrient media, whereas others have particular nutritional requirements, e.g., *Haemophilus infleunzae* requires the specific growth factors factor X (hemin) and factor V (nicotinic adenine dinucleotide [NAD]).

Colonial morphology

Bacterial colonies of a single species, when grown on specific media under controlled conditions, are described by their characteristic size, shape, texture, and color.

Colonies may be flat or raised, smooth or irregular, and pigmented (e.g., *Pseudomonas aeruginosa* is green/blue or *Serratia marcescens* is red) or nonpigmented. Experienced laboratory technicians can often provisionally identify an organism using colonial appearance alone.

Hemolysis

Some organisms produce hemolysins that cause lysis of red blood cells in blood containing media. This hemolysis may be:

- β-hemolytic—a clear zone of complete hemolysis around the colony
- α-hemolytic—a green zone of incomplete hemolysis
- Nonhemolytic or γ-hemolytic

This feature is often used in the initial identification of streptococci.

Biochemical tests

A variety of biochemical tests may be used for the identification of bacteria in the diagnostic laboratory.

Catalase test

Many aerobic and facultatively anaerobic organisms are catalase positive, whereas streptococci and enterococci are catalase negative. Hydrogen peroxide solution is drawn up into a capillary tube and the tip is then touched onto a colony. Vigorous bubbling indicates the presence of catalase.

Coagulase test

This test is used to differentiate the staphyloocci. Coagulase exists in two forms: bound coagulase/clumping factor (detected by the slide coagulase test) and free coagulase (detected by the tube coagulase test).

Slide coagulase test

A colony is emulsified in a drop of distilled water on a slide. A loop or wire is dipped into plasma and then mixed into the bacterial suspension. A positive test result occurs if agglutination is seen within 10 seconds.

Tube coagulase test

A colony is emulsified in a tube containing plasma and incubated at 37°C for 4 hours. A visible clot indicates a positive result. If negative at 4 hours, the tube should be reincubated overnight. Some species, e.g., MRSA, may give a negative result at 4 hours.

Deoxyribonuclease (DNase) test

This test is used to identify pathogenic staphylococci (e.g., *S. aureus* and *S. schleiferi*) that produce large quantities of extracellular DNase. A colony is streaked onto a DNase plate and incubated at 37°C for 18–24 hours. The following day, the plate is flooded with hydrochloric acid—unhydrolysed DNA is precipitated, producing a white opacity in the agar.

Cultures surrounded by a clear zone (hydrolysed DNA) are DNase positive. Some strains of MRSA are DNase negative, and *S. epidermidis* may be weakly positive.

Optochin test

This test is used to differentiate *S. pneumoniae* (optochin sensitive) from other α-hemolytic streptococci (optochin resistant). Optochin (ethylhydrocupreine hydrochloride) is a chemical that causes lysis of the cell wall of *S. pneumoniae*.

An optochin disc is placed in the center of the bacterial inoculum and incubated at 37°C in 5% CO_2 for 18–24 hours. A zone of inhibition ≥5 mm indicates a positive result.

Esculin hydrolysis test

This test is used to differentiate enterococci (esculin positive) from streptococci (esculin negative). It tests the ability of the organism to hydrolyse esculin to esculetin and glucose in the presence of 10–40% bile. The esculetin combines with ferric ions in the medium to form a black complex. The organism is inoculated onto a bile esculin plate or slant and incubated at 37°C for 24 hours. Presence of a dark brown or black halo indicates a positive result.

Indole test

The indole test is used to differentiate the *Enterobacteriaceae*. It detects the ability of an organism to produce indole from the amino acid tryptophan. A colored product is obtained when indole is combined with certain aldehydes. There are two methods:

- *Spot indole test:* a piece of filter paper is moistened with the indole reagent and a colony is smeared onto the surface. A green/blue color indicates a positive result.
- *Tube indole test:* the organism is emulsified in a peptone broth and incubated at 37°C for 24 hours. Then 0.5 mL of Kovac's reagent is added; a pink color in the top layer indicates a positive result.

ONPG (β-galactosidase) test

This test is used as an aid to differentiate the *Enterobacteriaceae*. Two enzymes, permease and β-galactosidase, are required for lactose fermentation. Late lactose fermenters do not possess permease but do have β-galactosidase.

Tubes containing ortho-nitrophenyl-β-D-galactopyranoside (ONPG) are inoculated with the organism and incubated at 37°C for 24 hours. If present, β-galactosidase hydrolyses ONPG to produce galactose and o-nitrophenol, a yellow compound.

Urease test

This test is used to differentiate urease-positive *Proteus* spp. from the other *Enterobacteriaceae*. Some strains of *Enterobacter* and *Klebsiella* spp. are urease positive. A slant of Christensen's medium is inoculated with the test organism and at 37°C for 24 hours. A pink/purple color indicates a positive result.

Oxidase test

This test determines if an organism has the cytochrome oxidase enzyme and is used as an aid in the differentiation of *Pseudomonas, Neisseria, Moraxella, Campylobacter,* and *Pasteurella* spp. (oxidase positive). Cytochrome oxidase catalyses the transport of electrons from donor compounds (e.g., NADH) to electron acceptors (usually oxygen).

The test reagent, *N, N, N', N'-tetra-methyl-p-phenylenediamine dihydrochloride,* acts as an artificial electron acceptor for the enzyme oxidase. The oxidized reagent forms the colored compound indophenol blue.

Overview of Gram-positive cocci

Gram-positive cocci are commonly isolated from clinical specimens. They are widely distributed in the environment and are found as commensals of the skin, mucous membranes, and other body sites. Because of their ubiquitous nature, recovery of these organisms from specimens should always be interpreted in the context of the clinical presentation.

Classification

Gram-positive cocci can be classified into a number of groups. The family *Micrococcaceae* includes four genera:
- *Planococcus:* marine cocci, nine species
- *Micrococcus:* large cocci 1–1.8 micrometer in diameter, three species
- *Stomatococcus:* upper respiratory tract commensal, one species
- *Staphylococcus:* human and animal commensals and pathogens, 0.5–1 micrometer in diameter, many species

The other important group of Gram-positive cocci is the streptococci and similar organisms. They belong to a number of families:
- *Staphyococcaceae,* genus *Gemella*
- *Lactillobacillaceae,* genus *Pediococcus*
- *Aerococcaeceae,* genus *Aerococcus, Abiotrophia,* etc.
- *Carnobacteriaceae,* genus *Alloiococcus*
- *Enterococcaceae,* genus *Enterococcus*
- *Leuconostocaceae,* genus *Leuconostoc*
- *Streptococcaceae,* genus *Streptococcus, Lactococcus*

Staphylocci

Staphylococci are nonmotile, non–spore-forming, catalase-positive, Gram-positive cocci. They occur as single cells, pairs, tetrads, or grape-like clusters (most common). Most species are facultative anaerobes, except *S. aureus* subsp. *anaerobius* and *S. saccharolyticus,* which are anaerobic.

Staphylococci are normally found on the skin and mucous membranes of animals. In some cases, their location may be very specific, e.g., *S. capitis* subsp. *capitis* on the scalp or *S. auricularis* in the external auditory canal.

S. aureus, S. epidermidis, and *S. saprophyticus* are the main human pathogens. They may be differentiated on the basis of the coagulase test (see Box 3.1) into coagulase positive (e.g., *S. aureus*) and coagulase negative (CoNS, e.g., *S. epidermidis*).

In addition, *S. aureus* produces DNase (deoxyribonuclease) whereas other staphylococci are usually DNase negative.

There are 30 or so species of CoNS, but it is rarely necessary to identify them at the species level.

Streptococci

The streptococci are nonsporing, nonmotile organisms, catalase-negative Gram-positive cocci that grow in pairs and chains. Some species are capsulated. They are facultative anaerobes and often require enriched media to grow.

The streptococci are subdivided on the basis of their classic appearance on sheep blood agar into α-, β- and γ (non)-hemolytic streptococci.

The α-hemolytic streptococci (incomplete hemolysis on blood agar, resulting in a greenish tinge) include *Streptococcus pneumoniae* (p. 190) and the viridans streptococci. The β-hemolytic streptococci (complete hemolysis and clear zone on blood agar) are grouped on the basis of their Lancefield carbohydrate antigens. The medically important ones are Groups A, B, C, F, and G.

The enterococci (*E. faecalis* and others, p. 192) were originally called *Streptococcus faecalis* and often react with group D antisera but are now a separate genus.

Nonhemolytic streptococci make up the remainder and include the viridans streptococci (*S. mutans, S. salivarus, S. anginosus, S. mitis,* and *S. sanguinis* groups), the anaerobic, and the nutritionally variant streptococci.

For a comprehensive review of taxonomic and nomenclature changes of the streptococci, see Facklam (2002).[1]

Other Gram-positive cocci

These include *Peptococcus, Peptostreptococcus, Leuconostoc, Pedioccoccus, Abiotrophia, Micrococcus,* and *Stomatococcus.*

Reference

1. Facklam R (2002). What happened to the streptococci: overview of taxonomic and nomenclature changes. *Clin Microbiol Rev* 15(4):613–630.

Staphylococcus aureus

S. aureus is a facultatively anaerobic, nonmotile, non–spore-forming, catalase-positive, coagulase-positive, Gram-positive coccus.

It is a major human pathogen and can cause a wide variety of infections ranging from superficial skin infections to severe life-threatening conditions, e.g., toxic shock syndrome.

Epidemiology

S. aureus is a skin colonizer and is found in the anterior nares of 10–40% of people. Chronic carriage is associated with an increased risk of infection, e.g., in hemodialysis patients. Nasal carriage has contributed to the persistence and spread of methicillin-resistant *S. aureus* (MRSA).

Pathogenesis

S. aureus possesses a wide array of virulence factors:

- *Biofilm* is an extracellular polysaccharide network produced by staphylococci (and other organisms) that result in colonization and persistence on prosthetic material. Polysaccharide intracellular adhesin (PIA) is synthesized by the *ica* operon.
- *Capsule:* more than 90% of *S. aureus* isolates have a capsule, with 11 serotypes reported.
- *Surface adhesions:* also known as microbial surface components reacting with microbial surface components recognizing adherence matrix molecules (MSCRAMMs). These include protein A, clumping factor A and B, collagen-binding protein, fibronectin-binding protein, serine aspartate repeat protein, plasmin-sensitive protein, and surface proteins A to K.
- *Techoic and lipotechoic acids* are components of the cell wall. Lipotechoic acids trigger release of cytokines by macrophages.
- *Peptidoglcan* is the scaffold for anchoring the MSCRAMMs. It also triggers release of cytokines. Modification of peptidoglycan synthesis is associated with antimicrobial resistance.
- *Hemolysins:* *S. aureus* possesses four hemolysins (A, B, G, and D).
- *Panton–Valentine leukocidin* (PVL) is a hemolysin encoded by two genes (*lukS* and *lukF*) that are carried on a mobile phage (ΦSLT). PVL-producing strains are often community acquired and associated with furunculosis, severe hemorrhagic pneumonia, and clusters of MRSA skin infections
- *Exfoliative toxins:* ETA and ETB are encoded by the *eta* and *etb* genes, respectively. They cause staphylcococcal scalded skin syndrome.
- *Superantigens:* this group includes the toxic shock syndrome toxin (TSST-1) and staphylococcal enterotoxins (SEs). TSST-1 is associated with toxic shock syndrome; the SEs are associated with food poisoning.
- *Pathogenicity (genomic) islands* are structures that vary in size from 15 to 70 kB and harbor virulence and drug-resistance genes, e.g., SaPI1 and SaPI2 carry the gene for TSST-1.
- *Resistance islands:* MRSA contains a resistance island called SCC*mec*, which confers resistance to methicillin.

Clinical features

S. aureus can cause a wide spectrum of clinical infections:

- Skin and soft tissue infections, e.g., impetigo, folliculitis, furuncles, and carbuncles, hidradenitis suppuritiva, mastitis, wound infections, erysipelas, cellulitis, pyomyositis, necrotizing fasciitis
- Necrotizing pneumonia
- Bone and joint infections, e.g., septic arthritis, ostemyelitis
- Systemic infections, e.g., bacteremia, endocarditis, meningitis
- Prosthetic device–related infections, e.g., intravascular catheter-associated infections, pacemaker infections, prosthetic joint infections
- Toxin-mediated diseases, e.g., scalded skin syndrome, toxic shock syndrome

Diagnosis

In some cases, e.g., skin and soft tissue infections, the diagnosis is clinical. In others, appropriate samples, e.g., pus, tissue, or blood, should be taken and submitted to the lab for microscopy, culture, and identification:

- *Gram stain:* Gram-positive cocci in clusters
- *Culture on blood agar or liquid media:* growth usually occurs within 18–24 hours. Prolonged incubation detects small-colony variants.
- *Biochemical tests:* catalase-positive, coagulase-positive, DNase-positive
- *Identification:* Staphaurex (Remel) is a latex agglutination test for the detection of clumping factor and protein A associated with *S. aureus,* and API Staph (bioMérieux)
- *Typing methods* include pulsed field gel electrophoresis (PFGE), toxin typing, SCCmec typing, and spa typing
- *Molecular diagnosis,* e.g., 16S or 23S rRNA polymerase chain reaction (PCR) or *mecA* gene PCR (for methicillin resistance)

Treatment

Treatment depends on the type of infection and drug susceptibility of the organism.

- Dicloxacillin or first-generation cephalosporins (e.g., cefazolin) PO (orally) or nafcillin or cefazolin IV (intravenous) are used for methicillin-sensitive *S. aureus* (MSSA) isolates.
- Vancomycin IV is used in suspected *S. aureus* infections where MRSA is a possibility, e.g., a hospitalized patient with an intravascular catheter.
- Aminoglycosides exhibit synergism and are used in endocarditis to help sterilize the blood cultures.
- Other agents active against *S. aureus* include clindamycin, doxycycline, trimethoprim-sulfamethoxazole, quinupristin/dalfopristin, daptomycin, and linezolid.
- Duration of treatment depends on the cause: 7 days for skin and soft tissue infection and 4–6 weeks for endocarditis. In bacteremia if the source is removable, e.g., intravascular catheter, 2 weeks of treatment is adequate.

Prevention

Prevention of S. aureus infections is based on bacterial decolonization of carriers with local antiseptics, e.g., nasal mupirocin and chlorhexidine soap. This is usually only done for MRSA carriers.

A conjugate vaccine has been shown to reduce S. aureus bacteremia rates in hemodialysis patients.[1]

Reference

1. Shinerfield H, et al. (2002). Use of Staphylococcus conjugate vaccine in patients receiving hemodialysis. N Engl J Med 346:491–496.

Methicillin-resistant *S. aureus*

Methicillin-resistant S. aureus (MRSA) was first detected in 1961, a few months after methicillin was introduced into clinical practice. However, it was not until the 1980s that endemic strains of MRSA with multi-drug resistance became a global nosocomial problem.

The epidemic strains of MRSA have been classified as E-MRSA 1 to 17. These strains have different genetics from those of the other epidemic strains and produce different toxins. They are also resistant to the macrolides, clindamycin, and ciprofloxacin ± other agents.

Mechanism of resistance

MRSA strains are resistant to all β-lactams because of alteration in the penicillin-binding protein PBP2' and, consequently, the structure of the cell wall. Methicillin resistance is due to the *mecA* gene, which codes for the low-affinity penicillin-binding protein PBP2'. *mecA* is usually located on a mobile genetic element called SCC-*mec* (staphylococcal cassette chromosome).

There are five SCC-*mec* elements, defined by class of *mecA* gene and type of CCR complex (cassette chromosome recombinase). SCC-*mec* types I to III are usually found in hospital strains, while type IV is more common in the community strains.

Epidemiology

Risk factors for MRSA include increasing age, prior antibiotics, indwelling catheters, severe underlying disease, and intensive care unit (ICU) stay.

MRSA rates vary in different parts of the world. Countries like Finland, Denmark, and the Netherlands with very low levels of MRSA (<5%) have strictly enforced contact precautions, take surveillance cultures of patients and personnel, and limit the use of broad-spectrum antibiotics. By contrast, some Asian countries (e.g., Japan, China) have high MRSA rates, probably because of antibiotic overuse. Many middle-income (e.g., Turkey) and some high-income countries (e.g., UK, U.S.) have hyperendemic MRSA and usually focus available resources on high-risk patients. Some countries with endemic MRSA (e.g., Australia, France, Belgium) have managed to stabilize or even lower MRSA prevalence in defined areas.

Recent changes in the epidemiology of MRSA include the following:
- Increase in MRSA bacteremia rates
- Emergence of new community-acquired MRSA strains, which are genetically different from previous health care–associated strains and tend to be more virulent

Clinical features

MRSA causes similar infections to those of methicillin-sensitive strains of S. aureus (see Staphylococcus aureus, p. 182). Community-acquired MRSA (CA-MRSA) was originally seen in people with a previous history of hospitalization or who were related to health care workers. Since the late 1990s, however, serious infections caused by CA-MRSA have been reported in previously healthy individuals.

CA-MRSA is several times more likely to cause skin and soft tissue infections, often complicated by deep abscesses or necrotizing fasciitis.[1] There have been community outbreaks of severe CA-MRSA pneumonia.[2]

CA-MRSA is defined genetically (type IV SCCmec; distinct PFGE profile) and has evolved from community MSSA, rather than from hospital MRSA. This genotype is often sensitive to non-β-lactam antibiotics and is PVL positive.

The highly successful USA-300 clone has caused considerable morbidity and mortality in the United States.[3]

Laboratory diagnosis of MRSA

- Criteria for methicillin resistance are presence of mecA gene or oxacillin minimum inhibition concentration (MIC) >2 mg/L or methicillin MIC >4 mg/L or cefoxitin MIC >4 mg/L.
- Molecular detection of the mecA gene is the diagnostic gold standard but is not available in many routine laboratories.
- Conventional methods for detecting MRSA rely on the use of selective media (oxacillin mannitol salt agar with 7% NaCl, incubated at 37°C for 18–48 hours). Broth enrichment in 7% NaCl prior to plating on selective media increases the diagnostic rate but increases the time for diagnosis by 24 hours.
- Chromogenic agars are routinely used for MRSA screening.
- Latex agglutination tests to detect PBP2' are also commercially available (Hardy Diagnostics).

Treatment of MRSA

Vancomycin is the treatment of choice. Drug concentrations should be monitored, and current practice is tending toward greater serum antibiotic levels (e.g., trough of >10 mg/L).[4]

There is variable susceptibility to trimethoprim, rifampin, tetracycline, doxycycline, clindamycin, and the aminoglycosides (e.g., gentamicin). These may provide alternative treatment choices if oral therapy or a second agent is required.

Newer agents active against MRSA include linezolid, quinupristin with dalfopristin (Synercid®), and daptomycin. These are all licensed for treating skin and soft tissue infections. In addition, linezolid and synercid may be used for pneumonia.

Infection control issues

The main strategies for controlling MRSA are isolation and cohorting of patients, appropriate hand hygiene by health care workers, and effective cleaning of shared equipment.

References

1. Miller LG, et al. (2005). Necrotizing faciitis caused by community-associated methicillin-resistant *Staphylococcus aureus* in Los Angeles. *N Engl J Med* 352:1445–1453.

2. Francis S, et al. (2005). Severe community-onset pneumonia in healthy adults caused by methicillin-resistant *Staphylococcus aureus* carrying the Pantone–Valentine leukocidin genes. *Clin Infect Dis* 40:100–107.

3. Moran GJ, et al. (2006). Methicillin-resistant *S. aureus* infections among patients in the emergency department. *N Engl J Med* 355:666–674.

4. Rybak M, et al. (2009). Therapeutic monitoring of vancomycin in adult patients. *Am J Health System Pharm* 66:82–98.

Glycopeptide resistance in *S. aureus*

Mechanism of resistance

The mechanisms of vancomycin resistance in *S. aureus* are as follows:
- Increase in cell wall turnover that leads to an increase of non–cross-linked D-alanyl-D-alanine side chains that bind vancomycin outside the cell wall and inhibit binding to target peptides
- Transfer of the enterococcal *vanA* determinant from *E. faecium* to *S. aureus*

Intermediate resistance

Strains of *S. aureus* with homogenously reduced susceptibility to glycopeptides (vancomycin MIC ≥8 mg/L) have been reported in several countries, e.g., Japan, France, and the United States. These organisms have been termed *vancomycin-intermediate S. aureus* (VISA), or *glycopeptide-intermediate sensitivity S. aureus* (GISA) on the basis of U.S. Clinical Laboratory Standards Institute (CLSI) vancomycin MIC breakpoints:
- Susceptible   ≤4 mg/L
- Intermediate 8–16 mg/L (VISA)
- Resistant   ≥32 mg/L (VRSA)

Heteroresistance

A much more common situation is for a strain to yield a small proportion of daughter cells (1 in 10^5) able to grow in the presence of 8 mg/L of vancomycin. Such heterogeneously resistant strains are called *hetero-VISA* and there is considerable debate about their clinical significance.

Vancomycin resistance

The first clinical VRSA infection was reported in the United States in 2002. VRSA (vancomycin MIC >128 mg/L) was isolated from a hemodialysis catheter tip and a chronic foot ulcer of a patient in Michigan. Vancomycin-resistant *E. faecalis* was also isolated from the ulcer, raising the possibility of transfer of the *vanA* determinant.

Clinical and epidemiological characteristics

The first GISA infection occurred in 1995 in France in a child with leukemia and catheter-associated MRSA bacteremia.

The second GISA infection occurred in 1996 in Japan in a 4-month-old infant with an MRSA sternal wound infection.

Seven VISA infections were reported in the United States between 1997 and 2000. These all had several features in common:

- Prolonged vancomycin exposure (3–18 weeks)
- Prior MRSA infection
- Underlying disease, especially renal failure
- Prosthetic devices, e.g., intravascular catheters, peritoneal dialysis (PD) catheter

The first VRSA infection was reported in the U.S. in 2000. Since then, six further VRSA infections have been reported in the United States.

Laboratory detection

The detection of glycopeptide resistance in S. aureus is problematic, as both VISA and hetero-VISA isolates appear susceptible to vancomycin by routine susceptibility tests. Furthermore, there have been conflicting recommendations regarding methods of detection:

U.S. guidelines

All laboratories should have an algorithm by which they can identify strains of S. aureus that may need additional testing. Laboratories should use acceptable confirmatory testing methods, e.g., 24-hour incubation and MIC susceptibility testing method. Any S. aureus with a vancomycin MIC ≥4 mg/L should be referred to a reference laboratory or the Centers for Disease Control and Prevention (CDC) for confirmatory testing.

Infection control issues

MRSA is known to be highly transmissible in health care settings, and it seems reasonable to assume that VISA and VRSA will be likewise highly transmissible. Although infection control experience with VRSA is limited, implementation of rigorous infection control procedures is crucial for containing an outbreak of VRSA in a hospital setting.

The U.S. Hospital Infection Control Practices Advisory Committee (HICPAC) has published infection control guidelines for all staphylococci with a vancomycin MIC ≥8 mg/L:

- Use contact precautions as recommended for multi-drug-resistant organisms (handwashing, gloves, gowns ± masks). Monitor and enforce compliance with contact precautions.
- Isolate the patient in a private room. Minimize the number of people in contact with and caring for the patient. Begin one-to-one care with specified personnel.
- Initiate epidemiological and laboratory investigations with the help of the state health department and CDC. Determine the extent of transmission within the facility. Assess the efficacy of precautions by monitoring the acquisition of VISA/VRSA by personnel.
- Educate all health care personnel about the epidemiology of VISA/VRSA and appropriate infection control precautions.

- Consult with state health departments and CDC before transferring or discharging the patient.
- Inform appropriate personnel about the presence of VISA/VRSA, e.g., emergency department personnel, admitting medical team.

Prevention

The appropriate use of antimicrobials, especially vancomycin, is paramount in preventing the continued emergence of VISA and VRSA. Several studies have shown that vancomycin is frequently used for inappropriate reasons.

Strategies to reduce inappropriate vancomycin use are essential, e.g., minimizing use of temporary central venous catheters, use of diagnostic techniques to avoid prolonged empiric use of vancomycin, and prompt removal of S. aureus–infected prosthetic devices.

Coagulase-negative staphylococci

The coagulase-negative staphylococci (CoNS) may present as culture contaminants or be true pathogens. Infection is often associated with the presence of prosthetic material, e.g., intravascular catheters, cardiac valves, and joint implants.

Infections are often indolent, but treatment may require removal of the foreign material. These organisms are often resistant to multiple antibiotics, which can make therapy difficult.

Epidemiology

CoNS are ubiquitous and are natural inhabitants of the skin. S. epidermidis is the most common species, accounting for 65–90% of all isolates, followed by S. hominis. S. saprophyticus is a urinary pathogen. S. saccharolyticus is the only strict anaerobe.

Other less frequent species include S. haemolyticus, S. warneri, S. xylosus, S. cohnii, S. simulans, S. capitis, S. auricularis, S. lugdunensis, and S. schleiferi (some spp. are coagulase positive).

Pathogenesis

Plasmid DNA is abundant in all species of CoNS, but only a few of the plasmid-encoded genes have been identified. Plasmid-mediated antibiotic resistance to a wide variety of antibiotics can occur and may be transferred by conjugation with other organisms.

CoNS also produce polysaccharide intracellular adhesin (PIA), resulting in biofilm formation, particularly on prosthetic devices. This biofilm protects the organisms from antibiotics and host defense mechanisms.

S. saprophyticus produces a number of substances that enable it to attach and invade the uroepithelium.

Clinical features

- Nosocomial bacteremia (most common cause)
- Endocarditis
- Intravascular catheter-related infections, e.g., lines, pacemaker wires
- Cerebrospinal fluid (CSF) shunt infections
- Peritoneal dialysis catheter-associated peritonitis
- Urinary tract infections (UTIs) (S. saprophyticus)
- Bacteremia in immunocompromised patients
- Sternal osteomyelitis (post–cardiothoracic surgery)
- Prosthetic joint infections
- Vascular graft infections
- Neonatal nosocomial bacteremias
- Endophthalmitis (after surgery or trauma)

Diagnosis

Appropriate samples, e.g., blood, pus, tissues, should be taken and submitted to the laboratory for microbiological examination. The following tests may be performed:

- Gram stain: Gram-positive cocci in clusters
- Culture on blood agar or liquid media: growth usually occurs within18–24 hours
- Catalase-positive
- Coagulase-negative (exceptions: S. schleiferi)
- DNase test-negative, or weakly positive
- Antimicrobial susceptibility testing
- Biochemical tests, e.g., API Staph
- Typing, e.g., PFGE
- Molecular diagnosis, e.g. 16S or 23S rRNA PCR or mecA gene PCR (for methicillin resistance)

Treatment

Infections usually require the removal of prosthetic material, if present. CoNS are often resistant to multiple antibiotics; >70% are resistant to methicillin. Most CoNS are sensitive to vancomycin, linezolid, quinupristin/dalfopristin, and daptomycin.

S. saprophyticus urinary tract infections may be treated with trimethoprim, nitrofurantoin, or a fluoroquinolone.

Streptococci—overview

For an introduction to streptococci, see Overview of Gram-positive cocci, p. 180.

Table 3.1 Classification of streptococci

Hemolysis	Lancefield group	Species name	Clinical syndromes
α		S. pneumoniae	Pneumococcal pneumonia, bacteremia, meningitis, otitis media, sinusitis
α		Viridans streptococci	Dental caries, endocarditis
β	A	S. pyogenes	Invasive (necrotizing fasciitis, GAS toxic shock syndrome, bacteremia); pharyngitis, skin infections
β	B	S. agalactiae	Neonatal meningitis and bactermemia
β	C	S. dysgalactiae subsp. dysgalactiae S. dysgalactiae subsp. equisimilis S. equi subsp. equi S. equi subsp. zooepidemicus	Pharyngitis, cellulitis
β or γ	D	S. bovis and others	S. bovis endocarditis, S. suis bacteremia and meningitis
β	G		Cellulitis
β or γ	F	S. milleri (reclassified as S. constellatus, S. intermedius, and S. anginosus)	Infective endocarditis, abscesses
γ	–	Viridans streptococci	Infective endocarditis

Streptococcus pneumoniae

S. pneumoniae was first isolated in 1881 by Sternberg in the United States and by Louis Pasteur in France. It became recognized as the most common cause of lobar pneumonia and was given the name pneumococcus. S. pneumoniae is an important bacterial pathogen of humans, causing meningitis, sinusitis, otitis media, endocarditis, septic arthritis, peritonitis, and a number of other infections.

It is a Gram-positive coccus that grows in pairs (diplococci) or chains. It produces pneumolysin, which causes α-hemolysis (green discoloration due to breakdown of hemoglobin) of blood agar. It is catalase negative, inhibited by ethyl hydrocupreine (optochin sensitive) and lysed by bile salts.

Epidemiology

S. pneumoniae colonizes the nasopharynx of 5–10% of healthy adults and 20–40% of healthy children. The rate of colonization is seasonal, with an increase in winter.

The rate of invasive pneumococcal disease is 15/100,000 persons/year. The incidence is up to 10-fold higher in certain populations, e.g., African Americans, Alaskans, and Australian aboriginals. Invasive pneumococcal disease is more common at the extremes of age (<2 years or >65 years).

Risk factors for pneumococcal infection include antibody deficiencies, complement deficiency, neutropenia or impaired neutrophil function, asplenia, corticosteroids, malnutrition, alcoholism, chronic diseases (liver, renal, diabetes, asthma, chronic obstructive pulmonary disease [COPD]), and overcrowding.

Antimicrobial resistance is increasing. Rates are high in European countries, e.g., Spain, and Hungary, and in Asia, e.g., Thailand, Hong Kong, Vietnam, and Korea. The major source of resistance is the worldwide geographic spread of a few clones that harbor resistance determinants.

Pathogenesis

A number of virulence factors have been identified:
- Capsular polysaccharide >90 serotypes (prevents phagocytosis, activates complement)
- Cell wall polysaccharide (activates complement and cytokine release)
- Pneumolysin (activates complement and cytokines)
- PspA (inhibits phagocytosis by blocking activation and deposition of complement)
- PspC (inhibits phagocytosis by binding complement factor H)
- PsaA (mediates adherence)
- Autolysin (causes release of bacterial components)
- Neuraminidase (possibly mediates adherence)

Antimicrobial resistance mechanisms

Penicillin resistance is mediated by alterations in PBP2a (low-level resistance) and mutations in PBP2X (high-level resistance).

Macrolide resistance is mediated by acquisition of *ermB* (ribosomal methylase) and *mefA* (efflux pump) genes.

Clinical features

S. pneumoniae may cause infection either by direct spread of the organism from the nasopharynx to contiguous structures (e.g., middle ear, sinuses, and lungs) or by hematogenous spread (to the central nervous system [CNS], heart valves, bones, joints, peritoneum).

Clinical syndromes include the following:
- Otitis media
- Sinusitis
- Meningitis
- Exacerbation of chronic bronchitis
- Pneumonia
- Meningitis

- Endocarditis
- Septic arthritis
- Osteomyelitis
- Peritonitis
- Others: percarditis, epidural abscess, cerebral abscess, skin and soft tissue infections. Unusual infections should prompt investigation for HIV.

Diagnosis

- Grows on routine media—causes α-hemolysis of blood agar
- Gram-positive lanceolate diplococci, often with visible capsule
- Identification: catalase negative, optochin sensitive, soluble in 10% bile salts. Commercial identification tests (e.g., latex agglutination tests, and serotyping tests) are available.
- Penicillin MIC should be determined for invasive isolates.

Treatment

Treatment depends on the nature and severity of the presenting infection and drug susceptibility results.

- Penicillin MIC <0.1 mg/L: penicillin or amicillin
- Penicillin MIC >0.1 ≤1.0 mg/L: ceftriaxone or cefotaxime for meningitis. High-dose penicillin or ampicillin is likely to be effective for non-meningeal sites of infection, e.g., pneumonia.
- Penicillin MIC ≥2.0 mg/L: vancomycin ± rifampin. If non-meningeal site, also consider ceftriaxone or cefotaxime, high-dose ampicillin, carbapenem, active fluoroquinolone, e.g., moxifloxacin

Prevention

- *Immunization:* the 7-valent pneumococcal conjugate vaccine (PCV) is approved for use in children. The 23-valent unconjugated polysaccharide vaccine is given to 'at-risk' adult groups, e.g., those >65 years old or with homozygous sickle cell disease, asplenia/severe splenic dysfunction, chronic renal disease or nephrotic syndrome, celiac disease, immunodeficiency or immunosuppression due to disease or treatment, including HIV infection, chronic diseases (cardiac, respiratory, liver, renal), or diabetes mellitus, or patients with cochlear implants.
- *Antimicrobial prophylaxis:* oral penicillin VK is recommended for the prevention of pneumococcal disease in asplenic patients.

Enterococci

Enterococci are environmental organisms found in the soil, water, food, and the gastrointestinal (GI) tract of animals. They are Gram-positive cocci that occur singly, in pairs, or in chains and thus resemble streptococci. Until fairly recently they were classified among the Lancefield group D streptococci. In the 1980s they were reclassified as a separate genus, *Enteroccoccus*, because of different pathogenic, biochemical, and serological profiles.

At least 12 different species exist. *E. faecalis* is the most common clinical isolate (80–90%), followed by *E. faecium* (5–10%). Others include *E. avium, E. casseliflavus, E. durans, E. gallinarum, E. hirae,* and *E. raffinosus.*

Epidemiology

Enterococci are part of the normal gut flora and can cause endogenous or exogenous infections, both in and out of hospital. In the hospital setting, enterococci are readily transmissible between patients and institutions. In the United States, enterococci are a common cause of nosocomial infections.

Risk factors for nosocomial enterococcal infections include GI colonization, severe underlying disease, prolonged hospitalization, prior surgery, renal failure, neutropenia, transplantation, urinary or vascular catheters, and ICU admission.

Pathogenesis

Enterococci are less intrinsically virulent than organisms such as *S. aureus* and group A streptococci. They do not have classical virulence factors but are able to adhere to heart valves and renal epithelial cells. Several extracellular molecules play an important role in colonization and adherence, e.g., aggregation factor and extracellular surface protein. Other virulence factors include extracellular serine protease and gelatinase (GelE) and hemolysins.

Enterococci are frequently found in cultures of intra-abdominal and pelvic infections. Their role in this setting has not been clearly defined.

Enterococcal bacteremia carries a high mortality (42–68%), but it is not clear whether this is due to the organism itself or a marker of severe debilitation. However, epidemiological studies have calculated an attributed mortality of 31–37% in patients with enterococcal bacteremia.

The intrinsic resistance of enterococci to many antibiotics enables them to survive and multiply in patients receiving broad-spectrum agents and accounts for their ability to cause superinfections.

Clinical features

- Urinary tract infections (most common)
- Bacteremia and endocarditis
- Intra-abdominal and pelvic infections
- Skin, wound, and soft tissue infections
- Meningitis (associated with anatomical defects, trauma, or surgery)
- Respiratory infections (rare)
- Neonatal sepsis

Diagnosis

- *Gram stain:* elongated Gram-positive cocci (cigar-shaped), often in pairs and short chains
- *Culture:* facultative anaerobes that can grow under extreme conditions, e.g., 6.5% NaCl, pH 9.6, temperatures of 10°C to 45°C
- *Biochemical tests:* enterococci hydrolyse esculin and L-pyrrolidonyl-B-naphthylamide (PYR)
- They usually agglutinate with group D in streptococcal grouping kits.

- Intrinsically resistant to aminoglycosides (low levels), β-lactams (high MICs), lincosamides (low level), co-trimoxazole (in vivo), and quinupristin/dalfopristin (E. faecalis)
- Isolates should be tested for susceptibility to ampicillin, high-level gentamicin and streptomycin resistance (blood stream infections), vancomycin, linezolid, daptomycin, quinupristin/dalfopristin, and nitrofurantoin (UTIs).

Treatment

Enterococci are intrinsically resistant to many agents (e.g., cephalosporins, ciprofloxacin), and readily acquire new resistance mechanisms.

Ampicillin is the usual first-line agent for E. faecalis infections, with vancomycin as an alternative. E. faecium is usually resistant to ampicillin.

When bactericidal therapy is needed (e.g., endocarditis, meningitis), combination synergistic therapy of a cell-wall agent plus aminoglycoside is standard.

Ciprofloxacin may be active in vitro but is not usually recommended clinically (apart from occasionally for UTIs). Newer fluoroquinolones are said to be more active against the enterococci but not against ciprofloxacin-resistant strains, which may preclude their usefulness.

E. gallinarum and E. casseliflavus have intrinsic low-level resistance to glycopeptides (pentapeptide terminates D-alanine-D-serine).

High-level resistance to aminoglycosides and vancomycin resistance (VRE) are increasing problems. VRE bacteremia has a worse prognosis than vancomycin-sensitive enterococcal bacteremia, but this may be related to comorbidity and delay in receiving appropriate antibiotic therapy.

Streptococcus bovis

S. bovis bacteremia and endocarditis are associated with gastrointestinal disease (primarily colonic malignancy). There are two biotypes of S. bovis: S. bovis biotype 1 (i.e., S. gallolyticus subsp. gallolyticus) bacteremia has a higher correlation with underlying GI malignancy and endocarditis (71% and 94%, respectively, in one study) than S. bovis biotype 2.

Pathogenesis

It is not clear whether S. bovis is a marker for malignancy or has an etiological role. In some cases, S. bovis bacteremia is the only pointer to the GI disease. There are also reports of the malignancy being found up to 2 years after the initial S. bovis infection. There seems to be an increase in stool carriage of S. bovis in patients with malignancy or premalignancy compared to that in healthy subjects.

Some investigators have suggested that biotype I has a type-specific adherence mechanism, which enables adherence to both cardiac valves and abnormal colonic mucosa.

Clinical features

The main clinical infections due to S. bovis are bacteremia and endocarditis. Occasionally, S. bovis causes other infections such UTIs, meningitis, or neonatal sepsis. The GI tract is the usual portal of entry for bacteremia, and there is a strong association of bacteremia with endocarditis.

Most patients with endocarditis have an underlying valve abnormality or prosthetic valve. They tend to have a subacute course, indistinguishable clinically from endocarditis due to the *Streptococcus viridans* group, but studies suggest that *S. bovis* endocarditis has a higher mortality rate (45%) than that of non–*S. bovis* endocarditis (25%).

Diagnosis

S. bovis may be misidentified as enterococci or viridans streptococci (notably *S. salivarus*).

Biochemical tests

S. bovis shares a number of properties with enterococci, e.g., they agglutinate with group D antisera, hydrolyse esculin, and are bile tolerant. However, they differ from enterococci by not growing in 6.5% salt, are PYR negative, and do not grow at 10°C.

Identification

The API Rapid Strep reliably identifies *S. bovis* and differentiates it to the biotype level, which is important for association with malignancy and endocarditis. Generally, *S. bovis* biotype 1 strains produce extracellular glucan from sucrose, hydrolyse starch, and ferment mannitol; *S. bovis* biotype 2 strains are usually negative for these tests. A PCR to differentiate the biotypes has been developed.

Treatment

S. bovis is highly susceptible to penicillin (MICs 0.01–0.12 mcg/mL). It is also susceptible to ampicillin, the antipseudomonal penicillins, erythromycin, clindamycin, and vancomycin.

Penicillin is the treatment of choice for *S. bovis* infections. Vancomycin is an alternative in β-lactam-allergic patients.

Although penicillin/aminoglycoside combinations show synergy against *S. bovis*, combination therapy is no more effective than penicillin alone for treatment of endocarditis.

All patients with *S. bovis* bacteremia should have a comprehensive work-up to exclude colonic malignancy and endocarditis.

Viridans streptococci

The viridans streptococci, sometimes known as the oral streptococci, are important in dental caries and endocarditis, bacteremia, and deep-seated infections. They include *S. sanguis*, *S. mutans*, *S. mitis*, and *S. salivarus*. This heterogenous group has been reclassified into five distinct groups on the basis of 16S rRNA gene sequence analysis:

- The *S. mutans* group is now divided into seven species collectively known as the *mutans streptococci*. The most common are *S. mutans* and *S. sobrinus*.
- The *S. sanguinis* group is now divided into *S. sanguinis*, *S. gordonii*, *S. parasanguis*, and *S. crista*.

- The S. milleri group is now divided into three species: S. constellatus; S. intermedius, and S. anginosus, now called the S. anginosus group or group F.
- The S. mitis group includes S. mitis, S. mitior, and S. oralis.
- The S. salivarus group includes S. salivarus and S. vestibularis.

Epidemiology

The viridans streptococci are commensals of the human upper respiratory tract, femal genital tract, and gastrointestinal tract, with large numbers present in the mouth. Each species has its own particular ecological niche.

Pathogenesis

These organisms seem to possess few virulence factors.

The ability to produce acid, especially by S. mutans, is thought to be important in dental caries. Production of various carbohydrates, which aid adherence to tooth enamel and gums, is important in the establishment and maintenance of colonization.

Extracellular dextran production is important in the adherence of organisms to heart valves and in resistance to antimicrobial therapy. Fibronectin production also mediates adherence to heart valves.

Clinical features

- Endocarditis (common cause in patients with abnormal valves)
- Bacteremia (especially in neutropaenic patients)
- Meningitis
- Pneumonia
- Other infections include abscesses, pericarditis, peritonitis, sialadenitis, odontgenic infections, and endophthalmitis.

Diagnosis

- Facultatively anaerobic Gram-positive cocci, catalase negative
- Most are α-hemolytic on blood agar; some are nonhemolytic.
- Resistant to optochin and lack bile solubility (unlike pneumococci)
- Unable to grow in 6.5% NaCl (unlike enterococci)
- Can be identified by biochemical tests or API STREP

Treatment

Community-acquired infections are usually sensitive to penicillin, which is the treatment of choice. Other β-lactams, e.g., ceftriaxone, also have good in vitro activity against viridans streptococci.

Nosocomial infections are associated with increased resistance to penicillin and other β-lactams.

Some strains, e.g., S. sanguis and S. gordonii, exhibit tolerance. They are inhibited at low concentrations of antibiotic, but high levels are required for bactericidal activity.

They are often resistant to aminoglyocides (when traditional breakpoints are applied) but exhibit synergy in combination with β-lactam antibiotics. This principle underlies combination treatment for bacterial endocarditis.

Vancomycin is used in penicillin-allergic patients and for penicillin-resistant infections.

Group A *Streptococcus*

Group A *Streptococcus* (GAS), also known as *Streptococcus pyogenes*, is responsible for a variety of conditions ranging from sore throat to severe invasive infections, such as necrotizing fasciitis, which have a mortality approaching 10%. There are also a number of postinfectious "immunological" conditions, such as post-streptococcal glomerulonephritis and rheumatic fever.

Epidemiology

Group A streptococci are upper respiratory tract commensals in 3–5% of adults and up to 10% of children. Transmission is mainly via droplet spread. Some people develop pharyngitis or tonsillitis, others are asymptomatic, and a handful will become carriers of GAS in the throat.

In the 1990s, the number of reports of invasive GAS increased globally, probably because of a re-emergence of more virulent strains.

Risk factors for sporadic disease include people >65 years old, those with recent varicella zoster (VZV) infection, HIV-positive individuals, those with diabetes, heart disease, cancer, or injecting drug use, or those on high-dose steroids.

Over time, the epidemiology of GAS infection in terms of clinical manifestation of disease has changed; e.g., scarlet fever and acute rheumatic fever have become less common and toxic shock has become more common over the last few decades.

Pathogenesis

Group A streptococci possess a number of virulence factors:
- *Somatic constituents:* hyaluronic capsule, M protein, serum opacity factor, lipotechoic acid, fibronectin-binding proteins
- *Extracellular products:* streptolysin O, streptolysin S, DNases A to D, hyaluronidase, streptokinase, streptococcal pyrogenic exotoxins (SpeA, SpeB, SpeC, SpeF), C5a peptidase, and streptococcal superantigens

Clinical features

- Pharyngitis is the most common infection. Suppurative complications include tonsillitis, peritonsillar abscess, retropharngeal abscess, suppurative cervical lymphadenitis, mastoiditis, sinusitis, and otitis media.
- Scarlet fever is a notifiable disease. It is similar to pharyngitis but associated with scarlatinal rash due to erythrogenic toxin production.
- Rheumatic fever may occur 1–5 weeks after pharyngitis. Relapses may occur.
- Post-streptococcal glomerulonephritis may occur after throat infections (commonly M types 12, 1, 25, 4, and 3) and skin infections (commonly M types 49, 52, 53–55, and 57–61) and is due to immunological cross-reactions between components of the glomerular basement membrane and cell membranes of nephritogenic streptococci.
- Impetigo, erysipelas, cellulitis, necrotizing fasciitis, pyomyositis
- Bacteremia: recent increase in group A streptococcal bacteremia in previously healthy adults. Also associated with intravenous drug users

- Puerperal sepsis is historically associated with group A streptococci.
- Streptococcal toxic shock syndrome, a fulminant disease with a high mortality, is mainly associated with types M1 and 3, but types 12 and 28 are also involved. It is differentiated from the other types of invasive disease by the occurrence of shock and multi-organ failure early in the course of the infection
- Others include meningitis, osteomyelitis, and septic arthritis.

Diagnosis

GAS are facultative anaerobic, catalase-positive, Gram-positive cocci, that tend to form long chains. They are nonsporing, nonmotile, and usually noncapsulate.

Culture on blood agar produces smooth, circular colonies of 2–3 mm diameter, which are usually β-hemolytic. Strains that produce hemolysin O and not hemolysin S will only demonstrate β-hemolysis when cultured anaerobically.

Lancefield grouping will reliably and accurately identify GAS. Most GAS are sensitive to bacitracin.

Serology is used to diagnose immunological complications, e.g., rheumatic fever, rather than in caute disease. A rise in anti-streptolysin O (ASO) titer confirms recent group A streptococcal disease. ASO titer is reliable in throat-associated disease, whereas anti-DNAase B is higher and more frequently raised in pyoderma-associated disease.

Treatment

The treatment of choice is oral phenoxymethylpenicillin (mild infections) or IV benzylpenicillin (severe infections). Pharyngitis is treated for 10 days.

In penicillin-allergic patients, options include azithromycin (which has comparative clinical and bacteriological response rates to those with phenoxymethylpenicillin but higher GI side effects), clindamycin, or a fluoroquinolone. GAS isolates may be resistant to macrolides, tetracycline, and/or fluoroquinolones, so sensitivity testing is required.

Treatment of more severe infections, e.g., toxic shock syndrome, usually requires addition of a second agent to the penicillin. Options include clindamycin (prevents toxin secretion).

Urgent surgical debridement is required in necrotizing fasciitis.

Prevention

- *Infection control:* GAS can spread from infected patients to close contacts, so isolate patients with invasive disease and involve the infection control team early.
- *Antimicrobial prophylaxis:* The available evidence suggests that routine administration of prophylactic antibiotics for close contacts of invasive disease is not justified. All household contacts should be informed of clinical manifestations of invasive disease and instructed to seek medical attention immediately if they develop any symptoms. Antibiotics are only given to certain high-risk groups.

Group B *Streptococcus*

Group B streptococci (GBS, *Streptococcus agalactiae*) were first reported as causes of puerperal sepsis in 1938. By the 1970s, group B streptococci had become the main cause of neonatal sepsis in infants aged <3 months.

Epidemiology

From 5% to 40% of women are colonized with GBS (genital tract or lower GI tract). Colonization of neonates usually occurs via the mother's genital tract. Risk factors are being African American and having diabetes.

Risk factors for early-onset neonatal GBS disease (≤7 days) include GBS bacteriruria, premature rupture of membranes, delivery <37 weeks, intrapartum fever or amnionitis, and prolonged rupture of membranes.

Risk factors for late-onset neonatal GBS disease (7–90 days) include overcrowding, poor hand hygiene, and increased length of hospital stay.

Over the past 20 years, there has been an increase in invasive group B streptococcal disease in nonpregnant adults, most of whom had underlying medical conditions. Risk factors include diabetes, chronic diseases (liver, renal, cardiovascular, pulmonary, GI, urological), neurological impairment, malignancy, HIV, corticosteroids, and splenectomy.

Pathogenesis

Bacterial virulence factors influencing the outcome between exposure and development of colonization/invasive disease include the polysaccharide capsule (in particular, high amounts of sialic acid and type III virulent strains).

Clinical features

Early-onset neonatal disease (defined as systemic infection in the first 6 days of life; mean age of onset = 12 hours, ± pneumonia or meningitis) tends to result from vertical transmission in utero or at the time of delivery.

Late-onset neonatal disease (onset 7 days to 3 months of age, mean = 24 days) arises from either horizontal transmission (often nosocomial, due to suboptimal nursery conditions) or vertical transmission.

GBS infection in adults and older children, especially those with underlying disease, includes bacteremia, postpartum infections, pneumonia, endocarditis, meningitis, arthritis, osteomyelitis, otitis media, conjunctivitis, UTI, skin and soft tissue infections, and meningitis.

Diagnosis

- GBS are facultative anaerobic, catalase-positive, Gram-positive cocci. They are nonsporing and nonmotile and usually capsulate.
- Culture on blood agar produces smooth, circular colonies of 2–3 mm diameter, which are usually surrounded by a very small zone of β-hemolysis.
- Selective media (e.g., Todd Hewitt broth) containing antimicrobials are used to enhance recovery of group B streptococci.

- *Identification:* Lancefield group B, resistant to bacitracin, hydrolyse sodium hippurate, do not hydrolyse esculin hydrolysis, production of CAMP factor (results in synergistic hemolysis with the B-lysin of *S. aureus* on sheep blood agar plate)
- *Typing:* GBS may be classified as serotypes I to VIII, on the basis of capsular polysaccharide and surface protein antigens. Other typing methods include multi-locus sequence typing (MLST) and PFGE.
- *Susceptibility:* like GAS, isolates of GBS remain susceptible to penicillin G. Some isolates, however, may be resistant to erythromycin and/or clindamycin.

Treatment

Neonatal infections are usually treated with IV ampicillin + gentamicin initially, then penicillin G.

Adults usually receive 10–14 days of IV penicillin G (+2 weeks gentamicin for endocarditis), vancomycin if penicillin-allergic.

Prevention

Consensus guidelines recommend that obstetrical health care providers adopt either a culture-based or risk-based strategy for antimicrobial GBS prophylaxis during labor and delivery.

Intrapartum antibiotics should be given if the previous child had GBS disease. Newborns with signs of sepsis should be treated with broad-spectrum antibiotics that cover GBS.

If chorioamnionitis is suspected, treat with broad-spectrum antibiotics active against GBS.

Capsular polysaccharide vaccines are under development, including a vaccine conjugated with tetanus toxoid.

Other β-hemolytic streptococci

Group C streptococci

There are four species in this group: *S. dysgalactiae* subsp. *dysgalactiae, S. dysgalactiae* subsp. *equisimilis, S. equi* subsp. *equi,* and *S. equi* subsp. *zooepidemicus.* They are primarily animal pathogens, but *S. equisimilis* and *S. zooepidemicus* can cause a range of infections in humans. The most common problem in humans is outbreaks of tonsillitis, especially in schools and institutions.

The group C streptococci can cause syndromes similar to those of group A streptococci, such as postpartum sepsis, septicemia, meningitis, pneumonia, skin, and wound infections, but group C infections are usually less severe.

Group C streptococci are usually sensitive to the penicillins.

Group F streptococci

These were formerly known as *Streptococci milleri,* which has a characteristic caramel odor when cultured in the laboratory. However, *S. milleri* has been reclassified within the viridans streptococcus group into *S. constellatus, S. intermedius,* and *S. anginosus.*

Group G streptococci

These produce infections similar to those of group A and C streptococci, such as sore throat, erysipelas, cellulitis, bone and joint infection, pneumonia, and septicemia.

Occasionally, group G streptococci bacteremia is associated with underlying malignancy.

Other Gram-positive cocci

Leuconostoc

Leuconostoc are catalase-negative, Gram-positive cocci or coccobacilli, which occasionally cause opportunistic infections. They are usually found on plants and vegetables or, rarely, in dairy products and wine. There are only a few case reports of human infections, including bacteremia (± indwelling line infection), meningitis, and dental abscess.

Leuconostoc are intrinsically resistant to the glycopeptides, because the pentapeptide cell wall precursors terminate in D-alanine-D-lactate. The usual agent of choice for these infections is penicillin or ampicillin, but they are generally susceptible to most agents with activity against streptococci.

Abiotrophia

Abiotrophia is the new name for the nutritionally variant streptococci (NVS). These organisms have been classified in various ways, but 16S rRNA sequencing defined the new genus *Abiotrophia* to be distinct from the streptococci. NVS are defined by the need for pyridoxal or thiol group supplementation for growth and thus appear as satellite colonies around bacteria such as *S. aureus*.

Gram staining tends to show pleomorphic variable-staining cells. The two main species, *A. defectiva* and *A. adiacens*, are resistant to optochin and susceptible to vancomycin. However, because they grow poorly on solid media, they are easily overlooked if not grown in broth or subcultured appropriately.

Abiotrophia are normal flora in the upper respiratory, urogenital, and GI tracts and are clinically important, as they cause approximately 5% of cases of endocarditis. *Abiotrophia* endocarditis responds less well to antibiotics and has higher morbidity and mortality than that of endocarditis due to other streptococci.

Correlation of in vitro antibiotic susceptibility testing and clinical outcome is a specialist field, and the general recommendation is for long-term combination therapy (e.g., penicillin and gentamicin for 4–6 weeks). Bacteriological failure and relapse rates are high.

Anaerobic Gram-positive cocci

Anaerobic Gram-positive cocci have undergone multiple taxonomic changes. Nucleic acid sequencing (particularly 16S rRNA) resulted in most species formerly classified as *Peptococcus* being transferred to the genus *Peptostreptococcus*. Other species include *Coprococcus*, *Ruminococcus*, *Sarcina*, and *Streptococcus saccharolyticus*.

Peptostreptococcus is an obligate anaerobe that is part of normal flora in the mouth, upper respiratory tract, GI tract, vagina, and skin. The most common species are *P. magnus*, *P. micros*, *P saccharolyticus*, and *P. anaerobius*, and they make up 20–40% of anaerobes isolated clinically.

They cause abscesses (e.g., brain abscess, often associated with otitis media, mastoiditis, chronic sinusitis, and pleuropulmonary infections), anaerobic pleuropulmonary disease, and bacteremia (notably due to oropharyngeal, pulmonary, and female genital tract sources).

When mixed with other bacteria, they may be involved with serious soft tissues infections such as necrotizing fasciitis. *Peptostreptococcus* causes anaerobic osteomyelitis and arthritis at all sites, including bites and cranial infections.

Little is known about virulence factors or pathogenesis of infection. Regarding treatment, anaerobic Gram-negative cocci are often mixed with aerobes and anaerobes on culture plates. Obtaining appropriate specimens may be difficult, culture can be prolonged, and anaerobic sensitivity testing can also be challenging.

Usually a combination of surgery (e.g., drainage and debridement) and antibiotic therapy is required. Most anaerobic Gram-positive cocci are sensitive to metronidazole, penicillin, and clindamycin.

Aerococcus

Aerococcus viridans, and the recently described *Aerococcus urinae*, are catalase negative, Gram-positive cocci. They tend to form tetrads and may resemble staphylococci on Gram stain, but their biochemical and growth characteristics are more characteristic of α-hemolytic streptococci.

Aerococcus viridans is generally considered a contaminant on culture, but occasionally may be implicated in bacteremia and endocarditis. It is a low-virulent organism and only causes systemic infections in immunocompromised patients. Optimal treatment of such cases is unclear, so consult an infection specialist.

Aerococcus urinae, first reported in 1989, has been implicated as a cause of approximately. 0.5% of UTIs. Most patients were elderly with predisposing conditions. It has also been found in patients with urogenic bacteremia/septicemia with or without endocarditis. *A. urinae* is usually susceptible to penicillin and resistant to sulfonamides and aminoglycosides.

Overview of Gram-positive rods

The Gram-positive rods can be divided into a number of groups (Table 3.2):
• Aerobic Gram-positive rods
• Anaerobic Gram-positive rods
• Branching Gram-positive rods

Table 3.2 Classification of Gram-positive rods

Group	Examples
Aerobic	*Bacillus* spp.
	Corynebacterium spp.
	Listeria spp.
	Erysipelothrix rhusiopathiae
	Rhodococcus equi
Anaerobic	*Clostridium* spp.
	Propionobacterium spp.
Branching	*Actinomyces*
	Nocardia spp.
	Actinomadura
	Streptomyces

Bacillus species

Bacillus spp. are environmental saprophytes found in water, vegetation, and soil. They are Gram-positive (or Gram-variable) aerobic or facultatively anaerobic rod-shaped bacilli with rounded or square ends.

They form endospores that tolerate extremes of temperature and moisture. The ubiquitous nature of *Bacillus* spp. means that isolation from clinical specimens may represent contamination.

Members of the group include the following:

- *B. anthracis* (see *Bacillus anthracis*, p. 204)
- *B. cereus*
- *B. circulans*
- *B. licheniformis*
- *B. megaterium*
- *B. pumilis*
- *B. sphaericus*
- *B. subtilis*
- *B. stearothermophilus*.

Clinical features

- *Food poisoning*: *B. cereus* is the most common cause. It may also be caused by *B. licheniformis* and *B. pumilis*. It occurs within 24 hours of ingestion of the preformed toxin in food. The emetic form presents after 1–5 hours with nausea, vomiting, and abdominal cramps. The diarrheal form occurs 8–24 hours after ingestion of food. Production of a heat-labile toxin results in profuse diarrhea and abdominal cramps (fever and vomiting are rare). Symptoms usually resolve within 24 hours.
- *Bacteremia* is the most common systemic infection and is often associated with presence of an intravascular catheter. *B. cereus* is the

most common isolate, but other species, e.g., *B. licheniformis,* have been reported. Bacteremia or endocarditis may occur in injecting drug users.

- *Disseminated infection* has been reported in neonates and young children. Neonatal infection is acquired perinatally. Multisystem involvement may occur. Immunocompromise, e.g., neutropenia, is associated with severe and sometimes fatal infections.
- *CNS infections* may occur following trauma or neurosurgery or in association with a CSF shunt. Removal of hardware is required. Lumbar puncture may result in *Bacillus* spp. meningitis.
- *Eye infections:* endophthalmitis may occur following trauma, eye surgery, or hematogenous dissemination. *B. cereus* is the most common cause. Keratitis may occur after corneal trauma.
- *Soft tissue and muscle infections* may occur after injuries or wounds, e.g., from road traffic accidents or after orthopedic surgery.

Diagnosis

Bacillus spp. grow readily on ordinary culture media at environmental temperatures (25–37°C). All species may form spores, but they vary in their colonial morphology, motility, and nutritional requirements.

Microscopically, they are large bacteria and are usually Gram-positive (older cultures may be Gram-variable or Gram-negative). Most *Bacillus* spp. are β-hemolytic and motile (unlike *B. anthracis*). They also lack the glutamic acid capsule (thus negative McFadyean's stain).

Treatment

There is no specific treatment for food poisoning syndromes, and most cases settle in 24 hours.

For intravascular catheter– or prosthetic device–related infections, removal of the catheter or device is required for cure.

Most *Bacillus* spp. isolates are susceptible to vancomycin, clindamycin, fluoroquinolones, aminoglycosides, and carbapenems.

Serious infections are usually treated with vancomcyin or clindamycin ± an aminoglycoside.

Bacillus anthracis

The name *anthrax* is derived from a Greek word for coal and refers to the eschar seen in cutaneous anthrax. Anthrax occurs most commonly in wild and domestic animals in Asia, Africa, South and Central America, and parts of Europe. Humans are rarely infected, and the most common form of infection is cutaneous anthrax, associated with occupational exposure to animal products, e.g., wool, hair, meat, bones, and hides.

Anthrax was used as an agent of bioterrorism in the United States in 2001 when *B. anthracis* spores were sent in contaminated letters.

Pathogenesis

B. anthracis has a number of virulence factors.

Capsule

Under anaerobic conditions, a polypeptide capsule consisting of poly-D-glutamic acid is produced. Synthesis of the capsule is by three enzymes encoded by the *capA*, *capB*, and *capC* genes on the pX-02 plasmid. A fourth protein, encoded by the *dep* gene, catalyses the formation of low-molecular-weight polyglutamates that inhibit phagocytosis.

Toxin

Two binary toxins, edema factor (EF) and lethal factor (LF), bind a third toxin component, protective antigen (PA), before entering the target cell. The three toxin components are also encoded on a plasmid pX-01.

The cellular receptor for PA, the anthrax toxin receptor, was identified in 2001. LF is a zinc-dependent metallopeptidase that inhibits dendritic cell function. EF converts adenosine monophoshpate (AMP) to cyclic AMP (cAMP), resulting in dysregulation of water and ions.

Clinical features

There are four forms of human disease.

Cutaneous anthrax

More than 95% of cases are usually acquired by direct contact with infected animals. The incubation period is 1–12 days, and the initial lesion is a pruritic papule, which becomes a vesicular or bullous lesion surrounded by non-pitting edema. The central part becomes necrotic and hemorrhagic and may develop satellite vesicles.

Finally, there is a classic black eschar which falls off in 1–2 weeks, unless systemic disease ensues.

Gastrointestinal anthrax

This accounts for <5% of case. Oropharyngeal anthrax presents with febrile neck swelling due to cervical adenopathy and soft tissue edema after ingestion of contaminated meat. Intestinal anthrax is more common and presents with fever, syncope, and malaise followed by abdominal pain, nausea, and vomiting.

Examination shows abdominal distension and a mass in the right iliac fossa or periumbilical area. The third phase is characterized by paroxysmal abdominal pain, ascites, facial flushing, red conjunctivae, and shock.

Inhalational anthrax

This is very rare. It occurs after inhalation of spores. The incubation period is <1 week. It presents as a flu-like illness with nonproductive cough, hemorrhagic mediastinal lymphadenopathy, and multilobar pneumonia ± pleural effusions and bacteremia. Chest X-ray (CXR) typically shows a widened mediastinum. It has a high mortality rate (45–85%).

CNS disease

This is very rare. It presents with a hemorrhagic meningoencephalitis and has a 95% mortality rate.

Diagnosis

Specimens
B. anthracis may be isolated from wound swabs (if cutaneous disease), nasal swabs, and blood cultures. Anthrax is a select agent; when clinically suspected the clinical laboratory, the state's health department, and the CDC should be notified. Laboratory safety is of the utmost importance (i.e., biosafetly level 2 precautions).

Microscopy
Gram-positive rods are 4 × 1 micrometer in "box car"– or cigar-shaped chains. The spore is oval and is central or subterminal. McFadyean's stain shows capsulated, dark, square-ended bacilli in short chains.

Culture
B. anthracis grows readily on ordinary media (optimal incubation temperature 35°C) after 2–5 days incubation. Colonies are white or gray-white with a characteristic "medusa head" appearance. In contrast to most other Bacillus spp., B. anthracis is nonhemolytic, nonmotile, and almost always penicillin susceptible.

Identification
B. anthracis can be identified by PCR or phage lysis.

Treatment
- Cutaneous anthrax: ciprofloxacin or doxycycline for 60 days
- Inhalational anthrax: initial therapy: IV ciprofloxacin or doxycycline and one or two additional antimicrobials (e.g., rifampicin, vancomycin, penicillin, ampicillin, chloramphenicol, imipenem, clindamycin, clarithromycin). This is followed by ciprofloxacin or doxycycline until day 60.

Prevention

Vaccines
Human and animal vaccines are available to prevent anthrax. Vaccination is recommended for workers at risk of cutaneous anthrax. Vaccination is also recommended postexposure to inhalational anthrax.

Antibiotic prophylaxis
Oral ciprofloxacin or doxycycline is indicated for postexposure prophylaxis of inhalational anthrax.

Corynebacterium diphtheriae

The name for C. diphtheriae is derived from the Greek korynee, meaning "club" and diphtheria, meaning leather hide (for the leathery pharyngeal membrane it provokes). Diphtheria is rare in the United States but remains a common problem in developing countries and the former Russian states.

The organism spreads via nasopharyngeal secretions and can survive for months in dust and contaminated dry fomites. Incidence is highest in young children (>3–6 months old), when protective maternal antibodies wane.

Pathogenesis

C. diphtheriae exerts its effects by production of a potent exotoxin that inhibits protein synthesis in mammalian cells. It consists of two fragments: fragment A (which inhibits polypeptide chain elongation at the ribosome) and fragment B (which helps transport fragment A into the cell). Inhibition of protein synthesis probably accounts for the toxin's necrotic and neurotoxic effects, which are mainly on the heart, nerves, and kidneys.

Clinical features

Respiratory tract

Asymptomatic upper respiratory tract carriage is common in countries where diphtheria is endemic and is an important reservoir of infection. Anterior nasal infection presents with a serosanguinous or seropurulent nasal discharge often associated with a whitish membrane. Faucial infection is the most common site for clinical diphtheria.

Clinical features include fever, malaise, sore throat, pharyngeal injection, and development of a pseudomembrane that is initially white, then gray with patches or green or black necrosis. Cervical lymphadenopathy may result in a characteristic "bull neck" and inspiratory stridor.

Cardiac disease

Myocarditis occurs after 1–2 weeks, usually as the oropharngeal disease is improving. Patients should be monitored by ECG, which may show ST segment changes, heart block, and arrhythmias. Clinical features include dyspnea, cardiac failure, arrhythmias, and circulatory collapse.

Neurological disease

Local paralysis of the soft palate and posterior pharynx leads to nasal regurgitation of fluids. Cranial nerve palsies and ciliary muscle paralysis may follow. Peripheral neuritis occurs 10–90 days after onset of pharyngeal disease and presents with motor deficits.

Skin infections

In the Tropics, chronic nonhealing ulcers with gray membranes may be due to C. diphtheriae. Outbreaks have been described in homeless alcoholics in the United States.

Invasive disease

Endocarditis, mycotic aneurysms, septic arthritis, and osteomyelitis have been described, caused by nontoxigenic strains.

Diagnosis

Culture

Nasopharyngeal, throat, or skin swabs should be immediately transported to the laboratory and cultured on suitable culture media (e.g., Loeffler's, Hoyle's tellurite, Tinsdale media). The colonies are black on tellurite media. C. diphtheriae shows a halo effect on Tinsdale's agar.

Microscopy
Gram staining of *C. diphtheriae* shows characteristic palisades, resembling Chinese letters. The beaded appearance obtained by Neisser or Albert stains, whereby the volutin/metachromatic granules are dark purple compared to brown/green counterstain, is characteristic.

Identification
C. diphtheriae is a nonmotile, nonsporing, and noncapsulate Gram-positive rod. It is catalase-positive, urease-negative, nitrate-positive, pyrazinamidase-negative, and cystinase-negative.

It can be identified with API Coryne. Isolates should be submitted to the local health department for toxigenicity testing. Several methods are available: Elek plate, rapid enzyme immunosorbent assay (EIA), or PCR.

Biotyping
Colonial appearance on tellurite, and biochemical tests (e.g., Hiss serum sugars) subdivide *C. diphtheriae* into biotypes var. *gravis*, *intermedius,* and *mitis*. These biotypes correspond to clinical severity. *Gravis* and *intermedius* (and some *mitis*) biotypes are usually toxigenic. The fourth biotype, var. *belfanti,* is rare and cannot produce the lethal exotoxin.

Treatment
- *Antibiotics:* if high clinical suspicion, treat immediately with IV penicillin for 14 days. Alternatives are erythromycin, azithromycin, or clarithromycin. Confirm elimination by nasopharyngeal swab; if cultures are positive, give a further 10 days of antibiotics.
- *Antitoxin* may be given at different doses, depending on the site and severity (see the CDC website[*]).
- *Infection control:* isolate and barrier nurse the patient. Identify close contacts, take nose and throat swabs, and arrange clinical surveillance for 7 days. Provide prophylactic antibiotics (single dose of benzylpenicillin or 7-day course of erythromycin) and booster vaccination for close contacts.
- *Notification:* diphtheria is a notifiable disease. Therefore, contact the local health department.

Prevention
Diphtheria toxoid is part of the triple vaccine TDaP (tetanus, diphtheria, acellular pertussis), which is given initially to children at 2, 4, 6, 15–18 months, and 4–6 years. See the CDC Web site for a review of vaccine-preventable diseases and vaccination schedules.[1] Note that diphtheria can occur in immunized individuals.

Non-diphtheria corynebacteria

Corynebacteria are also known as coryneforms or diphtheroids. They are environmental organisms found in water and soil, and commensals of the skin and mucous membranes of humans and other animals.

*. http://www.cdc.gov/vaccines/vpd-vac/diphtheria/dat/dat-main.htm

In the hospital environment, they may be cultured from surfaces and equipment. Thus corynebacteria are frequently considered contaminants but may cause severe disease in hospitalized or immunocompromised patients.

Classification

Corynebacteria are classified according to cell wall composition and biochemical reactions into the following groups:

- Nonlipophilic fermentative, e.g., *C. ulcerans, C. pseudotuberculosis, C. xerosis, C. striatum, C. minutissium, C. amycolatum, C. glucuronolyticum*
- Nonlipophilic nonfermentative, e.g., *C. pseudodiptheriticum*
- Lipophilic, e.g., *C. jeikeium, C. urealyticum*

Clinical features

Infections may be classified into two groups:

- Community-acquired infections, e.g., pharyngitis, native valve endocarditis, genitourinary tract infections, periodontal infections
- Nosocomial infections, e.g., intravascular catheter–associated bacteremia, endocarditis, prosthetic device–related infections, surgical site infections

Diagnosis

- *Microscopy:* club-shaped Gram-positive rods. Cells have variable size and appearance, from coccoid to bacillary forms, depending on the stage of their life cycle. Corynebacteria typically aggregate to form "Chinese letter" arrangements.
- *Culture:* corynebacteria grow readily on blood agar and blood culture media. Thioglycolate broth may be used for wound cultures. Special media used for species identification include tryptic soy agar with or without 1% Tween-80 to assess lipid-enhanced growth.
- *Identification:* corynebacteria are catalase-positive, nitrate-positive, and urease-positive. They can be identified to species level by the API CORYNE system. The CAMP test (named after Christie, Atkins, and Munch–Petersen) may be used. In this test, a streak of B-lysin-producing *S. aureus* is plated onto blood agar, and the test strain is plated perpendicular to it. A positive reaction is seen if CAMP factor (a hemolysin secreted by some corynebacteria) enhances the hemolysis produced by *S. aureus.*
- *Susceptibility testing* is problematic, but isolates are uniformly sensitive to vancomycin and daptomycin.

Infections caused by various corynebacteria

C. ulcerans is primarily a cause of bovine mastitis. However, it has the potential to produce diphtheria toxin and cause an exudative pharyngitis indistinguishable from *C. diphtheriae.* Several reported outbreaks of diphtheria have been found to be due to *C. ulcerans.*

C. pseudotuberculosis is an animal pathogen that causes caseous lymphadenitis in sheep. Human disease is rare, but granulomatous lymphadenitis and pneumonia has been seen in farm workers and vets.

C. xerosis is a commensal of the human nasopharynx, conjunctiva, and skin. It may cause severe invasive disease in immunocompromised patients.

C. striatum is a commensal of the skin and mucous membranes. It can rarely cause severe invasive disease in hospitalized patients. It may not be correctly identified by the API CORYNE.

C. minutissimum is a skin commensal that was previously thought to cause erythrasma. Bacteremia and endocarditis may occur in patients with indwelling catheters or immunocompromise.

C. amycolatum is another skin commensal. There are case reports of invasive disease. It may not be correctly identified by the API CORYNE.

C. glucuronolyticum occurs as normal flora of the genitourinary tract. It may cause urinary tract infection and prostatitis.

C. pseudodiphtheriticum occurs as normal flora of the upper respiratory tract. It is primarily associated with respiratory tract infections in immuno-compromised patients.

C. jeikeium colonizes the skin of hospitalized patients. It may cause severe nosomial infections, e.g., bacteremia, endocarditis, meningitis, CSF shunt infections, and prosthetic joint infections. Risk factors include immuno-compromise (malignancy, neutropenia, and AIDS), indwelling catheters and devices, prolonged hospital stay, use of broad-spectrum antibiotics, and impaired skin integrity. *C. jeikeium* is resistant to many antibiotics, and vancomycin is the treatment of choice.

C. urealyticum colonizes the skin of hospitalized patients. It causes chronic and recurrent urinary tract infections mainly in the elderly or immunosuppressed.

Listeria

Listeria monocytogenes is the main species in this genus and affects preg-nant women, their babies, the immunocompromised (especially those with impaired cell-mediated immunity), and the elderly. *L. ivanovii* occa-sionally causes human infection. Generally, *L. innocua*; *L. welshimeri*, and *L. seeligeri* are nonpathogenic to humans. Up to 5% of healthy adults carry *Listeria* spp. in the gut.

While *Listeria* infections are rare in the general population, they can cause life-threatening bacteremia and meningoencephalitis in susceptible groups. Clinical infections have high mortality rates.

Epidemiology

Disease is mainly sporadic but may be part of an epidemic associated with contaminated foodstuffs such as pâté, unpasteurised milk, chicken, or soft cheese. Hospital outbreaks have been reported. Vets or farmers may become infected through direct animal contact. Human–human transmis-sion occurs vertically (i.e., mother–baby), and cross-infection in neonatal units has been reported.

While the number of pregnancy-associated cases of listeriosis has been relatively stable, there was a dramatic rise in non–pregnancy-associated listeriosis between 2001 and 2004, especially in people over 60 years old. The reasons for this are unclear.

Pathogenesis

Animal studies have identified listeriolysin O: this is important for bacterial survival after phagocytosis, and its production is related to extracellular iron. In rodents, T lymphocytes are important in protective immunity, rather than antibodies. T cells attract monocytes to the infection, activate them, and destroy the *Listeria,* resulting in granuloma.

The organisms themselves show tropism for the brain, particularly the brainstem and meninges. In humans, gastrointestinal disease (e.g., low gastric pH or disrupted normal flora) may help establish *Listeria* infection in the bowel.

Clinical features

Pregnancy

Maternal listeriosis is rare before 20 weeks' gestation. After this, infection may be asymptomatic or present with mild symptoms such as fever, back pain, sore throat, and headache. Fever may result in reduced fetal movements, premature labor, stillbirth, abortion, or early-onset neonatal disease.

Neonate

Early neonatal disease occurs <5 days post-delivery, usually presents with septicemia, and has a mortality of 30–60%. Late neonatal disease occurs >5 days post-delivery, usually presents as meningitis, and may be hospital acquired. Mortality in late disease is lower (approximately 10%).

Adults

The main syndromes are CNS infection and meningitis, septicemia, and endocarditis. Rare manifestations include other CNS disease (such as encephalitis, cerebritis, CNS abscesses), arthritis, hepatitis, endophthalmitis, continuous ambulatory peritoneal dialysis (CAPD) peritonitis, gastroenteritis, and pneumonia.

Risk factors include immunosuppression due to steroids, cytotoxic therapy, and HIV. In *Listeria* meningitis, CSF biochemistry may be indistinguishable from bacterial meningitis. The Gram stain is often negative for organisms, but *Listeria* may sometimes be cultured from blood.
- *Neonatal disease:* early = 30–60% (20–40% survivors develop long-term sequelae such as lung disease or CNS defects); late = 10%
- *Adult disease:* CNS = 20–50%; bacteremia = 5–20%; endocarditis = 50%. Up to 75% survivors of CNS infection have sequelae such as hemiplegia or CNS defects.

Diagnosis

- *Microscopy:* *Listeria* are short, intracellular Gram-positive rods. However, in clinical specimens they may appear Gram-variable and look like diphtheroids, cocci, or diplococci.
- *Culture:* *Listeria* grow on blood agar, but selective media are available. Colonies are sometimes β-hemolytic on blood agar and can be mistaken for group B streptococci.

- *Identification:* they exhibit tumbling motility at 25° C. They are non-sporulating, and catalase-positive, esculin-positive, and oxidase-positive. They grow optimally at 30–37°C but better than most bacteria at 4–10°C (refrigeration temperature). *L. monocytogenes* and *L. seeligeri* show enhanced hemolysis in the presence of *S. aureus* (positive CAMP test). *L. ivanovii* produces a positive CAMP test. Species can also be differentiated by fermentation of D-xylose, L-rhamnose, and A-methyl-D-mannoside.
- *Typing techniques* include phage typing, serotyping, PFGE, and multi-locus enzyme electrophoresis (MLEE). Serotyping of *L. monocytogenes* with rabbit antisera results in 13 serovars: serovar 4 is most common in human infections (but serovars 1/2a and 1.2b are also important).

Treatment

Ampicillin ± gentamicin is the usual regimen for meningitis, with co-trimoxazole or meropenem as an alternative for patients who are penicillin allergic. There are no randomized controlled trials to establish the most effective drug or duration of therapy. In meningitis, antibiotics are usually given for at least 14 days (longer in the immunocompromised).

Most other clinical syndromes should be treated with ampicillin, with consideration given to adding gentamicin for synergy. Vancomycin may be given for bacteremia but has been associated with relapse of disease. Cephalosporins should never be used to treat listeriosis.

Prevention

Give health education and dietary advice to pregnant women, immunocompromised patients, and others who are at risk of disease. Co-trimoxazole prophylaxis prevents *Listeria* infections.

Erysipelothrix rhusiopathiae

E. rhusiopathiae is a thin, pleomorphic, nonsporing, Gram-positive rod. It was first isolated in mice by Robert Koch in 1878 and from swine by Louis Pasteur in 1882. It was identified as a human pathogen in 1909.

Epidemiology

E. rhusiopathiae is found in a wide variety of animals and invertebrates— the reservoir is thought to be swine. The organism in transmitted to humans by direct contact. Most human cases are associated with occupational exposure, e.g., fishermen, fish handlers, farmers, vets, and butchers.

Clinical features

There are three clinical presentations:
- *Erysipeloid:* a localized skin lesion. The organism enters the skin through trauma, and after an incubation period of 2–7 days, pain and swelling of the affected digit occur. The lesion is well defined, slightly raised, and violaceous. It spreads peripherally with central fading. Regional lyphadenopathy and lymphangitis may occur.
- *Diffuse cutaneous eruption* is rare and caused by progression of the primary lesion. Fever and arthralgia may occur. Recurrence is common.
- *Bacteremia* is also rare but frequently associated with endocarditis.

Diagnosis

- *Microscopy:* E. rhusiopathiae is a straight to slightly curved Gram-positive rod (1–2.5 micrometer in diameter). It decolorizes readily and may appear Gram-negative. Rods may be arranged singly, in V-shaped pairs, short chains, or nonbranching filaments.
- *Culture:* colonial and microscopic appearances vary with the medium, pH, and incubation temperature. Incubation in 5–10% CO_2 improves culture.
- *Identification:* E. rhusiopathiae is catalase-, oxidase-, indole-, Vosges–Proskauer-, and Methyl-red-negative.
- *Drug susceptibility:* E. rhusiopathiae is usually susceptible to penicillins, cephalosporins, clindamycin, imipenem, and ciprofloxacin. It is resistant to vancomycin, sulfonamides, co-trimoxazole, and aminoglyocisides.

Treatment

Penicillin is the treatment of choice. Alternatives include ampicillin, cephalosporins, and ciprofloxacin.

Rhodococcus equi

R. equi (previously known as *Corynebacterium equi*) was identified in 1923 as an animal pathogen causing pneumonia in horses. Since then it has been found in a wide variety of animals.

The first human case was reported in 1967, in an immunosuppressed patient who presented with a cavitatory pneumonia. Since the 1980s, the rise in the numbers of immunosuppressed patients (AIDS and transplantation) has been mirrored by an increase in R. equi infections.

Clinical features

Necrotizing pneumonia is the most common clinical presentation (80%) and is characterized by a cavitation on CXR. Blood cultures are positive in 50% of HIV patients and 25% of solid-organ transplant recipients.

Extrapulmonary infection may affect the brain or present as subcutaneous or organ abscesses. Bacteremia may also occur, usually associated with intravenous catheters.

Diagnosis

R. equi is a Gram-positive obligate aerobe that is a nonsporing and non-motile.
- *Microscopy:* it may appear coccoid or bacillary on Gram stain, depending on growth conditions. It can be acid-fast.
- *Culture:* R. equi grows optimally at 30°C and produces salmon-pink colonies. Selective media include colistin nalidixic acid agar (CNA), phenyl ethanol agar (PEA), or ceftazidime novobiocin agar.
- *Identification:* R. equi is catalase-, lipase-, urease-, and phosphatase-positive. It differs from other coryneforms in its lack of ability to ferment carbohydrates or liquefy gelatin. It can be identified using the API CORYNE, ribotyping or PCR RFLP (restriction fragment length polymorphism).

Treatment

Optimal treatment has not been determined by clinical trials. *R. equi* is susceptible to vancomycin, erythromycin, fluoroquinolones, rifampin, imipenem, and aminoglycosides. Combinations of two or three antimicrobials are usually used until antimicrobial susceptibility results are available.

Arcanobacterium haemolyticum

Arcanobacterium haemolyticum is a β-hemolytic, catalase-negative Gram-positive rod that pits the agar when a colony is removed. Identification can be confirmed by the API CORYNE test.

It causes acute pharyngitis and has also been associated with infective endocarditis and skin sepsis. It is sensitive to most antibiotics, except trimethoprim/sulfamethoxazole.

Treatment is usually with penicillin or erythromycin.

Clostridium botulinum

C. botulinum is widespread in the soil and environment. It produces one of the most potent toxins known, which causes botulism.

Pathogenesis

Toxins A–G have identical pharmacological effects, despite possessing different antigens. All can cause human disease, but A, B, and E are most common. Note that the type-specific antibody must be given to a patient with suspected botulism (see Treatment below).

Clinical features

Food-borne botulism

The preformed toxin is ingested from foods such as hams, sausages, tinned fish, meat, and vegetables (particularly home-preserved) and honey. The food itself may not appear spoiled. Botulinum toxin is absorbed from the human GI tract and blocks the release of acetylcholine mainly in the peripheral nervous system.

Initial symptoms include nausea and vomiting, diplopia, and bilateral ptosis (due to oculomotor muscle involvement), followed by progressive descending motor loss with flaccid paralysis. Speech and swallowing become difficult, but the patient maintains consciousness and has normal sensation.

Botulism is fatal in 5–10% cases. Death is usually due to cardiac or respiratory failure.

- *Wound botulism* causes a similar clinical picture, but is due to growth of the organism. Outbreaks have occurred in intravenous drug users.
- *Intestinal botulism* is also due to organism proliferation in the gut and toxin production in vivo.
- *Infant botulism* presents as the "floppy child syndrome" usually in babies <6 months, because the gut is not yet resistant to colonization.

Box 3.1 Botulinum toxin as a potential agent of bioterrorism

Several countries have attempted to weaponize the potent toxin for airborne dispersal, which would result in toxin inhalation. Contamination of food would also be possible. Water dispersal is unlikely, as standard water treatment protocols neutralize the toxin.

There is a vaccine against botulism, but it is not widely used because of concerns regarding effectiveness and adverse effects.

Diagnosis

If there is a suspected clinical case, involve experts and always alert lab staff, as the toxin is dangerous. Human samples and food should be tested for the organism and the toxin at a reference laboratory such as the CDC. *C. botulinum* is a motile strictly anaerobic rod, with optimal growth at 35°C, but some strains are able to grow as low as 1–5°C.

The oval subterminal spores are very hardy: some spores persist despite boiling at 100°C for several hours. Moist heat at 120°C for 5 minutes usually destroys spores.

Treatment

Involve the ICU, as the patient is likely to need organ support. A polyvalent antitoxin is available to neutralize unfixed toxin. In food-borne disease, any unabsorbed toxin should be removed from the stomach and GI tract.

In wound botulism, give benzylpenicillin (penicillin G) and metronidazole, and surgical debridement. Antibiotics are not recommended for food-borne or intestinal botulism.

Prevention

The canning industry must ensure that food in all parts of the can is adequately heated. Avoid home-canning of food. People who have eaten food suspected of causing botulism should be given one dose of polyvalent antitoxin prophylactically.

Clostridium tetani

This vaccine-preventable disease still causes considerable morbidity and mortality in the developing world. Tetanus is a notifiable disease.

Pathogenesis

Resilient spores survive in soil and GI tract of horses and other animals for a long time. Transmission usually occurs via introduction of spores into open wounds (particularly in injecting drug users), patients with recent abdominal surgery, patients with ear infections (otogenic tetanus), and neonates after cutting of the umbilical cord (tetanus neonatorum).

C. tetani produces tetanospasmin (powerful neurotoxin that diffuses to the CNS and causes localized or generalized disease) and tetanolysin (oxygen-labile hemolysin).

Clinical features

Localized tetanus involves muscle rigidity and painful spasms near the wound site. Usually, there is a prodrome of generalized tetanus, with symptoms summarized by the mnemonic ROAST (rigidity, opisthotonus, autonomic dysfuction, spasms, and trismus).

Diagnosis

Tetanus is a clinical diagnosis. There are three microbiological tests:
- Isolation of *C. tetani* from the infection site. *C. tetani* is a motile, obligate anaerobe that classically produces "drumstick" terminal spores.
- It often stains Gram-negative. *C. tetani* produces a thin spreading film on enriched blood agar, due to the motility by peritrichous flagella.
- Low or no antibody levels to tetanus toxin support the diagnosis.
  Treatment

Involve the ICU early. Give tetanus immunoglobulin (TIG). Perform wound debridement and give antimicrobials including metronidazole or penicillin.

Vaccination with tetanus toxoid following recovery is important to prevent future episodes. See Table 3.3.

Tetanus-prone wound risk factors
- Puncture-type wound
- Contact with soil or manure
- Clinical evidence of sepsis
- Significant degree of devitalized tissue
- Any wound with delay of >6 hours before surgical treatment

Prevention

Tetanus immunization involves the combined tetanus, diphtheria, acellular pertussis vaccine (Tdap) or the tetanus/low-dose diphtheria preparation (Td). See the CDC Web site for a review of vaccine-preventable diseases and vaccination schedules for children and adults.*

Table 3.3 Recommendations for vaccination

Immunization status	Clean wound	Tetanus-prone wound	
	Vaccine	Vaccine	TIG
Full, i.e., 5 doses	No	No	Only if high risk
Primary immunization complete, boosters incomplete but up to date	No	No	Only if high risk
Primary immunization incomplete, boosters not up to date, never immunized, or status unknown or uncertain	Yes – 1 dose and plan to complete schedule	Yes – 1 dose and plan to complete schedule	Yes – 1 dose in a different site

* www.cdc.gov/vaccines/recs/schedules/default.htm

Table 3.4 Diseases caused by *Clostridium* spp.

Organism	Clinical syndrome	Toxin production
C. botulinum*	Botulism	Neurotoxin
C. tetani*	Tetanus	Neurotoxin
C. difficile	Antibiotic-associated diarrhea/pseudomembranous colitis	Toxins A and B
C. perfringens*	Type A causes gas gangrene	Histiotoxic
C. novyi*	Type A causes gas gangrene	Histiotoxic
C. sporogenes	Debate re pathogenicity	
C. septicum	Gas gangrene	Histiotoxic
C. histolyticum	Gas gangrene	Histiotoxic
C. sordellii	Gas gangrene	Histiotoxic

*Clusters in injecting drug users in Europe in the last 5 years.

Other clostridia

These anaerobic Gram-positive, spore-forming organisms are responsible for a variety of conditions, many of which involve toxin production (see Table 3.4). The rods are pleomorphic, but are typically large, straight, or slightly curved, with rounded ends.

C. perfringens causes gas gangrene. It is occasionally isolated from blood cultures and may be associated with food poisoning (enterotoxin production). In developing countries it may cause enteritis necroticans ("pigbel").

C. histolyticum and *C. sordellii* may be associated with gas gangrene.

C. novyi gas gangrene is due to *C. novyi* type A (*C. novyi* types B, C, and D are differentiated by toxin permutation and soluble antigen production and do not cause human disease). Compared to *C. perfringens*, *C. novyii* bacilli are larger and more pleomorphic. It is a stricter anaerobe and has peritrichous flagella, but motility is inhibited in the presence of oxygen. The oval spores are central or subterminal. There are at least four toxins that possess hemolytic, necrotizing, lethal, lipase, and phospholipase activities. There was a large outbreak among injecting drug users in Scotland in 1999–2000.

C. sporogenes is probably not pathogenic in its own right. It is usually encountered in a mixed wound culture containing accepted pathogens and may have a role in enhancing local conditions and accelerating an established anaerobic infection.

C. septicum usually lives in the soil, human, or animal gut and can cause gas gangrene in humans and animals. *C. septicum* bacteremia is seen with breakdown of gut integrity, e.g., in leukemia. Gram stain appearance of the organism may be variable, with long, short, and filamentous Gram-positive rods, together with some older Gram-negative cells. Spores start off as swollen Gram-positive "citron bodies" then tend to be oval, bulging, and either central or subterminal.

C. septicum grows well on ordinary media at 37°C and has numerous peritrichous flagella, hence is actively motile. Colonies are often initially transparent and droplet-like, with projecting radiations, then become gray and opaque with time. The A exotoxin has lethal, hemolytic, and necrotizing properties and can be demonstrated in cultures.

C. difficile is an increasing nosocomial infection. It can cause *C. difficile*–associated diarrhea (CDAD) and pseudomembranous colitis. Clinical features vary, and diagnosis is usually by toxin tests or PCR rather than culture. Infection control measures and rational antimicrobial use are paramount to control the spread of this organism.

Mobiluncus

Mobiluncus is a genus of anaerobic, Gram-positive, rod-shaped bacteria. These organisms are found in the female genital tract in association with *Gardnerella vaginalis*. There are two named species: *M. curtisii* (smaller, Gram-variable, and slightly bent) and *M. mulieris* (larger, Gram-negative, and crescent-shaped).

Pathogenesis
Adherence to vaginal squamous epithelial cells is important and may be caused by a glycocalyx.

Clinical features
Mobiluncus spp. has been detected in >97% of women with bacterial vaginosis (together with mixed anaerobic flora) and ~5% of healthy controls. It has also been found in other sites, such as breast abscesses and mastectomy wounds.

Diagnosis
These curved Gram-variable rods grow slowly under anaerobic conditions. Electron microscope studies have described a Gram-positive cell wall. Their characteristic corkscrew motility is due to multiple flagella.

They need an enriched media for growth and are oxidase-, catalase-, and urease-negative. Gram stain morphology can reliably differentiate the two species.

Treatment
Metronidazole is an appropriate treatment for bacterial vaginosis so is used regardless of whether *Mobiluncus* is isolated or not.

Mobiluncus is usually susceptible to penicillin, erythromycin, clindamycin, and vancomycin.

Actinomyces

Actinomyces species are mouth commensals that may cause the chronic granulomatous infection actinomycosis. The main species of human importance are *A. israelii* and *A. gerencseriae*. Others include *A. meyeri* (isolated from brain abscesses), *A. viscosus* (found in dental caries), and *A. naeslundii* and *A. odontolyticus*.

Pathogenesis

Actinomycosis is endogenously acquired, and those with dental caries are at increased risk. It is unclear why males are affected more than females. Historically, rural farm workers were affected more than those living in towns, purportedly because of poor dental hygiene.

Abscesses, tissue destruction, fibrosis, and sinus formation are typical findings. The masses of mycelia in relatively young lesions may be visible as yellow sulfur granules; later on they form dark brown, hard granules through calcium phosphate deposition.

Clinical features

Most human cases of actinomycosis are in the cervicofacial area, especially around the jaw. Infection may follow dental procedures. Hematogenous spread to the liver, brain, and other organs is well recognized.

In addition to facial disease, clinical presentations include thoracic actinomycosis (due to aspiration of oral actinomyces, characterized by chest wall sinuses and bony erosion of the ribs and spine), appendix or colonic diverticula actinomycosis, pelvic actinomycosis (linked with intrauterine contraceptive devices [IUDs]), cerebral actinomycosis, and punch actinomycosis (knuckle infection due to human bite).

Diagnosis

Tissue biopsies of suspect lesions are stained with fluorescein-conjugated specific antisera to demonstrate characteristic sulfur granules and mycelia. Any sulfur granules available should be crushed and stained with Gram stain, which will show branching Gram-positive rods.

Actinomyces often fail to grow aerobically, so plates should be incubated anaerobically and under microaerophilic conditions (5–10% CO_2).

A. israelii form large molar teeth–shaped colonies at 2 to 10 days. Further identification can be confirmed at a reference laboratory by biochemical tests, fluorescent antisera staining, gas chromatography of metabolic products of carbohydrate fermentation, or 16S rRNA sequencing. Sputum often contains oral actinomyces.

Treatment

Surgical involvement is vital, and debridement reduces scarring, deformity, and the recurrence rate. Removal of the IUD is the primary treatment for pelvic disease.

Actinomycosis is usually treated with penicillin or ampicillin, for up to 6 months. Broad-spectrum antibiotics, e.g., ampicillin-sulbactam or ceftriaxone and metronidazole may be needed if there are concomitant pathogens.

Despite large doses of antibiotics given for long periods, recurrence is common. The issue seems to be one of tissue penetration, rather than drug resistance.

Nocardia

Nocardia species are environmental saprophytes that occasionally cause chronic granulomatous infections in humans and animals. The main organisms responsible for human disease are *N. asteroides* (colonies appear star shaped), *N. brasiliensis*, and *N. caviae*.

Pathogenesis

Pulmonary nocardiasis is acquired through inhalation of the bacilli. Cutaneous nocardiosis occurs as a result of inoculation injury.

Disseminated or CNS nocardiosis occurs following hematogarneous spread. Pulmonary and disseminated disease is more common in immunosuppressed patients.

Clinical features

Pulmonary nocardiasis is more common in the immunosuppressed and those with pre-existing lung disease, particularly alveolar proteinosis. Presentation and clinical and radiological findings are variable, making the diagnosis difficult. Patients tend to develop multiple lung abscesses, and the course may be acute or chronic.

Secondary abscesses, mainly in the brain, occur in approximately one-third of patients with pulmonary nocardiasis. Other clinical presentations include cutaneous disease (e.g., post-trauma) with lymphatic involvement (sporotrichoid), which may progress to a fungating mycetoma.

Diagnosis

These branching, aerobic, Gram-positive rods are weakly acid-fast when decolorized with 1% sulfuric acid (modified Ziehl–Neelsen stain). Colonies of *Nocardia* may be colored (orange/cream/pink) and the surface may be dry or chalky. Nocardia can take up to a month to grow on standard media (e.g., Lowenstein–Jensen media, brain–heart infusion agar, and trypticase–soy agar with blood enrichment).

Nocardia organisms can be differentiated from *Actinomyces* because they are strict aerobes (whereas *Actinomyces* organisms are facultative anaerobes), and *Nocardia* grow over a wide range of temperatures (whereas *Actinomyces* only grow at 35–37°C).

Treatment

Seek expert advice. Usually, a long course (e.g., >3 months in normal host, >6 months if immunocompromised) is required. Susceptibility patterns are species specific. Thus identification to the species level along with antibiotic susceptibility testing is an important part of management.

Trimethoprim/sulfamethoxazole has activity against most isolates. Alternatives include minocycline, imipenem, and amikacin.

Actinomadura and *Streptomyces*

Actinomadura and *Streptomyces* species are aerobic, filamentous actino-mycetes implicated in mycetoma, also known as Madura foot. This is a chronic granulomatous condition that mainly occurs in Africa, Asia, and Central America. Mycetoma can be divided into actinomycetoma (bacte-rial) or eumycetoma (fungal); this categorization has important treatment implications.

The important subspecies of *Actinomadura* and *Streptomyces* are *Actinomadura madurae*, *Actinomadura pelletierii*, and *Streptomyces soma-liensis*. Other causal organisms include species of *Madurella*, *Exophila*, *Acremonium*, *Pseudallescheria*, and *Nocardia*.

Diagnosis

Clinically, grains seen within host tissues or in the discharge from sinus tracts are diagnostic of mycetoma. These grains are colonies of the organ-ism and should be crushed in KOH and Gram stained in order to distin-guish between actinomycetoma (which have Gram-positive filaments) and eumycetoma (septate fungi). These grains should be rinsed in 70% alcohol before culture, to try to eliminate any surface contaminants, and appropri-ate plates set up at 26°C and 37°C.

Macroscopically, grains are often red. *Actinomadura* spp. show many sim-ilar properties to those of the *Actinomyces* spp., but strictly *Actinomadura* are not acid-fast when decolorized with 1% sulfuric acid.

Clinical features

Mycetomas usually involve the hand or foot and arise from traumatic inoc-ulation from soil or plants, usually via thorns or splinters. They are chronic granulomatous infections of the skin, subcutaneous tissue, and bone, and may progress to sinus formation.

Treatment

Actinomycetoma tend to respond to therapy better than eumycetoma, which usually requires surgery. Seek expert advice, as the regimen depends on the cause, and courses may be up to 9 months long.

A combination of streptomycin with dapsone, rifampin, trimethoprim-sulfamethoxazole, or sulfonamides is used.

Overview of Gram-negative cocci

The Gram-negative cocci include a variety of pathogenic and non-patho-genic species (Table 3.5).

Acinetobacter spp. are Gram-negative rods that may appear coccoid or bacillary. Unlike *Neisseria* spp., they are oxidase-negative. They are dis-cussed further on p. 245.

Table 3.5 Gram-negative cocci

Organism	Microbiology	Syndrome
Neisseria meningitidis	Aerobic Gram-negative diplococci, oxidase-positive, grow at 37°C on blood and chocolate agar, glucose- and maltose-positive	Meningitis
		Septicemia
Neisseria gonorrheae	Aerobic Gram-negative diplococci, oxidase-positive, grow at 37°C on blood and chocolate agar, glucose-positive	Gonorrhea
Nonpathogenic Neisseria spp.	Aerobic Gram-negative diplococci, oxidase-positive, grow at 22°C on nutrient agar	Oral commensals; can rarely cause invasive infections
Moraxella catarrhalis	Aerobic Gram-negative cocci, oxidase-positive, grow at 37°C on blood and chocolate agar	Respiratory pathogen
Anaerobic Gram-negative cocci, e.g., Veillonella spp.	Anaerobic Gram-negative cocci	

Neisseria meningitidis

Epidemic cerebrospinal fever was first described in 1805 by Vieusseaux. In 1887, Weichselbaum isolated *N. meningitidis* from CSF. In the late 19th century, meningococcal carriage was described. In 1909, different serotypes of *N. meningitidis* were recognized.

Epidemiology
Humans are the only known reservoir of *N. meningitidis*, and ~20% of the population carry the organism in their throat. However, half of these carriage strains are noncapsulate and thus nonpathogenic. During outbreaks, the carrier rate of an epidemic strain may reach 90%.

Risk factors for meningococcal disease include the following:
• Lack of bactericidal antibody
• Age—bimodal distribution: 3 months to 3 years and 18–23 years
• Travel to endemic areas, e.g., Africa, Mecca
• Complement deficiencies
• Splenectomy
• Host genetic polymorphisms, e.g., *MBL, TNFA, Fc/RIIa,* and *PAI-1*

Pathogenesis
To cause infection, the organism must cross the nasopharyngeal mucosa and enter the circulation. The type IV pilus (encoded by *pilC*) is involved in mucosal colonization. The polysaccharide capsule is important in avoiding host immunity (and defines the serogroup of the isolate in Table 3.5). Various secretion systems help deliver toxins.

Clinical features

- Meningitis and septicemia
- Other acute infections: purulent conjunctivitis (which occasionally becomes systemic), purulent monoarthritis, endocarditis, pericarditis and pneumonia
- Chronic septicemia with joint and skin involvement is also recognized.

Diagnosis

- *CSF examination:* in meningitis, the CSF pressure is elevated and the CSF appears turbid. The CSF white cell count and protein are normally raised and the CSF glucose level is low (compared to serum glucose). In very early infection, CSF results may be normal, as the meningeal reaction has not had time to take place.
- *Microscopy:* Gram-negative intracellular diplococci. In meningococcal meningitis, CSF usually has a higher yield than blood cultures. If the Gram stain is negative, a methylene blue stain may pick up scanty meningococci.
- *Culture:* transparent, nonpigmented, nonhemolytic colonies. May be mucoid if capsule production. Oxidase positive. Identified by API NH or other biochemical panels
- *Serogrouping:* capsular polysaccharide antigens are identified by slide agglutination test using polyclonal antibodies. There are at least 13 serogroups; the most common ones are summarized in Table 3.6.
- *Serotyping:* identification of (PorB) class 2/3 outer membrane protein by a dot-blot enzyme-linked immunosorbent assay (ELISA) using monoclonal antibodies
- *Serosubtyping:* identification of (PorA) class 1 outer membrane protein by a dot-blot ELISA using monoclonal antibodies
- MLST is being evaluated for routine surveillance.
- Meningococcal PCR (send to a reference lab)

Microbiology

N. meningitidis is a fastidious Gram-negative diplococcus. It produces a capsule that forms the basis of the serogroup typing system. There are now at least 13 serogroups, but the most common ones are summarized in Table 3.6.

Table 3.6 Major serogroups of *N. meningitis*

Serogroup	Pattern of disease	Vaccines
A	Epidemic meningitis, associated with different clones	Yes
B	Epidemic strains (and outbreaks)	A meningitis B vaccine is currently undergoing clinical trials
C	Local outbreaks	MenC vaccine introduced in 1999
W-135	Pilgrims returning from the Haj	Yes
X, Y, Z, 29E, Z'	Rare	

Treatment

See management of acute bacterial meningitis (see Acute meningitis, p. 644) and septicemia. Reduced susceptibility to penicillin in some countries has resulted in empirical therapy for meningitis being a third-generation cephalosporin.

After treatment, rifampin (or ciprofloxacin) should be given for nasopharyngeal eradication.

Infection control issues

Inform public health authorities, who will arrange chemoprophylaxis of household or kissing contacts of the case.

Rifampin is only effective in eradiating carriage in 80–90% of people treated, and rifampin-resistant strains, which have caused disease in contacts, have been reported. The alternatives are ciprofloxacin or ceftriaxone.

Neisseria gonorrhoeae

N. gonorrhoeae only infects humans and causes the sexually transmitted infection (STI) gonorrhea (see Gonorrhea, p. 638). This is the second-most common bacterial STI in the United States.

Increasing rates of antimicrobial resistance, together with its persistence and association with poor reproductive health outcomes, have made it a major public health concern.

Pathogenicity

Gonococci are divided into four Kellogg types, by colonial appearance, ability to auto-agglutinate, and virulence. Kellogg types T1 and T2 are more virulent and possess many fimbriae, while types T3 and T4 are non-fimbriate and avirulent. In gonococci, the fimbriae are associated with attachment to mucosal surfaces and resistance to killing by phagocytes.

Epidemiological typing of gonococci uses both auxotyping (nutritional requirements of arginine, proline, hypoxanthine, uracil, etc.) and monoclonal antibodies against specific proteins.

Clinical features

Gonorrhea commonly presents as a purulent disease of the urethral mucous membrane and also of the cervix in females. Secondary local complications (e.g., epididymitis, salpingitis, pelvic inflammatory disease, p. 639) and metastatic complications (e.g., arthritis) may occur if the primary infection is inadequately treated.

Other manifestations of disease include disseminated gonococcal infection (skin lesions, painful joints, and fever), ophthalmia neonatorum (purulent conjunctivitis of the newborn), perihepatic inflammation (Fitz-Hugh–Curtis), and, rarely, endocarditis or meningitis.

Rectal or pharyngeal infection is often asymptomatic and identified through contact tracing. If cultured, gonococcus should always be treated, as it is never a commensal.

Diagnosis

Culture

The only definitive test for legal purposes is culture. Urethral swabs from males and endocervical swabs from females should be Gram stained and then immediately inoculated onto selective media and placed in enriched CO_2 conditions.

Typical Gram stain appearance of *N. gonorrhoeae* (Gram-negative diplococci in association with neutrophils) from urethral or endocervical swabs, together with a consistent clinical presentation, is regarded as adequate for treatment in many cases. However, culture is critical for legal cases and for antimicrobial sensitivity testing. After 24–48 hours, oxidase-positive colonies appear, and identification can be confirmed by testing for acid production from sugars (APINH).

Many laboratories still test for β-lactamase production by means of the chromogenic cephalosporin (nitrocefin), acidometric, and paper strip methods, although all patients are likely to be treated with a third-generation cephalosporin according to current guidelines.

Nonculture methods

Rapid nonculture tests are increasingly available and are based mainly on detection of nucleic acid by hybridization or amplification. These are generally very sensitive and specific, and ligase chain reaction (LCR) has the advantage of being performed on urine.

If gonococcus is isolated from a prepubertal girl with vulvovaginitis, it may indicate sexual abuse. The case should be dealt with sensitively by a pediatrician, and senior laboratory staff should be involved. Thorough documentation is required, since evidence may be needed in court.

Treatment

The 2006 CDC guidelines (www.cdc.gov/std/treatment) recommend ceftriaxone, cefixime, or a fluoroquinolone as first-line therapy for uncomplicated infections of the cervix, urethra, or rectum. Cephalosporins have replaced the fluoroquinolones, however, for infections in men who have sex with men (MSM) or in those with a history of recent foreign travel or partners' travel, infections acquired in California or Hawaii, or infections acquired in other areas with increased quinolone resistance.

Treatment for *Chlamydia* should also be administered empirically unless coinfection has been ruled out.

Control

- Prompt and adequate diagnosis and treatment
- Effective contact tracing
- Prevention: condoms and barrier methods
- Prevent ophthalmia neonatorum by putting 1% aqueous silver nitrate into all newborn babies' eyes, in areas of high prevalence
- Screening of high-risk individuals
- Sex education and awareness of STIs

Nonpathogenic *Neisseria*

The nonpathogenic *Neisseria* species are upper respiratory tract commensals and include *N. lactamica, N. polysaccharea, N. subshara,* and *N. cirerla.* If invasive infection does occur, full susceptibility testing should be performed, as penicillin resistance is increasing.

Microbiology

N. lactamica and *N. polysaccharea* are the species most commonly isolated from nasopharyngeal swabs during meningococcal surveys. Colonies appear similar to *N. meningitidis*, and they also grow on selective media, unlike the nasopharyngeal commensals. *N. lactamica* is easy to distinguish, as it produces acid from glucose, maltose, and lactose and gives a positive ONPG (orthonitrophenyl-B-D-galactopyranoside) test result for B-galactosidase.

Clinical features

Nonpathogenic *Neisseria* spp. rarely cause invasive disease but have been associated with meningitis, endocarditis, bacteremia, ocular infections, pericarditis, osteomyelitis, and empyema. *Neisseria* spp. in general are naturally competent for DNA uptake, so the pathogenic *Neisseria* can take up DNA encoding for virulence factors or antibiotic resistance from the nonpathogenic *Neisseria* that are part of the normal flora.

For example, one mechanism by which *N. meningitidis* and *N. gonorrhoeae* have acquired penicillin resistance is the interspecies transfer of *penA* from the nonpathogenic *Neisseria* in the throat. Studying exactly what constitutes "normal flora, not just in the throat but also the GI tract, skin, and vagina, is likely to increase our understanding of the evolution of pathogens.

Moraxella

For decades, *M. catarrhalis* was regarded as an upper respiratory tract commensal. However, since the 1970s, it has been recognized as an important and common respiratory tract pathogen.

Microbiology

M. catarrhalis grows well on many media, including blood and chocolate agar. It shows the "hockey stick" sign, in that it slides across the agar surface when pushed and can be difficult to pick up onto a loop. *M. catarrhalis* is oxidase-, catalase-, and DNase-positive and produces butyrate esterase.

Clinical features

M. catarrhalis causes otitis media; lower respiratory tract infections in COPD patients; pneumonia, particularly in the elderly; nosocomial respiratory tract infections; sinusitis; and, occasionally, bacteremia.

Outer membrane proteins (OMPs), lipo-oligosaccharide (LOS), and pili are probably important in pathogenesis.

Treatment

Almost all strains of *M. catarrhalis* produce β-lactamase, which is inducible. Regardless of the results of ampicillin susceptibility testing, ampicillin should not be used.

Suitable agents include amoxillin-clavulonic acid, cephalosporins, fluoroquinolones, tetracyclines, and macrolides.

Anaerobic Gram-negative cocci

Veillonella spp. organisms are part of the normal flora of the gastrointestinal tract of humans and animals. *Veillonella* may be isolated from a variety of clinical conditions, though their role in causing infection is unclear.

The most common species is *Veillonella parvula*, which fluoresces red under ultraviolet (UV) light. *Veillonella* are able to use some of the lactic acid produced by streptococci, lactobacilli, and other bacteria that may induce dental caries. They are associated with supragingival dental plaque and also found as part of the tongue microflora. They are generally regarded as minor components of mixed anaerobic infections.

Acidominococcus spp. and *Megosphora* spp. are other anaerobic Gram-negative cocci found in the human gut. They are considered non-pathogenic.

Escherichia coli

E. coli is the type species of the genus *Enterobacteriaceae* and contains a variety of strains ranging from commensal organisms to highly pathogenic variants. Infections tend to infect the gut and urinary tract, but almost any extraintestinal site may be involved.

E. coli is often used as a marker of fecal contamination, e.g., in food and water testing, as it does not otherwise exist outside the animal body.

Pathogenesis

- *O and K polysaccharide antigens* protect *E. coli* from complement and phagocytic killing, unless antibodies are present. Phagocytosis is usually successful if there are antibodies to K antigens present alone, or to both O and K antigens.
- *Hemolysin* is more commonly produced by strains causing extra-intestinal infections and is thought to increase virulence.
- *The ColV plasmid*, harbored by some *E. coli,* encodes an aerobactin-mediated iron uptake system. This is more common in strains isolated from cases of septicemia, pyelonephritis, and lower UTIs than in commensal fecal strains.
- *Fimbriae:* type 1 fimbriae adhere to cells containing mannose residues, possibly contributing to pathogenicity, but their role in UTIs is debated. Other filamentous proteins may cause a mannose-resistant haemagglutination, e.g., colonization factor antigens (CFAs) in human enterotoxigenic *E. coli* (ETEC), K88 in pigs, and K99 in calves and

lambs. *P. fimbriae* bind specifically to receptors on P blood group antigens of human erythrocytes and uroepithelial cells.
- *Other:* enteric strains demonstrate specific interactions with the intestinal mucosa and release toxins and may harbor plasmid-encoded virulence factors.

Epidemiology

Serotyping of *E. coli* is based on O (somatic), H (flagellar), and K (surface/capsular) antigens, as detected in agglutination reactions.

There are >160 O antigens, and cross-reactions occur between *E. coli* O antigens and O antigens of other species, e.g., *Citrobacter* and *Salmonella*.

H antigens are usually monophasic and are determined from cultures in semi-solid agar.

K antigens traditionally were those that prevented O agglutination (thus agglutination tests are done on boiled samples). K antigens are the acidic polysaccharide capsular antigens and divided into groups I and II.

Clinical features

UTIs

E. coli is the most common cause of community-acquired uncomplicated UTIs (see Urinary tract infections: introduction, p. 610) and also causes nosocomial UTIs. Clinical manifestations range from urethritis and cystitis to pyelonephritis and sepsis. Many uropathogenic strains originate in the patient's own gut and cause infection by the ascending route.

Specific P fimbriae, or pili associated with pyelonephritis (known as the PAP pilus), which attach to uroepithelial cells, are important in pathogenesis. These uropathogenic strains may contain additional virulence factors, such as hemolysin and ColV plasmids, and resistance to complement-dependent bactericidal effect of serum.

Enteric infections

E. coli is responsible for many cases of diarrheal disease, ranging from acute gastroenteritis, particularly in the tropics (traveler's diarrhea, see Viral gastroenteritis, p. 354), to life-threatening hemorrhagic colitis. The strains involved fall into four to five groups, each with different pathogenic mechanisms (see below and Table 3.7).

Bacteremia

The usual sources of nosocomial *E. coli* bacteremia are the urogenital, gastrointestinal, and respiratory tracts, and foreign bodies such as IV lines and endotracheal tubes. The hallmark of cases of Gram-negative bacteremia is the systemic reaction to lipopolysaccharide or endotoxin, which may be fatal.

Neonatal sepsis

E. coli may cause neonatal meningitis and septicemia, especially in premature babies. The strains responsible may express the K1 or K5 surface/capsular antigens, which have enhanced virulence.

Table 3.7 Clinical features and pathogenic mechanisms of various E. coli

Abbreviation	Full name	Clinical features	Pathogenesis
EHEC/VTEC/STEC	Enterohemorrhagic E. coli Verotoxin-producing E. coli Shigatoxin-producing E. coli Enterotoxigenic E. coli	Hemorrhagic colitis/hemolytic uraemic syndrome (HUS)	**Verotoxins** (VT1 and 2), also called shiga-like toxins (SLT1 and 2), are phage-encoded toxins thought to target vascular endothelial cells. The A subunit mediates biological activity, while the B subunit is responsible for binding and toxin uptake. Risk of developing HUS depends on type of shigatoxin, plus host and environmental factors.
ETEC		Traveler's diarrhea	**ST (heat-stable enterotoxin)** causes ↑cGMP, thus altering ion transport and ↑fluid secretion by mucosal cells of small intestine. **LT (heat-labile enterotoxin)**: B polypeptide binds to mucosal surface of small intestine, allowing the A polypeptide to enter the cell and catalyse adenosine diphosphate ribosylation of the guanine nucleotide component of adenylate cylase, thus ↑cAMP and ↑fluid secretion (as with V. cholerae). Colonization/adherence factors—see text
EIEC	Enteroinvasive E. coli	Disease similar to Shigella-like dysentery	
EPEC	Enteropathogenic E. coli	Childhood diarrhea	
EAEC	Enteroaggregative E. coli	Traveler's diarrhea, especially in Mexico and N. Africa	

Other nonenteric infections
E. coli may cause postoperative wound infections and deep abscesses. Respiratory tract infection is usually opportunistic, often in debilitated patients such as diabetics or alcoholics. Nosocomial pneumonia (±empyema) is usually due to aspiration rather than hematogenous spread, and may be associated with high mortality.

Diagnosis

E. coli are usually smooth, colorless colonies on nonselective media and may appear hemolytic on blood agar. Most *E. coli* ferment lactose (and produce acid and gas in 24–48 hours), but approximately 5% are non-lactose fermenters (NLFs). *E. coli* are usually motile, and those responsible for extraintestinal infections often have a polysaccharide capsule.

E. coli are usually positive for indole production, ornithine decarboxylase, lysine decarboxylase, and methyl red. They are usually negative for urease, citrate utilization, H_2S production, and the Voges–Proskauer (VP) test.

Treatment

The management of *E. coli* depends on the site and severity of the infection. Simple *E. coli* UTIs may respond to trimethoprim/sulfamethoxazole or ampicillin. Many hospital-acquired *E. coli* infections are due to multi-resistant organisms and may require treatment with a cephalosporin, fluoroquinolone, aminoglycoside, piperacillin-tazobactam, or carbapenem.

Susceptibility data often vary geographically (because of prior antibiotic usage), so follow your hospital antibiotic policy. Be guided by antibiotic susceptibility results, and use targeted therapy when possible.

Antibiotics may be harmful in cases of *E. coli* O157.

Klebsiella

Klebsiella species are usually harmless colonizers of the human gut. The classification can be confusing, but the main species defined by DNA hybridization studies are *Klebsiella pneumoniae* subsp. *aerogenes* (formerly *Klebsiella aerogenes*), *Klebsiella pneumoniae* subsp. *pneumoniae* (formerly *Klebsiella pneumoniae*), and *Klebsiella oxytoca*.

Other rare respiratory subspecies include *Klebsiella ozaenae* and *Klebsiella rhinoscleromatis*. They belong to the tribe Klebsiellae.

Pathogenesis

Klebsiella organisms that express capsular K antigens are resistant to complement-mediated serum killing. No particular capsular subtype has been linked to a greater risk of infection. Those with O antigens are resistant to phagocytosis.

Klebsiella spp. have two iron uptake systems: one system uses aerobactin (related to virulence) and the other uses enterochelin (plasmid encoded).

Epidemiology

Common capsular (K) types are K2, K3, and K21. There are about 80 K antigens recognized overall, some of which cross-react with *H. influenzae* and *S. pneumoniae*. There are also five different somatic O antigen types, but these are rarely used for typing.

There is an association between antigenic structure, habitat, and biochemical reactivity; for example, capsular types 1–6 are most common in the human respiratory tract. For epidemiological investigations, capsular serotyping, bacteriocin typing, and phage typing may be useful.

Clinical features

Klebsiella infections are rare in the immunocompetent normal host. They tend to cause nosocomial and opportunistic infections, such as UTIs, pneumonia (lobar), other respiratory infections (bronchitis, bronchopneumonia), surgical wound infections, and bacteremia in those with risk factors such as diabetes, COPD, or alcoholism.

The likely focus in cases of nosocomial bacteremia is the urinary tract, intravascular lines, lower respiratory tract, biliary tract, and surgical wound site. Severe pneumonia with "red currant jelly" sputum and multiple lung abscesses is called *Friedlander's pneumonia* and has a high mortality.

Diagnosis

Klebsiella spp. are facultatively anaerobic, catalase test–positive, and oxidase test–negative and ferment glucose. Organisms are capsular, which may give colonies a mucoid appearance. The capsule is made of glucuronic acid and pyruvic acid, and there are ~80capsular K antigens.

On Gram stain, organisms may look thicker than other Gram-negative rods because of the prominent polysaccharide capsule. They are lactose-fermenters and usually fimbriate but nonmotile.

They are H_2S- and indole-negative (except *K. oxytoca*, which is indole-positive), and VP-positive, and they can use citrate as a sole carbon source. Different species of *Klebsiella* are usually recognized by different biochemical tests (Table 3.8).

Treatment

Klebsiella species are inherently resistant to ampicillin and most other penicillins. Many are now multiresistant, including cephalosporin resistance due to extended-spectrum β-lactameses (ESBLs).

In parts of the United States, *Klebsiella pneumonia* carbapenemase (KPC)-producing stains have become problematic. KPC resistance can coexist with other Gram-negative resistance mechanisms, including ESBL, fluoroquinolone, and aminoglycoside resistances.

Treat according to local hospital policy and sensitivity data.

Table 3.8 Biochemical reactions useful to distinguish *Proteus*, *Providencia*, and *Morganella*

	Proteus mirabilis	Proteus vulgaris	Providencia alcalifaciens	Providencia rettgeri	Providencia stuartii	Morganella morganii
Ornithine decarboxylase	+	–	–	–	–	+
Gas from glucose	+	+	V	–	–	+
H_2S production	+	V	–	–	–	–
Indole formation	–	+	+	+	+	+
Urease formation	+	+	–	+	–	+

+ = Most strains positive; – = most strains negative; V = variable.

This table was published in Greenwood et al. *Medical Microbiology: A Guide to Microbial Infections. Pathogenesis, Immunity, Laboratory Diagnosis and Control*, 15th ed, p.281. Copyright Elsevier 2000.

Proteus

P. mirabilis is most commonly isolated from community UTIs, whereas *P. vulgaris* and *P. myxofaciens* tend to cause nosocomial infections. *Proteus* belongs to the tribe Proteae.

Epidemiology

Proteus is probably the second-most common enterobacteria encountered in many diagnostic laboratories (after *E. coli*). This is because of the huge numbers isolated from urine samples: approximately 10% of uncomplicated UTIs are due to *Proteus* (usually *P. mirabilis*).

Pathogenesis

Factors that contribute to the ability of *Proteus* to colonize and infect the urinary tract include the following:
- Production of the enzyme urease, which splits urea into ammonium hydroxide. This increases urinary pH and encourages struvite stone formation. These stones act as a nidus for persistent infection and also obstruct urinary flow.
- Fimbriae help uroepithelial colonization.
- Flagella-dependent motility helps spread in the urinary tract.
- Uropathogenic *Proteus* synthesizes several hemolysins.

Clinical features

In addition to urine infections, *Proteus* also causes bacteremia, wound infections, and respiratory infections in debilitated hospital patients. The human GI tract is the main reservoir of infection for patients who subsequently become infected.

Diagnosis

Proteus organisms rapidly hydrolyse urea. The presence of hundreds of flagella on each organism makes them extraordinarily motile, which appears as swarming on agar plates and can produce the Dienes phenomenon (a line of inhibited growth where two strains meet).

Proteus organisms give positive methyl-red reactions, are usually VP-negative (except some strains of *P. mirabilis*). Most *P. mirabilis* strains are indole-negative; the other subspecies are indole-positive (see Table 3.8).

Phage typing, bacteriocin typing, and serotyping schemes have been developed. The Dienes phenomenon may be exploited for typing, in that two test organisms are viewed as identical if they show no line of demarcation where the swarming growths meet (after inoculation onto the surface of an agar plate).

Treatment

Antibiotic resistance is increasing, but the indole-negative *P. mirabilis* is generally more sensitive than the indole-positive species. Prescribe according to local policy until sensitivity results are available.

Some organisms carry the AmpC β-lactamase, which is inducible by cephalosporins. Amikacin, new quinolones, and carbapenems may be the only options. *Proteus* is inherently resistant to colistin.

Table 3.9 Appearance of *Salmonella* spp. on various media

Agar	Salmonella spp.
MacConkey agar	Non-lactose fermenters (NLF) appear white or clear
Cysteine lactose electrolyte deficient (CLED)	NLFs appear blue
DCA deoxycholate	Yellow or colorless, often with a dark center
Xylose lysine deoxycholate (XLD) agar	*Salmonella* appear red, some with black centers
Salmonella Shigella agar (SSA)	NLFs appear colorless, some with black centers
Hektoen agar	*Salmonella* are blue-green. S. Typhimurium and others that reduce sulfur produce a black precipitate
Brilliant green agar	Red-pink colonies surrounded by brilliant red zones
Selenite broth	Growth of *Salmonella* results in a cloudy tube
Tetrathionate broth	Tetrathionate-reducing bacteria (*Salmonella* and *Proteus*) can grow

Enterobacter

The genus *Enterobacter* includes *E. aerogenes*, *E. cloacae*, *E. sakazakii*, *E. taylorae*, *E. gergoviae*, *E. asburiae*, *E. hormaechei*, *E. camerogenus*, and *E. agglomerans*. The genus was previously known as *Aerobacter* species and belongs to the tribe Klebsiellae.

Epidemiology

Enterobacter organisms are common human gut commensals, which rarely cause infection in the normal host.

Clinical features

E. aerogenes and *E. cloacae* (and occasionally *E. taylorae*) colonize hospital inpatients and cause nosocomial opportunistic infections, such as wound infections, burn infections, pneumonia, and UTIs.

Risk factors for infection include indwelling lines, frequent courses of antibiotics, a recent invasive procedure, diabetes, and neutropenia. They can often be isolated from diabetic ulcers.

Enterobacter infections have been associated with IV fluid contamination. *E. sakazakii* has been implicated in severe neonatal meningitis (mortality rate 40–80%), and there have been outbreaks associated with dried infant formula.

Diagnosis

In common with the other *Enterobacteriaceae*, *Enterobacter* species are facultative anaerobes that give a positive catalase result and a negative oxidase result, ferment glucose (with the production of acid and gas) as well as lactose, and reduce nitrates to nitrites.

They do not produce H_2S on triple-sugar iron media. They are indole-negative, methyl red–negative, and VP-positive. They use citrate as a sole carbon source and are ONPG-positive. Unlike *Klebsiella*, they are usually motile and are less likely to be heavily capsulated.

The two most important clinical species are *E. aerogenes* (which usually decarboxylates lysine but not arginine) and *E. cloacae* (which usually decarboxylates arginine but not lysine).

Treatment

Enterobacter organisms (except *E. sakazakii*) are usually resistant to first generation cephalosporins and readily develop resistance to second- and third-generation cephalosporins because of inducible β-lactamases such as AmpC. Carbapenems are the mainstay of treatment.

E. sakazakii tends to be more sensitive to antibiotics overall.

Ampicillin and gentamicin in combination are the usual treatment of *E. sakazakii* neonatal meningitis.

Citrobacter

C. diversus, *C. freundii*, and occasionally *C. amalonaticus* are associated with nosocomial respiratory and urinary tract infections. Their role as primary pathogens or secondary infections or colonizers is debated.

C. koseri is a synonym for *C. diversus*. *C. diversus* has also been associated with outbreaks of neonatal meningitis.

Pathogenesis
Animal studies on neonatal meningitis showed that pathogenic strains of *C. diversus* were more virulent and had an extra outer membrane protein compared to nonpathogenic strains.

Clinical features
The clinical significance of isolation of *Citrobacter* species from the urinary and respiratory tracts of debilitated hospital patients is often unclear. When isolated from blood cultures, it is usually one of a number of species present, and such polymicrobial infections are often associated with a poor clinical outcome (probably because of the patient's general debilitated state rather than the organisms' virulence).

However, *Citrobacter* is a recognized cause of endocarditis, and in neonates, *Citrobacter* organisms (particularly *C. diversus*) can cause severe meningitis and brain abscesses.

Diagnosis
Citrobacter is so named because the organisms can grow on Simmons citrate media. They are usually motile, methyl red–positive, and VP-negative and slowly hydrolyse urea. They are usually non-lactose fermenters, but may appear as late lactose fermenters.

C. freundii may be mistaken for *Salmonella,* as it is produces H_2S.

There is considerable cross-reactivity with the O antigens of other *Enterobacteriaceae*.

Treatment
Like many of the other *Enterobacteriaceae* that cause nosocomial infections, *Citrobacter* spp. tend to be multiresistant, so reliance on laboratory antimicrobial susceptibility testing is paramount. *Citrobacter freundii* organisms have the inducible AmpC β-lactamase.

Plasmid-mediated ESBLs are becoming more common. Treatment options may include aminoglycosides, antipseudomonal penicillins, carbapenems, and quinolones.

Serratia

There are many named species of *Serratia*, which belong to the tribe Klebsielleae. *S. marcescens* is the main one that causes human disease. Infections with *S. liquifaciens, S. rubidaea,* and *S. odorifera* are much less common.

Epidemiology
Unlike the other *Enterobacteriaceae, Serratia* is more likely to colonize the respiratory and urinary tracts of hospital patients (rather than the gut). However, in neonates, the GI tract may be the reservoir for cross-contamination.

Clinical features

Serratia species are opportunistic pathogens, particularly in the health care setting, and cause respiratory and urinary tract infections, bacteremias, and skin and wound infections. Patients with intravascular catheters and urinary catheters are at increased risk.

Serratia infections have been associated with contaminated IV therapy and with septic arthritis in patients who have had intra-articular injections. *Serratia* also causes endocarditis and osteomyelitis in IV drug users and cellulitis in patients on hemodialysis.

Diagnosis

Serratia can be recognized by production of a characteristic red or deep pink pigment. They are slow or non-lactose fermenters and usually motile. They have the characteristics of the *Enterobacteriaeceae*.

Like *Enterobacter*, most *Serratia* do not produce H_2S or lactose on triple sugar iron media, are VP-positive, and use citrate as a sole carbon source. *Serratia* can be differentiated from the other *Enterobacteriaceae* by production of an extracellular DNase.

Treatment

Serratia are often multiresistant to antibiotics. Treat according to local epidemiology until sensitivity results are available. Options are often limited to amikacin, piperacillin-tazobactam, and carbapenems.

Efforts focused on good infection control practice, especially handwashing, are vital in reducing horizontal transmission between patients. *Serratia* organisms are inherently resistant to colistin.

Salmonella

Salmonella spp. belong to the family *Enterobacteriaceae*. There are seven subspecies and over 2400 serovars. The correct nomenclature is *Salmonella enterica*, followed by the serotype (e.g., *Salmonella enterica* serotype Typhimurium). This is commonly abbreviated to *S. enterica* ser. Typhimurium (serotype not italicized).

Epidemiology

Salmonella are commensals and pathogens of a wide range of domesticated and wild animals. Some species, e.g., *S. enterica* ser. Typhi and *S. enterica* ser. Paratyphi, are well adapted to humans and have no other host. Others are more adapted to animals and rarely affect humans, e.g., *S. arizonae*, and reptiles.

In humans, salmonellae can be divided into those that cause enteric fever (*S. enterica* ser. Typhi and *S. enterica* ser. Paratyphi) and the nontyphoidal *Salmonella* spp. (NTS). Salmonellae are usually transmitted via the feco-oral route.

Pathogenesis

Infection begins with ingestion of organisms in contaminated food and water.

Salmonellae express an array of distinct fimbriae that help them to adhere to the intestinal wall. They also encode a type III secretion system (T3SS) within *Salmonella* pathogenicity island 1 (SPI-1) that is needed for bacteria-mediated endocytosis and intestinal epithelial evasion.

A number of SPI-1 translocated proteins (SipA, SipC, SopE and SopE2) promote membrane ruffling and *Salmonella* invasion.

Salmonellae are also adapted to survival and replication in the intracellular environment.

Clinical features
- Gastroenteritis (p. 354)
- Enteric fever (p. 587)
- Bacteremia and endovascular infection
- Salmonellosis in HIV has a 20- to 100-fold increased risk. More likely to have severe invasive disease (enterocolitis, bacteremia, meningitis)
- Localized infections
- Chronic carrier state

Diagnosis
Salmonellae are facultative anaerobic Gram-negative rods, which grow readily on routine media. Their growth on specialized media is summarized in Table 3.9. They are motile, oxidase-negative, and urease-negative and are non-lactose fermenters.

Salmonellae possess lipopolysaccharide somatic (O) heat-stable antigens and flagellar (H) heat-labile antigens. Usually the H antigens exhibit diphasic variation so can exist in phases 1 and 2 (Table 3.10).

S. enterica ser. Typhi, *S. enterica* ser. Paratyphi C, and some strains of *S. enterica* ser. Dublin and *Citrobacter* produce the Vi polysaccharide capsule, which may mask the O antigens. If only the Vi antiserum is positive, heat the bacterial suspension in boiling water to remove the capsule and test it again using the same antisera. Rough strains, in which the O antigens are absent, tend to cross-agglutinate with different antisera.

Table 3.10 Antigenic structure of some *Salmonella* spp.

Serotype	O antigen	H (phase 1)	H (phase 2)
Typhi	9, 12 (Vi)	d	–
Paratyphi A			
Paratyphi B	1, 4, 5, 12	b	1, 2
Paratyphi C	6, 7 (Vi)	c	1, 5
Typhimurium	1, 4, 5, 12	i	1, 2
Enteritidis	1, 9, 12	g, m	1, 7
Virchow	6, 7	r	1, 2
Hadar	6, 8	Z10	e, n, x
Heidelberg	1, 4, 5, 12	r	1, 2
Dublin	1, 9, 12 (Vi)	G,p	–

Most diagnostic laboratories identify the organism as *Salmonella* with biochemical tests (e.g., API 20E or shorter panel) and partially determine the antigenic structure with different Poly-O and Poly-H antisera (Table 3.10). This identifies causes of enteric fever or invasive serotypes.

All *Salmonella* should be submitted to the local health department laboratory for confirmation of serotype and further epidemiological investigations as necessary.

Treatment

Enteric fever

First-line treatment for imported cases of typhoid fever in the United States is now ceftriaxone. When susceptibility results are available, options may include ciprofloxacin, azithromycin, ampicillin, or trimethoprim/sulfamethoxazole.

Nontyphoidal salmonella

Gastroenteritis does not usually require treatment, except in the immunosuppressed, neonates, the elderly, and those at risk of bacteremia. Suitable antibiotics include ampicillin, ciprofloxacin, and trimethoprim/sulfamethoxazole, depending on susceptibility results.

Invasive disease due to NTS (e.g., bacteremia, meningitis) always requires therapy. Cefotaxime and ceftriaxone penetrate the CSF well so are often used for *Salmonella* meningitis.

Chronic asymptomatic carriers

Management of chronic asymptomatic carriers is debated. Good personal hygiene should prevent spread of disease. In the absence of biliary disease, prolonged use of antibiotics (e.g., ampicillin, ciprofloxacin) may cure 80% of carriers.

Cholecystectomy may be considered for patients with gallstones or chronic cholecystitis, but there is a risk of spreading the organisms during surgery.

Shigella

The genus *Shigella* is divided into four species: *S. dysenteriae, S. flexneri, S. boydii,* and *S. sonnei,* on the basis of serology and biochemical reactions (Table 3.11). The organisms cause bacillary dysentery by an invasive mechanism identical to enteroinvasive *E. coli* (EIEC).

Shigella belongs to the tribe Escherichiaeae, and DNA hybridization studies show that *E. coli* and *Shigella* are a single genetic species.

Epidemiology

There are 10 serotypes of *S. dysenteriae* and 15 serotypes of *S. boydii*. *S. flexneri* can be divided into six serotypes by group- and type-specific antigens, and each serotype can be further subdivided.

S. sonnei must be typed by other means, such as colicine production or plasmids, as they are serologically homogenous.

Most cases of shigellosis in occur in young children, although infection occurs in any age after travel to areas where hygiene is poor.

Table 3.11 Biochemical reactions of Shigella

Shigella spp.	Gas from glucose	ONPG	Indole	Catalase	Acid from Lactose	Acid from Mannitol	Acid from Dulcitol
dysenteriae 1	–	+	–	–	–	–	–
dysenteriae 2–10	–	V	V	+	–	–	–
flexneri 1–5	–	–	V	+	–	+	–
flexneri 6	V	–	–	+	–	V	V
boydii	–	–	V	+	–	+	V
Sonnei	–	+	–	+	(+)	+	–

ONPG, ortho-nitrophenyl-ß-galactoside; V, variable; (+), positive after incubation for ≥48 hours.

Pathogenesis

The infecting dose of Shigella is only 10–100 organisms, so the illness can be transferred from person to person (feco-oral). When one member of a family has acquired the disease, the secondary attack rate is high. Infection can spread rapidly in institutions, especially among young children. It is commonly spread by food and water.

Dysentery results from invasion of the wall of the large bowel, with accompanying inflammation and capillary thrombosis. As the organisms invade and multiply within epithelial cells, cell death results in ulcer formation. Invasiveness is linked to the presence of a 140 MDa plasmid. The organisms rarely invade deeper than the mucosa, hence positive blood cultures are uncommon.

Some strains also produce an exotoxin, which results in water and electrolyte secretion from the small bowel (and has some similarities with the cholera toxin). This may explain the brief watery diarrhea that can precede bloody diarrhea.

Clinical features

See Gastroenteritis (p. 354). S. dysenteriae usually causes a more severe illness, possibly with marked prostration and pediatric febrile convulsions. S. dysenteriae may also be associated with toxic megacolon and the hemolytic uremic syndrome (HUS). S. flexneri and S. boydii may also cause severe disease, while S. sonnei usually causes mild symptoms.

The severity of S. dysenteriae infection may be due to an exotoxin (previously thought to be a neurotoxin), but its exact role in pathogenesis is uncertain. Shigella rarely invades other tissues, hence septicemia and metastatic infection are unusual.

Diagnosis

Shigella organisms are nonmotile, noncapsulated Gram-negative rods. Most appear as non-lactose fermenters after 18–24 hours' incubation on MacConkey or desoxycholate citrate agar (DCA), but S. sonnei is the only late lactose fermenter. Shigella is urease-, citrate-, and H_2S-negative. S. dysenteriae is the only one that cannot ferment mannitol.

Box 3.2 Positive leukocyte test

Remember, this indicates invasive diarrhea/colitis from a number of causes. Consider the following:

- *Shigella*
- *Salmonella*
- *Campylobacter* enteritis
- Idiopathic ulcerative colitis
- *C. difficile* diarrhea (but poor sensitivity in addition to poor specificity)

Suspicious colonies should be confirmed with species-specific antisera, followed by type-specific antisera for all except *S. sonnei*.

Direct microscopy of a stained fecal smear (usually methylene blue) will reveal numerous polymorphonuclear leukocytes (Box 3.2).

Treatment

Most cases of shigella are mild and self-limiting, so are treated with oral rehydration therapy rather than with antibiotics. Antibiotics may be indicated in severe infections, in patients at extremes of age, or in the immunocompromised.

Options include ciprofloxacin, ampicillin, trimethoprim/sulfamethoxazole, tetracycline, or cephalosporins, according to in vitro susceptibility testing.

Antibiotics are unlikely to reduce the period of excretion.

Other *Enterobacteriaceae*

Hafnia alvei

Hafnia alvei (formerly an *Enterobacter*) belongs to the tribe Klebsielleae. *Hafnia* is found in human and animal feces, sewage, soil, water, and dairy products. It usually produces gray colonies on blood agar and ferments fewer sugars than *Enterobacter*.

All *H. alvei* are lysed by a single phage, which does not act on any other *Enterobacteriaceae*. *H. alvei* occasionally causes opportunistic or nosocomial infections, and antibiotic sensitivities are usually similar to those of the *Enterobacter* group.

Pantoea agglomerans

Pantoea agglomerans (previously known as *Erwinia herbicola* or *Enterobacter agglomerans*) is similar to many plant pathogens. It occasionally causes opportunistic infections in humans (UTIs, bacteremia, and chest infections) and in the past has contaminated IV fluids.

Colonies are yellow and may be isolated from superficial skin swabs and respiratory specimens, when they are usually regarded as normal flora.

Edwardsiella tarda

Edwardsiella tarda infections in humans probably originate from contact with cold-blooded animals. These organisms are motile and ferment glucose to produce gas. Because they are H_2S-positive and do not ferment lactose, they may be mistaken for *Salmonella* species on enteric media.

Edwardsiella species rarely cause disease but are occasionally associated with a *Salmonella*-like gastroenteritis, which usually resolves without antibiotics. There are case reports of bacteremia, liver abscess, soft tissue infection, and meningitis.

Treatment should be guided by disc susceptibility testing.

Morganella morganii

This belongs to the tribe Proteeae. Thus they are motile, deaminate phenylalanine rapidly, give positive methyl-red reactions, and are usually VP-negative. Most are indole-positive and hydrolse urea rapidly (Table 3.8). *Morganella* organisms cause hospital-acquired infections, which are often multiresistant, so treatment is with carbapenems.

Providencia alcalifaciens, Providencia stuartii, and Providencia rettgeri

These also belong to the tribe Proteeae. Thus they are motile and deaminate phenylalanine rapidly. They give positive methyl-red reactions and are usually VP-negative and indole-positive.

Most *P. rettgeri* hydrolse urea rapidly, while the others are urease-negative (Table 3.8). *Providencia* causes nosocomial infections in debilitated patients. Treatment is with carbapenems.

Overview of Gram-negative rod nonfermenters

These organisms derive energy from carbohydrates through oxidative (rather than fermentative) metabolism.

Pseudomonads

The pseudomonads are a large and diverse group of aerobic, oxidative, Gram-negative rods (GNRs). Most are saprophytes found in soil, water, and moist environments. *Pseudomonas aeruginosa* is the species most commonly associated with human disease, particularly nosocomial infections.

Other opportunistic species of *Pseudomonas* include *P. putida*, *P. fluorescens* (which has been associated with blood transfusions), and *P. stutzeri*. Organisms that have been allocated to new genera include *Burkholderia* (*B. cepacia* and *B. pseudomallei*), *Stenotrophomas* (*S. maltophilia*), *Comamonas* (discussed later), and *Brevundimonas* (discussed later).

Delftia acidovorans

Formerly known as *Comamonas acidovorans* or *Pseudomonas acidovorans*, this rare organism may cause endocarditis in drug users. Confusion about its identity can arise, as it may grow on *B. cepacia*–selective media and may be resistant to colistin and gentamicin.

Brevundimonas
B. diminuta and *B. vesicularis* are rare and of doubtful clinical significance.

Glucose nonfermenters

This diverse group is taxonomically distinct from the oxidative pseudomonads and the carbohydrate-fermenting *Enterobacteriaceae*. They are mainly opportunistic pathogens and often multiresistant to antibiotics. Identification difficulties arise because they tend to be biochemically inert.

Eikenella corrodens

This oral commensal can cause endocarditis (*E* in HACEK; see HACEK organisms, p. 255), meningitis, skin and soft tissue infections (particularly from human bites), and pneumonia. It is a facultative anaerobe, requiring incubation in CO_2. The colonies pit (corrode) the surface of the agar.

Flavimonas
F. oryzihabitans is found in soil, water, and damp environments and most commonly causes central line–associated bacteremias in immunocompromised patients.

Flavobacterium
This group of yellow-pigmented organisms is so genetically diverse that many have been reclassified. *F. meningosepticum* is now *Chryseobacterium meningosepticum* and has caused epidemics of adult and neonatal meningitis with high mortality. Other flavobacteria now belong to the genus *Sphingobacterium* (see below).

Chryseobacterium

Other than *C. meningosepticum* (see above), isolation of these organisms from clinical samples usually reflects colonization rather than infection. As noted earlier, *C. meningosepticum* has caused epidemics of adult and neonatal meningitis with high mortality.

In vitro testing may not correlate with antibiotic clinical efficacy. There is evidence for treatment with vancomycin ± rifampicin, or ciprofloxacin, or levofloxacin.

Sphingobacterium

These contain high amounts of sphingophospholipid compounds in their cell membrane. Most human isolates of this genus are *S. multivorum* and *S. spiritivorum*, which can cause nosocomial infections in various sites.

Shewanella

S. putrefaciens (formerly *Pseudomonas putrefaciens*) is commonly isolated from water and the environment but rarely causes human disease. It is usually found as part of a polymicrobial infection, typically from cellulitis complicating a leg ulcer or burn.

Roseomonas

These are also known as the "pink-pigmented coccoid" group. *R. gilardii* is the most common species isolated from humans and has been reported to cause community-acquired bacteremia.

Chryseomonas

Infection with the rare *C. luteola* is usually associated with peritoneal dialysis catheters or indwelling lines and may result in peritonitis, endocarditis, bacteremia, or meningitis.

Ochrobactrum

Previously called *Achromobacter*, *Ochrobactrum anthropi* causes nosocomial opportunistic infections, particularly catheter-related bacteremia.

Oligella

O. urethralis (formerly *Moraxella urethralis*) is a genitourinary tract commensal, while *O. ureolytica* is usually found in patients with long-term indwelling urinary catheters. They are of low pathogenicity.

Alcaligenes

There are three clinically relevant species: *A. xylosoxidans* (sometimes called *Achromobacter xylosoxidans*), *A. faecalis* (formerly *Alcaligenes odorans*), and *A. piechaudii*. They are found in soil and water and in the GI and respiratory tracts of hospital patients.

Nosocomial outbreaks have occurred (generally, but not exclusively in immunocompromised patients) with a wide range of clinical manifestations.

A. xylosoxidans is often multiresistant to antibiotics, and carbapenems or trimethoprim/sulfamethoxazole may be required as therapy.

Agrobacterium

These plant pathogens are usually nonpathogenic to humans, with <50 case reports of human disease in the literature. These are mainly due to *A. radiobacter* and *A. tumifaciens*.

Sphingomonas

S. paucimobilis (the only species) has been implicated in nosocomial outbreaks associated with contaminated water. It may be confused with flavobacteria, as it produces a nondiffusible yellow pigment.

Pseudomonas aeruginosa

P. aeruginosa is widespread in soil, water, and other moist environments. Humans may be colonized with *P. aeruginosa* at moist sites such as the perineum, ear, and axilla. It is a highly successful opportunistic pathogen, especially in the hospital setting.

This success is largely due to its resistance to many antibiotics, its ability to adapt to a wide range of physical conditions, and its minimal nutritional requirements.

Epidemiology

P. aeruginosa is found almost anywhere in the environment, including surface waters, vegetation, and soil. It usually colonizes hospital and domestic sink traps, taps, and drains. It also colonizes moist areas of human skin, leading to "toe web rot" in soldiers stationed in swampy areas and otitis externa in divers in saturation chambers.

Pathogenesis

The broad range of conditions caused by *P. aeruginosa* may be explained by the fact that the pathogen is both invasive and toxigenic. *P. aeruginosa* has low intrinsic virulence in humans and animals.

Infection occurs when host defenses are compromised or the skin or mucous membranes are breached (e.g., neutropenia, burn patients, ICU patients, indwelling devices), or when a relatively large inoculum is introduced directly into the tissues.

The process can be divided into three stages:
- Bacterial attachment and colonization
- Local invasion
- Dissemination and systemic disease

Different virulence factors are produced, depending on the site and nature of the infections, and include the followng:
- Exotoxins: exotoxin A and exoenzyme S
- Lipopolysaccharide (endotoxin)
- Cytotoxic substances: proteases (elastase and alkaline phosphatase), cytotoxin (previously called leukocidin), hemolysins, phospholipases, rhamnolipids, pyocyanin
- Porins
- Pili and fimbriae (important in epithelial adherence, e.g., respiratory)

Clinical features

P. aeruginosa causes a wide spectrum of conditions:
- Community-acquired infections are rare and tend to be mild and superficial. Examples include otitis externa, varicose ulcers, and folliculitis associated with jacuzzis.
- Nosocomial infections with *P. aeruginosa* tend to be more severe and more varied than community infections. *P. aeruginosa* may account for ~10% of all hospital-acquired infections. Examples include pneumonia, urinary tract infections, surgical wound infections, bloodstream infections, and respiratory infections.
- Cystic fibrosis patients (see Box 3.3), burn patients, and mechanically ventilated patients are at particular risk.
- Other conditions associated with *P. aeruginosa* include endocarditis (in IV drug users and with prosthetic valves), eye infections, bone and joint infections, postoperative neurosurgical infections, and eye and ear infections.

Diagnosis

This nonsporing, noncapsulate, motile Gram-negative rod is a strict aerobe (hence often used in testing anaerobic cabinets). However, it can

Box 3.3 *P. aeruginosa* **inpatients with cystic fibrosis (CF)**

P. aeruginosa colonizes up to 80% of CF patients and causes chronic lung infection. Once established, it is refractory to treatment.

Many *P. aeruginosa* isolates appear mucoid, which is due to production of an alginate-like exopolyscaaharide capsule (glyocalyx). This may form a biofilm, which renders the infection less amenable to antibiotic treatment.

Isolates may have atypical growth requirements, such as appearing auxotrophic for specific amino acids, nonmotile, and susceptible to semisynthetic penicillins. Primary culture plates often show mixtures of colonial forms, but these variants are usually genetically identical.

grow anaerobically in the presence of nitrate. It grows on many different culture media and produces a characteristic freshly-cut grass odor.

The typical green-blue color is due to the diffusible pigments pyocyanin (blue phenazine pigment) and pyoverdin (yellow-green fluorescent pigment; principle siderophore). Other pigments include pyorubrin (red) and pyomelanin (brown). Note that ~10% do not produce detectable pigments even on pigment-enhancing media.

P. aeruginosa is oxidase-positive (usually within 10 seconds) and appears relatively inactive in carbohydrate fermentation tests (only glucose is used). It grows best at 37°C and also at 42°C, but not at 4°C. Confusion occasionally arises in differentiating *P. aeruginosa* from other *Pseudomonas* spp. with commercial kits: growth at 42°C; flagella stains; and differential sugar fermentation tests may prove useful.

For epidemiological studies, serotyping may be useful; however, of the 21 internationally accepted O serotypes, 4 account for ~50% of clinical and environmental isolates.

PFGE may help discriminate between serotypes. Other typing schemes are based on phage susceptibility and bacteriocin production.

Treatment

Antipseudomonal agents include the fluoroquinolones (these are the only oral option), ceftazidime, ticarcillin, piperacillin, carbapenems (imipenem, meropenem), aminoglycosides (gentamicin, tobramycin, amikacin), polymyxins (colistin), and aztreonam.

Theoretically, the use of dual therapy should reduce the development of antibiotic resistance and may also have the potential for bacterial synergy, but there is little clinical evidence for this.

Acinetobacter

Acinetobacter spp. are becoming increasingly important as a cause of nosocomial infections and are often multiresistant to antibiotics. Increasing antibiotic-selective pressure and the ability to survive well in the hospital environment (including on curtains and in dust) have contributed to its success as an opportunistic pathogen.

Table 3.12 Genomic species of *Acinetobacter*

Genospecies	Species name
1	A. calcoaceticus
2	A. baumannii
4	A. haemolyticus
5	A. junii
7	A. johnsonii
8	A. lwoffi
12	A. radioresistens
Other	A. species unnamed (>14)

There are ~19 genospecies, based on DNA–DNA hybridization studies; 7 of these have species names (Table 3.12).

Epidemiology

Nosocomial spread in ICUs is common and may occur via equipment (particularly ventilators), gloves, contaminated solutions, and colonized health care workers.

There are reports of *Acinetobacter baumanii* infections in casualties returning from Iraq.

Risk factors

Risk factors include the following:
- *Community-acquired infections:* alcoholics, smokers, chronic lung disease, diabetes, and living in a tropical developing country
- *Hospital-acquired infections:* intensive care, ventilation, urinary catheter, IV lines, increased length of stay, treatment with broad-spectrum antibiotics, total parenteral nutrition (TPN), surgery, wounds
  Pathogenesis

This organism has very few virulence factors, which explains why it only causes opportunistic infections. It occurs naturally as a saprophyte in soil and water, and occasionally colonizes moist human skin. The ability to survive in the environment is probably related to the capsule, the production of bacteriocin, and prolonged viability under dry conditions.

Clinical features

Acinetobacter spp. are able to infect almost every organ system, though it is vital to distinguish true infection from pseudoinfection (e.g., pseudobacteremia due to skin colonization). The most common site of infection is the respiratory tract, where it causes nosocomial pneumonia, particularly ventilator-associated pneumonia (VAP), adult community-acquired pneumonia, and community-acquired tracheobronchitis and bronchiolitis in children.

Other sites include the urinary tract, intracranial (usually post-neurosurgery) tissue, soft tissue (burns, wounds, and line-associated cellulitis), eye infections, endocarditis, and bone.

Nosocomial bacteremia is usually associated with the respiratory tract or intravenous catheters and has a reported mortality rate of 17–46%.

A. baumannii bacteremia tends to be more severe.

Diagnosis

Acinetobacter spp. classically appear as Gram-negative coccobacilli, although they may retain crystal violet so appear Gram-positive. They are generally encapsulated, nonmotile organisms, which readily grow on routine media as white, mucoid, oxidase-negative, catalase-positive colonies.

Misidentification may arise using API profiles, as they are biochemically relatively unreactive, but acidification of glucose, hemolysis of red blood cells, and ability to grow at 44°C are reliable characteristics.

Treatment

Treatment may require several different approaches:
- Localized cellulitis associated with a foreign body or indwelling line may respond to removal of the foreign body alone (antibiotics not needed).
- Choice of antibiotics for more serious infections is becoming limited—e.g., cerain clones are resistant to virtually all antibiotics including carbapenems. Susceptibility testing should include carbapenems, aminoglycosides (including amikacin), sulbactam, polymixins (e.g., colistin), and tigecycline. There is some evidence to support combination therapy with rifampicin and colistin, +/– imipenem.
- Liason with reference laboratories aboot typing and antibiotic options
- Review of infection control practices and antibiotic prescribing in the case of an outbreak
- *Multi-drug-resistant Acinetobacter* (MDRAB) is defined as an isolate of *Acinetobacter* spp. that is resistant to any aminoglycoside *and* to any third-generation cephalosporin.
- *MRDAB-C* is defined as an MRDAB that is also resistant to the carbapenems. These harbor metallocarbapenemases, such as VIM and IMP (see Carbapenems, p. 33) and are thought to have originated in Korea.

Stenotrophomonas maltophilia

Previously called *Pseudomonas maltophilia* or *Xanthomonas maltophilia*, this organism is becoming increasingly seen as a cause of nosocomial infection. It is an opportunistic pathogen, of relatively low virulence, but has an amazing ability to survive in a wide range of environments. It is frequently multiresistant to antibiotics.

Epidemiology

Ubiquitous in the environment, *S. maltophilia* has been isolated from multiple sources in hospitals, including water (tap and distilled), nebulizers, dialysis machines, solutions, intravenous fluids, and thermometers.

Transmission of nosocomial infection has been associated with hospital water or contaminated disinfectant solutions. Studies have shown that most outbreaks result from antibiotic-selective pressure (especially the extensive use of imipenem, to which S. *maltophilia* is resistant) and exposure to multiple environmental strains, rather than cross-infection.

Risk factors

Risk factors for nosocomial infection include intensive care, increased length of stay, treatment with broad-spectrum antibiotics, malignancy (especially if immunosuppressed), instrumentation (e.g., urinary catheter, intravenous lines, intubation, TPN, CAPD), patients with COPD, IV drug users, and neutropenia.

Pathogenesis

Potential virulence factors include those involved in adherence to plastics and production of exoenzymes such as elastase and gelatinase.

Clinical features

S. *maltophilia* can cause a variety of infections, ranging from superficial to deep-tissue to disseminated disease. It is most commonly isolated from the respiratory tract, and distinguishing true infection from colonization can be difficult. S. *maltophilia* pneumonia has a high mortality, especially when associated with bacteremia or GI obstruction.

Other common sites of S. *maltophilia* infection include skin and soft tissue, intra-abdominal, the urinary tract, the eyes (especially in contact-lens wearers), and implants. Endocarditis is also reported.

Diagnosis

This motile, non-lactose-fermenting, Gram-negative aerobic rod grows readily on standard media. It is often pale yellow on blood agar, with an ammonia-like smell. Most are oxidase-negative, catalase-positive, anDNase positive and can hydrolyse esculin and ONPG. It is the only pseudomonad that gives a positive lysine decarboxylase reaction.

Resistance to imipenem may be a useful marker.

S. *maltophilia* is increasingly isolated from sputum from patients with cystic fibrosis. It grows well on colistin-containing media, so may be misidentified as B. *cepacia*.

Treatment

Unfortunately, results of antibiotic susceptibility testing correlate poorly with treatment outcome. The drug of choice is trimethoprim- sulfamethoxazole (see Co-trimoxazole, p. 56). Other options to consider include ticarcillin-clavulanate, doxycycline, minocycline, newer-generation quinolones, and third-generation cephalosporins (e.g., ceftazidime).

There is clinical evidence that trimethoprim/sulfamethoxazole and moxifloxacin are synergistic.

Most strains are resistant to aminoglycosides.

Burkholderia cepacia

Previously classified as *Pseudomonas cepacia,* this opportunistic pathogen is a particular problem in patients with CF. Other risk factors for infection include chronic granulomatous disease (CGD) and sickle cell hemoglobinopathies.

There are 10 phylogenetically similar but genomically distinct species, known as the *Burkholderia cepacia* complex (Table 3.13).

Epidemiology

B. cepacia is ubiquitous in the environment and has been isolated from multiple sources in hospitals. Environmental transmission may occur via contact with respiratory equipment, water supplies, or disinfectants.

However, transmission by close contact with colonized patients to other CF patients is more significant, and patients should be segregated into separate groups (e.g., for outpatient clinics and summer camps), which can be a highly emotional issue.

Pathogenesis

This is a relatively poorly virulent organism, which can survive in a wide range of environments. Virulence factors include adherence to plastics and production of elastase, gelatinase, adhesin (a mucin-binding protein), siderophores, hemolysin, and exopolysaccharide.

Resistance to nonoxidative neutrophil killing may be important. One successful epidemic strain had giant cable pili to help attach to respiratory mucin.

Table 3.13 *Burkholderia cepacia* complex

Genomovar	Name	Notes
I	*B. cepacia*	*Type species*
II	*B. multivorans*	Common in CF, associated with epidemic spread in a number of CF centers worldwide
III*	*B. cenocepacia*	Most common in CF*
IV	*B. stabilis*	
V	*B. vietnamiensis*	
VI	*B. dolosa*	
VII	*B. ambifaria*	
VIII	*B. anthina*	
IX	*B. pyrrocinia*	
IX	*B. ubonensis*	

*Genomovar III has been linked to increased transmissibility between patients and with a poorer prognosis and higher mortality for some patients.

Clinical features

This is a significant pathogen in CF patients, with mortality rates >50% in the first year post-infection. The three main patterns of infection are

- Chronic asymptomatic carriage
- Progressive deterioration over months, with frequent hospital admissions, recurrent fevers, and weight loss
- Necrotizing pneumonia and bacteremia, associated with rapid deterioration, which is occasionally fatal. Risk factors for this pattern include females with poor lung function and severe CXR changes.

In other patients, *B. cepacia* can cause a range of other infections, from superficial to deep tissue to disseminated, but these are rare.

Diagnosis

B. cepacia are motile, non-lactose fermenting, Gram-negative, aerobic rods. Selective media are necessary for culture, and the color and shape of the colonies vary with the particular strain and media.

Treatment

Although agents such as trimethoprim/sulfamethoxazole, chloramphenicol, minocycline, and the carbapenems show good in vitro activity against *B. cepacia*, their activity against strains from CF patients is decreased. Also, clearance of these drugs is increased in the CF population, and monitoring of serum levels should be considered to ensure adequate dosing. Use of combination therapy is debated, and specialist units usually produce strict antibiotic treatment protocols.

Almost all *B. cepacia* are constitutively resistant to polymyxin. Immunotherapy with specific *B. cepacia* antigens may prove beneficial.

Burkholderia pseudomallei

Burkholderia pseudomallei (formerly known as *Pseudomonas pseudomallei*) causes melioidosis, which is endemic in parts of Southeast Asia, northern Australia, and the Caribbean. It is a major cause of community-onset septicemia in northeast Thailand.

Epidemiology

In endemic areas, *B. pseudomallei* can be cultured from moist soil, surface water (rice paddies), and the surface of many fruits and vegetables. It is also carried by rodents.

Pathogenesis

B. pseudomallei can survive and multiply within phagocytes. Thus a long course of antibiotics is recommended; antibiotics active in vitro do not always lead to clinical cure.

Clinical features

B. pseudomallei is usually acquired through inhaling contaminated particles or cutaneously through skin abrasions. This organism has been called the "great imitator," as it can cause suppurative infections of almost any organ.

Manifestations range from subclinical infection to localized lung infection (cavitating pneumonia with profound weight loss, resembling TB) to overwhelming septicemia. Bone and joint infections are common, as is parotid gland infection in children. Symptoms may occur years after exposure, because of the intracellular nature of the organism.

Diagnosis

B. Pseudomallei laboratory-acquired cases may occur, so all specimens should be handled under biosafety level 2 or 3 precautions (depending on the type of laboratory activity) if meliodosis is suspected clinically. *B. Pseudomallei* is considered a select agent.

Culture

B. pseudomallei colonies grow well on blood or Ashdown medium nutrient agar, after 1–2 days. They appear either wrinkled and dry, or mucoid, and after prolonged incubation may turn orange. Gram staining often shows small, bipolar, Gram-negative rods.

B. pseudomallei is a strict aerobe and oxidizes glucose and breaks down arginine. Isolates are characteristically resistant to gentamicin and colistin.

The API 20NE reliably identifies most isolates, but early involvement of the reference laboratory is recommended for confirmatory tests, e.g., indirect hemagglutination, PCR, IgM- and IgG-specific ELISAs, and serology (but there are problems with sensitivity and specificity).

Treatment

The antibiotic of choice is ceftazidime IV for 10–14 days or until clinical improvement occurs (with imipenem or meropenem as alternatives). This should be followed by prolonged oral therapy (e.g., trimethoprim/sulfamethoxazole plus doxycycline for 20 weeks, plus chloramphenicol for the first 4 weeks) or amoxicillin-clavulonic acid to prevent relapse.

Resistance to these oral agents may develop during treatment: seek expert advice. In case of β-lactam allergy, this oral regimen may be given IV in cases of sepsis, but is less effective than ceftazidime.

Burkholderia mallei

B. mallei causes glanders, which is a rare disease of horses in Asia, Africa, and the Middle East. In humans it causes symptoms similar to meliodosis.

Overview of fastidious Gram-negative rods

These organisms often require specialist supplements or media for culture. They can be divided by appearance on Gram stain as follows:

Coccobacilli
• *Haemophilus*
• HACEK organisms

- *Gardnerella*
- *Bordetella*
- *Brucella*
- *Yersinia*
- *Pasteurella*
- *Francisella*

Rods with pointed ends
- *Legionella*
- *Capnocytophaga*

Curved rods
- *Vibrio*
- *Aeromonas, Plesiomonas*
- *Campylobacter*
- *Helicobacter*

Streptobacillus moniliformis causes rat bite fever, as does *Spirillium minor*.

Haemophilus influenzae

Haemophilus influenzae is a small, fastidious, Gram-negative coccobacillus belonging to the family *Pasteurellaceae*. It is highly adapted to humans and found in the nasopharynx of 75% of healthy children and adults.

It was first isolated in 1890 by Pfeiffer and mistakenly thought to be the cause of influenza. It was also the first living organism to have its genome fully sequenced.

Epidemiology

Haemophilus influenzae capsular type 3 (Hib) used to be a common cause of meningitis in childcare. The annual incidence of invasive Hib disease dropped dramatically after introduction of the Hib conjugate vaccine in 1993 but started to rise again in 1999. In 2003, a booster campaign was implemented for children aged 6 months to 4 years.

Pathogenesis

H. influenzae inhabits the upper respiratory tract of humans; 25–80% of healthy people carry noncapsulate organisms, and 5–10% carry capsulate strains (~50% of which are capsular type b).

In addition to the polysaccharide capsule that facilitates invasion, virulence factors of capsular type b include fimbriae (involved in attaching to epithelial cells), IgA proteases (help colonization), and outer-membrane proteins (involved in invasion also). There is evidence that simultaneous viral infection may initiate invasion.

Clinical features

- *Invasive infections*: e.g., meningitis, epiglottitis, bacteremia with no clear focus, septic arthritis, pneumonia, cellulitis. These are mostly caused by capsular type b, but types e and f and noncapsulate strains can also cause serious disease. Infections generally occur in children between 2 months and 2 years of age. Babies <2 months are protected by maternal antibody.

- *Noninvasive infections:* e.g., otitis media, sinusitis, purulent exacerbations of COPD. These local infections are usually associated with non-capsulate organisms. There may be an underlying abnormality (anatomical or physiological). Intercurrent virus infection may precipitate infection.

Diagnosis

Culture

These organisms only grow in the presence of X and V factors. X factor (hemin) is needed to synthesize some respiratory enzymes that contain iron (e.g., cytochrome c, cytochrome oxidase, catalase, peroxidase). V factor is NAD(P): nicotinamide adenine dinucleotide (phosphate), and is required for oxidation–reduction processes in metabolism.

Blood agar (BA) contains both X and V, but *H. influenzae* grows poorly. NAD supplementation improves growth on BA, as will streaking an organism that excretes NAD, e.g., *S. aureus*. This phenomenon is called satellitism.

H. influenzae grows well on chocolate agar, which is made by heating BA at 70–80°C for a few minutes to lyse the red cells and inactivate the NADase, which normally limits utilization of V factor.

Growth is also better in CO_2-enriched conditions. Antibiotic susceptibility testing with discs may be unreliable: nitrocefin strips are recommended to test for β-lactamases.

Antigen detection

In addition to culture, *H. influenzae* may be diagnosed by antigen detection (e.g., with latex agglutination, but beware of cross-reactions with *S. pneumoniae* and *E. coli*, so culture is needed for confirmation).

Molecular tests, e.g., PCR, are available but not yet widely used.

Capsule detection

Encapsulated strains of *H. influenzae* are responsible for most invasive infections (e.g., meningitis and epiglottitis), while respiratory infections and otitis media are usually associated with nonencapsulated strains. The polysaccharide capsule can be demonstrated by the Quellung reaction with type-specific antisera.

- *Antigenic type:* there are six antigenic types (a–f). *H. influenzae* type b (Hib), which is a polymer of ribosyl ribitol phosphate, causes the most severe invasive infections.
- *Biotypes:* there are eight biotypes of *H. influenzae* (I–VIII), based on indole, ornithine decarboxylase, and urease reactions. The most common are biotypes I–III, and the most invasive (type b) organisms are biotype I.

Treatment

First-choice antibiotics for life-threatening *H. influenzae* infections are third-generation cephalosporins, e.g., ceftriaxone. They are bactericidal, penetrate the CSF, and are clinically effective. Less serious *H. influenzae* infections can be treated with oral ampicillin (β-lactamase-negative), amoxicillin-clavulonic acid, or clarithromycin.

Prevention
- *Hib conjugate vaccine:* for detailed information about use of the Hib vaccine, refer to the CDC guidelines posted at: www.cdc.gov/vaccines/recs/schedules/default.htm
- *Household contacts:* chemoprophylaxis is no longer recommended to household contacts of an invasive case of *H. influenzae* if all children <4 years old in the household have been fully vaccinated against *H. influenzae*. If one child <4 years old has been unvaccinated or incompletely vaccinated, then ALL household contacts should receive chemoprophylaxis with rifampin regardless of age or vaccination status.
- *Playgroup/nursery school contacts:* chemoprophylaxis should be offered to all room contacts (teachers and children) if two cases of Hib occur within 120 days. Unvaccinated children <4 years old should be vaccinated.
- *Cases of Hib <4 years old* should receive vaccine and chemoprophylaxis before they are discharged from the hospital, to eliminate carriage, as there are reports of infection failing to induce immunity.

Reference

Fleischmann RD, Adams MD, While O, et al. (1995). Whole-genome random sequencing and assembly of *Haemophilus influenzae* Rd. *Science* 269(5223):496–512.

Other *Haemophilus* spp.

Haemophilus species other than *H. influenzae* have been considered rare causes of human disease. However, they may cause infections more commonly than was previously believed. Most are normal flora of the human mouth and upper respiratory tract. They are associated with infections such as endocarditis, respiratory tract infection, septicemia, brain abscess, meningitis, and soft tissue infection.

H. parainfluenzae

H. parainfluenzae is increasingly recognized as a cause of human infection. Clinical infections are similar to those caused by *H. influenzae*, but *H. parainfluenzae* tends to be less virulent than *H. influenzae*.

H. parainfluenzae has been reported as a cause of pharyngitis, epiglottitis, otitis media, conjunctivitis, dental abscess, pneumonia, empyema, septicemia, endocarditis, septic arthritis, osteomyelitis, meningitis, abscesses elsewhere, and urinary and genital tract infections.

H. Parainfluenzae differs from *H. influenzae* in that it is V factor dependent only and catalase-positive.

H. haemolyticus and H. parahaemolyticus

It is commonly thought that these species rarely cause human disease. However, recent work suggests that standard methods do not reliably distinguish *H. haemolyticus* from *H. influenzae*, so it may be more common than previously considered.

Aggregatibacter aphrophilus

The species *H. aphrophilus* and *H. paraphrophilus* have been recently reclassified as a single species, *Aggregatibacter aphrophilus*. Both of these species require CO_2 for growth.

H. aphrophilus is V factor independent and has been linked with sinusitis, otitis media, pneumonia, empyema, bacteremia, endocarditis, septic arthritis, osteomyelitis, meningitis, soft tissue abscesses elsewhere, and wound infections.

H. paraphrophilus is V factor dependent and has been documented as a cause of laryngitis, epiglottitis, endocarditis, brain abscess, hepatobiliary infection, osteomyelitis, and paronychia.

H. ducreyi

This causes chancroid, a sexually transmitted infection, common in Africa and Southeast Asia. It presents as a painful penile ulcer associated with inguinal lymphadenopathy. Microbiological diagnosis is made when Gram-negative coccobacilli are isolated from a lymph node aspirate or from ulcer swabs.

The organisms may appear in loose clusters (i.e., "school of fish") or clustered coils of Gram-negative bacilli that line up in parallel. Treatment options include third-generation cephalosporins, quinolones, and macrolides. Resistance to tetracyclines and trimethoprim-sulfamethoxazole has been observed in vitro.

H. influenzae biogroup aegyptius

H. influenzae biogroup *aegyptius* was previously known as *H. aegyptius* or the Koch–Weeks bacillus. It is very similar biochemically to *H. influenzae* biotype III but can be differentiated by PCR. It causes Brazilian purpuric fever (conjunctivitis leading to fulminant septicemia, with high mortality) and epidemic purulent conjunctivitis. Combination therapy with ampicillin and chloramphenicol is recommended.

HACEK organisms

The HACEK organisms are rare causes of endocarditis (see Infective endocarditis, p. 569), which tends to be insidious in onset (mean time to diagnosis ~3 months). Most HACEK organisms are part of normal human mouth flora and are occasionally associated with periodontitis and infections elsewhere (e.g., joints).

Recommendations for the extended incubation of blood cultures to increase the recovery of HACEK bacteria are based on studies performed before improvements in blood culture media and implementation of automated blood culture instruments. Recent data show that extended incubation is unnecessary when using automated methods.[1]

Aggregatibacter actinomycetemcomitans

A. actinomycetemcomitans, a mouth commensal, is the major pathogen of the genus *Aggregatibacter*. There are two other *Aggregatibacter* species:

Aggregatibacter aphrophilus (includes *H. aphrophilus* and *H. paraphrophilus*) and *Aggregatibacter segnis* (formerly *H. segnis*).

Diagnosis

Aggregatibacter may be difficult to culture. Growth is enhanced by CO_2 supplementation (5–10%). *Aggregatibacter* may form granules in blood cultures and broth (the media remains clear). On Gram stain, they look coccoid or coccobacillary, resembling *Haemophilus*.

A. *actinomycetemcomitans* is urease-negative, indole-negative, and catalase-positive and reduces nitrate. They do not grow on MacConkey and are biochemically similar to *Pasteurella* spp.

Pathogenesis

Periodontal disease caused by A. *actinomycetemcomitans* is associated with the ability to invade and multiply within gingival epithelial cells and the production of a leuokotoxin that lyses neutrophils.

Other potential virulence factors include a bacteriocin, endotoxin, chemotaxis-inhibiting factor, and fibroblast-inhibiting factor.

Clinical

A. *actinomycetemcomitans* can cause endocarditis, joint infections, and severe periodontal disease. *Aggregatibacter* has also been found (together with some *Haemophilus* spp. fusiforms and anaerobic streptococci) in actinomycotic lesions. Their contribution to the pathogenesis of actinmy-coses is unclear.

Cardiobacterium hominis

C. hominis is the only species in the genus. It is normal flora in the human mouth, nose, and throat and occasionally other mucous membranes and the GI tract. Unlike the other HACEK organisms, it rarely causes diseases other than endocarditis.

Diagnosis

This Gram-negative rod has a pleomorphic appearance and may be difficult to decolorize during Gram staining. Culture is enhanced in 5–10% CO_2 and high humidity. It grows well on blood agar and chocolate, with slight β-hemolysis, but poorly on MacConkey agar.

It is catalse-negative and oxidase-positive. It produces indole (although positivity is weak with many strains), which differentiates it from other HACEK organisms.

Eikenella corrodens

E. corrodens exists as normal mouth and upper respiratory tract flora.

Diagnosis

This facultative anaerobic Gram-negative rod is oxidase-positive, catalase-negative, urease-negative, and indole-negative and reduces nitrate to nitrite. About 50% of strains create a depression in the agar (corroding bacillus).

As with the other HACEK organisms, culture may be slow and enhanced in 5–10% CO_2.

Clinical features

E. corrodens causes subacute endocarditis, but is more commonly found as part of mixed infections (e.g., human bite wounds, head and neck infections, respiratory tract infections). It often coexists with *Streptococcus* spp.

There are reports of *E. corrodens* causing a variety of other infections. Infections are usually indolent, taking >1 week from time of injury to clinical symptoms of disease. Suppuration is common and may smell like an anaerobic infection.

Antibmicrobial susceptibility

E. corrodens is usually susceptible to the β-lactams, tetracyclines, and fluoroquinolones. It is uniformly resistant to clindamycin, erythromycin, and metronidazole and often resistant to aminoglycosides.

Kingella kingae

There are four species of *Kingella*, which all colonize the respiratory tract and rarely cause human disease: *K. kingae* (previously known as *Moraxella kingae*), *K. indologenes*, *K. denitrificans*, and *K. oralis*. *K. kingae* is the most common one, and a recent increase in cases is likely to be due to increased awareness of the organism and improved diagnostics.

Diagnosis

Kingella organisms have been misidentified as *Moraxella or Neisseria* in the past. They are short Gram-negative rods with tapered ends, which sometimes appear coccoid. They tend to resist decolorization so may look Gram-positive.

Kingella is catalase-negative, oxidase-positive, and urease-negative, and ferments glucose. *K. kingae* grows on blood and chocolate agar but not MacConkey.

To increase the chance of recovering *K. kingae* from joint fluid, the fluid should be inoculated into blood culture bottles rather than plated out directly onto agar plates.

Clinical features

Most cases of invasive disease due to *K. kingae* occur in children aged between 6 months and 4 years. *K. kingae* most commonly causes bacteraemia, endocarditis (of native and prosthetic valves), and skeletal infections, e.g., septic arthritis.

K. indologenes and *K. denitrificans* also cause endocarditis. *K. oralis* is found in dental plaque, but its relation to periodontal disease is unknown.

HACEK treatment

Although most HACEK organisms were susceptible to ampicillin in the past, many species have aquired the ability to produce β-lactamase.

Virtually all of these organisms remain highly susceptible to third-generation cephalosporins such as ceftriaxone.

For native valve endocarditis, the American Heart Association recommends treatment with ceftriaxone or ampicillin-sulbactam for 4 weeks. Prosthetic valve disease should be treated for 6 weeks.

Fluoroquinolones are an alternative for those unable to tolerate β-lactam.[2]

References

1. Petti CA, et al. (2006). Utility of extended blood culture incubation for isolation of *Haemophilus, Actinobacillus, Cardiobacterium, Eikenella,* and *Kingella* organisms: a retrospective multicenter evaluation. *J Clin Microbiol* 44(1):257–259.

2. Baddour LM, et al. (2005). Infective endocarditis: diagnosis, antimicrobial therapy, and management of complications: a statement for healthcare professionals from the Committee on Rheumatic Fever, Endocarditis, and Kawasaki Disease, Council on Cardiovascular Disease in the Young, and the Councils on Clinical Cardiology, Stroke, and Cardiovascular Surgery and Anesthesia, American Heart Association: endorsed by the Infectious Diseases Society of America. *Circulation* 111:e394–e434.

Gardnerella

Gardnerella vaginalis is found in the female genital tract and is associated with bacterial vaginosis (BV)/nonspecific vaginitis (see Bacterial vaginosis, p. 626). It is usually classified with GNR, although it is usually susceptible to vancomycin.

Electron microscope studies have shown the cell wall to be Gramnegative or Gram-positive or have an atypical laminated appearance.

Epidemiology

There is debate whether specific biotypes have been associated with BV. Newly acquired strains of *G. vaginalis* may precipitate BV, rather than overgrowth of previously colonizing biopsies.

Pathogenesis

Adherence of *G. vaginalis* to vaginal and urinary epithelial cells may play a role in the pathogenesis of BV and UTIs. Pili have been seen on *G. vaginalis*, and hemagglutinating activity has been shown. *G. vaginalis* also produces a cytolytic toxin (hemolysin).

It is serum resistant, which may aid survival during bloodstream invasion at childbirth.

Clinical featues

- *BV*: *G. vaginalis* is almost universally present in women with BV, along with mixed anaerobic flora.
- *UTI*: *G. vaginalis* is isolated from <1% of UTIs, and because of its presence in the femal genital tract could represent vaginal contamination. However, it has been found from suprapubic aspirates and also in association with renal disease and interstitial cystitis.
- *Bacteremia*: this rare event is associated with female genital tract conditions, such as chorioamnionitis, postpartum endometritis, and septic abortion. Neonatal infection has also been reported.

Diagnosis

Gardnerella is a facultative anaerobe, which appears as a pleomorphic Gram-variable rod. It is oxidase- and catalase-negative, nonencapsualted, and nonmotile. It needs enriched media for growth. It is also urease-, indole-, and nitrate-negative.

G. vaginalis is susceptible to sodium polyanetholesulfonate (SPS), which is found in most blood culture bottles, so bacteremia figures may be underestimated.

In clinical practice, BV is diagnosed using the Amsel criteria.

Treatment

G. vaginalis is usually susceptible to penicillin, clindamycin, and vancomycin, and resistant to colistin, cephalexin, the tetracyclines, and nalidixic acid. Metronidazole is usually the preferred treatment for BV.

Bordetella

Bordetella pertussis and *B. parapertussis* cause whooping cough, which is a notifiable disease in the United States. The other species cause human infections only under special circumstances: these are *B. bronchiseptica* (causes kennel cough in dogs and snuffles in rabbits), *B. avium* (bird pathgoen), *B. hinzii*, *B.holmesii*, and *B. trematum*.

Epidemiology

The organism is spread by droplet infection and is highly infectious. Pertussis has the highest incidence in infants but also occurs in adolescents and adults.

Morbidity and mortality are higher in females than males, and in those <6 months old.

Pathogenesis

B. pertussis produces a number of biologically active substances that are thought to play a role in disease:

- Surface components, e.g., filamentous hemagglutinin (FHA), pertactin, and fimbriae
- Toxins such as pertussis toxin (PT), adenylate cyclase toxin (ACT), tracheal cytotoxin (TCT), and dermonecrotic toxin (DNT).
- Other products, e.g., tracheal colonization factor and BrKA (*Bordetella* resistance to killing)

Clinical features

Classic (severe) pertussis is defined by the World Health Organization (WHO) as ≥21 days cough with paroxysms, associated whoops or post-tussis vomiting, and culture confirmation.

Mild pertussis is any laboratory-confirmed disease that does not meet the criteria for classic disease.

Diagnosis

These tiny coccobacilli occur singly or in pairs. *B. pertussis* and *B. parapertussis* are nonmotile.

- *Bordet–Genou agar:* pearly colonies on days 3–4
- *CCBA agar* (charcoal cephalexin): *B. pertussis* produces glistening gray-white colonies on CCBA. It does not grow on nutrient agar and grows poorly on BA. *B. parapetussis* colonies are larger and duller and become visible sooner.
- *Culture for B. pertussis* lacks sensitivity. Enhanced diagnostic methods are available at the HPA Respiratory and Systemic Infection Laboratory.
- *PCR:* one PCR targets the toxin promoter, while another PCR targets the insertion sequence IS481 (occurs in *B. pertussis*; *B. holmesii*, and some *B. bronchiseptica*). A nasal swab or nasopharyngeal aspirate (NPA) is appropriate for testing. Given the potential for asymptomatic colonization, the ability to amplify and detect nonviable organisms, and false-positive results due to specimen contamination, pertussis PCRs should only be performed for patients with a compatible illness.
- *Serology:* anti-pertussis toxin IgG antibody levels are determined using an EIA, on paired sera or single samples taken >2 weeks after onset for any individuals with prolonged cough.

Treatment

A Cochrane review on antibiotics for pertussis (2007) found that short-term antibiotics (azithromycin 3–5 days, or clarithromycin/erythromycin 7 days) were as effective as long-term antibiotics (erythromycin 10–14 days) in eradicating *B. pertussis* from the nasopharynx, but had fewer side effects.[1] Trimethoprim/sulfamethoxazole x7 days was also effective.

There were no differences in clinical outcome or microbiological relapse between short- and long-term antibiotics. In 1994, an erythromycin-resistant strain was reported from the United States, but this has not become a clinical problem.

Antibiotic prophylaxis to contacts >6 months old did not significantly improve their clinical symptoms or the number of cases developing culture-positive *B. pertussis*. The Cochrane authors concluded that there is insufficient evidence to determine the benefit of prophylactic treatment of pertussis contacts.

Vaccine

There were major epidemics of whooping cough in 1977/79 and 1981/83, after immunization coverage dropped from >80% to 30%, following a report linking the vaccine to brain damage. Coverage is now back up at ~95%. Acellular pertussis (ap) vaccine is given in the primary immunization course as Tdap/IPV/Hib.

A further booster as TdaP–IPV is given with preschool, adolescent, and adult boosters, as vaccine immunity wanes over time.

Reference

1. Altunaiji S, Kukuruzovic R, Curtis N, Massie J (2007). Antibiotics for whooping cough (pertussis). *Cochrane Database Syst Rev* Issue 2:CD004404.

Brucella

Brucella spp. (Table 3.14) cause brucellosis, which is also called undulant fever, Mediterranean fever, or Malta fever (or contagious or infectious abortion in cattle). This zoonosis is transmitted via contaminated or untreated milk and milk derivatives or direct contact with infected animals or their carcasses.

Brucella species survive well in aerosols and resist drying so are candidates for agents of bioterrorism (see Bioterrorism, p. 753).

Epidemiology

Brucellosis is still endemic in Africa, the Middle East, central and Southeast Asia, South America, and in some Mediterranean countries. It has been virtually eliminated from most developed countries.

Human–human transmission has been documented but is rare. Vehicles include breastmilk, sexual transmission, and congenital disease. Most human cases seen in the United States are due to *B. melitensis* from unpasteurized goat milk and cheeses.

Brucellosis also occurs through occupational exposure of laboratory workers, vets, and slaughterhouse workers. A careful epidemiological patient history of travel, dietary habits, and possible exposure is crucial.

Pathogenesis

After ingestion (or entry via skin abrasions, or inhaling infected dust), the bacteria live in the regional lymph nodes during the incubation period (usually 2–8 weeks). They then enter the circulation and subsequenlty localize in different parts of the reticuloendothelial system, forming granulomatous lesions that may result in complications in many organs.

Brucella organisms surviving within granuloma may cause relapses of actue disease or result in chronic brucellosis.

Clinical features

Brucellosis has a wide variety of clinical presentations. The undulant or wave-like fever rises and falls over weeks in ~90% of untreated patients. Malodoros perspiration is said to be pathognomonic. Osteoarticular disease occurs in ~20%, with epididimo-orchitis in ~6%.

Table 3.14 Main species of *Brucella**

Brucella spp.	Animal infected	Human manifestations
B. abortus	Cattle; bison and elk in North America	Brucellosis
B. suis	Pigs (swine brucellosis)	Brucellosis
B. melitensis	Goats and sheep	Brucellosis
B. canis	Dogs (mainly beagles in U.S.)	Mild disease only
B. ovis	Sheep (Australia and New Zealand)	No evidence that this species infects humans

*The host relationship is not absolute, and humans and domestic animals may be susceptible to infections by different species.

Other symptoms are weakness, headaches, depression, myalgia, and bodily pain. Sequelae are variable and include granulomatous hepatitis, anaemia, leukopenia, thrombocytopenia, meningitis, uveitis, and optic neuritis.

Diagnosis

Select agent, biosafety level 2 organism for routine culture from blood or bone marrow. These coccobacilli or short bacilli may occur singly, in chains, or in groups and can take up to 8 weeks to grow. They are non-motile, nonsporing, and noncapsulate. They are aerobic, and *B. abortus* requires 5–10% CO_2 to grow.

The three main species (*B. melitensis*, *B. abortus*, *B. suis*) can be differentiated biochemically and by antigenic structure. Each of these three species can be further divided into biotypes: there are >9 biotypes of *B. abortus*, >3 of *B. melitensis*, and >5 of *B. suis*.

However, many *Brucella* spp. are not included in the databases of commercially available kits for the identification of Gram-negative organisms. Inoculation of *Brucella* into some kits has resulted in misidentification of the organisms as *Moraxella* spp. or *Haemophilus influenzae*.

- *Molecular techniques:* real-time PCR has been developed.
- *Serology:* raised (1:160) or rising antibody titer in symptomatic patients suggests diagnosis of active *Brucella*. Demonstration of antibodies by various tests—standard agglutination test (SAT), mercaptoethanol test, classic Huddleson, Wright, and/or Bengal Rose reactions
- *Histological evidence* of granulomatous hepatitis (hepatic biopsy)
- *Radiological alterations in infected vertebrae:* the Pedro Pons sign (preferential erosion of anterosuperior corner of lumbar vertebrae) and marked osteophytosis are suspicious of brucellic spondylitis.
- *Dye inhibition test* (basic fuschin and thiamin dyes) can differentiate individual *Brucella* spp.

Treatment

Drugs must penetrate macrophages and be active in an acidic environment. Doxycycline and either gentamicin, streptomycin, or rifampin are suitable regimens. The combination is usually given for at least 6 weeks. Fluoroquinolones or tetracyclines may also be used in combination.

Intensive treatment of the acute disease is recommended, to prevent progression to chronic forms, which are more difficult to treat. Antibody levels may be measured to monitor response to therapy. A triple combination of doxycycline together with rifampin and trimethoprim/ sulfamethoxazole has been used successfully to treat neurobrucellosis.

Prevention

Good standards of hygiene in the production of raw milk and its products, or pasteurization of all milk, will prevent brucellosis acquired from ingestion of milk. Also avoid contact with infected animals.

Vaccination of young cattle helps to protect animals against *B. abortus*, but is not completely effective. However it helps to limit the spread of disease and thus aids eradication. Only by testing all animals and slaughtering those with positive results can the disease be truly eradicated.

Yersinia pestis

Y. pestis causes plague. There are three clinical syndromes: bubonic, pneumonic and septicemic (Table 3.15).

Epidemiology

Y. pestis occurs worldwide, but most cases of plague are reported from developing countries of Africa and Asia. There are ~10 cases annually from rural areas of the United States. The last outbreak of plague acquired in the UK was in 1918.

Pathogenesis

The somatic (heat-stable) and capsular (heat-labile) antigens are important in virulence and immunogenicity. Somatic antigens V and W help resist phagocytosis, and the capsular antigen containing the immunogenic fraction (F1) is antiphagocytic also.

Other virulence factors include a lipopolysaccharide endotoxin, the ability to absorb iron as haemin, and temperature-dependent coagulase and fibrinolysin.

Diagnosis

- Select agent. Biosafety level 2 organism.
- *Culture* – this short Gram-negative coccobacillus occurs singly or in pairs (or as chains in fluid culture). Old cultures are pleomorphic and may even resemble yeast cells. They are non-sporing and non-motile, and often capsulate at 37°C. Methylene blue shows bipolar staining.

Table 3.15 Features of the main clinical forms of plague

	Bubonic	Pneumonic	Septicemic
Transmission	Rat flea bites *Xenopsylla cheopis*	Respiratory aerosols from rat fleas Person-to-person spread in crowded unhygienic conditions, during epidemics May arise as a complication of bubonic or septicaemic plague	Primary infection Complication of bubonic or pneumonic plague
Diagnostic specimen	Fluid from buboes	Sputum	Blood culture/blood films
Clinical symptoms	Fever, painful buboes, inguinal lymphadenopathy	Cough or hemoptysis bubo	Fever, hypotension, no buboes
Incubation period	2–8 days	1–4 days (maximum 6 days)	2-8 days
Mortality if untreated	~60%	High mortality (approaching 100%)	High mortality (approaching 100%)

Yersinia spp. grow between 14°C and 37°C, with optimal growth at 27°C. Small nonhemolytic colonies are seen on blood agar at 24 hours, which are catalase-positive and oxidase-negative. Although *Y. pestis* grows on MacConkey, it tends to autolyse after 2–3 days. Organisms are citrate-, indole-, and urease-negative. It is usually cultured from a bubo aspirate, but may also grow from blood, CSF, or sputum. Cefsulodin Irgasan Novobiocin (CIN) agar is selective for *Yersinia* (and *Aeromonas* species).

- Direct immunofluorescence is a more-rapid diagnostic method.
- PCR testing may be available through the local Health Department
- Serological tests for yersiniosis (acute and convalescent) include the complement fixation test and haemagglutination of tanned sheep red cells to which F1 capsular antigen has been adsorbed.

Treatment

Early antibiotic therapy for suspected cases (e.g., streptomycin, gentamicin, or doxycycline) reduce the otherwise high mortality to ~10%. Contacts may also be given antibiotic prophylaxis.

Patients with pneumonic plague should be isolated until they are sputum smear-negative (usually ~3 days since starting treatment). There is no vaccine currently available.

Control

Flea and rodent control are important.

Yersinia enterocolitica

Y. enterocolitica resembles *Y. pestis* and *Y. pseudotuberculosis* on culture and morphologically, but differs antigenically and biochemically. The most common serotypes causing human infection the US. Serotypes cultured from healthy individuals are probably nonpathogenic.

Epidemiology

Y. enterocolitica is acquired from eating infected meat or milk. Patients with conditions associated with iron overload (e.g., hemochromatosis) and the immunosuppressed are at increased risk of *Yersinia* infections.

Clinical features

Y. enterocolitica usually presents as a febrile illness associated with bloody diarrhea and may mimic salmonellosis, shigellosis, or appendicitis. Other presentations include mesenteric lymphadenitis and septicemia, which may be fatal in the elderly.

Secondary complications include erythema nodosum, polyarthritis, peritonitis, Reiter's syndrome, meningitis, osteomyelitis, and hepatic, renal, and splenic abscesses. *Y. enterocolitica* has been cultured from pseudotuberculous lesions in animals.

Treatment

Gastroenteritis usually resolves without antibiotics. In severe infection, the recommended regimen is doxycycline plus an aminoglycoside.

Alternatives include cefotaxime, trimethoprim/sulfamethoxazole, and fluoroquinolones.

Note resistance to penicillin. If the patient is on desferrioxamine, this should be stopped, as it may increase the severity of infection.

Yersinia pseudotuberculosis

Epidemiology

Strains of *Y. pseudotuberculosis* can be differentiated by somatic and flagellar antigens, some of which are shared with *Y. pestis*. Most human infections with *Y. pseudotuberculosis* are due to serotype 1.

Pathogenesis

See *Yersinia*, p. 263.

Clinical features

Y. pseudotuberculosis causes a fatal septicemia in animals and birds. Humans usually acquire the infection from contact with water polluted by infected animals or by eating contaminated vegetables; infection due to direct contact with animals is rare.

In humans, yersiniosis infection ranges from asymptomatic to a fatal typhoid-like illness with fever, purpura, and hepatosplenomegaly.

Mesenteric adenitis ± erythema nodosum may mimic appendicitis and tends to infect males aged 5–15 years.

Diagnosis

This small Gram-negative rod is slightly acid fast. It grows poorly on MacConkey agar (like *Y. pestis*) but can be differentiated from *Y. pestis* because *Y. pseudotuberculosis* can produce urease and is motile at 22°C.

Treatment

Y. pseudotuberculosis shows in vitro susceptibility to ciprofloxacin, tetracyclines, aminoglycosides, sulfonamides, and penicillin. Mesenteric adenitis is usually self-limiting.

Pasteurella

The genus *Pasteurella* includes the species *P. multocida*, *P. haemolytica*, *P. canis*, *P. stomatis*, and *P. pneumotropica*. *Pasteurella* live in the mouth, and GI and respiratory tracts of many animals (especially dogs and cats) ± humans. *P. multocida*, the most frequent species causing human infections, usually causes skin and soft tissue infections.

Epidemiology

Fifteen serotypes of *P. multocida* have been identified on the basis of 4 capsular antigens and 11 somatic antigens. PFGE can be used to compare strains. In addition to acquiring infection through animal bites, humans can also become infected through inhaling air that has become contaminated by infected animals' coughing.

Pathogenesis

In animals, *P. multocida* causes hemorrhagic septicemia, which is usually fatal. Most virulent *Pasteurella* strains have a polysaccharide capsule, which is antiphagocytic and protects against intracellular killing by neutrophils. Some strains produce a leukotoxin, and some bind transferrin.

Clinical features

P. multocida causes skin and soft tissue infections after animal bites, most commonly a localized abscess with cellulitis and lymphadenitis. *P. multocida* has also been associated with upper and lower respiratory tract infections. Other sites of infection are uncommon—these include meningitis after head injury, bone and joint infections, septicemia, endocarditis, and intra-abdominal infections.

P. haemolytica is nonpathogenic for humans. It causes pneumonia in sheep and cattle and septicemia in lambs and infects poultry and domestic animals.

P. pneumotropica may be isolated from the respiratory tract of laboratory animals. There are reports of it causing human infections, e.g., animal bite wound infections, septicemia, and upper respiratory tract infections.

Diagnosis

P. multocida is a facultative anaerobic Gram-negative coccobacillus, which appears pleomorphic in culture and does not grow on MacConkey agar. At 37°C, organisms are capsulate, non-sporing, and non-motile. They show bipolar staining with methylene blue. Most are fermentative, and oxidase-positive, catalase-positive, and indole-positive.

P. haemolytica can be differentiated from *P. multocida,* as it is hemolytic on blood agar and can grow on MacConkey agar.

Treatment

Penicillin is the mainstay of treatment, and there is a wealth of clinical experience to support this. It is resistant to oral first-generation cephalosporins, clindamycin, and erythromycin. It is often sensitive in vitro to fluoroquinolones, tetracyclines, macrolides, and trimethoprim/ sulfamethoxazole, which may be appropriate in penicillin-allergic patients.

Francisella

Francisella tularensis is primarily an animal pathogen (rabbits and hares), which occasionally infects humans as accidental hosts. The resulting infection is called *tularemia* and may be either ulceroglandular or typhoidal/pulmonary.

Only two of the four *F. tularensis* subspecies are clinically important type A is highly virulent and type B, less virulent). It is also a potential agent of bioterrorism (see Bioterrorism, p. 753).

Epidemiology

Tularemia is endemic in North America and parts of Europe, Asia, northern Australia, and Japan. Most cases in humans are sporadic, though outbreaks have been reported.

It may survive for days in moist soil and in water polluted by infected animals, and for years in culture at 10°C. Organisms are killed in 10 minutes after exposure to moist heat at 55°C.

For epidemiological investigations, the most discriminatory typing system is based on multiple-locus variable-number tandem repeats (VNTR).

Pathogenesis

There is evidence from animal experiments of intracellular multiplication of *F. tularensis*. Virulence has been associated with the capsule and also citrulline ureidase activity.

Clinical features

Infection ranges from asymptomatic to septic shock, depending on virulence of particular strain, host immune response, route of entry, and degree of systemic involvement. There are two main forms:

- *Ulceroglandular* form of tularemia (due to *direct contact* with infected animal): acute-onset fever, headache, and rigors, usually followed by glandular lesions and skin ulceration, ± eye involvement
- *Typhoidal/pulmonary* form of tularemia (results from *indirect contact* through bites from ticks, mosquitoes, or biting flies; inhaling infected dust; or eating contaminated food or water): acute-onset fever, headache, and rigors, usually followed by respiratory or typhoid-like symptoms

Diagnosis

F. tularensis is a select agent. Laboratory personnel should be informed of the possibility of tularemia when samples are submitted for diagnostic tests. Biosafety level 2 practices, containment equipment, and facilities are recommended for activities involving specimens suspected or known to contain *F. tularensis*.

It is a small, nonmotile, non-sporulating, capsulate Gram-negative coccobacillus, which shows characteristic bipolar staining with carbol fuchsin (10%). It stains poorly with methylene blue. It is a strict aerobe, and culture requires the addition of egg yolk or rabbit spleen to agar. After culture, the bacilli may appear filamentous and larger.

Traditional microbiological methods are slowly being replaced by immunological and molecular tests, including ELISA and immunoblots for antibodies (but tests relying on antibody detection are limited in early clinical stages of disease).

If a case is suspected, involve the state health department.

Treatment

Seek expert advice. Streptomycin or gentamicin is the antibiotic of choice with the addition of chloramphenicol for meningitis.

Relapse is more common if tetracycline or chloramphenicol is used, a these are bacteriostatic for *F. tularensis*. The live vaccine (LVS) is based o an attenuated strain of *F. tularensis*.

Postexposure prophylaxis with doxycycline or ciprofloxacin may be considered after potential inhalation.

Legionella

This organism is named after the outbreak of pneumonia affecting >18C members of the American Legion at a convention in Philadelphia in 1976 The *Legionellaceae* naturally live in water and only accidentally infec humans. This may result in either Legionnaires' disease or Pontiac fever.

There are 52 different genetically defined species of *Legionella*, of which ~50% infect humans. *Legionella pneumophila* serogroup 1 is the most pathogenic and accounts for ~95% of human cases.

Epidemiology

Legionella is acquired via inhalation of contaminated aerosols (e.g., from spas, showers, air-conditioning systems, water-storage tanks, nebulizers' or drinking water. Water systems are more likely to be contaminated with *Legionella* if the temperature is outside the recommended range (it should be <20°C or >55°C), flow is obstructed, or biofilms have formed.

Legionella is an intracellular organism and can survive in amoebae, within the environment. The incubation period is 2–10 days, and occasionally symptoms may develop up to 3 weeks post-exposure.

It is not transmitted person to person. Most cases are isolated, but outbreaks can occur.

Pathogenesis

After the infection is established, pneumonic consolidation develops, characterized by proteinaceous fibrinous exudates pouring into the alveoli The mechanism of distant toxic changes (e.g., confusion, hallucinations focal neurology) is poorly understood.

Legionella organisms are engulfed by monocytes and may survive intracellularly for prolonged periods of time.

Clinical features

In addition to the two main clinical syndromes below, rare conditions (e.g. prosthetic valve endocarditis, wound infections) have been reported:

- *Legionnaires' disease*: this rapidly progressive pneumonia is characterized by fever, respiratory distress, and confusion and has a mortality rate of >10% in healthy people. Risk factors include age >50 years, hospital admission, immunosuppression, and smoking. Men are affected more than women.
- *Pontiac fever*: this is a brief flu-like illness, which has a high attack rate but low mortality.

Diagnosis

Microscopy and culture

These short rods/coccobacilli may be difficult to see by Gram stain, so fluorescent antibody stains or silver impregnation may help. *Legionella* grows best on media such as buffered charcoal yeast extract (BCYE), which contains iron plus cysteine as an essential growth factor.

Some strains prefer 2.5–5% CO_2 at 35–36°C. *L. pneumophila* colonies usually appear by day 5, but other species may require 10 days. Colonies may autofluoresce under ultraviolet (UV) light.

Serogroups can be differentiated by slide agglutination or fluorescent antibody tests, which are available at reference laboratories.

Antigen detection

Legionella urinary antigen test (ELISA) only detects serogroup 1 of *L. pneumophila*.

Antibody detection

Fluorescent antibody test (FAT), rapid microagglutination test (RMAT), or ELISA is used. A >4-fold rise, or titre 1:256, is usually diagnostic.

Antibody may take >8 days to develop after onset of infection and may persist for months to years post-infection. Also note that there is some cross-reactivity with *Campylobacter*.

Treatment

Conventional susceptibility tests in broth and agar are unreliable, and methods have not been standardized. In addition, many antibiotics with excellent in vitro activity against *Legionella* (e.g., β-lactams and aminoglycosides) are ineffective. Essentially, the macrolides, quinolones, tetracyclines, and rifampin are effective as they have good intracellular penetration.

There are no randomized, controlled trials comparing macrolides to quinolones for the treatment of *Legionella* infections. Outcomes appear to be similar with both groups of agents; however, quicker defervescence and fewer complications and/or shorter hospital stays have been observed with quinolones.

In severe infections, the addition of rifampin may be considered.

Control and prevention

This relies on good design and maintenance of water systems to prevent growth of *Legionella* organisms, and subsequent treatment of the source (e.g., contaminated water systems) if a case occurs. The main approaches to control are as follows:

- *Physical:* heat, UV light, sonication: use of compressed air to drain and flush pipes
- *Chemical:* inhibit scale formation, use of biocides to kill the amoebae (such as sodium hypochlorite, ozone), use of charcoal filters
- *Plumbing:* regular maintenance, no dead legs in the system, pumps should be in series and not in parallel, no dead spaces in the heaters, regular flushing of the system, use of correct components

Capnocytophaga

The genus *Capnocytophaga* in the family *Flavobacteriaceae* may be divided into two groups:

- Species associated with dog-bite infections (and occasionally bites from other animals such as rabbits or cats) and normally found in dogs' mouths: *C. canimorsus* (formerly known as dysgonic fermenter, 2 DF2) and *C. cynodegmi*
- Species found in the human mouth: *C. ochracea* (these were the dysgonic fermenter group[1] [DF1]), *C. gingivalis*, *C. sputigena*, *C. haemolytica*, and *C. granulosa*

Epidemiology

While *C. canimorsus* and *C. cynodegmi* are most commonly associated with bites, there are reports of infections occurring merely after exposure to dogs, with no bites or scratches.

Pathogenesis

Species found in the human mouth produce a variety of enzymes that help in the invasion of periodontal tissue (e.g., acid and alkaline phosphotases, aminopeptidases, IgA, proteases, and trypsin-like enzymes). These are thought to be important in periodontitis.

Clinical features

All species may cause a wide range of infections in normal and immuno-compromised hosts. Among animal bite infections, *C. canimorsus* is more common and more severe than *C. cynodegmi*, with a mortality approaching 30%.

Those at particular risk include asplenic patients, alcoholics, and those on steroids. Asplenic patients with *C. canimorsus* infection may present with shock, disseminated purpuric lesions, and disseminated intravascular coagulation (DIC). Fulminant infections with *C. canimorsus* may also occur in healthy people, although infections tend to be milder. Meningitis, endocarditis, pneumonia, corneal ulcer, cellulitis, and septic arthritis due to *C. canimorsus* have also been reported.

Species found in the human mouth may be important in localized juvenile periodontitis. They have also been found in the female genital tract and associated with intrauterine infection, amnionitis, and neonatal infections in premature babies.

Rarely, they cause severe infections as opportunistic pathogens (e.g., endocarditis, eye infections, bacteremia, peritonitis) in both immunocompent and immunosuppressed patients.

Diagnosis

These long, thin, delicate GNRs are typically fusiform, but older cultures often show pleomorphic sizes and shapes. They are facultative anaerobes and grow best with CO_2 enrichment. On blood or chocolate agar they may appear yellowish, with a spreading edge with finger-like projections due to the typical gliding motility.

They do not grow on MacConkey agar and do not produce indole. Differentiating each individual species is more difficult and generally requires reference laboratory assistance. In general, species from the human mouth are oxidase-negative and catalase-negative, while those from animals' mouths are oxidase-positive and catalase-positive.

C. canimorsus is more fastidious than the others and may be difficult to grow from blood cultures (even when organisms have been seen on Gram stain). In this situation, culture on enriched agar (e.g., heart infusion agar with rabbit or sheep blood) for 14 days in 10% CO_2 may help.

Treatment

Amoxillin-calvulonic acid or ampicillin-sulbactam is usually recommended for these infections. Asplenic patients should be given prophylaxis after a dog bite, as the organism may take a while to grow and be identified, and the mortality rate is high.

While the animal bite–associated species are sensitive to penicillin, resistance to the β-lactams has been reported in the human-mouth species. For instance, *C. haemolytica* and *C. granulosa* are often resistant to β-lactams and aminoglycosides. All species are usually sensitive to clindamycin, erythromycin, tetracyclines, and the quinolones.

Vibrios

The genus *Vibrio* (family *Vibrionaceae*) includes over 30 species. The most important ones that result in human infections are *V. cholerae, V. parahaemolyticus* and *V. vulnificus*.

Other species, such as *V. alginolyticus, V. damsela, V. fluvialis, V. hollisae,* and *V. mimicus,* occasionally cause opportunistic infections.

Vibrio cholerae

A few cases of cholera (see Cholera, p. 589) are imported into the United States every year. These are most commonly O1-El Tor. In the mid-1990s, a new serogroup (O139) appeared in the Bay of Bengal; this was the first time a non-O1 serogroup had resulted in epidemic cholera.

Epidemiology

Cholera is prevalent in Central and South America, Africa, and Asia.

There are more than 130 different O (somatic antigen) serogroups of *V. cholerae*. Serogroup O1 (the cholera vibrio) causes epidemic cholera, and some strains of non-O1 (the non-cholera or nonagglutinable vibrios) can also cause diarrhea. Serogroup O1 is usually acquired via the fecal–oral route, while non-O1 *V. cholerae* may be associated with consumption of seafood or exposure to saline environments.

The two biotypes of serogroup O1 (El Tor, which is most common, and classical) can be distinguished by susceptibility to phage and the fact that El Tor is hemolytic and resistant to polymyxin B. The subtypes of serogroup O1 are Ogawa (most common), Inaba, and Hikojima (which possesses determinants of both other subtypes).

Pathogenesis

The potent cholera enterotoxin, produced by serogroup O1 and some non-O1 strains, comprises five B (binding) subunits and one A (active) subunit. Insertion of the B subunits into the host cell membrane forms a channel for subunit A to enter the cell. By causing transfer of ADP ribose from NAD to another protein, adenylate cyclase is irreversibly activated and cAMP is overproduced. The resulting hypersecretion of Cl^- and HCO_3^- causes loss of massive water and electrolytes (rice-water stool).

Other features important in the pathogenesis of serogroup O1 include production of mucinase and other proteolytic enzymes (which help the organism reach the enterocytes), the motility of the organism, and adhesive hemagglutinins (which aid close adherence to enterocyte surface). Non-O1 strains may produce other enterotoxins, cytotoxins, hemolysins, and colonizing factors.

Cholera is transmitted via contaminated food or water and requires a large infective dose. Humans are the only host. Only a handful of those infected are symptomatic (ratios quoted are 40 asymptomatic carriers to 1 symptomatic individual for El Tor and 5:1 for classical), which underscores the need for good hygiene.

Clinical features

V. cholerae usually causes the typical profuse watery diarrhea of cholera, which may rapidly lead to hypovolumic shock and death from dehydration. Milder cases are similar to other causes of secretory diarrhea, and asymptomatic infections also occur.

Non-O1 *V. cholerae* usually causes mild, sometimes bloody diarrhea, but may occasionally be severe and resemble cholera.

Patients exposed to aquatic environments may suffer from wound infections, and bacteremia and meningitis have been reported.

Diagnosis

During an epidemic, cholera is a clinical diagnosis. Otherwise, diagnosis is based on high clinical suspicion together with culture or dark-field microscopy of stool (comma-shaped organisms are seen moving around, which ceases when diluted O1 antisera is added).

Vibrios are short, curved, or comma-shaped, aerobic Gram-negative rods, which are motile by a single polar flagellum. They ferment both sucrose and glucose but not lactose, and reduce nitrate to nitrite. Most are oxidase-positive and produce indole.

The growth characteristics of vibrios are summarized in Table 3.16.

V. cholerae is nonhalophilic (can grow on media without added salt) if the necessary electrolytes are present. *V. cholerae* can grow at 42°C (along with *V. parahaemolyticus* and *V. alginolyticus*). Vibrios are tolerant to alkali but have low tolerance to acid. *V. cholerae* is usually VP-positive.

Vibrios accumulate on the surface of alkaline peptone water. If a loopful is inoculated onto thiosulfate citrate bile salts (TCBS), *V. cholerae* appear as a yellow sucrose-fermenter, which is oxidase-positive. *V. cholerae* is killed by most detergents and by heating at 55°C for 15 min. However, it can survive for up to 2 weeks in salt water at ambient temperatures and also on chitinous shellfish for 2 weeks, even if refrigerated.

Table 3.16 Growth characteristics of *Vibrio* spp.

Species	TCBS	Biochemistry	Salt requirement	Growth at 42°C
V. cholerae	Yellow	Oxidase-, nitrate-, lysine-, ONPG-positive	Not halophilic (0–3% NaCl)	Yes
V. parahaemolyticus	Green	Lysine-, indole-positive	Halophilic (3–6% NaCl)	Yes
V. vulnificus	Green (85%), yellow (15%)	Lactose-, lysine-, salicin-positive	Halophilic (3–5% NaCl)	No
V. alginolyticus	Yellow	Lysine-, VP-positive	Halophilic (3–10% NaCl	Yes

Treatment

Rehydration is key. Antibiotics (e.g., azithromycin, ciprofloxacin) reduce the duration of disease and period of excretion of *V. cholerae* in the stool of infected patients. Results of trials of a live oral vaccine (Peru-15) are promising. However, the most important preventative strategies are improvement of sanitation and food and water standards.

Vibrio parahaemolyticus

V. parahaemolyticus is ubiquitous in fish and shellfish and the waters they inhabit.

Epidemiology

V. parahaemolyticus infection is common in Southeast Asia, particularly Singapore and Japan. However it also occurs in the UK and United States, particularly during summer months.

Pathogenesis

Kanagawa-positive strains (see below) of *V. parahaemolyticus* adhere to human enterocytes and produce a heat-stable cytotoxin.

Clinical features

V. parahaemolyticus is usually acquired through ingesting seafood and causes acute explosive diarrhea. Extraintestinal infections arise from handling contaminated seafood or exposure to the aquatic environment, the most common being wound infections.

Diagnosis

This organism is halophilic, hence will not grow on cysteine lactose electrolyte deficient (CLED) agar. Clinical strains of *V. parahaemolyticus* usually appear as green, non-sucrose-fermenting colonies on TCBS agar, but isolates from estuary and coastal waters may ferment sucrose. Stool samples should be enriched in alkaline peptone water containing 1% NaCl.

The *Kanagawa phenomenon* refers to hemolysis of human erythrocytes on Wagatsuma's agar, by strains of *V. parahaemolyticus* that cause gastroenteritis.

Treatment and prevention

Rehydration is the main intervention for patients with diarrhea. Severe infections require treatment with fluoroquinolones, doxycycline, or third-generation cephalosporins. Antibiotics do not shorten the duration of symptoms.

Prevention strategies involve good food hygiene standards.

Vibrio vulnificus

V. vulnificus has been called the "terror of the deep" because of the severe fulminant infection it can cause.

Epidemiology

Infections are most common in areas with higher water temperatures, such as the mid-Atlantic and Gulf Coast states of the United States. Septicemia arises from eating contaminated raw shellfish, whereas wound infections are due to injuries sustained in aquatic environments.

Pathogenesis

The polysaccharide capsule helps resist phagocytosis and bactericidal effects of human serum. The association with liver disease (with increased serum iron levels) may be explained by the ability of virulent strains to use transferrin-bound iron. Toxin production is also important.

Clinical features

There are three main infections associated with *V. vulnificus*:
- Fulminant septicemia, followed by cutaneous lesions. This is associated with a high mortality (50%). Immunosuppressed patients are at increased risk, particularly elderly male alcoholics with liver dysfunction.
- Wound infection, rapidly progressing to cellulitis, edema, erythema, and necrosis. Patients may develop septicemia, and it may be fatal.
- Acute diarrhea, usually in those with mild underlying conditions. Mortality is rare.
  Diagnosis

This organism is also halophilic (see *V. parahaemolyticus,* above). See Table 3.16 for further growth characteristics.

Treatment

Early treatment with ceftazidime and doxycycline is key.

Other Vibrio species

V. alginolyticus is also found in seafood and seawater. It is a halophilic organism, which will not grow on CLED but grows in 10% NaCl. Colonies are large and yellow (sucrose fermenting) on TCBS agar, and there is swarming on nonselective media. It can cause opportunistic wound infections, with mild cellulitis and a seropurulent exudate. Most infections are associated with exposure to seawater and are self-limiting. Little is known about the pathogenic mechanisms.

V. fluvialis is phenotypically similar to *Aeromonas hydrophila* (see *Aeromonas*, p. 275). It has been implicated in outbreaks of diarrhea and is acquired from contaminated seafood.

V. damsela is a halophilic, marine organism that can cause severe wound infections. It is acquired in warm coastal areas.

V. hollisae is associated with diarrhea and bacteremia in areas of warm seawater in the United States. It is acquired from eating raw seafood.

V. mimicus is associated with gastroenteritis from eating raw oysters. There are also reports of ear infections. It occurs in environments similar to those of *V. cholerae*.

Aeromonas

Aeromonas spp. are aquatic organisms, which have been implicated in causing diarrhea. They also cause soft tissue infections and sepsis in the immunocompromised. *A. hydrophila*, *A. sobria*, and *A. caviae* are the main species, and *A. salmonicida* is an economically important fish pathogen.

The genus *Aeromonas* has undergone a number of taxonomic and nomenclature revisions recently and been moved from the family *Vibrionaceae* to the new family *Aeromonadaceae*.

Epidemiology

Aeromonas diarrhea is more common in the summer months when water concentrations of aeromonads are higher. Outbreaks may occur, and *Aeromonas* infection is being increasingly recognized as a cause of traveler's diarrhea.

Pathogenesis

Gastroenteritis is the most common disease associated with *Aeromonas*, but its role is debated (Box 3.4). It is unclear whether most fecal isolates

---

Box 3.4 Evidence supporting the causative role of *Aeromonas* in diarrhea

- Symptomatic people have a higher carriage rate of *Aeromonas* than that of asymptomatic individuals.
- Most symptomatic patients harboring *Aeromonas* do not have other enteric pathogens.
- *Aeromonas* produces an enterotoxin.
- Antibiotics active against *Aeromonas* usually improve patient symptoms.
- There is evidence of a specific secretory immune response coincident with diarrheal disease.

recovered from symptomatic patients actually cause diarrhea. It may be that only specific subsets of *Aeromonas* are pathogenic, and new biotyping schemes are needed to differentiate environmental from clinical strains.

Clinical features

Diarrhea tends to be watery and self-limiting but is occasionally more severe. Chronic colitis following diarrhea has been reported. In addition to gastroenteritis, there are reports of *Aeromonas* septicemia in the immuno-compromised, and wound infections in healthy people and those undergo-ing leech therapy.

The main skin-associated aeromonad is *A. hydrophila*. There are rare reports of nosocomial bacteremia, peritonitis, meningitis, and eye and bone and joint infections.

Diagnosis

This facultatively anaerobic GNR is usually β-hemolytic on blood agar and ferments carbohydrates to produce acid and gas. It grows readily on MacConkey agar, and lactose fermentation is variable. Growth on TCBS agar is also variable. It is oxidase-positive, so it can be distinguished from the oxidase-negative *Enterobacteriaceae*.

Selective techniques are needed to isolate it from a mixed culture. Suitable plates for detection of *Aeromonas* from stool include cefsulodin-irgasan-novobiocin (CIN) agar or blood agar containing ampicillin.

Not all laboratories routinely culture stools for *Aeromonas*, and some enteric media actually inhibit its growth.

Treatment

There are no controlled trials, but clinical improvement has been seen with antibiotics that are active in vitro, such as fluoroquinolones, trimethoprim-sulfamethoxazole, and aminoglycosides (except streptomycin). Resistance to the carbapenems has been reported.

Plesiomonas

Plesiomonas shigelloides, the only species in the genus, is associated with outbreaks of gastroenteritis in warm climates. In the literature it has been known as *Pseudomonas shigelloides*, C27, *Aeromonas shigelloides*, and *Vibrio shigelloides*. The taxonomic status has varied; it is related to *Proteus* but currently placed in the family *Vibrionaceae*.

Epidemiology

P. shigelloides is found in soil and water (mainly fresh water, but also salt water in warm weather). It is usually transmitted to humans via water or food (e.g., shrimp, chicken, and oysters) and also colonizes many animals. Most patients have recently traveled abroad.

Pathogenesis

There is no animal model, and no pathogenic mechanism has been identi-fied. Volunteer studies have been largely unsuccessful in causing disease. Hence, it has been difficult to prove a causal relationship.

Clinical features

Symptoms vary from mild self-limiting diarrhea to mucoid bloody diarrhea with features of enteroinvasive disease. It has occasionally resulted in serious extraintestinal infection such as osteomyelitis, septic arthritis, endophthalmitis, spontaneous bacterial peritonitis, pancreatic abscess, cellulitis, cholecystitis, and neonatal sepsis with meningitis.

Bacteremia is rare and usually in the immunocompromised.

Diagnosis

This motile, facultatively anaerobic GNR does not ferment lactose. It grows readily at 35°C on most enteric agars, such as MacConkey, but does not grow on TCBS. It appears nonhemolytic and is oxidase-positive. Selective techniques are needed to isolate it from a mixed culture.

Treatment

The role of antibiotics is unclear and results of studies conflicting. In vitro, it is usually sensitive to the quinolones, cephalosporins, and imipenem.

Campylobacter

Campylobacter organisms are spiral-shaped flagellate bacteria belonging to rRNA superfamily VI. *C. jejuni* is the most common cause of diarrhea in most developed countries. *C. coli* also causes diarrhea. *C. fetus* is the type species of the genus and causes abortion in sheep and cows.

It occasionally causes septic abortions in humans and bacteremia in the immunocompromised. Some species, including *C. lari* and *C. upsaliensis*, cause diarrhea in children in developing countries. Species such as *C. concisus* and *C. rectus* are associated with periodontal disease.

Pathogenesis

Campylobacter organisms are ingested (feco-oral transmission), then colonize (and usually invade) the jejunum, ileum, and terminal ileum, occasionally extending to the colon and rectum. Mesenteric lymph node involvement and transient bacteremia may occur.

Histological findings of acute inflammation ± superficial ulceration are the same as in *Salmonella*, *Shigella*, or *Yersinia* infections.

Clinical features

Campylobacter gastroenteritis is variable in symptoms and severity. In severe cases, GI hemorrhage, toxic megacolon, and hemolytic uremic syndrome (HUS) have been reported. Severe abdominal pain arising before the onset of diarrhea can mimic acute appendicitis. Other complications are meningitis, deep abscesses, cholecystitis, and reactive arthritis.

About 25% cases of GBS have documented preceding *Campylobacter* gastroenteritis. The LOS cell surface structures act as critical factors in triggering the syndrome through ganglioside mimicry.

Diagnosis

This small, spiral, or curved Gram-negative rod has a single unsheathed flagella at one or both poles and is extremely motile. It is micro-aerophilic and grows best at 42°C. Like *Helicobacter*, *Campylobacter* organisms undergo coccal transformation under adverse conditions and are biochemically inactive. However they are catalase- and oxidase-positive. *C. jejuni* is the only species that hydrolyses hippurate.

Typing methods include serotyping (Penner scheme for O antigens and Lior scheme for heat-labile surface and flagellar antigens), biotyping, phage typing, and newer molecular methods.

Treatment and prevention

Rehydration and symptom relief is usually adequate, as *Campylobacter* infection is usually self-limiting in 5–7 days. However, in severe dysenteric disease or for immunocompromised patients, a macrolide, quinolone, or aminoglycoside may be prescribed.

Treatment should be based on susceptibility test results, as quinolone resistance is increasing. Resistant strains, especially *C. coli*, may respond to trimethoprim/sulfamethoxazole. Good hygiene standards are important in prevention. Infective organisms may be excreted in the stool for ~3 weeks after resolution of diarrhea. There is no vaccine.

Helicobacter

The genus *Helicobacter* contains up to 17 species, which colonize the stomachs of various animals. *H. pylori* is a spiral-shaped flagellate bacteria belonging to rRNA superfamily VI, which colonizes humans (it is found in approximately 50% of the world's population).

H. pylori was discovered in 1983 in Australia by Warren and Marshall, who went on to receive the Nobel Prize for Medicine in 2005. Its importance in the pathogenesis of peptic ulcer disease soon became clear.

H. cinaedi and *H. fennelliae* are associated with proctitis in gay men.

Pathogenesis

As with other bacteria in rRNA superfamily VI, *H. pylori* is adapted to colonizing mucous membranes (in this case the gastric mucosa only) and penetrating mucus.

The cagA protein is important in virulence. After phosphorylation by tyrosine kinase, cagA is injected into epithelial cells by a type IV secretion system. This alters signal transduction and gene expression in host epithelial cells

Clinical features

H. pylori is associated with 95% of duodenal and 70% of gastric ulcers. Epidemiological studies have highlighted the association of *H. pylori* and gastric cancer, and the WHO classifies *H. pylori* as a group 1 carcinogen.

Diagnosis

This GNR is shaped like a helix (hence its name) and has a tuft of sheathed unipolar flagella. It is strictly microaerophilic and requires CO_2 for growth. It is relatively inactive biochemically, except for strong urease production. Under adverse conditions, it undergoes coccal transformation. Options for testing patients are as follows:

- *Serology:* if positive, this indicates that the patient has been infected
- *Biopsy* of stomach or duodenum for histology ± urease test ± culture
- *Urea breath tests:* the patient drinks ^{14}C- or ^{13}C-labeled urea, which is metabolized by *H. pylori*, producing labeled CO_2 that can be detected in the breath. This test is also used to assess effectiveness of treatment.
- *Rapid urease test* (The enzyme urease produced by *H. pylori* catalyses the conversion of urea to ammonia and bicarbonate, which is reflected by a rise in pH.): this is usually performed on a biopsy sample.
- *Fecal antigen tests*

The urea breath test or stool antigen test have greater sensitivity and specificity than that of serology for diagnosis and can also be used to confirm eradication. The patient should receive no antibiotics for 4 weeks before the tests and no proton pump inhibitor (PPI) for 2 weeks before tests. Molecular typing of *H. pylori* is more useful than serotyping.

Treatment

Guidelines for treatment have been proposed by the Amerrican College of Gastroenterology.[1] Primary "triple therapy" consists of a PPI, e.g., omeprazole, and two antibiotics (e.g., clarithromycin and amoxicillin, or metronidazole).

Eradication of *H. pylori* is beneficial in duodenal and gastric ulcers and low-grade MALToma (mucosal-associated lymphoid tissue) but *not* in gastroesophageal reflux disease (GERD).

In non-ulcer dyspepsia, 8% of patients benefit. Triple treatment achieves >85% eradication.

Essentially, any dyspeptic patient with no alarm symptoms should receive a PPI for 1 week. If symptoms relapse, the patient should be tested and treated for *H. pylori,* using the breath test or stool antigen test. First-line triple therapy is indicated for 1 week.

Clarithromycin or metronidazole should not be given if they have been used for any infection in the previous year. Approximately 10% of patients fail treatment, possibly because of antibiotic resistance (Box 3.5).

A Cochrane review (2006) of eradication therapy for peptic ulcer disease in *H. pylori*–positive patients found that treatment had a small benefit in initial healing of duodenal ulcers, and a significant benefit in preventing the recurrence of both gastric and duodenal ulcers, once healing had been achieved.[2]

Other treatment includes probiotics (which improved eradication rates and reduced adverse events in a recent meta-analysis) and bismuth compounds.

Box 3.5 Antibiotic resistance in *H. pylori*

Antibiotic resistance varies geographically. Metronidazole resistance varies from ~40% in the U.S. to 90% in developing countries. Clarithromycin resistance is ~10% in the U.S. but may be rising. A recent meta-analysis has shown that pretreatment clarithromycin resistance may reduce the effectiveness of therapy by 55%. Levofioxacin is being investigated as an alternative antibiotic in resistant strains.

References

1. Chey WD, Wong BC (2007). American College of Gastroenterology Guideline on the management of *Helicobacter pylori* Infection. *Am J Gastroenterol* 102(8):1808–1825.

2. Moaygedi P, et al. (2006). Eradication of *Helicobacter pylon* for non-ulcer dyspepsia. *Cochrane Database Syst Rev* 2.:CD002026.

Bacteroides

More than 30 genera of anaerobic GNR are recognized, but human infections are largely restricted to four of these: *Bacteroides, Prevotella, Porphyromonas,* and *Fusobacterium* (Table 3.17). These organisms are found in the mouth, gastrointestinal tract, and vagina and are among the most important constituents of normal flora.

They may cause a variety of infections in humans, particularly polymicrobial infections and abscesses. *Bacteroides fragilis* is the most important

Table 3.17 Characteristics of anaerobic Gram-negative rods

Organism	Growth in 20% bile	Pigmented	Fluorescence	Resistant to	Sensitive to
Bacteroides fragilis	Yes	No	No	Penicillin Vancomycin Kanamycin Colistin	Erythromycin Rifampin
Fusobacterium	Variable	No	No	Erythromycin Vancomycin	Colistin Penicillin Kanamycin
Prevotella	No	Brown/ black	Brick red	Erythromycin Vancomycin	Colistin Rifampin Colistin Penicillin
Porphyromonas	No	Brown/ black	Brick red	Erythromycin Vancomycin	Erythromycin Rifampin Penicillin Vancomycin

species; it is found in the gastrointestinal tract and is associated with a wide variety of infections.

Pathogenesis

Virulence factors of *Bacteroides* spp. include the following:

- Capsular polysaccharide inhibits opsonization and phagocytosis, promotes abscess formation, and promotes adherence to epithelial cells.
- Pili and fimbriae promote adherence to epithelial cells and mucus.
- Succinic acid inhibits phagocytosis and intracellular killing.
- Enzyme production contributes to tissue damage and promotes invasion and spread, e.g., heparinase, fibrinolysin, hyaluronidsase, and neuraminidase.
- Synergy between anaerobic and facultative bacteria—see Box 3.6

Clinical features

- *Intra-abdominal infections:* B. fragilis is the most common anaerobic isolate in intra-abdominal abscesses
- *Diarrhea:* enterotoxin-producing strains have been implicated in diarrhea in children.
- *Bacteremia:* B. fragilis is the most common isolate in anaerobic bacteremias. The source is usually intra-abdominal and associated with abscesses, malignancy, bowel performation, or surgery. Septic shock is less common in *B. fragilis* bacteremia than in bacteremia caused by aerobic Gram-negative bacilli; this is presumably related to the absence of lipid A in the endotoxin of *B. fragilis*.
- *Endocarditis* is associated with large vegetations and high frequency of thromboembolic complications.
- *Skin and soft tissue infections* are often found as part of mixed flora in diabetic and decubitus ulcers. *B. fragilis* has also been isolated from cutaneous abscesses of the lower limbs.
- *Bone and joint infections:* B. fragilis may rarely cause osteomyelitis and septic arthritis.
- *CNS infections:* anaerobic meningitis is rare, and most laboratories do not culture CSF anaerobically. In the cases of anaerobic meningitis that

---

Box 3.6 Synergy in anaerobic infections

- Infections involving anaerobes usually contain multiple anaerobic bacteria as well as facultative anaerobic bacteria.
- Evidence suggests true synergy between anaerobic and facultative bacteria, with formation of abscesses occurring more readily infections involving both groups of bacteria than either alone.
- Facultative organisms may lower the oxidation-reduction potential in the microenvironment promoting more favorable conditions for anaerobes.
- Anaerobic bacteria may inhibit phagocytosis of facultative bacteria
- *B. fragilis* produces β-lactamases in abscess fluid that may protect other normally susceptible bacteria from antimicrobials

have been described, *B. fragilis* is the most common isolate. In contrast, anaerobes are frequently implicated in brain abscesses.

Diagnosis

Bacteroides are non-spore-forming, nonmotile, anaerobic Gram-negative rods. On blood agar, *Bacteroides* appears as glistening, nonhemolytic colonies that are aerotolerant. Gram stain may reveal pale pink, pleomorphic coccobacilli, with irregular or bipolar staining. They can be differentiated from the other anaerobic GNRs by growth in 20% bile.

Identification is also based on sensitivity to rifampin and resistance to penicillin G and kanamycin.

Treatment

Drainage of abscesses and debridement of necrotic tissue is the mainstay of treatment for anerobic infections. However, some abscesses (e.g., brain, liver, and tubo-ovarian) have been managed with antimicrobial therapy alone.

The choice of antibiotics to treat anaerobic infections is usually empirical, as most of the infections are polymicrobial and require broad-spectrum therapy.

Bacteroides is usually sensitive to antimicrobials such as metronidazole, carbapenems, cefoxitin, and β-lactam/β-lactamase inhibitor combinations (e.g., ampicillin-sulbactam, piperacillin-tazobactam).

Prevotella and *Porphyromonas*

Prevotella and *Porphyromonas* formerly belonged to the genus *Bacteroides* (p. 280) but were reclassified in 1990.

The genus *Prevotella* includes *P. melaninogenica, P. bivia, P. oralis,* and *P. bucalis.*

The genus *Porphyromonas* includes *P. gingivalis P. endodontalis,* and *P. asaccharolytica.*

Pathogenesis

Virulence in *P. melaninogenica* is associated with the capsular polysaccharide, which inhibits opsonophagocytosis, promotes abscess formation and also promotes adherence to epithelial cells.

In *P. gingivalis,* pili and fimbriae aid adherence to epithelial cells and mucus. Production of various enzymes may also aid evasion of the host immune response, or promote tissue destruction.

Clinical features

Prevotella and *Porphyromonas* contribute to the formation of abscesses and soft tissue infections in various parts of the body. They also cause infections of the oral cavity (such as periodontal and endodontal disease), female genital tract infections, osteomyelitis of the facial bones, and human-bite infections.

Diagnosis

These are non-spore forming, nonmotile anaerobic GNR. They are usually isolated (along with other anaerobes) from abscesses and soft tissue infections. *Prevotella* and *Porphyromonas* may both appear pigmented, usually brown or black.

Young unpigmented colonies can show brick-red fluorescence under UV light. *Prevotella* and *Porphyromonas* are both inhibited by 20% bile. *Prevotella* are moderately saccharolytic, whereas *Porphyromonas* are asaccharolytic.

Treatment

The mainstay of treatment for anaerobic infections is surgical drainage of abscesses and debridement of necrotic tissue.

Prevotella and *Porphyromonas* are usually sensitive to agents such as metronidazole, clindamycin, and cefoxitin. Penicillin resistance is common, but isolates are usually susceptible to β-lactam/β-lactamase inhibitor combinations.

Fusobacterium

Fusobacterium spp. colonize the mucous membranes of animals and humans and occasionally cause infections of the oral cavity and head and neck. Clinically, the most important species are

- *F. nucleatum* (subspecies *nucleatum, polymorphum,* and *fusiforme*)
- *F. necrophorum* (subspecies *necrophorum* and *fundiliforme*).

Epidemiology

Fusobacteria are commensals of the oral cavity. As with other obligate anaerobes, the significance of these organisms is being increasingly recognized.

Pathogenesis

Fusobacterium spp. produces lipopolysaccharide (LPS) endotoxin, which is biologically active. They also produce metabolites that are important to oral spirochetes.

Clinical features

F. necrophorum causes severe systemic infections such as Lemierre's disease (see p. 535), post-anginal sepsis, and necrobacillosis.

Lemierre's disease is a severe systemic disease that occurs in previously healthy young adults and usually presents initially as severe sore throat, followed by fever, cervical lymphadenopathy, and unilateral thrombophlebitis of the internal jugular vein. Metastatic infection with spread to the lungs or bones or brain may occur. If left untreated, the condition leads to death in 7–15 days.

Other species commonly isolated from oral infections include *F. periodonticum, F. alocis, F. sulci,* and *F. naviforme.*

Species found in the gastrointestinal or genitourinary tracts (e.g., *F. mortiferum*, *F. necrogenes*, *F. varium*, and *F. gonidiaformans*) may cause intra-abdominal infections, osteomyelitis, ulcers, and skin and soft tissue infections.

F. ulcerans was originally isolated from tropical ulcers but may be found in other sites.

Diagnosis

Fusobacterium are long, thin, GNR with pointed ends (fusiform) that are often arranged in pairs. They are non–spore forming and nonmotile. They may be hemolytic on blood agar and may grow in the presence of 20% bile.

They can be identified using commercial tests, e.g., MASTRING™ ID (Mast Diagnostics) and the API 20A or Rapid ID 32A (bioMérieux).

Susceptibility testing is vital, as there have been reports of penicillin-resistant strains.

Treatment

The mainstay of treatment for anaerobic infections is surgical drainage of abscesses and debridement of necrotic tissue.

Lemierre's syndrome and other severe invasive disease are usually treated with a combination of penicillin and metronidazole for 2–6 weeks. Alternatives include clindamycin.

Spirochetes—an overview

The *spirochetes* are a group of helical organisms sharing many properties with Gram-negative bacteria. The vast majority are nonpathogenic, but a few are important causes of disease in humans (see Table 3.18). There are aerobic and anaerobic species, both free living and parasitic.

Axial filaments, fixed at each end of the organism, run along the outside of the protoplasm within the outer sheath and give the characteristic coiled appearance. These are similar to bacterial flagella and are capable of constricting, warping the cell body, and enabling the bacterium to move by rotating it in space.

Table 3.18 Overview of spirochetes of clinical significance

Genus	Species	Clinical disease	Morphology	Culture	Diagnosis
Treponema	T. pallidum subsp. pallidum	Syphilis	Morphologically identical Thin helical cells 10 × 0.15 micrometers Visible on dark-field microscopy	Cannot be cultured in vitro; remain motile in specific enriched media at 35°C for several days	Direct detection is only means in primary syphilis; mainstay is serology; cross-reactivity between species
	T. pallidum subsp. pertenue	Yaws			
	T. pallidum subsp. endemicum	Endemic syphilis			
	T. carateum	Pinta			
Borrelia	B. recurrentis	Louse-borne relapsing fever	Helical; 3–20 × 0.25 micrometers Can be stained with aniline dyes	Can be cultured but is not practical	Demonstration of spirochetes in peripheral blood smears; immunological and PCR-based tests available
	B. hermsii and others	Tick-borne relapsing fever			
	B. burgdorferi	Lyme disease		Culture possible from biopsy of rash	Serology: can remain positive for years
Leptospira	L. interrogans	Lepto-spirosis	Motile, 10 × 0.1 micrometers. Stain poorly; visible on dark-field or phase contrast	Specialized media. Allow a minimum of 6 weeks	Serology; molecular techniques available

Treponema species

Four members of the genus *Treponema* cause human disease: *Treponema pallidum* subsp. *pallidum* (syphilis) and three nonvenereal treponematoses.

Microbiology

Morphologically identical, *Treponema* species appear as motile helical rods on dark-field microscopy. They are thin, helical cells around 10 micrometers long and 0.15 micrometer wide. They cannot be cultured in vitro (unlike the nonpathogenic treponemes) but remain motile in specific enriched media for several days at 35°C.

Organisms remain viable after freezing. The organisms all share a significant degree of DNA homology and are very similar antigenically, thus all cause positive serological tests for syphilis.

Epidemiology and clinical features

Treponema pallidum subsp. *pallidum*

This is the causative agent of syphilis. An increasing incidence in the United States, beginning in the 1960s, plateaued in the mid-1990s, but several large outbreaks between 1998 and 2003 saw diagnoses of infectious syphilis in men rise 15-fold.

Transmission is via sexual contact, direct vascular inoculation (IV drug use, transfusions), and direct cutaneous contact with infectious lesions or transplacental infection (congenital syphilis, p. 642). It interacts with HIV in both acquisition and diagnosis. See p. 642 for clinical features.

Treponema pallidum subsp. *pertenue*

This is the causative agent of yaws, a chronic nonvenereal disease endemic in the humid tropics (Central Africa, South America, Southeast Asia, and parts of the Indian subcontinent). It is acquired in childhood through contact with infectious skin lesions. Incubation is 3 weeks.

Infection affects the skin (papular skin lesions, which may ulcerate) and bones (periosteitis, dactylitis).
- *Primary stage:* lesion at inoculation site
- *Secondary stage:* dissemination of treponemes, causing multiple skin lesions
- *Latent stage:* usually asymptomatic (most patients remain noninfectiously latent for their lifetime)
- *Tertiary stage* (<10% patients 5–10 years later): bone, joint, and soft tissue deformities

Treponema pallidum subsp. *endemicum*

This is the causative agent of nonvenereal endemic syphilis or "bejel." It is endemic in dry subtropical or temperate areas of the Middle East, India, Asia, and parts of Africa. Infection occurs in childhood and is associated with poor standards of hygiene.

Transmission is vai contact with mucosal lesions or contaminated eating utensils or water. The incubation period is 10–90 days.
- *Primary lesions* (1–6 weeks): patches in the mouth followed by skin lesions resembling the chancres of venereal syphilis

- *Secondary stage* (6–9 months): macerated patches on the lips and tongue, anogenital hypertrophic condyloma lata, painful osteoperiostitis of long bones
- *Tertiary stage:* destruction of cartilage and bone, gummata of skin, bones, and nasopharynx. CNS and cardiovascular system (CVS) disease is very rare.

Treponema carateum

This is the causative agent of pinta, the most benign of endemic treponematoses affecting only the skin. It is endemic to South and Central America. It is spread by contact with infected skin. Incubation 2–3 weeks.

- *Primary lesion:* papule or erythematous plaque on exposed surfaces of the legs, foot, forearm, or hands, which slowly enlarges, becoming pigmented and hyperkeratotic. May be associated with regional lymphadenopathy
- *Secondary lesions:* disseminated lesiosn of similar appearance developing 3–9 months later.
- *Late/tertiary pinta:* disfiguring pigmentary changes and atrophic lesions

Diagnosis

Direct detection is with culture (gold standard), which is expensive, time consuming, and used primarily in research. Direct detection of organisms via dark-field microscopy or, preferably, immunofluorescence of material scraped from a lesion, is the only means of diagnosis in primary syphilis.

Serological diagnosis is the mainstay. Serological tests fall into two groups. Both show cross-reactivity between the four *Treponema* species:

- *Nontreponemal tests* (e.g., Venereal Disease Research Laboratory [VDRL] detect antibodies to cardiolipin produced as a response to treponemal infection and are not specific but are very sensitive. Samples with very high antibody titers may give false-negative results (the "prozone" phenomenon), e.g., in early infection or HIV. Poor sensitivity occurs in late-stage infection. Antibody titer tends to decline to negativity, with adequate therapy.
- *Treponemal tests* (e.g., treponema enzyme immunoassay [TP-EIA] and fluorescent treponemal antibody absorption [FTA-ABS]) use specific treponemal antigens and are consequently more specific. They are able to detect late-stage infection and tend to remain positive after adequate therapy.

Traditional WHO recommendations for diagnosis are a sensitive non-treponemal screening test, with positive samples followed up using a more specific and equally sensitive treponemal assay. Enzyme-immunosorbent assays (EIAs) for treponemal IgG and IgM are beginning to supersede this technique because thay are more easily automated, more objective, and a useful method for detecting antibody in patients with HIV.

Seronegative patients at recent risk of acquiring disease should be followed up because of the seronegative window in early primary syphilis (see Syphilis, p. 642).

Molecular techniques include PCR tests; these are available but not widely used.

Treatment

- *Early syphilis and pinta, yaws, bejel:* prolonged antibiotic therapy is required because of the slow dividing rate of *T. pallidum* (averages one doubling in vivo per day). These are highly sensitive to penicillin and a long-acting depot injection of benzathine benzylpenicillin is the standard therapy. A single dose is sufficient for early infection. An alternative is a 15-day course of azithromycin (increasing reports of resistance), doxycycline, or ceftriaxone (limited data).
- *Late syphilis:* give weekly doses of benzathine penicillin over 3 weeks. Alternatives are doxycycline and ceftriaxone. Consider the possibility of reinfection in cases of treatment failure.
- *Neurosyphilis:* use IV penicillin, as benzathine benzylpenicillin achieves no measurable CSF levels and there are a number of reports of patients treated with benzathine benzylpenicillin developing neurosyphilis.
- *Jarisch–Herxheimer reaction:* patients may develop the Jarisch–Herxheimer reaction, which is an acute febrile reaction frequently accompanied by headache and myalgias within the first 24 hours of penicillin treatment. This reaction is most common among patients with early syphilis. Antipyretics can be used for symptomatic relief.

Borrelia species

These are helical bacteria around 0.25 micrometer in diameter and between 3 and 20 micrometers long. Those causing human disease are transmitted by insect vectors.
- Louse-borne relapsing fever: *B. recurrentis*
- Tick-borne relapsing fever: a variety of species
- Lyme disease: *B. burgdorferi*

Relapsing fever

Relapsing fever is caused by several *Borrelia* species transmitted by arthropods, characterized by recurring episodes of fever. Two distinct clinical forms were recognized as far back as ancient Greece: epidemic louse-borne and endemic tick-borne relapsing fever.

The presentation of abrupt fever, muscle aches, and joint pains with crisis, remission, and then relapse are similar for both forms, but the periodicity tends to be characteristic (e.g., 5.5 days for louse-borne vs. 3.1 days for tick-borne). The recurrent nature is thought to be due to antigenic variation of the spirochetal outer-membrane proteins.

Epidemiology

Tick-borne relapsing fever is worldwide and transmitted by soft-bodied *Ornithodorus* ticks. Most tick species carry a distinctive borreliae. Epidemiology depends on the local vector, e.g., *O. hermsii* is the most commn vector in California and Canada and lives in dead trees and on rodents and transmits *B. hermsii*. Infection is passed down the tick generations, thus disease tends to be endemic.

Louse-borne relapsing fever has occurred in Africa, the Middle East, and Asia. The human body-louse inhabits only humans and *B. recurrentis* is not transmitted vertically within lice, thus is maintained by passage from louse to human and then back to another louse, which remains infective for its entire life. Therefore, infection is associated with poverty and overcrowding, and disease tends to be epidemic.

Clinical features

Incubation and symptoms are similar in both conditions: 3–8 days after exposure there is the abrupt-onset fever, headache, myalgia, arthralgia, chills, weakness, anorexia, epistaxis, cough/hemoptysis, and weight loss.

Examination findings include hypotension, hepatosplenomegaly, lymphadenopathy, nuchal rigidity, jaundice, photophobia, injected conjunctiva, and iritis.

- *Tick-borne disease:* the primary episode lasts 3–6 days and is followed by a critical episode than may cause fatal shock. The first relapse occurs 7–10 days later. Subsequent relapses are less severe. The average number of relapses experienced is 3 but can be as many as 10.
- *Louse-borne disease:* there are fewer relapses than with tick-borne infection, and hepatic or splenic involvement is more common, as are neurological manifestations (coma, hemiplegia, meningitis, seizures).

Diagnosis

Organisms can be cultured, but isolation is not practical. Serological tests are available, but cross-reactivities among related species and the time required to develop an antibody response affect diagnostic utility in real time. Approximately 5% of patients have a positive VDRL. Most useful is demonstration of spirochetes in peripheral blood smears (and other body fluids, e.g., marrow aspirates, CSF).

Unlike the other spirochetes, borreliae stain well with acid aniline dyes such as Giemsa. They are most likely to be found during febrile episodes when the sensitivity of blood smears is around 70% for louse-borne fever (less for tick). Multiple thin smears may need to be examined. Immunological and PCR-based tests are available. Other lab findings include deranged clotting tests and elevated liver function tests (LFTs).

Treatment

- *Tick-borne relapsing fever:* tetracycline is the drug of choice, given for 7–14 days. Other treatment is doxycycline for 7 days, or erythromycin for 10 days.
- *Louse-borne relapsing fever:* give a single dose of doxycycline (preferred), tetracycline, erythromycin, or penicillin G.
- *Jarisch–Herxheimer reactions* can occur (usually within the first 2 hours after antibiotic administration), particularly in louse-borne relapsing fever. Features include sweating, tachycardia, and hypertension followed by profound hypotension. It can be fatal and appears to be mediated partly by tumor necrosis factor (TNF)-α. Preadministration of steroids does not appear to limit the reaction significantly.

Lyme disease

This disease is caused by infection and the host immune response to *Borrelia burgdorferi*. It is acquired via the bite of ixodes (hard) ticks, and coinfection with other tick-borne organisms can occur (e.g., babesiosis).

Epidemiology

Ticks acquire a spread infection through feeding on infected animals (particularly deer). A tick must be attached to a person for 2–3 days to pass on infection, as only small numbers of bacteria are present in the tick until it feeds—the act of feeding sees bacteria multiply and pass to the salivary glands.

Until this multiplication occurs, ticks are rarely able to pass on infection; 85% of human infections occur while the tick is in the nymph stage (spring to summer), 15% when it is in the adult stage (autumn).

Cases are most common in children aged 5–9 years and adults aged 60–69 years; only 40% give a definite history of tick bite. Cases occur across Europe, China, Japan, Australia, and parts of the United States. It is relatively rare in the UK, with most cases occurring in the south (New Forest and Salisbury Plain), East Anglia, Cumbria, and the Scottish highlands.

Clinical manifestations

Like its cousin, syphilis, it is a great imitator. Clinical features may be a result of direct bacterial infection (particularly in the early stages of disease) or a consequence of an immune response leading to symptoms in many organs (e.g., arthritis). Asymptomatic infection occurs less than 10% of the time.

In general, Lyme disease has three overlapping stages, but symptoms may differ with the strain of *Borrelia* involved (see below):

- *Early localized:* around 7 days after tick bite <75% of patients develop erythema migrans; an expanding, painless, annular target-shaped skin lesion centered on the bite with or without local lymphadenopathy may occur. It is probably a result of the inflammatory response to the organism in the skin. Multiple lesions can occur and do not necessarily represent multiple bites. It lasts 2–3 weeks if untreated.
- *Early disseminated:* weeks to months after the bite, patients develop more severe constitutional symptoms, malaise, generalized lymphadenopathy, hepatitis, arthritis (50%—initially intermittent and migratory, it may evolve into a chronic monoarticular arthritis in 10% of those affected), neurological features (15%—these include meningitis, meningo-encephalitis, cranial nerve lesions, and neuropathy), or cardiac features (10%—atrioventricular [AV] block, pericarditis, congestive heart failure [CHF]).
- *Late persistent* (but can occur within the first year): arthritis, late neurological manifestations including focal deficits, fatigue, and neuropsychiatric problems. Acrodermatitis chronica atrophicans is a decoloration of the skin, seen in the extremities and similar to the skin changes of peripheral vascular disease.

Microbiology

Three members of the *Borrelia burgdorferi sensu lato* complex cause Lyme disease: *Borrelia garinii* and *afzelii* in Asia, and *Borrelia burgdoferi sensu stricto* in North America. *Borrelia garinii* and *afzelii* are the most common European clinical isolates.

These differences account for the variation in clinical manifestations across the world (*B. garinii* is associated with neurological disease, *B. afzelli* with cutaneous manifestations, and *B. burgdorferi sensu stricto* with joint symptoms).

Diagnosis

Culture of the organism is possible from skin specimens taken from those patients with erythema migrans. It is difficult to identify spirochetes in histological sections.

Serology is the diagnostic method of choice. The CDC recommends a screening ELISA for anti-Lyme antibody, with positive titers confirmed by Western blot. Specific response is sensitive but develops late (30% positive in the acute phase, 70% at 2–4 weeks, 90% at 4–6 weeks). Prompt antibiotic therapy may prevent a good antibody response.

Some patients remain positive for years after illness, thus active and inactive infection cannot be distinguished. Tests must be interpreted with caution in those without a positive travel history or a presentation consistent with Lyme disease.

Serology is nearly always positive in those with extracutaneous lesions. False positives may be seen in association with rheumatoid disease, infectious mononucleosis, and syphilis.

PCR for *Borrelia burgdorferi* DNA is more sensitive than culture or microscopy in the examination of blood or joint fluid but has not been standardized for routine diagnosis.

Spinal fluid should be obtained in those patients with neurological symptoms in whom the diagnosis is not obvious. CSF serology may be helpful.

Treatment

Patients with a good history and classic erythema migrans should be treated regardless of serology results. Patients probably remain at risk of infection even after treatment for one episode.

- *Early-stage skin manifestations, arthritis, or Bell's palsy:* doxycycline or amoxicillin PO for 28 days. If arthritis persists, repeat course or consider IV ceftriaxone for 14–30 days.
- *Third-degree heart block:* IV ceftriaxone for 14–28 days
- *Neurological disease*
  - Cranial nerve palsies: 30-day oral regime as above
  - Parasthesia/radiculopathy: 14 days IV ceftriaxone
  - Encephalitis/encephalopathy: 28 days IV ceftriaxone

Prevention

Avoid ticks and promptly remove any attached ticks. Some specialists recommend the use of a single dose of prophylactic doxycycline within 3 days of removal of a tick that has been attached for at least 24 hours in high-risk areas or hyperendemic regions.

Vaccines are no longer available in the United States.

Leptospira species

Leptospira are motile, obligately aerobic spirochetes measuring 0.1 micrometer in diameter and around 10 micrometers long. They stain poorly but can be visualized on dark-field or phase-contrast microscopy.

Two species are identified: *L. interrogans* (includes all human pathogens) and *L. biflexa* (a saprophytic species). *L. interrogans* has many serotypes, and antigenically related organisms are grouped into serovars (a synonym for *serotype*) for classification.

Although more recent DNA analysis does not correlate well with serological classification, serological classification will continue to be used for the foreseeable future. The type strain is *L. interrogans* serovar Icterohaemorrhagiae, and the type disease, leptospirosis.

Leptospirosis

This is a biphasic disease with initial septicemia and a secondary phase characterized by immune phenomena (vasculitis, aseptic meningitis). Weil's disease is a severe form characterized by jaundice and acute renal failure.

Epidemiology

Leptospira are found worldwide. The primary reservoirs of most leptospiral serovars are wild mammals. These continually reinfect domestic populations and at least 160 mammalian species are affected. The organism has been recovered from rats, pigs, dogs, cats, and cattle among others, but rarely causes disease in these hosts. Rodents are the most-important reservoir, and rats are the most common worldwide source.

There are associations between particular animals and serovars (e.g., *L. interrogans* serovar Icterohaemorrhagiae and rats). Humans are incidental hosts, and onward transmission is rare.

Transmission occurs when people come into contact with infected animal urine, e.g., while canoeing, swimming in lakes and rivers, or farming. It is primarily a disease of tropical and subtropical regions, and infection in temperate regions is uncommon.

Pathogenesis

After gaining entry via the skin or mucous membranes, the organism replicates in blood and tissue. Leptospiremia particularly affects the liver and kidneys, causing centrilobular necrosis and jaundice, or interstitial nephritis and tubular necrosis, respectively. Renal failure may occur, exacerbated by hypovolemia.

Other organs affected include muscle (edema and focal necrosis), capillaries (vasculitis), and eye (chronic uveitis).

Clinical features

Incubation is 7–12 days. Most patients (90%) develop mild disease without jaundice; 5–10% develop the severe form, Weil's disease. Disease is biphasic.

The first phase (septicemic—the organism can be cultured from blood, CSF, and most tissues) lasts 4–7 days and is characterized by a flu-like illness, fever, chills, weakness, myalgia, cough, hemoptysis, rash, meningism, and headache. A 1- to 3-day period of improvement follows and patients may become afebrile.

The second stage then starts (immune or leptospiruric phase, in which antibodies may be detected and the organism isolated from urine). Features are due to the immunological response to infection and may last up to a month. Disease may be anicteric or icteric.

Aseptic meningitis is the most important feature of anicteric disease and is seen in 50% of cases. Death is rare in this group. Icteric disease is characterized by jaundice, hepatosplenomegaly, nausea and vomiting, anorexia, and diarrhea or constipation. Organisms can be isolated from the blood <48 hours after jaundice onset.

Other features include uveitis (<10%; can occur up to a year after initial illness), subconjunctival hemorrhage is the most common ocular complication (92% of patients), renal impairment (uraemia, pyuria, hematuria, oliguria), and pulmonary manifestations.

Weil's disease is characterized by jaundice, renal failure, hepatic necrosis, lung disease, and bleeding. It starts at the end of stage 1. Overall mortality is 10% and up to 40% in those with hepatorenal involvement.

Diagnosis

Direct examination

Dark-field examination of blood, CSF, or urine may demonstrate leptospira, but there is a high false-positive rate (misinterpretation of fibrils and red cell fragments). It is notrecommended.

Culture

There has been little change in culture techniques over the years. It is difficult and insensitive and requires several weeks of incubation. Specialized culture media are required (e.g., Ellinghausen-McCullough-Johnson-Harris [EMJH], which contains 1% bovine serum albumin and Tween 80, a fatty acid source). They should be inoculated within 24 hours of specimen collection (either blood or CSF in heparin or sodium oxalate). Leptospiral culture can be established by subculture of routine blood culture samples.

Organisms can be isolated from blood and CSF in the first week of illness. In the second phase of illness they can be found only in the urine, where they may be isolated for up to 1 month. Cultures can be reported as negative after a minimum of 6 weeks; continuing for as long as 4 months is preferable.

Molecular techniques

Quantitative PCR assays to detect leptosiral DNA have been developed. They are sensitive, can distinguish different species, and allow early diagnosis, and organisms can be detected after antibiotic therapy has been initiated.

Serology

Serology is the mainstay of diagnosis. Commercial tests using genus-specific antigens are used to screen sera, and positive reactions are confirmed in a reference laboratory using the microagglutination test (MAT) with live leptospira (killed have lower sensitivity).

The MAT detects agglutinating antibodies in patient serum and is relatively serovar specific, so a large number of antigens must be tested. Interlaboratory variation is high. A positive MAT is considered to be a fourfold increase in antibody titer, or a switch from seronegative to a titer of 1/100 or over.

Early samples tend to cross-react; convalescent samples are more specific and diagnostic. Enzyme immunoassay for IgM is useful for diagnosing current infection, but cross-reactions occur.

Treatment
- *Mild disease:* doxycycline, ampicillin, amoxicillin
- *Severe disease:* ampicillin, penicillin G, ceftriaxone
- *Prophylaxis:* doxycycline reduces morbidity and mortality in endemic areas but has no impact on infection rates as measured by seroconversion. It is likely to be useful in cases of accidental lab exposure or military or adventure travel. Vaccines are available against specific serovars.

Overview of Rickettsia

Microbiology
The genus *Rickettsia* is a member of the *Rickettsiales* order, which also includes *Coxiella*, *Ehrlichia*, and *Bartonella*. All are maintained in a cycle involving mammal reservoirs and arthropod vectors.

Rickettsia organisms are fastidious, obligate, intracellular Gram-negative coccobacilli (0.3 micrometer by 1–2 micrometers). They survive only briefly outside a host (unlike *Coxiella*). Isolation is usually only performed in reference laboratories.

Epidemiology
Zoonotic reservoirs are varied and include wild rodents, dogs, and livestock. Humans are incidental hosts, with the exception of louse-borne typhus, for which humans are the main reservoir. *R. rickettsii*, *R. typhi*, *R. tsutsugamushi*, and *R. akari* can exist as vector commensals. *R. prowazekii*, however, kills its human body louse vector within 3 weeks.

See Table 3.19 for geographic distribution.

Diagnosis

Culture
Culture is usually only performed in reference laboratories. Blood or biopsy tissue from skin lesions should be frozen at −70°C. Organisms may be isolated in small lab animals or in embryonated eggs. They are highly infectious if aerosolized and have been responsible for lab-acquired infections (some fatal).

Detection of antigen
Direct immunofluorescence of skin lesions in cases of Rocky Mountain spotted fever (RMSF) can identify organisms at the time the rash appears (days 3–5 of illness). Sensitivity is around 70%, with specificity approaching 100%. Organisms are most likely to be in a blood vessel near the center of the lesion—the biopsy should include this to increase chances of detection. The availability of immunofluorescent stains in non-endemic areas, however, may be limited.

Table 3.19 Overview of rickettsial disease

Genus and species	Species syndrome	Vector (geography)	Clinical features
Spoted fever group			
R. rickettsii	Rocky Mountain spotted fever (RMSF)	Ixodid ticks (Western hemisphere)	Incubation ~7 days. Fever, headache, myalgia, eschar, rash. Multisystem involvement; 20% untreated mortality
R. conorii	Mediterranean spotted fever	Ixodid ticks (Mediterranean, Africa, and India)	Incubation ~ 5 days. Eschar and local lymphadenopathy. Rash. Mild.
R. akari	Rickettsial pox	Mite (U.S., Africa, Korea, and CIS [Commonwealth of Independent States])	Incubation ~7 days. Features as for R. conorii, plus vesicular rash resembling chickenpox
Typhus group			
R. prowazekii	Epidemic typhus	Body louse (S. America, Africa, and Asia)	Incubation ~10 days. Fever, headache, neurological and GI symptoms. Rash. 20–50% untreated mortality
	Brill–Zinsser disease	Nil—recurrence years after primary attack	Similar, milder illness than epidemic typhus develops years after recovery; in the West it was seen in E. European immigrants after World War II. Lasts around 2 weeks
R. typhi	Murine (endemic) typhus	Flea (worldwide, where humans and rats coexist)	Similar to epidemic typhus but much milder
R. tsutsugamushi	Scrub typhus*	Mite (S. Pacific, Asia, Australia)	Eschar is common. Similar to epidemic typhus

*So-called scrub typhus as the vector is harbored in scrub vegetation. The chigger mites stay within several meters of where they hatch and are transovarially infected. Infection therefore occurs in very focused rural "mite islands."

Serology
Serology is the main means of confirming diagnosis. Antibodies first appear around days 7–10 after infection. A fourfold rise on a convalescent sample is required for diagnosis, but a single titer over 1:64 is very suggestive of infection.

Box 3.7 Weil–Felix test

In 1915 in Poland, Weil and Felix found that serum from patients with typhus agglutinated certain strains of *Proteus vulgaris*. This test has been the mainstay of diagnosis for many years.

Currently, the most sensitive and specific serological assay is the micro-immunofluorescence test. It requires trained personnel and a fluorescent microscope.

Latex agglutination tests are available for the diagnosis of RMSF. A single positive test is considered diagnostic; these tests rarely produce positive reactions in convalescence.

Both complement fixation and the classic Weil–Felix test (see Box 3.7) are now considered to be neither sufficiently sensitive nor specific.

Cross-reactions among rickettsial species occur and vary from patient to patient. They tend to be strongest between rickettsial subgroups—e.g., it is difficult to distinguish spotted fevers from each other.

Rickettsial diseases

Rickettsiae replicate within the cytoplasm of infected endothelial and smooth muscle cells of capillaries and small arteries. They cause a necrotizing vasculitis with protean manifestations.

The classic triad of fever, headache, and rash with the appropriate exposure history should alert the clinician to the possible diagnosis. An eschar (black, ulcerated lesion) may develop at the bite site. Severity varies greatly with species—any organ can be involved.

Spotted fevers

Rocky Mountain spotted fever (RMSF)

Clinical features
RMSF is the most virulent spotted fever, with 20% mortality if untreated. Fever, myalgia, arthralgia, nausea, and headache follow a 2- to 14-day incubation.

GI involvement may suggest an acute surgical abdomen, especially in children. Maculopapular rash (90%) appears around days 3–5, often starting at the ankles and wrists.

Severe multisystem involvement is common, including lung (pneumonia, effusions, edema), nervous system (meningitis, focal deficits, e.g., deafness), and renal impairment. Thrombocytopenia and DIC can occur.

Antimicrobial therapy has a dramatic effect on case fatality.

Treatment
Doxycycline continued for at least 3 days after the patient becomes afebrile. It is recommended that doxycycline be used even in children with suspected RMSF, given the life-threatening nature of the disease. Chloramphenicol is preferred in pregnancy.

There is no demonstrated benefit from steroid therapy.

Other spotted fevers

Mediterranean spotted fever (also known as *boutonneuse fever*) and African tick bite fever are milder diseases; 5–7 days after inoculation patients develop an eschar with local tender lymphadenopathy and a generalized maculopapular rash. Severe disease can occur in patients with diabetes, cardiac disease, or G6PD deficiency and in the elderly.

Rickettsialpox is similar in presentation, with the addition of a vesicular rash that resembles chickenpox.

Treatment is as for RMSF. Antibiotics should generally be administered for 5–7 days.

Typhus group

Epidemic typhus

Clinical features

Humans are the reservoir, and outbreaks are associated with conditions of crowding, especially during winter and war. The louse feeds on an infected person, bites, and defecates. The infected feces are scratched into the bite.

After 1 week's incubation, abrupt onset of headache and fever is followed by maculopapular rash at day 5. This involves the entire body within a few days. Neurological features are common, as is multisystem involvement.

Mortality is 20–50% untreated. It is low in children, high in the elderly.

Treatment

Treatment is as for RMSF. Early therapy nearly eliminates fatal illness.

Murine typhus

- *Clinical features:* longer incubation (up to 2 weeks) and patients rarely recall flea exposure. Fever, headache, and myalgia are followed by rash in 50%. Some may develop multisystem features, but this is less common than with epidemic louse-borne typhus. Mortality is <1%.
- *Treatment:* as for Rocky Mountain spotted fever.

Scrub typhus

- *Clinical features:* not as severe as epidemic typhus. An individual is inoculated by the bite of the chigger mite and develops abrupt fever and headache 6–18 days later. Usually, there are tender lymph nodes and an eschar at the inoculation point. Severity varies widely; neurological features can occur. Untreated mortality varies—up to 30%. There are many serotypes (unlike the other organisms), so people may become infected again.
- *Treatment:* as for RMSF, but resistance to doxycycline and chloramphenicol has been seen in northern Thailand. Treatment may need to be prolonged to avoid relapse (2 weeks).

Coxiella burnetii (Q fever)

Q fever is the name coined by the medical officer in Queensland, Australia who first investigated the outbreak of febrile illness that hit 20 employees of a Brisbane meat works.

Microbiology

Coxiella burnetii is a short, pleomorphic rod previously characterized as a *Rickettsia* but more recently placed into the gamma subdivision of *Proteobacteria* on the basis of 16S rRNA sequencing.

It may be transmitted by aerosol or infected milk. It can form spores and is able to survive outside a host for some time—over 40 months in skimmed milk at room temperature! It grows in the phagosomes of infected cells rather than the cytoplasm (as other rickettsia), appreciating the more acidic environment the phagosome affords.

Epidemiology

Q fever is a worldwide zoonosis, typically acquired from occupational exposure to cattle or sheep or through exposure to parturient cats. Acquisition from unpasteurized dairy products has occurred, and person-to-person spread is possible but unusual. The reservoir in nature is large and includes mammals, birds, and ticks.

Infected ungulates are usually asymptomatic, although abortion or still-birth may result. Organisms from a heavily infected placenta may be found in the soil for 6 months, and in air for 2 weeks after parturition.

Clinical features

Humans are infected by inhalation of contaminated aerosols from parturi-ent fluids of infected livestock or occasionally by ingestion. Organisms proliferate in the lungs and bacteremia follows.

Acute presentation is 2–5 weeks after infection and ranges from a self-limited febrile illness (most common) to pneumonia with or without hepatitis. Acute Q fever can be complicated by behavioral disturbances, Guillain–Barré syndrome, myocarditis, arthritis, and glomerulonephritis, among others. Autoantibodies are often found (anti-mitochondria, smooth muscle). Mortality is around 1% and associated with myocarditis.

Chronic Q fever is defined as infection lasting more than 6 months. The most common manifestation is culture-negative endocarditis, which may be accompanied by many extracardiac manifestations. Hepatitis, osteomyelitis, vascular graft infection, and neurological infection are also recognized.

Immunocompromised hosts and pregnant women are at higher risk.

Diagnosis

- *Culture:* difficult and hazardous for lab staff—a biosafety level 3 organism
- *Serology:* the organism has two biological phases. Antibodies to phase II are produced first. Phase I antibodies appear weeks later. If antibodies to both phases are present simultaneously, chronic infection (specifically endocarditis) should be considered. Cross-reactions

occur with *Bartonella* infection. The complement fixation test is most widely used. Fourfold rise between acute and convalescent titers is considered diagnostic of Q fever
• *Molecular:* PCR tests exist but are not in widespread use.

Treatment
• *Pneumonia:* infection is nearly always self-limited. Even without therapy, recovery occurs at around 2 weeks. However, treatment is indicated in all cases to reduce chance of chronic disease: doxycycline for 14 days is recommended for acute Q fever and should be used in children with life-threatening disease. Chloramphenicol or trimethoprim-sulfamethoxazole has been used during pregnancy.
• *Endocarditis:* prolonged combination antibiotic therapy (e.g., minimum duration 18 months) is required. No consensus on the drugs or duration exists. Doxycycline with ciprofloxacin, rifampin, or hydroxychloroquine has been used. Valve replacement may be required.

Bartonella species

Microbiology
Bartonella are fastidious Gram-negative intracellular organisms. The three most important species causing human disease are highlighted below.

Clinical syndromes

Oroya fever (B. bacilliformis)
This develops 3–12 weeks after inoculation by the fly vector and may be mild or abrupt and severe (high fever, headache, confusion, anemia due to erythrocyte invasion, hepatomegaly, and lymphadenopathy). Complications include abdominal pain, thrombocytopenia, seizures, dyspnea, and hepatic and GI dysfunction, and angina can occur. Mortality rate is high.
    Survivors have a high incidence of opportunistic infections (e.g., salmonella, toxoplasmosis). Asymptomatic bacteremia with *B. bacilliformis* occurs in 15% of survivors.

Veruga peruana (B. bacilliformis)
This late-stage manifestation is characterized by crops of skin lesions weeks to months after untreated acute infection. Initially of a miliary appearance, they become nodular, then mular—erythematous round lesions, 5 mm in diameter. Lesions occur on mucosal surfaces and internally.
    Histology demonstrates neovascular proliferation with occasional organisms.

Cat scratch disease (B. henselae)
This can result from a cat scratch or bite as well as from a flea bite; 3–10 days after inoculation a papule or pustule may be visible at the site. Most cases present at 2–3 weeks with regional lymphadenopathy and low-grade fever. Rarer features include headache, sore throat, and skin rash. Lymphadenopathy settles over 2–4 months, even without treatment.

Complications (more common in the immunocompromised) include encephalopathy, retinitis, bone and skin involvement, and granulomatous hepatitis. Conjunctival exposure may present as the Parinaud's oculoglandular syndrome (ocular granuloma or conjunctivitis, preauricular lymphadenopathy). Other atypical presentations are fever of unknown origin (FUO), osteomyelitis, and hepatic and splenic granulomas.

Diagnosis is based on history but biopsy may be necessary to exclude lymphoma. Organisms may be visible on Warthin–Starry stain. Culture is possible from blood and tissue and should be attempted in cases of FUO, neuroretinitis, or encephalitis after cat exposure, especially in the immunocompromised.

Bacillary angiomatosis (BA)

BA is a unique vascular proliferation caused by *B. henselae* or *B. quintana* infection. It usually occurs in the immunocompromised, mostly HIV patients with CD4 <100/mm^3, but also transplant patients and those on chemotherapy.

Lesions begin as small papules that grow to form round red to purple nodules that can ulcerate. They can also appear as flat hyperpigmented plaques. They occur on the skin, liver, spleen, bone, mucosal surfaces, heart, CNS, and bone marrow.

The organism's outer membrane adhesin binds to endothelial cells and induces endothelial proliferation and new vessel formation.

Numerous organisms are visible in lesions stained with Warthin–Starry stain. Diagnosis is with lesion biopsy.

All patients should be treated with a prolonged course (3 months or longer) of erythromycin or doxycycline.

Bacillary peliosis (BP)

BP is characterized by blood-filled cystic lesions scattered throughout a visceral organ. Cases involving the liver (peliosis hepatic) and spleen present with weight loss, diarrhea, abdominal pain, nausea, fever, hepatosplenomegaly, and elevated liver enzymes.

BP is caused by *B. henselae* or *quintana* infection. Most patients also have bacillary angiomatosis and previous cat exposure.

Fever, bacteremia, endocarditis (B. quintana)

This syndrome is acquired by scratching infected louse feces into skin lesions. Epidemics have occurred across the world, usually in conditions of overcrowding and poor sanitation (e.g., soldiers in World War I—"trench fever"). Bacteremia has also been described in homeless alcoholics.

Incubation is 3–40 days, followed by a relapsing fever with headache, rash, and splenomegaly. It is a recognized cause of culture-negative endocarditis in those with HIV and in immunocompetent alcoholics. *B. henselae* bacteremia occurs in the immunocompetent and those with HIV.

Treatment is with macrolides and tetracyclines for 4–6 weeks. Endocarditis may need surgery and very prolonged antibiotic courses.

Diagnosis

Direct examination

Giemsa-stained blood films may be used to detect *B. bacilliformis* in areas of endemic Oroya fever because of the large number of organisms present. This is not feasible in the detection of *B. henselae* or *B. quintana* because of the low level of blood-borne organisms. They may be detected by silver staining of lesions in BA or BP and in lymph nodes in the early stages of cat scratch disease.

Culture

Bartonella are fastidious organisms that require specific laboratory conditions. Yield from blood culture is low but increases with the use of isolator tubes (Wampole). Subculture to chocolate agar or heart infusion agar supplemented with rabbit blood supports growth after 21 days' incubation at 37°C in 5% CO_2.

Colonies with the appropriate morphological characteristics can have their identity confirmed by cellular fatty acid analysis, immunofluorescent antibody, using commercial enzymatic substrate kits, or by 16S rRNA sequencing.

Molecular

PCR or DNA-hybridization techniques can be used to speciate isolates. Direct detection of *Bartonella* organisms in pus or tissue is possible using PCR, with wide-ranging sensitivity, depending on the technique and sample.

Serology

Enzyme immunoassay or immunofluorescence kits may be used to demonstrate anti-*Bartonella* antibodies in culture-negative endocarditis, those with cat scratch disease, or HIV-associated infection. There is substantial cross-reactivity between *B. henselae* and *B. quintana* as well as with certain *Chlamydia* species.

Mycoplasma

Microbiology

The term *mycoplasma* refers organisms within the class *Mollicutes*, which means "soft skin." They lack a rigid cell wall and are bound only by a trilaminar membrane. They have a small genome with consequent limited biosynthetic capabilities and require enriched media for growth. They can be distinguished by their differing phenotypic characteristics.

Mycoplasma are found in a wide range of animals and plants. Three species (*M. pneumoniae*, *M. hominis*, *Ureaplasma urealyticum*) are well-established human pathogens.

Mycoplasma pneumoniae

This is one of the most common causes of respiratory tract infections and atypical pneumonia (7–20%). Infection via droplet transmission occurs year round (peaks in winter) and affects all ages. Most significant clinical disease (e.g., pneumonia) is seen from age 5 years to young adulthood.

Once exposed, the organism attaches to respiratory tract epithelial cells and multiplies locally. Incubation is for 2–3 weeks, and presentation is usually insidious with flu-like symptoms. Multiple lobes may be involved but without consolidation and CXR-confirmed infection is usually more dramatic than clinical presentation suggests. Pleural effusions are in 20%.

Disease is usually self-limited with resolution over 3–10 days without antibiotics; CXR abnormalities may take 6 weeks to clear. Antibiotic therapy (e.g., macrolides) speeds resolution but rarely eradicates the organisms from the respiratory tract; recurrences can occur.

Rare complications include pleuritis, pneumothorax, lung abscess, hemolytic anemia (secondary to cold agglutinins), thrombocytopenia, arthritis, rashes (e.g., erythema nodosum and multiforme), and Guillain–Barré syndrome. Most complications are immune mediated, with the exception of neurological complications such as meningoencephalitis, which are thought to be due to direct invasion.

Humoral and cellular immunodeficiency predisposes to more severe disease.

U. urealyticum and M. hominis

These organisms may be part of the normal genital flora in sexually experienced men and women. They are implicated in endometritis and chorioamnionitis; are statistically linked with prematurity, low birth weight, and infertility; and are frequently recovered in culture along with other genital tract pathogens. Both may be isolated from blood cultures in women with postpartum fever (10% of cases). In men, they are causes of nongonococcal urethritis and a rare cause of epididymitis.

In neonates, they cause meningitis, and there is an association between neonatal U. urealyticum colonization of the respiratory tract and the development of chronic lung disease of the newborn.

Both may cause septic arthritis and subcutaneous abscesses in those with immunodeficiency.

Sternal wound infections with M. hominis have occurred in heart and lung transplant patients.

Other Mycoplasma organisms

M. genitalium is a cause of nongonococcal urethritis and may also have a role in respiratory tract disease. M. fermentans, M. penetrans, and M. pirum have been isolated in those with HIV and are unusual in their ability to actively invade cells.

Certain organisms found in animal hosts have caused human disease in cases of sufficient exposure and significant predisposing comorbidity (e.g., M. arginini—in many animals; M. canis—in, you guessed it, dogs).

Diagnosis

Direct detection

Indirect fluorescent antibody tests to detect M. hominis in genital samples have been developed (but not widely used).

Culture

M. pneumoniae can be recovered from respiratory tract specimens. Genital mycoplasmas can be isolated from many specimens. As they re fastidious organisms, they should be inoculated to culture media as soon as possible. Several media are used for culture of mycoplasma—most are diphasic (media with agar overlayed by media without agar). All species grow at 35–37°C but differ in their optimal pH and atmospheric conditions as well as their substrate utilization.

M. pneumoniae isolates should be kept for at least 4 weeks, initially in selective broth. Growth is indicated by change in pH. Positive isolates are subcultured to agar. Colonies should be visible by 1 week and identity confirmed by serological methods or by enzyme substrate tests (e.g., tetrazolium reduction).

Genital mycoplasma samples are inoculated into broth and onto agar and should be kept for 8 days (although *M. genitalium* and *M. fermentans* can take longer and are not routinely looked for). Broths that exhibit a change in color are plated to the appropriate agar. Plates are examined by microscope each day for colonies. Selective plates and colonial morphology are usually sufficient to allow identification.

Anti-sera are available to confirm *M. hominis*.

Molecular

PCR and DNA probe techniques have been developed but are not in wide use.

Serology

The time required to culture these organisms means that diagnosis is often made by serology. *M. pneumoniae* complement fixation tests detect mostly the early IgM—a fourfold rise between acute and convalescent (7–10 days) samples is diagnostic of recent infection.

Enzyme immunoassays are available and detect IgM and IgG.

Treatment

M. pneumoniae is sensitive to a wide range of agents—tetracyclines, quinolones, or macrolides.

M. hominis is usually resistant to erythromycin. Some genital mycoplasma isolates have been found to be tetracycline resistant and carry the *tetM* resistance determinant (also found in other genital-tract organisms, e.g., group B streptococci).

U. urealyticum is usually resistant to clindamycin and less susceptible to quinolones. Erythromycin is effective.

Chlamydia

These are small, obligate, intracellular (they are unable to produce ATP themselves) Gram-negative organisms. Outside a host cell they are tiny (300 nm diameter), inactive "elementary" bodies. They infect cells primarily by receptor-mediated endocytosis. They are able to inhibit lysosome fusion and reside in a membrane-protected inclusion body, where they activate and increase to a diameter of around 800 nm.

Three species produce human disease: *Chlamydia trachomatis*, *C. psittaci*, and *C. pneumoniae*. They differ antigenically, in host cell preference and in antibiotic susceptibility.

The family *Chlamydiaceae* was reorganized in 1999 on the basis of generic similarities. *C. trachomatis* remains in the genus *Chlamydia*, but *psittaci* and *pneumoniae* were moved to a new genus, *Chlamydiophila*.

Chlamydia trachomatis

Clinical features

There are 15 different serovars causing distinctive clinical syndromes. Natural infection confers only short-lived protection against reinfection.

Lymphogranuloma venereum
Serovar L1, L2, L3 is endemic in Africa, India, Southeast Asia, South America, and the Caribbean. It is sexually transmitted—the organism enters through skin abrasions (it cannot infect squamous epithelial cells) and causes a small papule or ulcer (primary lesion) on genital mucosa or nearby skin 3–30 days after infection.

It heals rapidly, and weeks later the patient may develop secondary symptoms: lymphadenopathy (inguinal or femoral), fever, headache, myalgias, proctitis (can resemble inflammatory bowel disease), and, occasionally, meningitis. Nodes may coalesce, forming abscesses and buboes.

Trachoma
Serovars A, B1, B2, and C cause chronic follicular keratoconjunctivitis, which leads to corneal scarring and is the most common cause of preventable blindness in the developing world (~9 million blind, 500 million affected).

First infections are usually acquired in childhood and resolve spontaneously, but multiple reinfections and the consequent host immune response result in conjunctival scarring and corneal damage. The inner surface of the eyelid scars, and in-turning eyelashes further abrade the cornea.

Inclusion conjunctivitis
Serovars D to K can cause sexually transmitted eye infection of adults (of whom slightly over half have concurrent genital tract infection) and neonatal conjunctivitis (probably from the mother's genital tract, but it can occur even if delivered by Caesarean section, 5 days to 6 weeks after delivery). There is no corneal scarring.

Neonatal pneumonia
With serovars D to K, most cases are acquired from the mother's genital tract. Pneumonia is seen in 10–20% of infants born to infected mothers. The infants are usually symptomatic by 8 weeks with nasal congestion, and cough and are only moderately ill.

Sexually transmitted infections (STIs)
Serovars D to K can cause epididymitis (along with *N. gonorrhoeae*, the common cause in those under 35), urethritis, salpingitis, cervicitis with

consequent pelvic inflammatory disease, and infertility. Reactive arthritis (formerly called Reiter syndrome) may follow.

Diagnosis

Trachoma may be diagnosed on clinical grounds. Other clinical presentations require lab identification for a definitive diagnosis.

- *Antigen detection:* monoclonal antibodies and immunofluorescence have high sensitivity with conjunctival specimens. Enzyme immunoassay can demonstrate chlamydial antigen in respiratory or genital secretions.
- *Culture:* being obligate intracellular organisms, the techniques for culturing are similar to those used in virus culture. The infective elementary bodies must first be extracted by centrifugation before infecting a cell line. Inclusion bodies containing the organism can be seen at 48–72 hours, and species-specific monoclonal antibodies are used to confirm identity.
- *Serology:* most useful for epidemiological studies. Chlamydial complement fixation tests do not distinguish between species; microimmunofluorescence does.
- *Molecular tests:* for chlamydial DNA, these are the preferred initial investigation for diagnosis of *C. trachomatis* in all specimen types. PCR- and ligase chain reaction (LCR)-based tests are available; sensitivity is a high as 99% for some of these but varies with specimen type and quality. The notable advantage is that it allows the diagnosis of urethritis on noninvasively acquired specimens.

Treatment

- *Trachoma:* transmission is via flies or eye-to-hand contact in endemic areas, thus hygiene is important for control (rates fall quickly with socioeconomic improvement). Systemic therapy (erythromycin or doxycycline) is effective in areas of low transmission (where reinfection is less frequent). Mass treatment at the village level has been shown to be effective. Eyelid surgery can prevent further mechanical damage.
- *Lymphogranuloma venereum:* buboes should be aspirated. Give doxycycline for 3 weeks.
- *Genital and ocular infections in adults:* single-dose azithromycin, or doxycycline for 7 days. Longer courses of amoxicillin may be effective in pregnant women.
- *Neonatal infections:* topical eye therapy is not recommended, as it does not eliminate carriage. Erythromycin is given orally for 14 days for both conjunctivitis and pneumonia. Prenatal screening of mothers and treatment of those infected with *Chlamydia* is 90% effective in preventing infants from acquiring the infection.

Chlamydiophila psittaci

C. psittaci can infect many kinds of birds. The classic term for infection caused by this bacterium, *psittacosis,* derived from the Greek word for parrot, is therefore not as accurate a description as *ornithosis*. It is an occupational disease of zoo workers, petshop workers, and poultry farmers.

Human-to-human transmission occurs but is very rare. Infection is primarily acquired by inhalation of organisms from aerosolized avian excreta or respiratory secretions from sick birds (mouth-to-beak resuscitation has been implicated in acquisition).

Transient exposure is sufficient (e.g., petshop customers). The disease is found worldwide.

Incubation is 5–14 days and presentation is with fever, chills, malaise, cough, headache, breathlessness, mild pharyngitis, and epistaxis. Less commonly, nausea, vomiting, and jaundice may be seen. Examination may demonstrate the features of an atypical pneumonia. Other features are bradycardia, peri- or myocarditis culture-negative endocarditis, splenomegaly, meningitis, encephalitis, Guillain–Barré syndrome, rashes, acute glomerulonephritis, severe respiratory failure, sepsis, and shock. Relapses can occur.

Diagnosis is by serology: the demonstration of a fourfold rise in CF antibody titer is considered diagnostic. Antibodies may cross-react with other chlamydial species.

Culture is possible but avoided because of the risks to lab staff. Other tests include ELISA and PCR.

Treatment is with tetracycline or doxycycline for 2–3 weeks (reduces the risk of relapse). Erythromycin may be used in children and pregnant women.

Chlamydophila pneumoniae

This is the cause of 3–10% of community-acquired pneumonia cases among adults. Adolescents tend to experience a mild pneumonia or bronchitis, whereas older adults can experience more severe disease and repeated infections. Fifty percent of young adults have serological evidence of previous infection.

Unlike *C. psittaci*, human-to-human transmission via respiratory secretions is the norm. In most populations, infection is more common in males; this may reflect cigarette use.

Incubation is 3–4 weeks, and symptoms of a upper respiratory tract infection are followed by bronchitis or pneumonia 1–4 weeks later. Most infections are asymptomatic or cause only mild symptoms. Other features are hoarse voice, nonproductive cough, and headache. Fever is often absent. Symptoms can be very prolonged, even with appropriate treatment.

Diagnosis is by serology (preferably microimmunofluorescence, if available, as compliment fixation tests cross-react with other chlamydial species). A definite case requires a fourfold rise in titer—single elevated IgG titers may be seen in the uninfected elderly as a consequence of repeated infections.

Antibody tests may be negative in the early weeks after infection; it can take as long as 8 weeks for a significant IgG response to develop after primary infection. Other tests include PCR and cell culture tests.

Treatment is with doxycycline or erythromycin.

Mycobacterium tuberculosis

The *Mycobacterium tuberculosis* complex comprises seven species: *M. tuberculosis*, *M. bovis*, *M. africanum*, *M. microti*, *M. canetti*, *M. caprae*, and *M. pinnipedii*. The term *tuberculosis* (TB) describes a broad range of clinical diseases caused by *M. tuberculosis* (and, less commonly, *M. bovis*).

Epidemiology

M. tuberculosis infects one-third of the world's population and is the most frequent infectious cause of death worldwide, accounting for 3 million deaths per year. Most cases occur in the developing world, with 13 countries accounting for 75% of cases. In the developed world, despite a general downward trend, there has been an increase in incidence in certain groups, e.g., immigrants from high-prevalence countries and HIV-infected patients.

Infection is acquired via inhalation of infectious droplet nuclei. Occasionally it is due to skin inoculation (e.g., pathologists, laboratory personnel) or sexual transmission. Ninety percent of primary infections are asymptomatic (a person clinically well with positive tuberculin skin test).

HIV infection increases the risk of developing all forms of TB. The risk of disease progression is highest at the extremes of age and in immunocompromised individuals. Immunocompetent people have a 5–10% lifetime risk of progression; this increases to 7–10% per year in HIV-infected patients.

Immunology

Tuberculosis is the prototype of infection that elicits a cellular immune response. CD4+ T lymphocytes recognize mycobacterial antigens in association with major histocompatibility (MHC) class II molecules, presented by macrophages. The T cells become activated and proliferate, resulting in the production of cytokines (interferon-gamma [IFN-γ], migration inhibition factor), which attract and activate more macrophages at the site of infection. Macrophages also secrete a number of cytokines (tumor necrosis factor-alpha [TNF-A], platelet-derived growth factor [PDGF], transforming growth factor-beta [TGF-B], fibroblast growth factor [FGF]).

The interplay of these factors determines the nature of the pathological and clinical features. The Langhan's giant cell consists of epithelioid cells (activated macrophages) oriented around mycobacterial antigens and is a characteristic feature of tuberculous granulomas.

When the population of activated lymphocytes reaches a certain size, a cutaneous delayed hypersensitivity reaction to tuberculin occurs.

Pathogenesis

Primary infection results from inhalation of infectious droplet nuclei that lodge in the alveoli and multiply, resulting in the formation of a Ghon focus. Involvement of the regional lymph nodes produces the Ghon complex.

Depending on the host's immune response, the infection becomes quiescent or progress and/or disseminates. Reactivation of disease may occur in later life, particularly in the immunosuppressed.

Clinical features

Pulmonary tuberculosis is the most common presentation. Tuberculosis may also disseminate (military TB) or affect almost any other organ (extrapulmonary TB): pleural cavity, pericardium, lymph nodes, GI tract, peritoneum, GU (genitourinary) tract, skin, bones and joints, and CNS.

Diagnosis

Diagnosis is based on a combination of compatible clinical syndrome, supportive radiological investigations, and detection of acid-fast bacilli or culture of *M. tuberculosis* from clinical specimens. The gold standard for diagnosis is culture. Patients are often treated on the basis of a presumptive diagnosis.

M. tuberculosis is an aerobic, non-spore-forming, nonmotile, weakly Gram-positive bacillus with a thick cell wall containing mycolic acid, which renders it acid-fast.

Samples of sputum or tissue are liquefied, decontaminated, neutralized, and centrifuged, and the deposit is inoculated into solid or liquid media. Normally sterile samples, e.g., CSF, need not be decontaminated, as loss of mycobacterial viability may occur.

Acid-fast stains include the following:

- Auramine stain (fluorochrome phenolic auramine or auramine-rhodamine stain, acid-alcohol decolorization, potassium permanganate counterstain)
- Ziehl–Neelsen (ZN) stain (carbol fuschin stain, decolorize with acid-alcohol, counterstain with methylene blue)
- Kinyoun stain (ZN stain modified to make heating unnecessary)

Molecular methods

- PCR-based tests may be used to detect *M. tuberculosis* in clinical specimens, e.g., Amplicor test (Roche), amplified *M. tuberculosis* Direct Tests (MDT, GenProbe), strand displacement amplification (BD ProbeTec-SDA), ligase chain reaction (Lcx, Abbott systems). Although specificity is high, sensitivity is lower: 90–100% and 60–70% for smear-positive and -negative specimens, respectively.
- Identification of mycobacterial species, e.g., high-pressure liquid chromatography (HPLC) of mycolic acids, DNA sequencing of 16S rRNA, PCR restriction enzyme assay (PRA), DNA probe hybridization (LiPA MYCOBACTERIA, Innogenetics)
- Identification of drug-resistant mutations, e.g., rpoB mutations (InnoLiPA Rif.TB assay, Innogenetics)
- Typing for epidemiological studies, e.g., IS6110 RFLP, MIRU, spoligotyping

Culture methods

- Solid media, e.g., Lowenstein–Jensen media, Middlebrook agar
- Liquid culture, e.g., BACTEC 460 system, MB/BacT (Organon Teknika), Mycobacterial Growth Indicator Tube (MGIT, Becton Dickinson)

Identification and susceptibility testing is usually done at the reference lab level. For definitions of drug resistance, see Box 3.8.

Box 3.8 Drug-resistant tuberculosis

- Monoresistant = resistance to one drug
- Polyresistant = resistance to >1 drug (but not MDR)
- Multi-drug resistant (MDR) = resistance to at least isoniazid and rifampin
- Extensively drug resistant (XDR) = resistance to rifampin, isoniazid, a quinolone, and an injectable agent.

Tuberculin skin test

Purified protein derivative (PPD) is a standardized protein precipitate of tuberculin. The Mantoux test is a quantitative tuberculin test that is performed by intracutaneous injection of 5 tuberculin units (TU) of PPD in 0.1 mL of solution. The reaction is usually read after 48–72 hours.

A positive result is defined as >10 mm of induration. Reactions of 5–10 mm may be due to BCG (bacilli Calmette–Guérin) vaccination but are also suspicious of TB in low-prevalence areas.

False-positive results can occur with nontuberculous mycobacteria (NTM) infections. False-negative reactions can occur in up to 20% of patients with TB and in HIV-infected patients.

Delayed reactivity (>10 mm induration after 6 days) may occur in certain populations, e.g., Indochinese immigrants.

Interferon gamma-release assays (IGRA)

IGRA this is a relatively new method of detecting T cells specific for M. tuberculosis antigens. It has a sensitivity >80% and is more specific than the tuberculin skin test. Sensitivity remains high in children <3 years and in HIV coinfection and is not confounded by BCG vaccination or infection with NTM.

The main limitation of the test is that it cannot distinguish active from latent infection.

Treatment

Treatment is with combination chemotherapy for several months. For most types of tuberculosis, the usual regimen is a 2-month intensive phase with three or four drugs, followed by a 4-month continuation phase. The choice of drugs and duration of treatment depend on the likelihood of drug resistance, site of infection, and patient's HIV status.

For details, see Anti-tuberculous agents—American Thoracic Society (ATS) or CDC guidelines (Box 3.9).

Prevention

BCG vaccine is a live attenuated vaccine derived from M. bovis. It is given to infants and children in high-prevalence areas and results in a 60–80% reduction in the incidence of TB. It should only be given to infants <12 weeks of age or children who are tuberculin skin test (TST) negative. Although it does not prevent infection, BCG vaccination reduces the risk of disseminated disease in children.

> **Box 3.9 Guidelines for tuberculosis treatment**
>
> - American Thoracic Society guidelines. ATS/CDC/IDSA: treatment of tuberculosis. *Am J Respir Crit Care Med* 2003;167:603–662. See also www.thoracic.org
> - World Health Organization guidelines. Treatment of tuberculosis: guidelines for national programmes. WHO/CDS/TB 2003.313. Geneva: World Health Organization, 2003. Available at: http://whqlibdoc.who.int/hq/2003/WHO_CDS_TB_2003.313_eng.pdf

BCG is contraindicated in HIV-infected individuals. Vaccination can occasionally cause disseminated BCG infection, usually in immunosuppressed patients. Intravesicular BCG (used to treat bladder cancer) can cause liver or lung granulomas, psoas abscess, or osteomyelitis.

Newer vaccines include modified vaccinia Ankara (MVA) DNA vaccines, which use a prime-boost strategy to induce *M. tuberculosis*–specific immune responses. These vaccines look promising in phase II clinical trials.

Chemoprophylaxis

Chemoprophylaxis is given to individuals at increased risk of tuberculosis, e.g., contacts of active cases, and those with recent TST conversion abnormal CXR, HIV infection, or certain medical conditions, e.g., transplant, myeloproliferative or hematological malignancies.

For detailed indications, see the ATS and CDC guidelines (Box 3.9). The usual regimen is isoniazid 300 mg for 6–12 months with pyridoxine (vitamin B_6). The risk of isoniazid hepatotoxicity increases with age and daily alcohol consumption.

In 2006, an outbreak of XDR tuberculosis was described in Tugela Ferry, South Africa. All patients tested for HIV were found to be positive and 52/53 died with a median survival of 16 days. Genotyping of the outbreak strains showed that 85% were similar, suggesting recent nosocomial transmission.

Mycobacterium leprae

Leprosy, or Hansen's disease, is caused by infection with *Mycobacterium leprae*, an obligate intracellular parasite whose only natural hosts are humans and armadillos. Experimental infections can be induced in the mouse footpad.

The clinical manifestations of leprosy include skin lesions, deformities and peripheral neuropathy, making it one of the most socially stigmatizing diseases. Leprosy exhibits a spectrum of clinical features ranging from lepromatous (multibacillary) to tuberculoid (paucibacillary) forms.

Epidemiology

Worldwide, there are an estimated 6 million people living with leprosy, million of whom are untreated. Although Africa has the highest prevalence

Asia has the greatest number of cases. Leprosy is associated with poverty and rural residence but not HIV infection. Distribution in endemic countries is nonhomogeneous, suggesting that genetic factors may play a role in disease expression.

The mode of transmission remains uncertain but is thought to be human-to-human, via nasal droplet infection. Leprosy may also be acquired by direct inoculation into the skin.

The incubation period is long, with an average of 5–7 years (range 2–40 years) and the peak onset is in young adults.

Pathogenesis

M. leprae has a dense, mainly lipid, capsule outside the cell wall, which is rich in *M. leprae*–specific phenolic glycolipid 1 (PGL-1). This has been implicated as a scavenger for free radicals, allowing intracellular survival and limiting antibiotic penetration.

PGL-1 and lipoarabinomannan have been implicated as causing immunological hyporesponsiveness of both lymphocytes and macrophages in the anergic, highly bacillary lepromatous form of leprosy.

Clinical features

Clinical manifestations of leprosy are largely confined to the skin, upper respiratory tract, and peripheral nerves. Most of the serious sequelae are a result of peripheral nerve damage resulting in deformities (e.g., ulnar, median, and peroneal nerve palsies), loss of peripheral parts of digits, and plantar ulceration.

Lepromatous leprosy

This is characterized by symmetric skin nodules, plaques, and a thickened dermis that typically occurs in cool areas of the body, e.g., earlobes and feet. This condition is multibacilliary (infectious) and associated with poor cell-mediated immunity.

Involvement of the nasal mucosa results in congestion, epistaxis and, rarely, septal collapse ("saddle nose" deformity). It may also cause loss of eyebrows and eyelashes, trichiasis, corneal scarring, uveitis, lagophthalmos, testicular dysfunction, and amyloidosis.

Tuberculoid leprosy

This is characterized by hypopigmented, anesthetic skin plaques and asymmetric peripheral nerve involvement. It is typically paucibacillary (noninfectious) and associated with a good cell-mediated immune response.

Borderline leprosy

Most patients have manifestations intermediate between the two polar forms, a condition termed *borderline leprosy*.

Reversal reactions

An abrupt increase in inflammation within previously quiescent skin lesions, as well as new skin lesions, neuritis, and low-grade fever may develop in borderline leprosy patients either before (down-grading reaction) or after (reversal reaction) the initiation of therapy. If the neuritis is not treated promptly, irreversible nerve damage may occur.

Erythema nodosum leprosum

This affects >50% of lepromatous and borderline leprosy patients after initiation of therapy. Clinical features include painful nodules (usually on extensor surfaces, which may pustulate or ulcerate), neuritis, fever, malaise, anorexia, uveitis, lymphadenitis, oorchitis, anemia, leucocytosis, and glomerulonephritis.

Diagnosis

A firm diagnosis of leprosy requires the presence of a characteristic peripheral nerve abnormality or the demonstration of acid-fast bacilli in skin biopsies or split skin smears. In atypical cases, two of the following three criteria are required: a clinically compatible skin lesion, dermal granuloma on skin biopsy, or hypoesthesia within the lesion.

Skin biopsies should be taken from skin plaques or nodules in lepromatous patients and from the periphery of lesions in tuberculoid patients. Nerve biopsies may result in loss of function and should only be performed if there is sufficient diagnostic uncertainty to warrant it.

Microbiology

M. leprae is a Gram-variable, acid-fast bacillus that is best visualized by a modified Fite stain (as it may be decolorized by the Ziehl–Neelsen stain). Viable bacilli stain brightly, whereas dead bacilli stain irregularly.
M. leprae grows best at temperatures <37°C in humans and armadillos. Unique properties of *M. leprae* include loss of acid-fastness by pyridine extraction, presence of dopa oxidase activity, and multiplication in the mouse footpad with a doubling time of 12–14 days.

Experimental infection of the mouse footpad can be used to assess antimicrobial susceptibility.

Treatment

Treatment requires combination therapy with two or more agents, e.g., dapsone, clofazimine, and rifampicin. Ethionamide, prothionamide, and certain aminoglycosides have also been used. Newer agents such as minocycline, clarithromycin, and certain fluoroquinolones look promising.

The National Hansen's Disease Clinical Center in Baton Rouge, Louisiana, provides free services for physicians, including: consultation, antimicrobials, pathologic review, educational materials, and surgical care and rehabilitation. See their Web site:
www.hrsa.gov/hansens/clinicalcenter.

Prevention

Dapsone prophylaxis of household contacts of leprosy patients is not recommended; it only forestalls development of lepromatous leprosy.

Nontuberculous mycobacteria

This group of organisms comprises about 100 species of mycobacteria, excluding those in the *M. tuberculosis* complex and *M. leprae*. Other names for nontuberculous mycobacteria (NTM) include *atypical mycobacteria* or *mycobacteria other than tuberculosis* (MOTT).

Classification

NTM were previously classified according to growth rate, colonial morphology, and pigmentation (Runyon classification). This has been superseded by molecular methods but nonetheless remains useful to separate NTM into three groups:

- *Rapidly growing mycobacteria* (≤7 days incubation), e.g., *M. fortuitum* complex, *M. chelonae/abscessus* group, *M. mucogenicum*, and *M. smegmatis*
- *Slow-growing mycobacteria* (>7 days incubation), e.g., *M. avium* complex, *M. kansasii*, *M. xenopi*, *M. simiae*, *M. szulgai*, *M. scrofulaceum*, *M. malmoense*, *M. terrae/nonchromogenicum* complex, *M. malmoense*, *M. haemophilum*, and *M. genavense*
- *Intermediately growing mycobacteria* (7–10 days), e.g., *M. marinum*, *M. gordonae*

Clinical features

The NTM can cause a wide spectrum of diseases (Table 3.20).

Diagnosis

Because the signs and symptoms of NTM lung disease are often variable and nonspecific, diagnosis requires multiple positive respiratory cultures. Diagnosis of NTM infections at other sites requires positive cultures from pus, tissue biopsies, or blood cultures.

- *Microscopy:* the acid-fast stains used for identifying *M. tuberculosis* also work well for identifying NTM.
- *Culture:* appropriate culture media include Middlebrook 7H10 or 7H11 agars or BACTEC broth. Samples from skin and soft tissue infections

Table 3.20 Clinical syndromes caused by NTM

Syndrome	Most common causes
Chronic bronchopulmonary disease (adults, CF patients)	*M. avium* complex, *M. kansasii*, *M. abscessus*
Cervical lymphadenitis (children)	*M. avium* complex
Skin and soft tissue infections	*M. fortuitum* group, *M. chelonae*, *M. abscessus*, *M. marinum*, *M. ulcerans*
Bone and joint infections	*M. marinum*, *M. avium* complex, *M. kansasii*, *M. fortuitum* group, *M. abscessus*, *M. chelonae*
Disseminated infection (HIV positive)	*M. avium*, *M. kansasii*
Disseminated infection (HIV negative)	*M. abscessus*, *M. chelonae*
Catheter-related infections	*M. fortuitum*, *M. abscessus*, *M. chelonae*

need to be plated at 28–30°C as well 35–37°C, as some species only grow at low temperatures, e.g., *M. chelonae*, *M. haemophilum*, and *M. marinum*. *M. xenopi* grows best at 42°C. Other species have special growth requirements, e.g., *M. genavense* (BACTEC broth for 6–8 weeks) and *M. haemophilum* (iron supplementation).

- *Identification:* although traditional biochemical and other standard tests may be performed, identification of NTM increasingly uses rapid molecular methods:
  - HPLC of mycolic acids
  - PCR-RFLP analysis of the heat-shock protein gene
  - Genetic probes for mycobacterial RNA
  - 16S ribosomal RNA gene sequencing
- *Drug susceptibility testing:* various methods are used:
  - Agar disk elution
  - Broth microdilution
  - E-test
  - BACTEC radiometric detection
- *Strain comparison:* for epidemiological studies, standard biochemical identification and susceptibility testing have been superseded by molecular methods.

Treatment

Treatment of NTM infections may be medical, surgical, or a combination of the two. The choice of drugs and duration of treatment depend on the causative organism, site of infection, and patient's HIV status.

- U.S. guidelines: ATS/IDSA guideline: Treatment of non-tuberculous mycobacteria. *Am J Respir Crit Care Med* 2007;175:367–416. Also see www.thoracic.org

Overview of virology

Table 3.21 Summary of viruses and common clinical syndromes

Group	Virus	Consider in the differential of...									Other
		Respiratory	Rash	Hepatic	Muscular	Diarrhea	Encephalitis	Meningitis	Shock		
DNA viruses											
Adenoviridae	Adenovirus (p. 379)	...				...	...	...			Cystitis, conjunctivitis
Herpesviridae	HSV-1 and -2 (p. 344)	-	...				1	2			Genital, eye, dissemination
	EBV (p. 347)	-	-	-	...	-	-				
	VZV (p. 343)	-	...	-			-				
	CMV (p. 351)	-	-	-	-	-	-				Congenital
	HHV-6 and -7 (p. 339-340)		...								Fever alone
	HHV-8 (p. 381)		-								Kaposi sarcoma
Poxviridae (also smallpox) (p. 388)	Molluscum		...								
	Orf		...								

Table 3.21 (Contd.)

Group	Virus	Consider in the differential of...								
		Respiratory	Rash	Hepatic	Muscular	Diarrhea	Encephalitis	Meningitis	Shock	Other
Parvoviridae	Monkeypox		---							
	Parvovirus B19 (p. 336)		---				-			Arthropathy, aplastic anemia, congenital
Papovaviridae	HPV (p. 383)									Warts, epithelial tumors of skin
	Polyomavirus (p. 386)	-								Progressive focal neurological deficits
Hepadnaviridae	Hepatitis B (p. 359)		---							
RNA viruses										
Orthomyxoviridae	Influenza (p. 320)	---			-		-			
Paramyxoviridae	Parainfluenza (p. 326)	---				-	-			
	Mumps (p. 332)						--	-		Parotitis, epididymoorchitis, GBS

Family	Virus					Disease
	Measles (p. 330)	--	-	-		SSPE
	RSV/ metapneumovirus (p. 327) (p. 330)	---				
Coronaviridae	Coronavirus (p. 329)	---		--		
Picornaviridae	Poliovirus (p. 390)	---	-			Paralysis, myocarditis
	Non-polio enteroviruses (p. 372)	-	---			Myopericarditis, conjunctivitis
	Hepatitis A (p. 358)	---				
	Rhinovirus (p. 530) ---					
Reoviridae	Rotavirus		---			
Retroviridae	HTLV-1 & -2 (p. 393)					Spastic paraparesis, leukaemia/ lymphoma
	HIV-1 & -2 (p. 368)	---		-		Immunodeficiency
Togaviridae	Rubella (p. 335)	---				Congenital
	Alphaviruses (p. 375)	-				Arthralgia

Table 3.21 (Contd.)

Group	Virus	Consider in the differential of. . .								
		Respiratory	Rash	Hepatic	Muscular	Diarrhea	Encephalitis	Meningitis	Shock	Other
Flaviviridae	Yellow fever (p. 399)		--	---			-	-		Hemorrhage
	Dengue (p. 401)		--	--			-	---		Hemorrhage
	Hepatitis C (p. 362)			---						
	Japanese encephalitis (p. 396)						---			
Bunyaviridae	Hantavirus (p. 378)	-						---		Hemorrhage, renal failure
	CCHF (p. 378)							---		
	Californian encephalitis (p. 378)						---			Hemorrhage

Arenaviridae	Lassa (p. 407)	--	-	-	Hemorrhage
	LCMV (p. 375)	---	--	-	Congenital
Filoviridae	Marburg, Ebola (p. 406)	--	--	--	Hemorrhage
Rhabdoviridae	Rabies (p. 408)	---			
Other	Astrovirus and calicivirus (p. 356)	--			

--- Very frequently seen; -- commonly seen; - occasionally seen.

"Congenital" indicates viruses with the potential to cause significant sequelae if infecting the developing fetus.

CCHF, Congo–Crimean hemorrhagic fever; CMV, cytomegalovirus; EBV, Epstein–Barr virus; GBS, Guillain–Barré syndrome; HHV, human herpesvirus HIV, human immunodeficiency virus; HPV, human papillomavirus; HSV, herpes simplex virus; HTLV, human T-cell lymphotrophic virus; LCMV, lymphocytic choriomeningitis virus; RSV, respiratory syncytial virus; SSPE, subacute sclerosing panencephalitis; VZV, varicella zoster virus.

[a] HIVmay of course present in a multitude of ways. However, the more common presentations of primary HIV infection (as opposed to a subsequent opportunistic infection) are rash and encephalitis.

Influenza: introduction

Influenza is one of the most common infectious diseases of humankind, causing primarily epidemics of upper respiratory tract infection. Global pandemics may follow dramatic antigenic changes—21 million people died in the 1918–1919 pandemic.

The virus

The influenza viruses are members of the family *Orthomyxoviridae*. These are negative sense single-strand (ss) RNA viruses.

The three types of influenza viruses are as follows:

- Influenza A causes the typical influenza syndrome and can precipitate pandemics
- Influenza B is similar clinically but does not cause pandemics.
- Influenza C causes an afebrile common cold–like syndrome and does not occur in epidemics.

All have host cell–derived envelopes embedded with glycoproteins important to viral entry and exit. These have hemagglutinin (HA) or neuraminidase (NA) activities, are key antigenic components, and may alter gradually by mutation (by antigenic drift—see Box 3.10).

At least 16 HA and 9 NA variants have been identified in influenza A viruses. Viruses are named by their type, place of initial isolation, strain, year, and antigenic subtype, e.g., A/Victoria/3/75/H3N2.

Box 3.10 Antigenic variation

Alteration of viral antigenic structure allows the production of variants to which there may be little or no herd immunity. This variation involves changes in the HA and NA glycoproteins and takes place by two mechanisms.

Antigenic drift

Relatively minor changes occur every year or so through a gradual accumulation of amino acid changes. There is a selective pressure for those changes that are less well recognized by host antibody, and these viruses begin to predominate.

Antigenic shift

This is a major antigenic change that may herald flu pandemics because of lack of population immunity. Type A viruses are able to infect a variety of species: humans, pigs, horses, birds. Fortunately, viruses adapted for birds are fairly limited in their ability to replicate in humans (on account of divergent evolution?).

However, evidence suggests that pandemics have been caused by viruses containing both human and avian viral sequences, probably facilitated by recombination within a third party (e.g., pig) easily infected by both human and avian viruses. This is consistent with the observation that pandemics often arise in Asia where humans, pigs, and birds all live in close proximity. Other pandemics may have been caused by direct viral adaptation to humans (the 1918 pandemic was probably due to a pig virus).

Epidemiology

The CDC and WHO track influenza activity throughout the world during flu season (http://www.cdc.gov/flu/weekly).

Outbreaks are associated with excess rates of pneumonia and influenza-related illness and mortality, typically peaking in the winter and varying with the viral type responsible. Not all influenza-related deaths present as pneumonia. Sporadic cases of severe disease have occurred in some countries as a result of human acquisition of viral strains adapted to birds (see Box 3.11).

Attack rates are highest in the young, and mortality is usually highest in the elderly. Rates for both groups are increased in those with pre-existing medical problems, e.g., cardiovascular, pulmonary, and renal impairment or immunodeficiency.

Box 3.11 Avian influenza H5N1

H5N1 has been around since the 1950s, when it killed a number of chickens in Scotland. No human cases occurred. In 1997, 18 people were infected and 6 died during an H5N1 outbreak among poultry in Hong Kong. From 2003, cases of H5N1 human infection have been reported, predominantly in Southeast Asia, most related to direct or close contact with H5N1-infected poultry or H5N1-contaminated surfaces.

Person-to-person spread has been reported extremely rarely. This is probably a consequence of differences in binding preference demonstrated by the avian and human flu viral HA molecules.

Avian HA tends to prefer sialic acid (2–3) galactose, which in humans is found in the terminal bronchi and alveoli. Human viruses prefer sialic acid (2–6) galactose, found on epithelial cells of the upper respiratory tract.

The case fatality rate has increased with time (well over 50%), although it is likely that many milder cases have gone unreported. Nonrespiratory symptoms (e.g., diarrhea) have been reported. Death is a result of respiratory failure probably due to a severe cytokine storm effect precipitated by the virus.

H5N1 remains much better adapted to birds than other hosts, and the precise nature of the genetic alterations necessary to produce a human flu strain capable of causing a pandemic cannot be known in advance.

The virus that has caused human illness and death in Asia is resistant to amantadine and rimantadine. Oseltamivir and zanamivir are probably effective, but there is evidence that resistance develops rapidly with their use. There is no human vaccine available.

Cases of H5N1 infection in wild birds and poultry have occurred across Europe, the Middle East, Asia, and parts of Africa. Human cases have occurred in parts of Europe and North Africa, as well as in Asia.

Up-to-date information is available at:
http://www.who.int/csr/disease/avian_influenza/en/

Person-to-person transmission occurs by dispersion in small-particle aerosols. Virus is present in large quantities in the secretions of infected people. One individual can infect a large number of others, contributing to the explosive nature of outbreaks. Outbreaks can occur in an epidemic or pandemic fashion:

- *Epidemics:* confined to a single location, e.g., a town or country, and occur almost exclusively in winter. They start abruptly, with cases seen initially in children and then adults, peak within 3 weeks, and last around 6 weeks. Different strains may circulate simultaneously.
- *Pandemics:* severe outbreaks that spread to all parts of the world. They are caused only by type A viruses. They are associated with the emergence of a new virus to which the population has no significant immunity, and characterized by rapid transmission across the world, often out of the usual patterns of seasonality and with high levels of mortality among healthy young adults. A case in point, pandemic 2009 H1N1 was unique in that infections were uncommon in persons ≥65 years, and activity peaked in October in the United States (see Box 3.12). Obesity and pregnancy were associated with increased morbidity and mortality.

Influenza viruses' capacity to continue to cause human disease on such a scale is a function of frequent antigenic changes (see Box 3.10). In the early years after a pandemic, disease is clinically severe, becoming milder as herd immunity improves. As of winter 2008, late in the interpandemic cycle, severe disease is rare.

Pathogenesis

Virus enters respiratory epithelial cells and replicates, and progeny are released—the cell dies. Viral shedding may start within 24 hours of infection; illness follows 24 hours later.

There is diffuse inflammation of the trachea and bronchi with an ulcerative, necrotizing tracheobronchitis in severe cases. Primary viral pneumonia is uncommon but is severe when it occurs. Bacterial superinfection is common, facilitated by damage to the mucociliary escalator and virus-induced defects in lymphocyte and leukocyte function.

Viral levels fall rapidly after 48 hours of illness, becoming undetectable by 5–10 days.

Box 3.12 The 2009 H1N1 swine influenza pandemic

In March 2009, an outbreak of H1N1 influenza A was detected in Mexico. By June 2009, WHO had issued its highest-level pandemic alert: widespread community transmission on at least two continents.

The virus was a reassortant of two swine strains, one human strain, and one avian flu strain. It quickly displaced the seasonal flu variant in Europe and the United States, accounting for over 99% of subtyped influenza A isolates at its peak. The rate of infections was highest in those <24 years of age, with infection proving uncommon in those over 65, possibly because of pre-existing immunity gained in pre-1957 infections.

Hospitalization rates among confirmed cases in the United States were around 2–5% at the peak of the 2009 outbreak; taking into account unreported mild cases, the overall rate is thought to be around 0.3%. The highest death rates among those once hospitalized were seen in adults over 50 years of age. Those most at risk of severe illness were individuals with comorbidities (chronic lung disease, immunosuppression, cardiac disease, diabetes), the obese, and pregnant women.

Prophylaxis and treatment guidelines have evolved rapidly as more data become available and as the level of transmission varies. The UK 2009/10 pandemic saw negligible oseltamivir resistance, although resistance was documented in the United States. Vaccination is the key prevention strategy and has been recommended for those at risk of severe disease, health care workers, and children aged between 6 months and 5 years. For the latest guidance, see www.cdc.gov.

The CDC's Advisory Committee on Immunization Practices (ACIP) voted to expand the influenza vaccination recommendations for the 2010–11 flu season to include all persons 6 months of age and older who do not have a contraindication to the vaccine. The recommendations are intended to remove barriers to flu immunization, such as the need to determine whether each person has a specific indication for vaccination, and to protect as many people as possible against the dangers of flu.

Hospitalized patients with suspected influenza should be considered for testing with an available influenza diagnostic test. Rapid influenza diagnostic tests (RIDTs) and direct immunofluorescence assays (DFAs) are widely available influenza diagnostic tests, but these tests have lower sensitivity than that of real-time reverse transcriptase polymerase chain reaction (rRT-PCR) tests. Since a negative RIDT or DFA test result does not exclude influenza virus infection, hospitalized patients with a negative RIDT or DFA result should have priority for further testing with rRT-PCR, if influenza infection is clinically suspected.

Specimens may be collected in a variety of ways, including nasopharyngeal swab; nasal aspirate, wash, or swab; endotracheal aspirate; bronchoalveolar lavage (BAL); and combined nasopharyngeal or nasal swab with oropharyngeal swab.

- The Infectious Diseases Society of America (IDSA) maintains an expert question and answer site at http://www.idsociety.org/Content.aspx?id=15743
- Clinician guidance is available at http://www.cdc.gov/h1n1flu/guidance/
- Current recommendations are in development and available at: http://www.cdc.gov

Influenza: clinical features and diagnosis

Clinical features

Uncomplicated disease

A 1- to 2-day incubation is followed by an abrupt onset of symptoms: fever, chills, headache, malaise, myalgia, eye pain, anorexia, dry cough, sore throat, and nasal discharge. After around day 3, respiratory features dominate as fever and other systemic features settle. Convalescence may take 2 or more weeks.

Elderly patients may present with fever and confusion and few respiratory features. Attack rates are highest in children, who may present with croup.

Respiratory complications

Outside of a pandemic these complications are more common in the elderly. Primary viral pneumonia occurs more commonly in those with pre-existing cardiac and lung disorders and presents with worsening cough, breathlessness, and cyanosis shortly after disease onset (resembles acute respiratory distress syndrome). Mortality is high.

Secondary bacterial pneumonia develops shortly after an initial period of improvement following the influenza syndrome. Pathogens include *Strep. pneumoniae, H. influenzae,* and, less commonly, *S. aureus.* Other respiratory complications include croup, COPD, and CF exacerbations.

Immunocompromised patients

More severe disease may occur in some groups of HIV-infected patients, but this has not been widely observed. HIV-infected children with low CD4 counts may shed virus for prolonged periods. Severe disease does occur in immunosuppressed children with cancer, bone marrow transplant recipients, and those with leukemia. Viral shedding may be prolonged in these groups.

Nonpulmonary complications

These include myositis, pericarditis, myocarditis, toxic shock syndrome, encephalitis, and Guillain–Barré syndrome.

Diagnosis

In the context of a community outbreak, the diagnosis of influenza can be made with some confidence on clinical criteria alone—85% accuracy in some studies. Outside of outbreaks or in the institutional setting, laboratory diagnosis is required.

- *Rapid tests* provide results within 10–30 minutes based on antigen detection by enzyme immunoassay. Performance varies by patient age, duration of illness, sample type, prevalence of virus in the community, and influenza type.
- *Immunofluorescence:* fluorescent antibody stains applied directly to cells in respiratory specimens have moderate sensitivity and high specificity.
- *Nucleic acid tests:* RT-PCR techniques are the most sensitive method.
- *Rapid culture:* antigen expression in cell culture that is detected using immunofluorescence has a turn-around time of 24–48 hours. Sensitivity approaches that of standard culture.

- *Standard culture:* virus is readily isolated from throat or nasal swabs, sputum, or bronchoalveolar lavage (BAL) fluid. It is cultured in cell lines and detected within 3–5 days by its cytopathic effect.
- *Serology:* acute and convalescent (10–20 days apart) samples showing a fourfold rise in antibody titer can be considered diagnostic but are not useful in clinical decision making.

Influenza: treatment and prevention

Treatment

The cornerstone of influenza management is an effective vaccination strategy.

- *General measures:* adequate hydration, antipyretics (not aspirin in children), and decongestants
- *Antivirals:* when initiated promptly (within the first 24–30 hours of symptoms), therapy can shorten symptoms by 1–3 days. Patients with severe disease and those at high risk for complications should be treated. The 2008 ACIP recommends oseltamivir or zanamivir for most cases. Amantadine should not be used because of high rates of resistance in the United States. The clinician must review local surveillance data to determine which types of virus are circulating and to understand unique susceptibility profiles.
- *Severe disease:* there is little information available on the effectiveness of antiviral agents in severe disease. The rapidly progressive nature of secondary bacterial infections argues for early presumptive use of antibiotics where suggested by the clinical scenario.

Prevention

Vaccines

Inactivated vaccines are the main control measure, and annual vaccination is recommended for certain risk groups, including those with diabetes or cardiac, lung, or renal disease; those who are immunocompromised; all people over 65 years of age; and health care workers.

The vaccines are prepared each year and are usually trivalent, containing two type A strains and one type B strain. Strains are collected continuously across the world, and those to be included in the year's vaccine are chosen by educated guess. It takes 6–9 months to produce a vaccine once its components are decided.

Two doses are required in children under 9 years who have not been previously vaccinated. Otherwise, a single dose is sufficient, usually given in October. The main contraindication to vaccination is hypersensitivity to hens' eggs.

Protection is around 70% and lasts for 1 year. Diminished responses are seen in organ transplant recipients receiving immunosuppressive therapy. Protection is reduced in the elderly.

Prophylaxis

Post-exposure antiviral therapy should be considered on a case-by-case basis, according to the individual's risk for influenza complications and the likelihood of acquisition from the specific exposure.

Parainfluenza

This is a group of five viruses causing a spectrum of respiratory illnesses, from upper respiratory tract symptoms in healthy children to severe pneumonia in the immunosuppressed.

The viruses
- *Paramyxoviridae* and members of either genus *Respirovirus* (parainfluenza types 1 and 3) or *Rubulavirus* (types 2, 4A and 4B)
- Negative-sense ssRNA viruses, spherical in appearance with a host cell derived envelope

Epidemiology
Sixty percent of childhood croup cases in which virus is isolated are due to parainfluenza. It is second only to RSV as a cause of childhood respiratory hospitalization; 10% of adult acute respiratory illness can be attributed to parainfluenza. Nosocomial and residential care outbreaks have occurred.

Parainfluenza type 3 is the most frequently isolated member, and like RSV is commonly seen in the first 6 months of life. It is endemic and may be isolated throughout the year, peaking in spring.

Types 1 and 2 occur in autumn, often alternating each year.

Type 4 viruses are rarely isolated.

Pathogenesis
Transmission is by droplet spread. Replication occurs in cells of the respiratory epithelium. Clinically, illness most frequently involves larger airways of the lower respiratory tract, causing croup.

Reinfection may occur and tends to cause milder upper airway disease, probably representing waning of immunity; antigenic variation is not progressive (unlike influenza virus). Mucosal immunity is most important for resisting infection. CD8 T cells are important in viral clearance.

Clinical features
- *Healthy individuals:* children: upper respiratory tract illness (those under 5 years), otitis media, croup, bronchiolitis (infants under 6 months); adults: upper respiratory tract infection
- *Immunocompromised:* severe disease in recipients of bone marrow or lung transplants in all age groups. May cause pneumonia with high rates of mortality. Other immunodeficiencies are associated with prolonged viral shedding.

Diagnosis
- Viral isolation by tissue culture and immunofluorescence is the standard.
- Multiplexed RT-PCR-based tests are faster and can distinguish viral type.
- Paired serology can confirm a diagnosis but is unhelpful.

Treatment
There is no specific antiviral therapy. Some advocate inhaled steroids for the clinical treatment of croup.

Respiratory syncytial virus

Respiratory syncytial virus (RSV) is a major cause of lower respiratory tract infection (LRTI) in young children.

The virus

The virus is a member of the *Paramyxoviridae* family. It is an enveloped (bilipid layer derived from the host cell) ssRNA virus that may survive up to 24 hours in patient secretions deposited on nonporous surfaces and around an hour on porous surfaces (tissues, fabric, skin).

RSV isolates fall into two antigen groups (A and B), which differ in envelope proteins and non-structural protein-1. Several strains from both groups may circulate in the same outbreak.

Epidemiology

RSV infection has been found worldwide. In temperate parts, outbreaks are annual, occurring in the winter months. Mild outbreaks may be followed by a more severe one the next year.

It is the major cause of childhood pneumonia and bronchiolitis (90% of children admitted with a LRTI in the peak of an epidemic); 95% of children are seropositive by age 2 years. Naturally acquired immunity to RSV is incomplete, but subsequent infections rarely produce severe illness.

Boys and those under 2 years of age experience the most severe illness. Severity is also affected by socioeconomic factors.

RSV is an important nosocomial infection; virus may spread from an infected infant (secretions, staff) or an infected adult with mild symptoms.

Pathogenesis

Incubation is between 2 and 8 days. Inoculation is by nose and eye, with infection confined to the respiratory tract. Infants often have evidence of pneumonia as well as bronchiolitis.

Lymphocytic infiltration of the areas around the bronchioles with wall and tissue edema is followed by proliferation and necrosis of the bronchiolar epithelium: bronchiolitis. Sloughed epithelium and mucus block small-airway lumens, leading to air trapping and hyperinflation. Air absorbed distal to obstructed airways leads to multiple areas of atelectasis.

Disease is due to the vulnerability of the small airways of the very young to inflammation and obstruction (resistance to air flow being inversely related to the cube of the radius), as well as immunopathology, perhaps immune complex formation.

The most severe forms are experienced by infants when maternally derived specific antibody is at a high level. Severe disease was seen in children vaccinated with a trial inactivated vaccine in the 1960s.

Clinical features

Young children

Pneumonia and bronchiolitis (see p. 550) are the most common manifestations of RSV infection in infants. Tracheobronchitis and croup are less common. All may occur in association with fever and otitis media (RSV is present in 75% of middle ear effusions from children with respiratory RSV infection). RSV infection is rarely asymptomatic.

Those with LRTI may have a preceding URTI with nasal congestion and pharyngitis. Cough and fever are common in young children.

Clinical findings include wheeze and crepitations. It is difficult to differentiate pneumonia from bronchiolitis, and many infants have both. There are minimal CXR changes regardless of severity. Hypoxia may be profound.

Duration of illness is 7–21 days. Acute complications include apnea and secondary bacterial infection. RSV has been shown to be a contributing factor to sudden infant death syndrome.

Long-term studies suggest that those hospitalized with RSV LRTI may have a higher rate of later reactive airway disease.

Older children and adults

Most commonly, a severe "common cold" develops, with nasal congestion, cough, fever, and earache (in children); <50% of infected older people develop pneumonia (particularly those in residential homes); 2–6% of hospitalized adults with pneumonia have RSV. Secondary infections cause URTI or tracheobronchitis.

Severe disease

Young infants, premature infants, and those with underlying disease (congenital and cardiopulmonary disease, e.g., cystic fibrosis) are at risk of severe RSV. Less than 66% of deaths occur in those with underlying disease. Prematurity is a risk into the third year of life.

Immunodeficient patients (including those with transplants and on chemotherapy) have extensive pulmonary infiltration and prolonged viral shedding.

Diagnosis

Clinical diagnosis can be made with some confidence in children during an outbreak. Serology is only useful epidemiologically.

Microbiologic tests

A nasopharyngeal aspirate (NPA) or swab provides the best sample with a high rate of virus isolation. Specimens can be applied to rapid antigen detection kits, stained directly with fluorescent monoclonal antibodies, or processed for RT-PCR.

Culture remains the standard for definitive diagnosis. The major advantage of culture is the ability to identify other viral pathogens. Specimens should be inoculated onto cell lines as soon as possible. Cytopathic changes are characterized by the typical syncytial appearance visible at around days 3–7, with confirmation by immunofluorescent staining.

Treatment

- *Supportive care:* oxygen to maintain saturation at 92% or above. No specific benefit is shown with bronchdilators, steroids, or antibiotics.
- *Ribavirin:* indicated for RSV LRTI in hospitalized infants considered at high risk of complicated or severe disease (underlying cardiac, pulmonary, or immunosuppressive conditions). Given as an aerosol for 2–5 days. Follow-up over a year shows better pulmonary function

and a reduced incidence of reactive airway disease at 1 year in those treated with ribavirin.

Prevention

- *Immunotherapy:* active immunization is not available. Palivizumab (RSV monoclonal antibody) reduces morbidity in infants at risk of severe RSV. Administered to those at risk once a month during outbreaks, it significantly reduces disease severity and hospital admissions for respiratory illness. It has a role in prophylaxis to those with high-risk exposure in the hospital.
- *Infection control* is vital in hospitalized cases. Handwashing, eye–nose goggles, and glove use reduce nosocomial infections. Infected patients should be isolated or cohorted, especially on wards with high-risk patients.

Other respiratory viruses

Coronavirus

These are enveloped viruses of the family *Coronaviridae* with a large positive-sense ss RNA genome. They are found worldwide.

The name derives from the Latin *corona* ("crown"), reflecting the electron microscopy (EM) appearance of the viral spike protein that populates the surface of the virus and determines its host tropism.

Human respiratory strains cause colds in adults, have been isolated from infants with pneumonia, are associated with bouts of wheeze in children with asthma or recurrent bronchitis, and may be a contributor to exacerbations of COPD. Enteric viruses may cause gastroenteritis in infants and have been associated with outbreaks of necrotizing enterocolitis.

SARS-coronavirus

Severe acute respiratory syndrome (SARS) was recognized in China in November 2002 and had spread to affect 29 countries across the world by February 2003. The epidemic died out by July 2003; 8422 cases were reported with a fatality rate of 11% (43% in those over 60 years of age). Between July 2003 and May 2004, there were four small and rapidly contained outbreaks of SARS, three of which were associated with laboratory releases and the fourth thought to be due to an animal source. The possibility of SARS re-emergence remains.

It is caused by a novel coronavirus. Animals are thought to be the main reservoir. Transmission is by droplets and contact with contaminated surfaces; nosocomial transmission was common in the early stages of the outbreak. Virus is present in the stool and may cause diarrhea. Incubation is 2–10 days.

Interepidemic case definitions proposed by the WHO define a possible case as an individual meeting the clinical criteria, within 10 days of onset of illness with *either* a history of travel to an area classified by the WHO as a potential zone of re-emergence of SARS (mainland China, and Hong Kong SAR) *or* a history of exposure to laboratories or institutes that have retained SARS virus isolates and/or diagnostic specimens from SARS patients.

Clinical criteria include fever of 38°C, one or more symptoms of lower respiratory tract illness (cough, difficulty breathing, shortness of breath), radiographic evidence of pneumonia or acute respiratory distress syndrome (ARDS), or autopsy findings consistent with the pathology of pneumonia or ARDS without an identifiable cause and no alternative diagnosis to fully explain the illness. Note that this definition is for public health, not diagnostic purposes.

Confirmation is by PCR, seroconversion, or virus isolation.

Details of these and further case definitions are available on the CDC Web site.[1]

Metapneumovirus

This is a newly identified virus (family *Paramyxoviridae*) first reported in June 2001 as a cause of respiratory tract disease in Dutch children.

Clinical features are indistinguishable from those caused by RSV, and it is now known to be a cause of respiratory tract disease in both children and adults worldwide; 98–100% of people are seropositive by age 10 years, it is a significant pathogen in LRTI of children and is implicated in nosocomial spread of infection in hospital wards.

Symptoms are identical to those of RSV in children (mild URTI to severe cough, bronchiolitis, and pneumonia) and older adults (cough, fever, respiratory distress).

Diagnosis is by immunofluorescent staining or PCR of respiratory secretions or using serology. Currently there is no specific treatment (experimental evidence suggests a role for ribavirin) or vaccine.

Reference

1 Centers for Disease Control. *Severe acute respiratory syndrome (SARS)*. http://www.cdc.gov. ncidod/sars/.

Measles

Measles is an acute, highly infectious disease of children that is characterized by cough, coryza, fever, and rash.

The virus

The virus is a member of the family *Paramyxoviridae*, genus *Morbillivirus*. It is an ssRNA, enveloped virus, covered with short surface projections: the hemagglutinin (H) and fusion (F) glycoproteins.

Humans are the only natural host.

Epidemiology

Meassles is found in every country in the world. Without vaccination, epidemics lasting 3–4 months would occur every 2–5 years.

It is airborne, spread by contact with aerosolized respiratory secretions, and one of the most communicable of the infectious diseases. It is sensitive to light and drying but can remain infective in droplet form for some hours. Patients are most infectious during the late prodromal phase when coughing is at its peak. Immunity after infection is lifelong.

Pathogenesis

Virus invades the respiratory epithelium, and local multiplication leads to viremia and leukocyte infection. Reticuloendothelial cells become infected and their necrosis leads to a secondary viremia. The major infected blood cell is the monocyte.

Tissues that become infected include the thymus, spleen, lymph node, liver, skin, and lung. Secondary viremia leads to infection of the entire respiratory mucosa with consequent cough and coryza. Croup, bronchiolitis, and pneumonia may also occur.

Koplik's spots and rash appear a few days after respiratory symptoms; they may represent host hypersensitivity to the virus.

Clinical features

Incubation is 2 weeks (longer in adults than in children). A prodromal phase (coinciding with secondary viremia) of malaise, fever, anorexia, conjunctivitis, and cough is followed by Koplik's spots (blue-gray spots with a red base classically found on the buccal mucosa opposite the second molars. Severe cases may involve the entire mucosa, then rash.

Patients feel most ill around day 2 of the rash. From late prodrome to resolution of fever and rash is around 7–10 days. Rash begins on the face and proceeds down, involving palms and soles last. It is erythematous and maculopapular and may become confluent. It lasts around 5 days and may desquamate as it heals.

Complications include bacterial superinfection (pneumonia and otitis media) and acute encephalitis, which is seen in 1 in 2000 and is probably due to host hypersensitivity to virus. It is characterized by fever recurrence, headache, seizures, and consciousness changes during convalescence. Subacute sclerosing panencephalitis (SSPE), a chronic degenerative neurological condition occurring years after measles, is due to persistent CNS infection with measles virus despite a vigorous host immune response.

Unlike rubella, there is no association with fetal malformations, but the disease can be more severe in pregnancy and infants can acquire it. Infants born to mothers with active infection should be given immunoglobulin at birth.

Prior to vaccination, measles was a common cause of viral meningitis and remains so in unvaccinated populations, usually occurring with rash.

Special conditions

Modified measles

This is a very mild form of the disease seen in people with some degree of passive immunity, e.g., those receiving immunoglobulin, or babies under 1 year of age.

Atypical measles

This is seen in those who received early killed measles vaccines and are later infected by wild-type virus. The rash is atypical and may resemble Henoch–Schönlein purpura (HSP), varicella, spotted fever, or a drug eruption. High fever, peripheral edema, pulmonary infiltrates, and effusions may occur.

The disease is more severe, has a longer course, and is thought to be due to hypersensitivity to virus in a partially immune host. It is rare now, but those who have received only killed vaccine should be offered live vaccine.

Immunocompromised patients

Such patients (including the malnourished) may experience severe disease, e.g., primary viral giant cell pneumonia, encephalitis, and SSPE-like encephalitis. They may not develop rash, making diagnosis difficult. Immunocompromised people should be passively immunized following exposure even if previously vaccinated.

Diagnosis

Diagnosis can usually be made clinically. However, the WHO recommends laboratory confirmation. In low-prevalence countries, use of culture and paired serologies is reasonable. A suspected case of measles in the United States should be reported to the local health department.

- *Virus isolation:* possible in renal cell lines, growth is slow. Useful in immunodeficient patients in whom antibody responses may be minimal.
- *Serology:* a fourfold increase in measles antibody titer between acute and convalescent specimens is diagnostic. ELISA is capable of detecting specific IgM on a single sample.

Treatment

- Supportive therapy and treatment of bacterial superinfection
- Vitamin A 200,000 IU given orally to children for 2 days has been shown to reduce severity but should be avoided at or after immunization, when it appears to reduce seroconversion.

Prevention

Measles vaccine is given as part of measles, mumps, rubella (MMR) (12 months and preschool). It can be given earlier in at-risk populations, but responses are suppressed and an additional dose should be given later.

Passive immunization with immunoglobulin is recommended for those exposed susceptible people at risk of severe or fatal measles. It must be given within 6 days of exposure to be effective. Such groups include the following:

- Children with defects in cell-mediated immunity
- Children with malignant disease, particularly if receiving chemo- or radiotherapy
- Children with HIV should be given immunoglobulin after exposure even if already vaccinated. Cases have occurred in vaccinated HIV-infected children.

Mumps

Mumps is an acute, generalized viral infection of children and adolescents that causes swelling and tenderness of the salivary glands and, rarely, epididymo-orchitis. More severe manifestations may occur in older patients.

Mumps was recognized as far back as Hippocrates. The name may derive from the English verb *to mump*—to be sulky.

The virus

The virus, a member of the *Paramyxoviridae* family, is a single-stranded RNA virus with an irregular, spherically shaped virion (average diameter 200 nm); the nucleocapsid is enclosed by a three-layer envelope.

The nucleocapsid contains the S (soluble) antigen; antibodies to it may be detected early in infection. Glycoproteins on the surface have hemagglutinin, neuraminidase, and cell-fusion activity and include the V (viral) antigen detected in late infection by complement fixation.

Epidemiology

Mumps is endemic throughout the world. Prior to vaccination, epidemics took place every 2–5 years, with 90% of cases occurring in those under 15 years of age. In the United States, one-third of cases occur in those over 15 years of age.

Passive immunity makes infection uncommon in children under 1 year.

Pathogenesis

Mumps is transmitted by droplet spread or direct contact. It is most infectious just before parotitis.

During incubation, the virus proliferates in the upper respiratory tract with consequent viremia and localization to glandular and neural tissue.

Parotid glands show interstitial edema and serofibrinous exudate with mononuclear cell infiltration. Cases of orchitis are similar with the addition of interstitial hemorrhage, polymorphonuclear infiltration, and areas of local infarction due to vascular compromise.

Clinical features

Incubation is 2–4 weeks. A 24-hour nonspecific prodrome of fever, headache, and anorexia is followed by earache and ipsilateral parotid tenderness. The gland swells over 2–3 days and is associated with severe pain. Swelling can lift the ear lobe up and outward. The other side follows within a couple of days in most cases; unilateral parotid involvement is seen in 25%.

Patients experience difficulty in pronunciation and mastication and may develop fever. Once swelling has peaked, recovery is rapid—within a week. Complications of parotitis (e.g., sialectasia) are rare. Other salivary glands may be involved.

CNS involvement

This is the most common extraglandular manifestation in children.

- *Meningitis* is seen in <10% of those with parotitis, although <50% of cases of mumps meningitis show evidence of glandular disease. Onset is 4–7 days after glandular symptoms but can occur 1 week before or 2 weeks later. Men are affected more than women. Symptoms resolve 3–10 days later and recovery is complete with no sequelae. CSF findings are typical of viral meningitis (p. 649). Hypoglycorrachia (CSF glucose <40 mg/100 mL) is seen in up to 30% of cases, more than in other viral meningitides.

- *Encephalitis* is seen in 1 in 6000 and takes two forms: early onset, representing direct neuron damage due to viral invasion, and a larger late-onset (7–10 days) group, representing a postinfectious demyelinating process. Recovery takes around 2 weeks and sequelae (e.g., psychomotor retardation) and death (around 1.4% of cases) may be seen.
- *Other neurological manifestations:* transient deafness, permanent deafness (1 in 20,000), ataxia, facial palsy, transverse myelitis, GBS

Other extraglandular manifestations

- Presternal pitting edema and tongue swelling (thought to be due to lymphatic obstruction by swollen regional glands) (6%)
- Epididymo-orchitis is the most common extraglandular manifestation in adults: 20–30% of postpubertal males with mumps develop it (1 in 6 of those bilateral). It is rare before puberty. It may be the only manifestation of mumps. Onset is abrupt with fever and a warm, swollen (up to four times normal) tender testicle with erythema of the overlying skin. Fever resolves at 5 days, with gonadal symptoms following. Some degree of atrophy may be seen in 50% once recovered. Infertility is rare.
- Oophoritis is seen in 5% of postpubertal women with mumps. Impaired fertility and premature menopause are reported but rare.
- Other manifestations include migratory polyarthritis, pancreatitis, myocarditis, nephritis, thyroiditis, mastitis, and hepatitis.

Diagnosis

Lab confirmation is required for epidemiology or when disease is atypical.

- *General features:* exposure history and symptoms; leukocytosis may be seen, particularly with meningitis, orchitis, or pancreatitis; serum amylase is elevated in parotitis or pancreatitis (isoenzyme analysis is required to differentiate the source).
- *Serology:* most reliably determined using ELISA for IgM. Hemagglutination inhibition (convalescent serum prevents the adsorption of chick red cells to mumps-infected epithelial cells) can be positive with antibodies to parainfluenza 3 (another cause of parotitis).
- *Virus isolation or nucleic acid detection:* present in saliva from 2 days before symptom onset to 5 days after. It may be present in CSF up to 6 days after onset.

Treatment

- Symptom control: antipyretics and fluids if persistent vomiting
- No benefit in steroid use has been demonstrated.
- Anecdotal evidence that interferon-alfa speeds resolution of orchitis

Prevention

Vaccination is more than 95% effective and takes place at 12–15 months and preschool as part of MMR vaccination.

Rubella

Rubella is an acute, mild, exanthematous viral infection of children and adults resembling mild measles but with the potential to cause fetal infection and birth defects.

The virus

The virus is a member of the *Togaviridae* family, in the genus *Rubivirus*. It is spherical in shape with a diameter of 60 nm and relatively unstable.

Epidemiology

Unlike measles, rubella is only moderately contagious. Prior to vaccination, incidence was highest in the spring among children aged 5–9 years. It was once termed "third disease," with measles and scarlet fever being the first and second exanthematous infections in childhood.

After infection or vaccination, most people develop lifelong protection against disease. Reinfection occurs (the majority asymptomatic) as demonstrated by rises in antibody titer in previously vaccinated people.

There have been rare cases of congenital rubella acquired through the reinfection of a vaccinated mother.

Pathogenesis

Spread is by droplets; patients are at their most contagious when the rash is erupting. Virus may be shed from 10 days before to 2 weeks after its appearance.

Rash may be immune mediated; it appears as immunity develops and viral titers fall. Primary viremia follows infection of the respiratory epithelium; secondary viremia occurs a few days later once the first wave of infected leukocytes release virions.

Infants with congenital rubella shed large quantities of virus for many months.

Clinical features

Incubation is 12–23 days. Postnatal rubella is a mild infection. Many cases are subclinical. Adults may experience a prodrome of malaise, fever, and anorexia. The main symptoms are lymphadenopathy (cervical and posterior auricular) and a maculopapular rash (starting on the face and moving down), which may be accompanied by coryza and conjunctivitis and lasts 3–5 days. Splenomegaly can occur.

Complications are uncommon: arthritis affecting the wrists, finger, and knees and resolving over a month may be seen as the rash appears (women more than men). Hemorrhagic manifestations occur in 1 in 3000 (children more than adults) and may be due to thrombocytopenia as well as vascular damage. Encephalitis occurs in 1 in 5000 (adults more than children), with a mortality of up to 50%.

Congenital rubella can be catastrophic in early pregnancy leading to fetal death, premature delivery, and many congenital defects. It is rare since the introduction of vaccination. The younger the fetus when infected, the more severe the illness.

In the first 2 months of gestation there is an up to 85% chance of being affected by either multiple defects or spontaneous abortion. In the third month, there is a ~30% chance of developing a single defect (e.g., deafness), dropping to 10% in the fourth month and nil after 20 weeks.

Temporary defects include low birth weight, low platelets, hepatosplenomegaly, hepatitis, meningitis, and jaundice. Permanent defects include hearing loss, cardiac abnormalities, microcephaly, inguinal hernia, cataract, and glaucoma.

Developmental defects may become apparent as the infant grows, e.g., myopia, mental retardation, diabetes, behavioral and language disorders.

Diagnosis

Its mild nature makes clinical diagnosis difficult.

- *Serology:* positive IgM on a single sample or a fourfold rise in IgG in paired sera is diagnostic. IgM may be positive in cases of reinfection. Serological diagnosis of congenital rubella in neonates may necessitate analysis of several samples over time to determine whether antibody titers are falling (maternal antibody) or rising (recent infection). Detection of rubella IgM in a newborn's serum indicates infection.
- *Intrauterine diagnosis* has been made by placental biopsy and by cordocentesis with detection by PCR.

Treatment

No treatment is indicated in most cases of postnatal rubella.

Immunoglobulin used to be given to exposed susceptible pregnant women; however, it does not prevent viremia despite suppressing symptoms.

All women of child-bearing age should be vaccinated before pregnancy.

Prevention

Vaccination achieves a seroconversion rate of 95%. Women should not become pregnant in the 3 months following vaccination.

Parvovirus B19

Parvovirus B19 has a wide variety of clinical manifestations, depending on the state of the host: in immunocompetent children, "slapped-cheek" disease; in those with underlying hemolytic disorders or HIV, an aplastic crisis. Parvovirus B19 was found in 1974 while evaluating assays for hepatitis B surface antigen using panels of serum samples: sample 19 in panel B gave a false-positive, and electron microscopy revealed the guilty virus.

The virus

The virus is a member of the family *Parvoviridae*, genus *Erythrovirus* (so called because replication occurs only in human erythrocyte precursors). B19 remains the only known human pathogenic parvovirus. They are non-enveloped and extremely resistant to physical inactivation.

Epidemiology

Infection is common in childhood—50% are IgG positive by 15 years, 90% are antibody positive by 90 years. Infected children pass virus on to uninfected members of their family. Patients are infectious 24–48 hours before viral prodrome until rash appearance.

In temperate climates, infection is most common from late winter to early summer. Rates peak every 3–4 years. Prevalence is higher in Africa.

Infection may be passed vertically, by respiratory secretions or from blood and blood products (standard thermal treatments and solvent-detergents are not completely effective), although viremia is rare.

Pathogenesis

Parvovirus B19 infects erythroid progenitors and erythroblasts. The receptor it uses to infect cells, P antigen, is found on megakaryocytes, endothelial cells, fetal myocardial cells, and erythroid precursors. Those who lack P antigen on their erythrocytes are resistant to infection.

Infected individuals may experience an acute, self-limited (4–8 days) halt in red blood cell manufacture as infected cells are destroyed. This may be unnoticed in those with normal erythroid turnover (falls in hemoglobin >1 g/dL are uncommon), but in those with a high turnover (e.g., hemoglobinopathies, hemolytic anemia), falls of 2–6 g/dL are not uncommon and aplastic anemia may develop.

The infected fetus may have severe manifestations due to high red cell turnover and the immature immune response: anemia, myocarditis, and heart failure can occur. These effects are reduced by the third trimester.

Rash and arthralgia associated with some forms of the disease are probably immune complex related.

Clinical features

Twenty percent of infections are asymptomatic.

- *Erythema infectiosum (EI):* the most common manifestation, also known as "fifth disease." The classic slapped cheek–appearing rash (fiery red eruption with surrounding pallor) follows a 5- to 7-day prodrome of fever, coryza, and mild nausea and diarrhea. A second erythematous maculopapular rash may follow on the trunk and limbs 1–2 days later, fading to produce a lacey appearance. Adults have milder manifestations. Pruritus (especially soles of the feet) can occur.
- *Arthropathy:* seen in adults, especially women. Symmetric, mainly small joints of hands and feet lasting for 1–3 weeks. It may persist or recur for months, may be confused with acute rheumatoid arthritis.
- *Transient aplastic crisis (TAC):* the first clinical illness associated with B19 infection—the abrupt cessation of erythropoiesis with absent erythroid precursors in bone marrow. It is described in a wide range of hemolytic conditions: sickle cell (nearly 90% of TAC episodes), thalassemia, pyruvate kinase (PK) deficiency, and autoimmune hemolytic anemia. It has also been seen after hemorrhage, in iron-deficiency anemia and in those who are otherwise well (who are likely to see deficiencies in other blood lineages: neutropenia, thrombocytopenia). Patients can be severely ill, with dyspnea,

confusion, or cardiac failure. It does not appear to cause true, permanent aplastic anemia.

- *Pure red cell aplasia (PRCA):* anemia in the immunosuppressed (HIV, congenital immunodeficiency, patients undergoing transplantation). Administration of immunoglobulin may be beneficial.
- *Virus-associated hemophagocytic syndrome:* usually occurs in healthy patients with cytopenia. It is characterized by histiocytic hyperplasia and hemophagocytosis and is self-limiting.
- *Fetal infection:* 10–15% of nonimmune hydrops fetalis. Where maternal infection occurs, fetal loss averages 9% and occurs within the first 20 weeks of pregnancy. There is no evidence of long-term abnormality in those who survive.
- *Other manifestations:* encephalitis, myocarditis, hepatitis, vasculitis, erythema multiforme, glomerulonephritis, idiopathic thrombocytopenia purpura, Henoch–Schönlein purpura

Diagnosis

Diagnosis is with IgM detection—90% of cases are positive by the time of the rash in EI or by day 3 of TAC. IgM remains detectable for up to 3 months.

IgG is detectable by day 7 of illness and remains detectable for life (50% of the population are IgG positive). It is not useful in diagnosing acute infection or in attributing manifestations such as chronic arthropathy to B19.

Immunocompromised people with chronic infection do not mount an immune response, and diagnosis relies on detecting DNA by PCR.

Fetal infection can be confirmed molecularly by amniotic fluid sampling, and investigations should include maternal B19 serology.

Those with aplastic anemia will show a fall of at least 2 g/dL from baseline hemoglobin (Hb).

Treatment

General measures include nonsteroidal anti-inflammatory drugs (NSAIDS) for arthritis and transfusions for TAC.

Immunosuppressed patients with persistent infection may benefit from reduction or temporary cessation of immunosuppression (if possible) to allow them to mount an immune response. If this is not feasible, IV IgG over 5 days may help. If disease recurs, they may require repeated infusions. Some HIV-infected patients will resolve chronic B19 infection with the initiation of highly active antiretroviral therapy.

Intrauterine blood transfusions may help some cases of hydrops.

Prevention

Unlike "slapped-cheek" patients, those with TAC and PRCA are infectious at presentation and should be separated from high-risk contacts (glove and gown, own room, mask) for 7 days or for the duration of the illness. Pregnant health workers should not care for such patients.

Human herpesvirus type 6

This lymphotropic virus is the single most common cause of hospital visits in infants with fever. It is the cause of roseola (also known as "sixth disease" and exanthem subitum).

The virus

The virus is a herpesvirus, originally called B-lymphotropic virus, now shown to grow in many different cell types (T cells, macrophages).

There are two subtypes (A and B), which differ in their epidemiology and growth.

Epidemiology

Nearly all humans are infected by age 2 years, probably by saliva exchange. Most isolates from healthy people are HHV-6B, the only variant to have been linked to specific clinical syndromes.

Pathogenesis

Primary infection is via the oropharynx. Regional lymph nodes and mononuclear cells are subsequently infected, and virus spreads throughout the body. Incubation is 5–15 days.

Like other herpesviruses, it causes an initial infection, a lifelong latency, and has the potential for clinical reactivation, especially in hosts who are immunocompromised (see Box 3.13). Asymptomatic carriers may continue to excrete the virus for months. Specific mechanisms for host immune evasion facilitate persistent infection.

Clinical features

- *Infantile fever*: fever without rash is the most common manifestation and may be accompanied by periorbital edema. 10% of cases in one series of acute febrile illnesses were attributed to HHV-6. Benign febrile convulsions may occur and are more frequent than fever alone, perhaps because of viral replication within the CNS.
- *Exanthem subitum* (sixth disease): an illness of infants and young children. 3–5 days of fever and upper respiratory tract symptoms are followed by development of rose-pink papules that are mildly elevated, nonpruritic, and blanche on pressure. Rash lasts around 2 days and

---

Box 3.13 HHV-6 and HIV

These viruses have an interesting relationship. Both infect and replicate in CD4+ cells, and HHV-6 induces CD4 expression in otherwise CD4-negative lymphocyte populations, rendering them susceptible to HIV infection. It also seems to accelerate HIV 1 transcription and replication. In turn, HIV-1 up-regulates *HHV-6* gene expression, and immune suppression permits HHV-6 spread. However, although there is evidence that HHV-6 disseminates widely in AIDS, there is no conclusive evidence that it either causes any opportunistic illness or affects AIDS progression.

may be associated with malaise, vomiting, diarrhea, cough, pharyngitis, and lymphadenopathy. Most infants are asymptomatic.

- *Encephalitis:* can occur alone or as complication of exanthem subitum. Virus is frequently detected in the CNS, even with no symptoms.
- *Immunocompromised hosts:* as with other herpesviruses, immune suppression permits replication with the potential for clinical illness. Viral DNA has been isolated in bone marrow transplant recipients with thrombocytopenia, pneumonitis, and encephalitis, but often in the presence of other pathogens (such as CMV) with better established pathological pedigrees. There are other anecdotal reports, including associations with certain leukemias and lymphomas, but no definitive links have been established.
- *Other:* infectious mononucleosis, hepatitis, chronic fatigue syndrome (causality unproven)

Diagnosis

Exanthem subitum does not need specific investigation or treatment because of its self-limiting nature. Diagnosis should be confirmed in those patients who are recipients of organ transplants or patients with immuno-deficiency, encephalitis, or hepatitis.

- *Serology* is rarely helpful, as nearly everyone is positive by age 2 years. IgM assays are in any case not good indicators of acute infection; paired sera may cross-react with HHV-6. CMV antibodies may cross-react with HHV-6.
- *Quantitative PCR* may be useful for active transplant-related infections. Aside from latent infection in mononuclear cells, HHV-6 can also be integrated into human chromosomes. The results of PCR performed in whole blood, for example, must be interpreted with caution.

Treatment

In vitro data indicate that acyclovir is inactive, ganciclovir responsiveness is variable, and foscarnet is inhibitory. There are no controlled trials.

Human herpesvirus type 7

Epidemiology

HHV-7 was first demonstrated in 1990 from the peripheral blood mono-nuclear cells of a healthy adult. Researchers are still looking for a role in human disease.

It infects nearly all humans by age 5 years. It is a commensal inhabitant of saliva.

Homology to HHV-6 is limited but confused earlier serological studies.

Pathogenesis

HHV-7 infects activated cord blood and CD4+ cells. CD4 is a receptor for the virus, thus HHV-7 interferes with HIV-1 infection.

Like HHV-6, it encodes genes, allowing it to evade the immune system.

Clinical features

Causation is difficult to establish given its ubiquitous nature. It probably causes fever and rash syndromes similar to those of HHV-6.

Herpes simplex virus

The virus

Herpes viruses are enveloped, containing dsDNA.

Nine known viruses are similar morphologically but differ clinically and biologically. They are classified on this basis into one of three groups:

- Alpha-herpesviruses (HSV-1, HSV-2, and VZV)
- Beta-herpesviruses (CMV, HHV-6 and HHV-7, Simian herpes B)
- Gamma-herpesviruses (EBV and HHV-8)

HSV genome encodes for around 80 gene products with around 50% sequence homology between HSV-1 and -2.

HSV is able to infect a wide variety of cells and is cytopathic to those cells in which it completes a full replication cycle, with the exception of certain neuronal cell types. In these cells, the virus is capable of establishing latent infection. Only certain viral proteins are produced, but reactivation of the viral genome can occur, resulting in the production and release of viral particles with consequent infection of adjacent cells.

Epidemiology

HSV exists worldwide. Humans are the only known natural reservoir.

Nearly all adults have antibodies to HSV-1 by their 40s; prevalence is highest in lower socioeconomic groups.

HSV-2 antibodies correlate with sexual activity, either that of the individual or their partners, appearing in puberty and being closely related to the number of partners and the presence of a history of STIs.

HSV-2 seroprevalence is around 22% in the United States (slightly higher in women than men) and is higher in developing countries.

Half of HSV-2 seroconversions are subclinical, with more occurring in those who have previously had HSV-1 infection. Many of these individuals will experience symptomatic reactivation.

Infection with one viral type confers partial immunity to the other.

Pathogenesis

Infection occurs via close contact with an individual who is shedding virus peripherally. Virus enters through mucosal surfaces or skin breaks and replicates locally, often with no clinical manifestations.

Viral progeny infect neurons and travel via the axon to the nerve ganglion (e.g., HSV-1 and trigeminal, HSV-2 and sacral nerve root ganglion) where a second phase of replication takes place, virus then spreading peripherally along sensory nerves. This accounts for the large areas that may be involved in clinical disease.

After primary disease resolution, infectious HSV cannot be detected, but viral DNA may be found in up to half of ganglion cells.

Reactivation mechanisms are not clear; viral subtype, route of infection, and host factors all contribute. Individuals infected with HSV-1 both orally and genitally experience reactivation more frequently orally. With HSV-2, by contrast, local reactivation is 8–10 times more frequent if acquired genitally.

Individuals with impaired cellular immunity (transplant recipients, patients with AIDS) may develop severe, possibly disseminated life-threatening disease.

Clinical features

Clinical manifestations are various, influenced by the site of infection, viral type, host age, and immune status. First infections tend to be more severe than reactivation, with more systemic features, longer symptom duration, and a higher rate of complications. Both viral subtypes can cause genital and orofacial infection.

- *Cutaneous manifestations* (see Cutaneous manifestations of systemic fungal infection, p. 685)
- *Visceral infection*: viremia usually results in multiple-organ involvement, but single organs may be affected. Severe disseminated disease is rare but occurs at increased frequency in women in the third trimester of pregnancy (see Maternal infections associated with neonatal morbidity, p. 711).
  - *HSV esophagitis* may follow disease extension from the pharynx or by viral reactivation via the vagal nerve. Ulceration usually involves the distal esophagus with retrosternal chest pain and dysphagia. Disease may be extensive and resemble invasive *Candida* infection.
  - *Pneumonitis* is rare. It tends to occur in the severely immunosuppressed; mortality exceeds 80%.

Encephalitis

More than 95% of cases are caused by HSV-1, incidence peaking in those aged between 5 and 30 years and those over 50 years old. Higher rates occur in the immunocompromised.

Primary infection may cause encephalitis in children and young adults, virus entering the CNS by neurotropic spread from the periphery. Most adults have evidence of previous infection, and disease can result from reactivation or reinfection with exogenous virus.

Onset is usually acute (may be insidious) with a prodrome of headache, behavioral change, and fever. Other symptoms include focal neurological signs (classically temporal lobe), seizures, and coma.

Diagnosis is by CSF PCR. Electroencephalogram (EEG) and computerized tomography (CT) may demonstrate characteristic temporal lobe localization but can be normal early in illness. MRI is more sensitive. Brain biopsy for culture and histology is rarely indicated.

Meningitis

Meningitis is more commonly caused by HSV-2. Cases may complicate genital herpes (women > men) with symptoms following genital lesions by 3–10 days. It is usually benign in the immunocompetent, lasting 2–4 days, resolving over 2–3 days.

CSF findings include raised white cells (majority lymphocytes, PMN cells in early infection). Glucose is usually over 50% blood levels but hypoglycorrhachia occurs and raised protein. PCR for HSV DNA is the most sensitive means of diagnosis. Mollaret's meningitis is a form of recurrent lymphocytic meningitis most commonly associated with HSV-2.

Other neurological features

These include sacral radiculopathy, autonomic nerve dysfunction (hyperesthesia/anesthesia of lower back and sacral area, constipation, urinary retention, transient impotence resolving over 4–8 weeks), transverse myelitis, with decreased tendon reflexes and reduced muscle strength in lower extremities, and autonomic features.

Diagnosis

Herpetic ulcerations resemble those of other causes. Lab diagnosis is important to guide therapy where there is doubt.

• *Histology* may demonstrate giant cells or intranuclear inclusions.
• *Viral isolation:* culture allows identification within 48 hours.
• *Antigen detection* is fast but not as sensitive as viral isolation in asymptomatic patients.
• *PCR to detect HSV DNA* is very sensitive, particularly when samples have been taken from late-stage lesions and using CSF in CNS infections where culture is less reliable.
• *Serology* may be used to identify asymptomatic carriers, but changes occur too late to be useful in the diagnosis of acute disease.

Treatment

Acyclovir, famciclovir, and valacyclovir have similar activity against HSV. Famciclovir and valacyclovir have improved bioavailability over that of acyclovir. Safety and tolerability are excellent with all three.

Oral therapy shortens the duration of primary attacks of cutaneous, oral, and genital herpes. It is less effective against recurrent disease but may be given prophylactically when recurrences are very frequent and in the immunocompromised.

• *Severe and disseminated HSV infection:* intravenous therapy
• *Encephalitis:* antiviral therapy (IV acyclovir for 10 days) should be given to suspected cases of HSV encephalitis until the diagnosis can be confirmed. It reduces the mortality from nearly 80% to around 25%.

Varicella zoster virus

Varicella zoster virus (VZV) causes two distinct diseases: a primary infection—chickenpox (varicella), and the localized recurrence—shingles (herpes zoster).

The virus

A dsDNA virus is around 200 nm in diameter and a member of the *Herpesviridae* family. The lipid-containing envelope is studded with glycoprotein spikes, which are the primary markers for humoral and cell-mediated immunity.

The virus spreads between cells by direct contact and may be isolated in many human cell lines. Virus can be detected by immunofluorescence 8–10 hours after infection.

Epidemiology

Humans are the only known reservoir. Infection is acquired via the respiratory tract, and over 90% of people are seropositive by 20 years of age. Exposure of a susceptible person to VZV results in chickenpox.

Infection is common in childhood (90% of cases in those under 13 years), peaking in late winter and early spring. Secondary attack rates in susceptible siblings within a household are around 80%.

Patients are infectious for 48 hours before rash appearance, and 4–5 days after vesicles crust over. After infection, the virus becomes latent within the dorsal root ganglia.

Reactivation, causing shingles, occurs in 20% of the population. All ages are affected; highest incidence is in the elderly and immunocompromised.

Mortality is under 2 per 100,000 for children, increasing 15-fold for adults.

Pathogenesis

After infection and local replication, patients become viremic.

Viral replication in the skin precipitates degenerative change of epithelial cells with ballooning and the appearance of multinucleated giant cells and eosinophilic intranuclear inclusions.

Vesicles contain a cloudy fluid (leukocytes, fibrin, and degenerate cells) and either rupture, releasing infectious virus, or slowly resolve.

Necrosis and hemorrhage may occur in the upper part of the dermis.

Histological findings of the skin in chickenpox and herpes zoster are very similar.

Clinical features

Chickenpox

Incubation is 10–14 days and may be followed by a 1- to 2-day febrile prodrome before the onset of constitutional symptoms (malaise, itch, anorexia) and rash.

Skin lesions start as maculopapules (up to 5 mm across), progressing to vesicles that quickly pustulate and form scabs that fall off 1–2 weeks after infection. Lesions appear in successive crops over 2–4 days, starting on the trunk and face and spreading centripetally. They may rarely involve the mucosa of the oropharynx and vagina.

Complications

These include secondary bacterial infection of lesions (Gram-positive organisms), such as the following:

- Streptococcal toxic shock, acute cerebellar ataxia: 1 in 4000 children under 15 years, onset 7–21 days after rash, resolves over 2–4 weeks
- Encephalitis: 0.2% cases, characterized by depressed consciousness, fever, vomiting, seizures; may be life threatening in adults; recovery over 2 weeks; 5–20% experience progressive deterioration and die
- Cerebral angiitis (after herpes zoster opthalmicus)

- Meningitis
- Transverse myelitis
- Pneumonitis: 1 in 400 adult VZV cases, often without symptoms; life-threatening in second and third trimester of pregnancy
- Myocarditis, bleeding
- Hepatitis

Pregnant women are at increased risk of complicated disease (Box 3.14)

Immunocompromised

Children (especially those with leukemia) have many more lesions, often hemorrhagic, with healing extended threefold. There is a greater risk of visceral involvement (lung, liver, CNS).

Those undergoing bone marrow transplantation are at increased risk of infection, and nearly half of cases have cutaneous or visceral dissemination. Risks are greatest in those requiring antithymocyte globulin or experiencing graft-versus-host disease (GVHD).

Herpes zoster

Unilateral vesicular eruption in a dermatomal distribution (most commonly thoracic and lumbar) is often preceded by 2–3 days of pain in the affected area. Maculopapular lesions evolve into vesicles with new crops forming over 3–5 days. Resolution may take 2–4 weeks.

Other manifestations include eyelids (first or second branch of the trigeminal); keratitis (herpes zoster opthalmicus, which is sight threatening and requires ophthalmic referral); intraoral—palate, tonsillar fossa, tongue (maxillary or mandibular branch of trigeminal nerve); Ramsay–Hunt syndrome, with pain and vesicles in the external auditory meatus; ipsilateral facial palsy; loss of taste to the anterior two-thirds of the tongue (geniculate ganglion); encephalitis; granulomatous cerebral angiitis (after zoster opthalmicus); and paralysis (anterior horn cell involvement).

- *Immunocompromised patients:* disease is more severe with prolonged lesion formation and recovery with higher risk of cutaneous

---

Box 3.14 Infection in pregnancy (p. 353)

Pregnant women with varicella are at increased risk of complications. Pneumonitis can be particularly severe and is most likely in the last trimester and in those with COPD, who smoke, are on steroids, or have extensive cutaneous disease.

- If there are signs of pneumonitis together with CXR changes or hypoxia, IV acyclovir should be given. When the CXR is normal and there are no symptoms, patients should be observed and oral aciclovir started if over 20 weeks' gestation.
- If there are no signs of pneumonitis and the rash is less than 24 hours old, oral aciclovir should be considered (but with expert advice in those under 20 weeks' gestation).
- If there are no signs of pneumonitis and the rash is over 24 hours old, aciclovir should be withheld but the patient reviewed daily.

dissemination and visceral involvement. Disease is rarely fatal. Those with HIV have an increased incidence of complications such as retinitis, acute retinal necrosis, and chronic progressive encephalitis and may develop chronic herpes zoster.

- *Postherpetic neuralgia* is uncommon in young people but occurs in up to 50% of those over 50 years old. Pain can be debilitating and may be constant or stabbing.

Diagnosis

- Vesicular fluid analysis allows differentiation from certain forms of impetigo (Gram stain of lesion fluid) and other viral infections (e.g., Coxsackie and HSV) that might present with either widespread or unilateral dermatomal vesicular lesions (direct fluorescent antibody stain, PCR, or culture of vesicle contents).
- Demonstration of seroconversion or titer rises between acute and convalescent samples may confirm diagnosis.
- PCR of CSF for VZV DNA can allow diagnosis of CNS infection.

Treatment

Chickenpox

General measures include hygiene to prevent secondary infection of lesions, management of pruritus to reduce scratching, and acetaminophen for fever.

Acyclovir

If given within 24 hours of onset, acyclovir significantly reduces the duration and severity of illness but is not recommended for routine use in immunocompetent children <12 years of age.

- Children >12 years and those with chronic skin or lung disease as well as adults presenting within 24 hours may benefit from oral acyclovir; IV therapy should be considered for patients who present late and show signs of complications or are failing to improve.
- Valacyclovir is not licensed for the treatment of chicken pox but is often used in preference to acyclovir.
- Immunocompromised individuals, neonates, and those with disseminated disease (ophthalmic, encephalitis, pneumonitis) should receive early IV therapy and may also require antibiotics to treat or prevent secondary bacterial infections.

Shingles

- General measures as for chickenpox
- Ophthalmic referral in cases involving the eye
- Antiviral treatment is recommended for patients over 50 years of age who present within 72 hours of symptoms. The benefit of antiviral treatment in younger patients is not as clear.
- Oral valacyclovir has better oral bioavailability than acyclovir and is indicated for treatment of herpes zoster.
- IV acyclovir may be necessary in the immunocompromised.
- Postherpetic neuralgia is unusual beyond 4 weeks, but such cases can be difficult to treat. They usually resolve over 6–24 months. Therapies include tricyclics, counterirritants, and gabapentin.

Prevention

Live-attenuated vaccines are available. They are recommended for healthy nonimmune children between 12 and 15 months with a second dose at age 4–6 years; persons >13 years without evidence of immunity; seronegative adult health care workers, including laboratory staff; and the healthy susceptible contacts of immunocompromised patients where continuing close contact is unavoidable (e.g., siblings of a leukemic child, or a child whose parent is undergoing chemotherapy).

A vaccine has been produced for the prevention of shingles in those over 60 (Zostavax®) reduced incidence of shingles by 64% in those aged 60–69 years and reduced postherpetic neuralgia by 39% in those vaccine recipients who developed shingles).

Varicella zoster immune globulin (VZIG) does not prevent infection but reduces disease severity. It is most effective if given within 72 hours. It is indicated for seronegative patients with a contact history who are at increased risk of complications: those with defects in cell-mediated immunity; those on significant doses of steroids; those who have received a bone marrow transplant, radiotherapy, or chemotherapy within the last 6 months; organ transplant recipients on immunosuppression; pregnant women; and infants under 1 month old whose mothers develop chickenpox between 1 week before and 4 weeks after delivery or who are exposed to chickenpox and whose mothers have no history of prior infection or are seronegative.

Infectious mononucleosis

Infectious mononucleosis is a syndrome of sore throat, fever, and lymphadenopathy with atypical lymphocytosis; 80–90% of cases are due to Epstein–Barr virus (EBV), which is generally associated with a positive heterophile antibody test (see next section).

Most of the remaining cases are caused by CMV. Young adults and adolescents are most frequently affected. Other conditionsthat should be considered are viral hepatitis, acute toxoplasmosis, rubella, streptococcal sore throat, primary HIV, and diphtheria.

Epstein–Barr virus

EBV is a human herpesvirus, the cause of heterophile-positive infectious mononucleosis, and associated with African Burkitt's lymphoma.

The virus

Enveloped hexagonal nucleocapsids contain dsDNA that encodes around 80 proteins.

The virus can be cultivated in human B cells and nasopharyngeal epithelial cells. The cell surface receptor for the virus is the receptor for C3d complement protein.

Early after infection, Epstein–Barr nuclear antigens (EBNA) are detectable in cell nuclei. Viral DNA may become incorporated into host DNA in transformed cells but most remains in a circular nonintegrated form.

The virus remains latent in most infected cells.

Epidemiology

EBV occurs worldwide. Infection is acquired earlier in tropical countries than in industrialized countries. By adulthood, 90–95% of most populations are antibody positive.

Infection does not occur in epidemics, and the virus is of relatively low transmissibility. Spread is by intimate contact.

Incidence is the same for men and women (but female peak age-specific incidence occurs 2 years earlier) but is 30 times higher in whites than blacks, reflecting the higher rate of early primary infection in blacks.

Pathogenesis

Virus infects epithelial cells and susceptible B lymphocytes. Incubation is 30–50 days, shorter in young children. It can persist in the oropharynx of those who have recovered from infectious mononucleosis <18 months.

EBV-related infectious mononucleosis prompts the synthesis of antibodies against viral antigen and unrelated antigens such as those found on sheep, horse, and beef red cells (heterophile antibodies, see p. 350) and, less frequently, platelets, neutrophils, and ampicillin.

In early illness there is a mononuclear lymphocytosis—most cells bear T-cell markers. The immune response includes both T cells and natural killer (NK) cells. Atypical lymphocytosis resolves by recovery; the virus is, however, not eliminated from the host.

Clinical features

Infection is usually asymptomatic in young children (perhaps mild changes in LFTs). When there are symptoms, children are more likely to experience rash, neutropenia, or pneumonia than adults; 50% of cases in adolescents are asymptomatic.

A typical case involves a triad of fever, sore throat, and lymphadenopathy (symmetric involvement of cervical, axillary, and sometimes inguinal nodes), which may be abrupt or follow a 1- to 2-week prodrome of anorexia and malaise; 5% develop rash (macular, urticarial, petechial, or erythema multiforme-like); 90–100% develop a pruritic maculopapular rash if given ampicillin (may appear after the drug has stopped).

Examination is for pharyngitis (exudative in 33%, with palatal petechiae in 25–60%), hepatomegaly, splenomegaly (50% of cases are maximal at day 8, resolving over 10 days), periorbital edema, and lymphadenopathy Tachycardia is unusual even in the presence of fever. Tonsillar enlargement can be so great as to threaten the airway. Abdominal pain, particularly in the left upper quadrant, may be related to hepatomegaly or splenic enlargement, which may be rapid. There is a danger of splenic rupture with minor trauma or even spontaneously.

Fever resolves over 10–14 days. Recovery from fatigue can take longer with good days interspersed with periods of symptom recrudescence.

Complications

Death is unusual in immunocompetent individuals but may follow neurological complications, airway obstruction (due to tonsillar hypertrophy, <1%), or splenic rupture.

- *Hematological:* thrombocytopenia (50%), autoimmune hemolytic anemia (0.5–3% cases, with 70% having cold agglutinins, usually IgM). Hemolysis is apparent days 7–14 and recovers over 6 weeks. Corticosteroids may help. Splenic rupture (0.2%, usually in the second or third week of illness and may be abrupt or insidious following rapid increase to 2–3 times normal size) is usually associated with left upper quadrant and shoulder pain; 50% of cases have associated trauma, therefore, it is recommended that patients avoid contact sports.
- *Neurological:* encephalitis, meningitis (may find atypical lymphocytes in CSF), Guillain-Barré syndrome, optic neuritis, Bell's palsy; 85% of cases with neurological features recover completely
- *other:* hepatitis (90%, jaundice in only 5%), renal (interstitial nephritis), cardiac (pericarditis, myocarditis), lung (rare pneumonia)

EBV associations with other diseases

- *Neoplastic disorders:* most patients with nasopharyngeal carcinoma and nearly all African cases of Burkitt's lymphoma have high EBV antibody titers, and EBV DNA has been detected in biopsy specimens from such patients. Associations have also been found between EBV and Hodgkin's lymphoma and both polyclonal B- and T-cell lymphomas (particularly in the setting of immunodeficiency and solid organ and bone marrow transplants).
- *Infection in immunocompromised children:* several congenital immunodeficiencies are associated with the development of EBV-associated lymphoproliferative disorders. X-linked immunoproliferative syndrome has a particular association with acute fatal infectious mononucleosis with hepatic necrosis and pancytopenia.
- *EBV and HIV:* EBV is associated with polyclonal B-cell lymphomas seen in AIDS patients and is the cause of oral hairy leukoplakia. Children with AIDS may develop a lymphoid interstitial pneumonitis.
- *Chronic fatigue syndrome (CFS):* there is no serological or epidemiological basis to suggest that EBV infection is the cause of CFS. Rare patients have chronic ongoing organ dysfunction due to EBV (fever, pulmonary involvement), but these are clearly identifiable.

Diagnosis

General findings

- *Hematological:* peripheral lymphocytosis representing activated T cells responding to virus-induced B-cell proliferation (peaks day 7–21 with lymphocytes/monocytes accounting for 70% of the total white cell count of 20–50,000 leucocytes/mm^3); atypical lymphocytes (about 3% of cells—large, vacuolated, basophilic, eccentric lobulated nucleus— also seen in CMV, rubella, mumps, and drug reactions); neutropenia (60–70% cases); thrombocytopenia (50% but bleeding is rare)
- *Biochemical:* LFT abnormalities (90% cases), mild elevation of bilirubin (45%), low-level cryoglobulins (IgG and IgM) in 90% of cases

Specific tests

Heterophile antibodies

EBV-infected B cells produce polyclonal IgM antibodies. Some of these (heterophile antibodies) agglutinate the red blood cells (RBCs) of other species. Such antibodies may be present in the sera of some healthy patients and those with lymphoma. Preincubation with guinea pig cells removes these.

Antibody titer is reported as the highest serum dilution at which sheep or horse (more sensitive) red cells are agglutinated; 40% of patients are positive by week 1, and 80% by week 3 of illness. Delayed appearance may be associated with prolonged convalescence. A test remains positive for up to 1 year.

The Paul–Bunnell test measures agglutination of sheep RBCs by patient sera. The Paul–Bunnell–Davidson test is similar but is performed after preabsorption of sera with guinea pig cells.

The monospot test measures the agglutination of formalinized horse RBCs after preabsorption of sera with guinea pig cells. Commercial monospot tests have slightly greater sensitivity than that of the classic tube test.

EBV-specific antibodies

Positive antiviral capsid antigen (VCA) IgM and negative EBNA is a sensitive and specific indicator of acute infection. Positive VCA-IgG, positive EBNA (appears late in illness), and negative VCA-IgM (remains positive for 4–8 weeks) suggest infection occurring between 3 and 12 months ago. VCA-IgG and EBNA remain positive for life.

PCR

PCR is rarely used in immunocompetent patients with suspected EBV. it is useful in the management of transplant patients with EBV-associated lymphoproliferative diseases.

Treatment

Most cases are self-limited and do not require specific therapy. The virus is poorly transmitted and isolation is unnecessary. The level of activity a patient undertakes depends on symptom severity. Some may require bed rest. Patients should not participate in contact sports or heavy lifting for 3 weeks to 2 months.

Admit to the hospital those patients with evidence of splenic rupture, airway compromise, dehydration, significant thrombocytopenia, or hemolytic anemia, and other major complications.

Corticosteroids may be indicated in cases of severe thrombocytopenia, hemolytic anemia and impending airway obstruction and for CNS or cardiac involvement. Response is usually rapid, and doses can be tailed of over 1–2 weeks.

Immunoglobulin has been used to treat severe immune thrombocytopenia.

Antiviral drugs show no evidence of benefit in uncomplicated infectious mononucleosis. Acyclovir has been used in the treatment of complicated disease associated with immunodeficiency. It has been shown to reduce the oral hairy leukoplakia in HIV-positive patients and been used to induce a temporary remission of a polyclonal B-cell lymphoma in renal transplant recipients.

Splenic rupture requires urgent surgical intervention, usually splenectomy.

Tracheotomy may be indicated in some cases of airway obstruction.

General malaise can persist for up to 3 months. Hematological and hepatic complications settle over 2–3 months. Adults with neurological complications may be left with residual deficits.

Cytomegalovirus

Cytomegalovirus (CMV) is a herpesvirus—the largest virus to infect humans—that is found across the world and is the cause of a wide spectrum of clinical syndromes from congenital disease to pneumonia.

The virus

This dsDNA virus encodes around 230 proteins, many of which are directly involved in down-regulating the host immune response (e.g., preventing class I HLA molecule transport to the surface). The genome is surrounded by a nucleoprotein core, which in turn is covered by matrix proteins and a lipid envelope.

It infects by endocytosis. CMV replication takes place in the nucleus of the cell, resulting in large nuclear inclusions useful in diagnosing infection.

After acute infection, CMV persists in a nonreplicating form, reactivating with immunosuppression or illness. Some cases of secondary infection can be reinfection as well as simply reactivation.

Clinical features

Mononucleosis

Primary infection in a young adult produces an infectious mononucleosis picture (fever, sore throat, lymphadenopathy). The heterophile agglutinin test is negative. Lymphadenopathy and sore throat are milder than with EBV. Virus is acquired by intimate contact and by transfusion.

Complications include interstitial pneumonia, which is seen in bone marrow transplant patients in whom there is a high mortality despite antiviral therapy. Rare occurrence is in healthy people in whom therapy is not required. Hepatitis is common and mild in the immunocompetent. In Guillain–Barré syndrome, CMV is the precipitant of around 10% of GBS cases. Meningoencephalitis, myocarditis, thrombocytopenia, hemolytic anemia (common in children with congenital CMV), and skin eruptions (usually mild and can be associated with ampicillin) can also occur.

Patients with AIDS

Coinfection with CMV is seen in over 90% of gay men with HIV-1, and there is an increased risk of serious CMV disease once CD4 cells fall below 100/mm^3. The incidence of end-organ CMV disease has now fallen by over 80% with the introduction of highly active antiretroviral treatment (HAART). CMV retinitis is the most common manifestation and was once seen in nearly one-third of HIV-infected patients.

Polyradiculopathy is the most common CNS manifestation, characterized by ascending weakness in the legs, and loss of bowel and bladder control.

Gastrointestinal manifestations include esophageal erosions, colitis (fever and diarrhea, which can be complicated by perforation or partial obstruction due to lesions resembling Kaposi sarcoma), pancreatitis, and cholecystitis. Characteristic inclusion bodies may be seen on biopsy.

Immunosuppressive therapy

Agents such as cyclophosphamide and azathioprine are sufficient in themselves to reactivate CMV. Corticosteroids, insufficient alone, act synergistically with these agents. Cyclosporin increases CMV disease only in combination with steroids.

Transplant recipients

Immunosuppressive regimes render such people prone to severe CMV. It is the most common pathogen isolated after solid-organ transplantation. Some cases represent reactivation of latent infection; many are acquired from the transplanted organ or transfused blood.

The severity of the end-organ disease caused by CMV reflects the degree of immunosuppression and type of infection (i.e., primary infections). The most important source of infection is the transplanted organ, or transfused blood:

- *Bone marrow:* an important life-threatening complication following allogeneic BMT is CMV interstitial pneumonia, which usually occurs in the first 4 months following the procedure. Onset is rapid—over the course of a few days with fever, nonproductive cough, and dyspnea. Severe cases will require ventilation, and that occurring in the context of BMT has a mortality of around 80%, even with antiviral therapy (ganciclovir and CMV immunoglobulin). This may reflect an element of GVHD in the lung
- *Liver:* CMV infection, particularly CMV hepatitis, is a leading cause of morbidity in the first 3 months following transplantation. CMV hepatitis has led to liver failure and repeat transplantation. Liver biopsy is required to distinguish it from graft rejection, a complication with the opposite management strategy. A prolonged course of ganciclovir at the time of transplantation may reduce the incidence of CMV disease in seronegative recipients.
- *Kidney:* the rate of CMV infection of seronegative recipients following transplantation of a kidney from a seropositive donor is over 80%. Such primary infections tend to be more symptomatic than reactivation secondary to immunosuppression. Primary infections may present with CMV syndrome: fever, leucopenia, atypical lymphocytes, lymphocytosis, hepatosplenomegaly, myalgia, and arthralgia. CMV pneumonia is less severe than that with BMT. Ganciclovir therapy can be life saving. Significant CMV hepatitis is rare.

Congenital infection

Intrauterine CMV infection (seen in 0.5–22% of live births) is less common than perinatal infection but is clinically more severe, with fulminant cytomegalic inclusion disease: jaundice, hepatosplenomegaly, petechial ash, multiple organ involvement with the possibility of CNS findings such as microcephaly and cerebral calcification.

Diagnosis is best made by confirmation of infant viruria within the first week of life. Such infections tend to be seen in infants born to primiparous mothers experiencing primary CMV infection during pregnancy. Asymptomatic congenital infection has been reported in infants born to CMV-immune mothers. Perinatal infection follows acquisition from virus carried in the cervix or breast milk.

Diffuse visceral and CNS disease does not occur and resembles mild CMV mononucleosis. Perinatal CMV infection may be associated with hearing loss.

Infection in pregnancy

During pregnancy, primary infection of the mother may present with a mild mononucleosis syndrome but is usually asymptomatic. CMV may colonize the cervix; the rate of cervical infection increases in the later stages of pregnancy.

Diagnosis

Classical tube culture is slow (up to 4 weeks). Shell vial culture combined with immunofluorescence to enable the early detection of viral antigens yields results within 24–48 hours. Culture of virus from saliva or urine does not necessarily indicate active infection (healthy seropositive people may asymptomatically shed virus intermittently). Culture from blood is highly suggestive of pathogenic infection; however, it is insensitive and rarely performed in the era of molecular diagnostics.

CMV viremia corresponds with active infection. PCR to detect CMV DNA correlates well with culture results and can detect virus in CSF, blood, and tissue.

Biopsy of infected tissue may reveal the distinctive appearance of CMV-infected cells (e.g., inclusion bodies).

Seroconversion suggests recent infection. Serology is not useful in most cases, outside of transplant donor and recipient screening.

Treatment and prevention

Infection in immunocompetent individuals does not require treatment.

Ganciclovir, foscarnet, and cidofovir (see Antivirals for cytomegalovirus, p. 81) inhibit the CMV DNA polymerase and are effective at treating CMV end-organ disease in the immunocompromised. AIDS-related retinitis responds to oral valganciclovir. Those with sight-threatening lesions should be considered for intravitreal (injection or implant) or IV ganciclovir. Intravitreal treatment should be accompanied by PO valganciclovir. Induction therapy should last at least 3 weeks. Those not on HAART should be initiated and maintenance valganciclovir continued until CD4 >100 and expert review confirms that retinitis is quiescent. Relapse may occasionally occur in those with CD4 counts above 100.

Serious CMV disease may be prevented after BMT and solid-organ transplantation with antiviral therapy. Both pre-emptive (initiation of therapy to those with evidence of viral replication in the absence of symptoms) and prophylactic (therapy to all those with positive CMV serology) strategies have shown benefit. Because of the risk of drug toxicity, many centers reserve prophylactic therapy for those most at risk (e.g., CMV-positive donors and CMV-negative recipients of solid organs).

Drug resistance

For antiviral activity, ganciclovir requires phosphorylation by both viral and cellular enzymes. Resistance may be conferred by mutations of either or both the viral enzyme responsible for phosphorylating the prodrug and the CMV DNA polymerase. Mutations in both these regions may render a virus resistant to both ganciclovir and cidofovir.

Cross-resistance between ganciclovir and foscarnet is rare. Foscarnet resistance has been reported.

Viral gastroenteritis

Viruses account for over half the diarrheal episodes in infants and young children, particularly in poorer, overcrowded parts of the world where viral diarrhea and dehydration account for millions of deaths each year.

Acute viral gastroenteritis is seen in three settings:
- Sporadic gastroenteritis of infants (usually rotavirus, see below; sometimes adenovirus, see p. 379)
- Epidemic gastroenteritis occurring in semiclosed communities (families, institutions, ships) or as a result of classic water- or food-borne infection (mostly caliciviruses, see p. 356)
- Sporadic acute gastroenteritis of adults (caliciviruses, rotaviruses, astroviruses, see p. 556; adenoviruses).

All are transmitted feco-orally, but droplet spread and food contamination can also occur. Asymptomatic infection is common. Electron microscopy is the only way to detect all known viruses. It is labor intensive, expensive, and insensitive unless the titer is extremely high.

Other methods include antibody-based methods (ELISA, immunofluorescence) and PCR. These are useful in identifying the cause of an outbreak rather than individual cases; patients have usually recovered by diagnosis.

Rotavirus

Rotavirus outnumbers other viral causes of diarrhea by 4:1, causing around 50% of those cases requiring hospitalization in the developed world.

The virus

The virus is from the family *Reoviridae*, genus *Rotavirus*. Three antigenically distinguishable groups (A to C) cause human disease. Virtually all outbreaks worldwide are caused by group A organisms.

On electron microscopy they have a wheel-like appearance (Latin *rota*). They have no envelope, just an outer capsid and core.

Epidemiology

An infectious dose is very small—100 organisms or even less. Transmission is feco-oral (contaminated food, water, direct contact, or inhalation of aerosol from vomit or feces), and virus is shed for up to a week after symptom onset. Many strains are avirulent.

Almost all children are infected within the first 3 years of life. There appears to be no difference in exposure risk in low-income countries (unlike bacterial causes of diarrhea). Antibody to virus is acquired by 80 to 100% of the population by age 3 years.

Highest incidence is between 6 months (maternal antibody wanes) and 24 months old. Severe disease may still occur in younger and older children; however, those under 2 months are more resistant to disease.

Infection is seasonal in temperate countries (peaking in winter), with attack rates around 20–30% for a child's first two seasons. Susceptibility continues throughout life; 50% of parents experience infection if they have an infected infant.

Pathogenesis

Viral capsid protein vp4 binds glycolipids on the surface of villous epithelial cells lining the small intestine, leading to virus entry.

Diarrhea is induced through several mechanisms: certain strains have nonstructural proteins that act as enterotoxins causing diarrhea directly, loss of villus tip cells decreases absorptive capacity, and a decrease in intestinal disaccharidases can cause an osmotic diarrhea. Rotavirus-induced lactase deficiency lasts up to 2 weeks.

Clinical features

Incubation is 1–2 days. Infants and young children experience fever, vomiting (duration is 2–3 days), and watery (bloodless) diarrhea (duration is 4–5 days).

More severe cases may have prolonged symptoms and develop an isotonic dehydration requiring hospital treatment. There is no clear evidence that rotavirus causes any other syndrome. Children with immunodeficiency can develop a gastroenteritis lasting many weeks.

Asymptomatic viral shedding occurs.

Diagnosis

Electron microscopy is now rarely used. Rapid diagnostic tests with high levels of specificity include ELISA for rotavirus-specific antigen and latex agglutination kits.

Other techniques include electrophoresis (no false positives and allows identification of strain-identical infections) and PCR (allows serotyping).

Treatment

See Infectious diarrhea (p. 585) for more information on the management of diarrhea.

Fluid replacement is fundamental. It should be administered orally in mild and moderate cases. Feeding early in illness (within 24 hours) promotes enterocyte regeneration and reduces gut permeability. Fruit juices and soft drinks should be avoided. Milk can be given to infants; lactose-free, carbohydrate-rich foods given to older children.

There is no role for antibiotics or antimotility drugs.

Prevention

Prevention by hygiene alone is difficult. Asymptomatic shedding is common. Rotavirus are relatively resistant to common handwashing agents and can survive for some time on hard surfaces and in water.

For management of hospital outbreaks, see Infection control in the community (p. 170).

There are currently two oral vaccines. Several other oral vaccines are in development for use in developing countries. The WHO recommends rotavirus vaccine introduction into the immunization schedules of those regions in which its efficiency has been demonstrated.

Caliciviruses

These ssRNA viruses are detected in a variety of animal species. Norwalk virus, first isolated in 1972, is the prototype of this group. The name *calicivirus* derives from cup-like indentations in the surface of the virus (from the Latin *calyx*).

They are associated with point-source outbreaks among adults (particularly in closed settings such as ships, hospitals, and the military) and are common causes of diarrhea in children worldwide.

Incubation is 24–48 hours; symptoms last 2–3 days. Vomiting is a dominant feature in most affected people. Secondary attack rates are high. Pathological changes are similar to those seen in rotavirus infection.

Vehicles for infection include water, food that has come into contact with contaminated water, and even contact with lakes or pools with which an infected individual has been in contact. They are relatively resistant to inactivation by chlorine.

Outbreaks last 1–2 weeks but recurrent episodes on ships are common despite efforts to disinfect the ship between cruises. Disease is self-limited. IV fluid replacement may be indicated in rare instances of severe dehydration.

Antibody may be detected in up to 90% of older children and adults. Resistance to a specific virus lasts a maximum of 2–3 years, and there is little if any cross-protection against infection by other caliciviruses.

Astroviruses

These RNA viruses are members of the family *Astroviridae* and are important causes of gastroenteritis in children and adults. The name is derived from its 5- or 6-pointed star appearance when examined by EM.

They cause diarrhea in schools, daycare institutions, and hospitals, usually in children under 3 years of age. Asymptomatic infection is common, and they appear to be less pathogenic in adults than Norwalk viruses.

Incubation is 3–4 days, with symptoms lasting up to 5 days. Diarrhea, malaise, and nausea are dominant, vomiting less so.

Disease is self-limited and treatment is directed at maintaining hydration.

Hepatitis viruses

Acute viral hepatitis is characterized by a necroinflammatory response in the liver. It can be caused by a number of viruses and may be mimicked by many other infectious diseases and noninfectious causes. It is usually a self-limiting disease but can progress to fulminant hepatitis (rare, but 1–20% mortality) or chronic liver disease (depending on the cause).

A flowchart for the investigation of acute hepatitis given in Fig. 3.1.

Hepatitis viruses

Over the past 30 years, at least five primarily hepatotropic viruses have been identified:
- Hepatitis A virus (p. 358)
- Hepatitis B virus (p. 359)

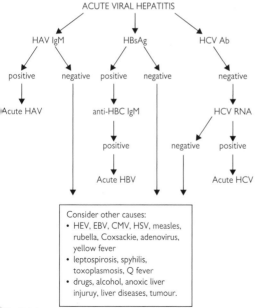

Fig. 3.1 Investigation of acute hepatitis.

Hepatitis A virus

Hepatitis A is usually a self-limiting illness caused by hepatitis A virus (HAV), an enterically transmitted picornavirus. Although outbreaks of infectious hepatitis have been recognized for centuries, the virus was only demonstrated in the stool of volunteers infected with HAV in 1973. Since then, the virus has been identified, transmitted to primates, propagated in culture, and sequenced.

The virus

HAV is a 27–28 nm spherical nonenveloped virus with a surface structure suggesting icosahedral symmetry.

Purification of the virus yields three distinct types of particle:
- Mature virions
- Empty capsids or particles with incomplete genome
- Less stable particles with more open structure

The HAV genome is a single-stranded, positive sense, linear RNA of 7478 nucleotides with a molecular weight of 2.25×10^6. As with other picornaviruses, the coding region is divided into three parts:
- P1, which encodes the four capsid proteins (VP1, VP2, VP3, and VP4)
- P2 and P3, which encode the nonstructural proteins

Although a variety of genotypes (I to VII) have been identified, there appears to be only one major serotype.

Epidemiology

HAV has a worldwide distribution. It is associated with overcrowding and poor sanitation, and endemic in the developing world where it is an infection of childhood. In developed countries, incidence increases with age. Epidemics are associated with food and waterborne transmission.

Certain groups are at increased risk:
- children and staff in childcare facilities
- patients and staff in mental health institutions
- men who have sex with men (MSM)
- intravenous drug users
- travelers to endemic areas.

The virus is usually transmitted via the feco-oral route, although outbreaks have been associated with contaminated blood products.

Clinical features

Subclinical infection is common in children (>90% in children <5 years of age).

Acute hepatitis occurs more frequently with increasing age. Symptoms include fever, headache, malaise, anorexia, vomiting, weight loss, dark urine, and pale stools. Occasionally, diarrhea, cough, coryzal symptoms, or arthralgia may occur (more common in children). Physical findings include jaundice, hepatomegaly, splenomegaly (5–15%), and spider nevi.

Complications include prolonged cholestasis, relapsing disease, fulminant hepatitis (rare, more common in older patients), extrahepatic disease, and triggering of autoimmune chronic active hepatitis.

Diagnosis

Liver function tests are elevated with high aspartate transaminase (AST) and alanine aminotransferase (ALT) levels. Bilirubin and alkaline phosphatase are usually only mildly elevated.

Serology is used for detection of anti-HAV IgM, which confirms the diagnosis and remains positive for 3–6 months. Anti-HAV IgG becomes positive at 2–3 months and persists for life.

Treatment

Acute hepatitis is treated symptomatically (alcohol).

For fulminant hepatitis, patients should be treated with supportive therapy and referred for consideration of liver transplantation.

Prevention

Passive immunization

Pooled immunoglobulin (gammaglobulin) was previously the mainstay of prophylaxis in travelers to endemic regions. However, there are concerns that waning antibody levels may not be adequate to confer protection and the duration of protection is short-lived.

Immunoglobulin is now only used for post-exposure prophylaxis and for unvaccinated individuals who will be in a high-risk situation in <2 weeks.

Active immunization

Several inactivated HAV vaccines exist, and these have largely superseded the use of immunoglobulin. Two doses of HAV vaccine are given, at 0 and 6–12 months, and provide protection for at least 10 years.

Indications for immunization include travelers to endemic areas, MSM, intravenous drug users, regular recipients of blood products, high-risk employment, and military personnel. Hepatitis A vaccine may also be given as post-exposure prophylaxis.

Hepatitis B virus

Hepatitis B virus (HBV) is a DNA virus that causes acute and chronic viral hepatitis in humans. Serum hepatitis has been recognized since 1833, when shipyard workers in Bremen developed jaundice following smallpox inoculation.

In 1965, Blumberg found a serum antigen in the blood of an Aboriginal, initially called the Australia antigen, which was associated with post-transfusion hepatitis. This was eventually identified as the hepatitis B surface antigen (HBsAg).

The virus

Virus structure

The HBV virion (Dane particle) has a diameter of 42 nm. It has an outer envelope that contains HBsAg proteins, glycoproteins, and cellular lipid. HBsAg proteins may also be released from HBV-infected cells as small spherical particles or filamentous forms.

Beneath the envelope is the internal core or nucleocapsid, which contains hepatitis B core antigen (HBcAg). The third antigen, hepatitis B e antigen (HBeAg), is a truncated form of the major core polypeptide. It is released from infected liver cells in which HBV is replicating.

Viral genome

HBV has one of the smallest viral genomes, consisting of a 3200 base pair circular DNA molecule. The genome has four long open reading frames:
• C (core or nucleocapsid) gene, which encodes HbcAg and HbeAg. Mutations in the pre-core region result in HBV mutants that lack HBeAg.
• S (surface or envelope) gene, which includes the pre-S1, pre-S2, and s regions, encodes HBsAg.
• P (pol or polymerase) gene, which encompasses 3/4 of the viral genome and overlaps part of the C gene, the S gene, and part of the X gene. It encodes a polypeptide with DNA polymerase and ribonuclease H activity.
• X gene, which encodes a polypetide, with several functions

Epidemiology

HBV infection is a global public health problem with an estimated 400 million people chronically infected and >500,000 deaths per year. HBV may be transmitted by the following routes:
• Vertical/perinatal
• Sexual
• Transfusion of contaminated blood or blood products
• Intravenous drug use
• Needlestick injury
• Horizontally between children in Africa

Clinical features
• Acute hepatitis
• Fulminant hepatic failure (0.1–0.5% of acute infections)
• Chronic hepatitis (5–10% of adult acute infections)
• End-stage liver disease (15–40% of chronic infections)
• Hepatocellular carcinoma
• Extrahepatic manifestations, e.g., arthropathy

Diagnosis

Initial evaluation should include the following:
• History and physical examination (risk factors for HBV, clinical evidence of cirrhosis, portal hypertension, liver failure)
• Liver function tests: bilirubin, AST, ALT, alkaline phosphatase (ALP), gamma-glutamyl transferase (GGT), prothrombin time (PT), albumin
• HBV markers: HBsAg, HBeAg, HbcAg, anti-HBs, anti-HBe, HBV DNA

- Screening for other blood-borne viruses, e.g., HCV, HIV
- Screening for hepatocellular carcinoma (HCC): alpha-fetoprotein (AFP), and liver ultrasound
- Screening for esophageal varies by upper GI endoscopy
- Liver biopsy to determine disease activity (necroinflammatory and fibrosis scores)

Treatment

General advice
- Avoid alcohol
- Safe sexual practices
- Hepatitis A vaccination (low-prevalence areas)
- Avoid occupations that may spread HBV (e.g., surgery, dentistry)
- HBV immunization of household contacts

Antiviral therapy
Refer to the 2009 Guideline approved by the American Association for the Study of Liver Diseases (www.aasld.org). Treatment depends on the stage of infection, HBeAg seropositivity, HBV DNA viral load, and ALT:
- Acute HBV: no treatment, refer for transplantation if fulminant hepatic failure
- Inactive HbsAg carrier: no treatment, monitor ALT every 6–12 months, screen for HCC every 2 years
- Chronic HBV with normal ALT: no treatment, monitor ALT every 3–6 months, screen for HCC every 2 years
- Chronic HBV with raised ALT: treat.
- Compensated cirrhosis: treat (but there is poor response)
- Decompensated cirrhosis: +/– treat, refer for transplantation

Approved medications include interferon-alpha (INF-A)/pegylated INF-A, adefovir (ADV), lamivudine (LAM), entecavir (ETV), tenofovir (TDF), and telbivudine (LdT), which may be used as initial therapy. However, ADV, LAM, and LdT are not preferred as initial treatment because of high rate of resistance development.
   INF is contraindicated in patients with decompensated cirrhosis.

End points for treatment of chronic HBV
- Biochemical: normalization of ALT
- Virological: HBV DNA level to <10^5 copies/mL
- Serological: loss of HbeAg and appearance of anti-HBe
- Histological: reduction in necroinflammatory score ≥2 points

Difficult-to-treat patients
- Patients coinfected with other viruses, e.g., HCV, HDV, HIV
- Decompensated cirrhosis
- Renal failure
- Immunodeficiency, e.g., chemotherapy

Prevention
- Education regarding modes of transmission
- Screening of blood products

- Pre-exposure immunization, e.g., neonates, health care workers
- Post-exposure vaccination, e.g., sexual contacts, needlestick recipients
- Hepatitis B immunoglobulin for neonates born to HBeAg-positive mothers and unvaccinated needlestick recipients from HBeAg-positive donor

Hepatitis D virus

Hepatitis delta virus (HDV) is a defective virus whose replication requires coinfection with HBV.

Virions of HDV consist of a core of delta antigen and RNA enclosed in an HBsAg-containing envelope.

The delta antigen was originally discovered by immunofluorescent staining, as an antigen distinct from HBsAg, HbcAg, and HBeAg in the hepatocytes of chronic HBV carriers in Italy. Most patients with delta antigen in the liver have anti-delta antibodies in their serum. Serological surveys have shown high anti-delta seroprevalence in southern Italy, Mediterranean countries, and North Africa.

There is a higher incidence of HDV infection in HBsAg-positive patients with acute and chronic hepatitis, compared with asymptomatic carriers.

Simultaneous infection with HBV and HDV is more likely to result in severe or fulminant hepatitis than with HBV infection alone.

Exacerbations of hepatitis may also occur in HBsAg carriers who subsequently acquire HDV. There is no specific treatment for HDV.

Hepatitis C virus

Hepatitis C virus (HCV) is an RNA flavivirus that was discovered and sequenced in the late 1980s. Prior to this, it was recognized as a major cause of post-transfusion hepatitis and called non-A, non-B hepatitis virus.

The virus

Virus structure

HCV is a spherical, enveloped, RNA virus, similar in structure to other flaviviruses. Its genome is a positive ssRNA molecule, approximately 9.7 kB in length, which contains a large open reading frame flanked by untranslated regions (UTRs). The open reading frame encodes a polyprotein that is processed into at least 10 proteins: core protein (C), envelope proteins (E1 and E2), NS2a, and six nonstructural proteins (NS2, NS3, NS4a, NS4b, NS5a, NS5b).

Little is known about the life cycle of HCV; it has only recently been propagated in cell culture.

Genetic diversity

The high level viral turnover and the absence of proofreading by the NS5b polymerase result in a rapid accumulation of mutations within the genome. Multiple closely related but distinct HCV variants (quasispecies) may be recovered from the plasma and liver of an infected patient at one time. There is also remarkable genetic heterogeneity among HCV sequences recovered from different patients.

At least seven major genotypes (genotypes 1–7) exist, and these may be further grouped into subtypes (e.g., 1a, 1b, 1c). Different subtypes predominate in different geographic locations.

Epidemiology

HCV infects an estimated 170 million people worldwide. In developed countries, HCV prevalence is generally low (0.5–2%), apart from in intravenous drug users. In certain geographic areas, HCV is more common, e.g., Egypt, Japan, Taiwan, and Italy, and may be related to reuse of needles for injection, acupuncture, or folk remedies.

Routes of transmission
- Transfusion of contaminated blood or blood products
- Intravenous drug use
- Nosocomial transmission, e.g., needlestick, hemodialysis, colonoscopy (inadequate sterilization of colonoscopes)
- Sexual transmission or mother-to-child transmission is rare.

Natural history and pathogenesis
Viral persistence
Fifteen percent of acutely infected people clear the virus in the 3–24 months after infection; 85% develop chronic infection. Because of limitations in experimental models and the infrequent recognition of acute infection, the mechanisms of viral clearance remain poorly understood. An HCV-specific cytotoxic T lymphocyte (CTL) response plays an important role in suppressing HCV RNA levels, but this does not appear to be sufficient to clear the virus.

Similarly, viremia persists despite a broad humoral response to HCV epitopes. This suggests that HCV has developed mechanisms to evade immune responses, e.g., changes in the viral envelope.

Disease progression
HCV leads to hepatic inflammation, steatosis, and, eventually, hepatic fibrosis and hepatocellular carcinoma (estimated risk is 5–25% after 10–20 years). A number of factors are associated with cirrhosis, including excessive alcohol ingestion, coinfection with HBV or HIV, human leukocyte antigen (HLA) B54, HCV genotype 1b, HCV quasispecies complexity, and higher levels of HCV viremia.

Clinical features
- *Acute HCV:* 75% of infections are anicteric. Symptomatic infection is similar to acute HAV and HBV, but with lower transaminases.
- *Fulminant HCV* is unusual in Western countries but occurs in 40–60% of cases in Japan.
- *Chronic HCV* occurs in 85% of patients and is associated with fatigue, malaise, and reduced quality of life indices. ALT levels fluctuate independent of symptoms, whereas HCV RNA levels remain fairly

constant. It eventually progresses to cirrhosis, decompensated liver disease, and HCC.
- *Extrahepatic manifestations:* essential mixed cryoglobulinemia, membranoproliferative glomerulonephritis, sporadic porphyria cutanea tarda, Mooren's corneal ulcers, Sjögren's syndrome, lichen planus, idiopathic pulmonary fibrosis, thyroid hormone abnormalities

Diagnosis

- *Serology:* laboratory diagnosis is based on detection of antibody to recombinant HCV peptides using an EIA. Third-generation EIAs have an estimated sensitivity of 97% and can detect HCV antibody within 6–8 weeks. Infection is confirmed using recombinant immunblot assay (RIBA), which identifies the specific antigens to which the EIA is reacting and is positive if ≥2 antigens are detected.
- *Detection of viral RNA* indicates ongoing infection. HCV RNA can be detected by RT-PCR (Roche AMPLICOR HCV detection kit) or bDNA assays (Chiron Quantiplex HCV-RNA assay). RT-PCR assays are generally more sensitive. Various methods have been used to genotype HCV, but phylogenetic analysis of cDNA remains the gold standard.
- *Liver biopsy* remains the best method for assessing the severity of hepatitis C. Various grading systems exist that quantify the extent of inflammation and fibrosis, e.g., Knodell score. These are used to influence the decision to treat the disease.[1]
- *Elastography/fibroscan* is a new ultrasound method that is used to assess hepatic fibrosis in a noninvasive manner.

Treatment

The treatment of chronic HCV depends on histological stage and HCV genotype. Histologically mild disease does not require treatment. Moderate disease is treated with combination therapy.

Cirrhosis may also be treated with combination therapy, but complication rates are higher and response rates lower. Decompensated liver disease is an indication for hepatic transplantation.

- *INF-A and pegylated INF-*A (p. 85) have combined antiviral and immunomodulatory activity. It was the first drug to be licensed for the treatment of chronic HCV but sustained virological response rates (SVR, defined as HCV RNA-negative 6 months after end of treatment) were disappointing. Problems with IFN-α include the need to administer it by SC injection three times a week and its side effects, e.g., flu-like symptoms, bone marrow suppression, mood disturbance, and thyroid hormone abnormalities. PEG-IFN may be given once a week and is now the standard of care (in combination with ribavirin).
- *Ribavirin:* the mechanism of action of ribavirin, a guanosine analog, is not fully understood, but it has been shown to be of benefit in combination with IFN-α and PEG-IFN. Its main side effect is a hemolytic anemia, which is reversible.
- *Combination therapy:* the combination of IFN-α with ribavirin has resulted in improved SVR. The use of PEG-IFN has further improved SVR (genotypes 1 and 4, ~40%; genotypes 2 and 3, 70–80%).

- *Other therapies* that have been tried are iron-reduction therapy, parenteral thymosin-A1, oral amantadine, *N*-acetylcysteine, and ursodeoxycholate, but none have become generally accepted.

Prevention

The main methods to reduce the transmission of HCV infection are
- Screening of blood and blood products for HCV
- Improving adherence to universal infection control precautions
- Needle exchange programs for intravenous drug users

After a documented exposure, e.g., needlestick injury, the recipient should be screened for HCV antibodies immediately and at 6 months. No vaccine currently exists, and treatment is not indicated.

Reference

1. 2009 AASLD Guidelines. http://www.aasld.org/practiceguidelines

Hepatitis E virus

Hepatitis E virus (HEV) is an unclassified virus that is enterically transmitted and causes acute hepatitis. It is the most common cause of acute hepatitis in certain parts of Asia.

Infection with hepatitis E may be asymptomatic or range in severity from mild to fulminant hepatitis; the latter is more common in pregnant women and older men. There is no specific treatment.[1]

The virus

- *Structure:* HEV is a spherical, nonenveloped particle (30–32 nm diameter) with a surface structure intermediate between the Norwalk agent (a calicivirus) and hepatitis A virus (p. 358).
- *Genome:* a single-strand positive-sense RNA molecule approximately 7.2 kB in length. It encodes three open reading frames (ORFs): ORF1 encodes nonstructural proteins, ORF2 encodes the capsid, and ORF3 encodes an immunogenic protein of unknown function.
- *Classification:* HEV was originally classified as a calicivirus because of its morphology and genomic structure. However, its genomic sequence most closely resembles the rubella virus, a togavirus. HEV is the sole member of the genus *Hepevirus*. Four genotypes have been reported.

Epidemiology

- *Geographic distribution:* HEV is important in the developing world and is endemic in Southeast and Central Asia, the Middle East, and North and West Africa. Epidemic hepatitis E has been reported in Mexico.
- *Host range:* HEV has a wide host range and has been shown to experimentally infect New and Old World monkeys, swine, rodents, and sheep.
- *Routes of transmission:* most epidemics of HEV have been waterborne, but a few food-borne outbreaks have been reported. The epidemiological risk factors associated with sporadic transmission have not been identified. Zoonotic transmission, e.g., from swine,

may occur. Recent evidence suggests that HEV may be transmitted by blood transfusions.

- *Seroprevalence:* the presence of anti-HEV antibodies is lower than might be expected in endemic countries (15–60%) and higher than expected in nonendemic regions (1–28%). HEV seroprevalence is also low in infants and children, which is surprising for a virus transmitted by the feco-oral route. The greatest incremental increase in anti-HEV occurs in young adults, who are also most at risk of clinical disease. In older adults the prevalence is relatively constant at 10–40%.
- *Peak incidence* in 15- to 35-year-olds: men are more commonly affected.

Pathogenesis

The incubation period is 2–9 weeks. The duration of infectivity is not known, but the virus has been detected in feces 1–5 weeks after experimental infection in nonhuman primates, and protracted viremia of 45–112 days has been detected by PCR in naturally infected patients.

The replicative pathway is not fully understood, as HEV does not replicate well in cell culture.

The histological changes are characteristic: hepatoctye ballooning, cytoplasmic cholestasis, focal cytolytic necrosis, and pseudoglandular alteration.

Clinical features

Infection with hepatitis E may be asymptomatic or range in severity from mild to fulminant hepatitis. Acute HEV is clinically indistinguishable from other causes of viral hepatitis, with fever, nausea, vomiting, jaundice, and abdominal tenderness. The only complication is fulminant hepatitis, which is more common in pregnancy and older men and carries a high mortality (up to 20%).

Outcome can be poor in those with chronic liver disease (up to 70%). Recently chronic HEV infection has been reported in organ transplant recipients.

Diagnosis

Specific IgM and IgG responses occur early in the infection, usually by the onset of clinical illness. These can be detected using commercial tests based on ELISA or Western blot assays. Anti-HEV IgM can be detected in up to 96% of cases 1–4 weeks after acute infection. This response wanes, so that by 3 months, anti-HEV is only detectable in 50% of patient.

Anti-HEV IgG is also detectable 2–4 weeks after onset of illness; a single high titer or rising titers suggest recent infection. Molecular tests have been used to study the epidemiology of acute HEV infection and seem to be more sensitive than serology.

Treatment

There is no specific therapy, and treatment is supportive. Patients who develop liver failure should be referred for transplantation.

Prevention

Despite the fact the HEV appears to be less prevalent and less easily spread than HAV in developing countries, improved sanitation is likely to be important in the control of an infection that is predominantly spread by the feco-oral route. Pork should be cooked properly to prevent possible zoonotic transmission.

Attempts at passive immunoprophylaxis with pooled immune globulin derived from endemic areas have been generally unsuccessful. Several HEV vaccines are under development.

Reference

1. Dalton HR, Bendall R, Ijaz S, Banks M (2008). Hepatitis E: an emergency infection in developed countries. *Lancet Inf Dis* 8:698–709.

Novel hepatitis viruses

Further efforts to identify novel viruses have led to the discovery of other candidate viruses, the significance of which is debated.

Hepatitis G virus (HGBV-C or HGV)

This virus was independently identified by two groups. It is an RNA flavivirus that is spread by the parenteral route, by sexual intercourse and, to a lesser extent, from mother to child. It does not appear to be pathogenic in humans.

Other viruses

Many other viruses can induce hepatitis as one feature of a wider clinical syndrome. These include the following:

- Epstein–Barr virus (p. 347)
- Cytomegalovirus (p. 351)
- Herpes simplex virus (p. 341)
- Measles virus (p. 330)
- Rubella virus (p. 335)
- Coxsackie B virus
- Adenovirus (p. 379)
- Yellow fever virus (p. 399).

Differential diagnosis

Other nonviral infectious diseases may cause an acute hepatitis:

- Leptospirosis (p. 292)
- Syphilis (p. 286)
- Toxoplasmosis (p. 468)
- Q fever (p. 298).

Finally, noninfectious causes may also mimic viral hepatitis:

- Drug-induced hepatitis
- Anoxic liver injury
- Alcoholic hepatitis
- Cholestatic liver disease
- Wilson's disease
- Budd–Chiari syndrome
- Liver tumors.

HIV virology and immunology

Human immunodeficiency virus (HIV) is an enveloped RNA virus belonging to the retrovirus family.

Types and subtypes

There are two HIV types.

HIV-1 accounts for the majority of infections worldwide. HIV-1 is divided into seven subtypes or clades, designated A–K (referred to as the "M" subtypes) and O. There are now also circulating recombinant forms (CRFs); the major ones are CRF01_AE and CRF02_AG.

A new group of viruses labeled "N" (for new) was reported in 1998. The majority of infections in Europe and North America are caused by subtype B, whereas subtypes A, C, and D dominate in Africa.

HIV-2

HIV-2 occurs primarily in West Africa. It is less readily transmissible than HIV-1 and is associated with lower viral loads, higher CD4 counts, and slower disease progression than that of HIV-1. Laboratory confirmation is difficult, as 20–30% of patients have negative HIV antibody tests and there are no commercially available HIV-2 viral load assays.

Treatment is complicated, as there are no specific treatment guidelines. HIV-2 is not susceptible to non-nucleoside reverse transcriptase inhibitors (NNRTIs) (p. 91) and may have multiple protease inhibitor (PI) (p. 93) mutations.

Virus structure

The HIV-1 virion is composed of the following (Fig. 3.2):
- Viral envelope, constructed from host cell membrane, into which are inserted HIV-1 envelope proteins (e.g., gp41 and gp120) and host proteins (e.g., MHC class II molecules)
- Matrix, predominantly protein p17
- Core, containing viral RNA associated with protein p7; the enzymes reverse transcriptase, protease, and integrase; and the major structural proteins p6 and p24

The genomic structure of HIV consists of *gag-pol-env* genes flanked by two complete viral long tandem repeats (LTRs):
- gag gene products: p24, p17, p7, p6, p2, p1
- pol gene products: protease, reverse transcriptase, and integrase
- env gene products: gp120, gp 41

The virus also encodes several other genes of diverse function, e.g., *vif*, *vpr*, *tat*, *rev*, *vpu*, *nef* (HIV-1 only), and *vpx* (HIV-2 only).

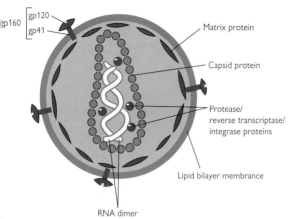

Fig. 3.2 HIV-1 virus structure.

Virus lifecycle

Infection is initiated by binding of the envelope protein gp120 to CD4 molecules found on some T cells, macrophages, and microglial cells. Binding is also mediated by a second receptor, usually CCR5 or CXCR4.

Fusion of the viral envelope with the host cell membrane results in release of the viral core into the cytoplasm.

Viral cDNA is produced by reverse transcription and integrated into the host genome to form proviral DNA.

In the presence of appropriate host cell stimulation, the viral 5' LTR produces viral mRNA transcripts.

New virions are released from the host cell membrane by budding.

Immunology

HIV infection is associated with a wide array of immune dysfunction:
• CD4+ T-cell depletion is the hallmark of disease and results in the development opportunistic infections.
• After primary infection, CD8+ T cells rebound and may remain elevated until late in disease.
• Cells of the monocyte–macrophage lineage serve as a reservoir of infection, are central to the pathogenesis of HIV-associated CNS disease, and contribute to impaired host defenses against intracellular pathogens, e.g., *M. tuberculosis*.
• HIV infection is usually associated with B-cell hyperactivation and hypergammaglobulinemia.
• Abnormalities of neutrophil function occur at all stages of HIV infection and predispose to *Candida* infections.
• Abnormalities of NK cells also increase with disease progression.

See p. 735–747 for clinical manifestations of HIV and drug treatment of HIV.

HIV laboratory tests

HIV infection may be established by a number of methods:
- Serology (detecting antibodies to the virus)
- Detection of viral antigens
- Detection of viral RNA/DNA
- Virus culture

HIV serology – the "HIV test"

This is the most commonly used diagnostic test. Indications include adult in populations with an estimated prevalence >1%, pregnant women, sexual assault victims, occupational exposure, and anyone who requests an HIV test.

The standard test consists of a screening EIA followed by a confirmatory Western blot; this has a sensitivity of 99.5% and a specificity of 99.9% in patients with established disease (>3 months after transmission).

False-negative results occur in <0.001% (low-prevalence populations) to 0.3% (high-prevalence populations). Causes include testing in the window period before seroconversion (up to 6 months), seroreversion (occurs rarely in advanced disease), atypical host response, agammaglobulinemia types N, O, or HIV-2 infection, and technical or clerical error.

False-positive results occur in 0.0004% to 0.0007%. Causes include autoantibodies, HIV vaccines, factitious HIV infection, and technical or clerical error.

Alternative serological tests include immunofluorescence assay (IFA), rapid tests (e.g., OraQuick, UniGold Recombigen, Reveal G2, Multispot HIV-1/HIV-2), and home kits (e.g., Home Access Express Test).

Viral detection

This may also be used to establish HIV infection when serological tests are likely to be misleading, e.g., early HIV infection (prior to seroconversion), agammaglobulinemia, and neonatal HIV infection.

- *HIV-1 DNA PCR:* qualitative DNA PCR is used to detect cell-associated proviral DNA, including HIV reservoirs in peripheral CD4 cells in patients on HAART. It is highly sensitive (>99%) and can detect 1–10 copies of HIV proviral DNA. It is not Food and Drug Administration (FDA) approved.
- *HIV-1 RNA PCR:* these assays are 95–98% sensitive; this depends on viral load, threshold of assay, and status of antiretroviral therapy. False-positive tests occur in 2–9%, usually at lower titers, e.g., <10,000 copies/mL.
- *p24 antigen* is sometimes used as an alternative to HIV RNA PCR to diagnose acute HIV infection. It is cheaper, but sensitivity is poor (30–90%) compared with that of quantitative HIV RNA tests. It is also sometimes used as a low-cost viral load test in resource-limited settings.

Quantitative plasma HIV-1 RNA (viral load)

Quantitative HIV RNA is useful for the following:

- Diagnosing acute HIV infection (in neonates and prior to seroconversion)
- Predicting rate of disease progression
- Monitoring treatment
- Predicting probability of transmission

There are multiple commercially available assays:
- *Standard RT-PCR assays* (Amplicor HIV-Monitor test version 1.5, Roche). Dynamic ranges are 400–750,000 copies/mL (standard assay) or 50–100,000 copies/mL (ultrasensitive assay).
- *Real-time RT-PCR assays:* COBAS AmpliPrep/TaqMan HIV-1 test (dynamic range 48–10,000,000 copies/mL); Abbot RealTime HIV-1 test (dynamic range 40–10,000,000 copies/mL).
- *Branched-chain DNA (bDNA) assay* (Versant RNA 3.0 assay, Bayer). Dynamic range is 75–500,000 copies/mL.
- *Nucleic acid sequence–based amplification (NASBA) assay* or Nuclisens HIV-QT, bioMérieux). Dynamic range is 176–3,500,000 copies/mL and it can be used on various body fluids or tissue.

Testing should be done at baseline and then usually every 3–4 months. The target of therapy is an undetectable viral load. The time to viral load nadir depends on pretreatment viral load, potency of the regimen, adherence, pharmacology, and resistance.

An expected response is a reduction in viral load by 1 $\log_{10}$ copies/mL at 1 week. Failure to achieve a reduction in viral load of 1 $\log_{10}$ copies/mL at 4 weeks suggests nonadherence, inadequate drug exposure, or pre-existing resistance. Failure to achieve a reduction in viral load of 1 $\log_{10}$ copies/mL at 8 weeks constitutes virological failure (U.S. guidelines).

CD4 T-lymphocyte count

The CD4 count is used to assess prognosis for progression to AIDS (see Table 4.20 p. 733) and to guide therapeutic decisions regarding antiretroviral treatment and prophylaxis for opportunistic infections.

The standard method involves flow cytometry, which relies on fresh cells and is expensive. An alternative system (TRAX CD4 Test Kit) uses EIA technology and may be more suitable for resource-limited settings.

The normal mean value is 800–1050 cells/mm³ (range 500–1400 cells/mm³). There is considerable analytical variability in CD4 test results, e.g., the 95% confidence interval for a true count of 200 cells/mm³ is 118–337 cells/mm³. CD4 counts may be influenced by seasonal and diurnal variation, intercurrent illnesses, and corticosteroids.

The CD4 count is usually tested every 3–6 months in untreated patients and every 2–4 months in patients on treatment. The CD4 count typically increases by ≥50 cells/mm³ at 4–8 weeks after viral suppression with HAART, and then 50–100 cells/mm³ per year thereafter. Factors that correlate with a good response include a high baseline viral load and low baseline CD4 count.

Resistance testing

The prevalence of ≥1 major resistance mutation in treatment-naive patients is 10–25% and in patients receiving HAART is about 50%.

Limitations of resistance testing
- Resistance assays measure only the dominant species at the time the test is performed; resistant variants that account for <20% in sequestered havens, e.g., CNS, latent CD4 cells, genital tract, will not be detected.
- There must be a sufficient viral load to perform the tests, usually ≥500–1000 copies/mL.
- Genotypic assays are often difficult to interpret because multiple mutations are required for agents other than lamivudine and NNRTIs.
- Phenotypic assays are difficult to interpret because of arbitrary thresholds used to define susceptibility, e.g., for ritonavir-boosted regimens. They are also less sensitive at detecting emerging resistance.
- Clinical trials with resistance tests compared with standard care for selection of salvage regimens have shown variable results.

Indications for resistance testing
- Acute HIV infection
- Chronic infection, treatment naive
- Virological failure
- Pregnancy

Genotypic assays
- Identify mutations associated with phenotypic resistance
- May be performed by commercial kits or in-house assays
- Methodology involves amplification of the reverse transcriptase, protease, and integrase genes by RT-PCR. DNA sequencing of amplicons is generated for the dominant species, as well as reporting of mutations for each gene using a letter-number-letter standard, e.g., K103N.
- Interpretation requires expertise—see http://www.iasusa.org or http://hivdb.stanford.edu for more information.

Phenotypic assays
- Measure the ability of HIV to replicate at different concentrations of tested drugs
- Methodology involves insertion of reverse transcriptase and protease genes from the patient's strain into a laboratory clone, and monitoring of replication at various drug concentrations compared with a reference wild-type virus.
- Interpretation is more straightforward, as results are reported as IC_{50} for the test strain relative to the reference strain.
- Phenotypic resistance testing is more expensive and time consuming than genotypic testing but useful in treatment-experienced patents.

Enterovirus

The genus *Enterovirus* includes polio, Coxsackie A and B, and the echoviruses. Here we consider the non-polio enteroviruses, causes of a large number of different clinical syndromes. They account for the majority of childhood fever-rash syndromes and are important causes of meningitis, myocarditis, and neonatal sepsis. For discussion of polio, see Poliovirus (p. 390).

The viruses

These small RNA viruses, family *Picornaviridae* (*pico* = very small), are identical in appearance to another genus of the same family, rhinoviruses.

Most are identified in stool during polio research. Historically they have been divided into subgroups: polioviruses, group A and B Coxsackie viruses, and echoviruses (**e**nteric **c**ytopathic **h**uman **o**rphan viruses). New enteroviruses are now simply numbered sequentially.

Some clinical syndromes are caused by many enteroviral types (e.g., rashes and meningitis); others are associated with specific enteroviruses (e.g., Coxsackie B and pericarditis).

Epidemiology

Enteroviruses are found worldwide throughout the year, but in temperate climates infections peak in the summer and autumn months.

Three-quarters of cases occur in those under 15 years old, with attack rates highest in those under 1 year. Over 90% of non-polio enteroviral infections are asymptomatic or cause only a mild febrile illness.

Pathogenesis

Infection may take place via the respiratory tract but is mainly feco-oral.

Viral replication occurs in respiratory and GI epithelium, passing to regional lymph nodes. Patients become viremic (usually undetectable).

Most individuals clear the infection and experience no symptoms. A minority experience further viral replication at distant reticulendothelial sites and a secondary viremia that coincides with their nonspecific illness. This major viremia sees dissemination to other organs, e.g., CNS.

Humoral immunity is the main host defense. People with an isolated cell-mediated immune deficiency are not predisposed to severe enteroviral illness. Virus is shed in feces for weeks after symptoms resolution.

Clinical features

Aseptic meningitis

Manifestations of enteroviral meningitis vary with host age and (particularly humoral) immune state.

Neonates

Fever, vomiting, rash, anorexia, upper respiratory tract symptoms, and altered mental state can occur. Meningeal signs are uncommon and presentation is usually nonspecific. Severe meningoencephalitis is a rare manifestation (death rate 10%) and may be associated with hepatic necrosis, myocarditis, and necrotizing enterocolitis.

Older children and adults

Severe disease is rare. It commonly manifests as sudden fever (may be biphasic, with a gap as long as 2–10 days), nuchal rigidity, headache, photophobia, and nonspecific features (e.g., vomiting, anorexia, diarrhea, upper respiratory tract symptoms). Those with humoral immune deficiency can develop a chronic meningoencephalitis that may last for years and is often ultimately fatal.

There may be general features of enteroviral infection (e.g., pharyngitis) as well as those specific to the infecting enterovirus (characteristic rashes, pericarditis. In uncomplicated disease, the illness usually lasts a week. Sequelae are rare in those beyond the neonatal period.

Other neurological syndromes
- *Encephalitis:* lethargy, drowsiness, seizures, paresis, coma. Features can be focal (particularly with Coxsackie A infection): focal motor seizures, cerebellar ataxia, hemichorea
- *Paralysis:* sporadic flaccid paralysis has been seen with Coxsackie A7 and enterovirus 71, among others. It is less severe than that seen with polio and rarely permanent. Guillain–Barré syndrome is associated with certain Coxsackie A and echovirus types. Other neurological manifestations include transverse myelitis and opsoclonus-myoclonus.

Other manifestations of enteroviral disease
Rashes include herpangina and hand-foot-and-mouth disease. Respiratory features are URTI and epidemic pleurodynia (spasmodic rib pain and fever). Cardiac manifestation is myopericarditis, and ophthalmological is acute hemorrhagic conjunctivitis.

Diagnosis
See above referenced sections for diagnosis of non-neurological disease.

CSF is clear and pressure is usually normal to slightly raised. White cell count is raised: initially neutrophils, but lymphocytes dominate within 6–48 hours of symptoms. Higher counts are associated with a greater likelihood of viral identification. A slight rise in CSF protein and depression in CSF glucose may be seen.

Viral identification by culture is not sensitive (around 30%) because of the low viral titer in CSF. RT-PCR is more sensitive (60–90%) and over 94% specific for diagnosing enteroviral meningitis.

Concomitant culture from sites other than CSF may aid diagnosis. However, virus is shed from some parts of the body for several weeks after infection has resolved, and during viral seasons enterovirus is produced by 7.5% of healthy controls.

Treatment
Exclude bacterial etiology of suspected meningitis. Otherwise, treatment rests on symptom relief.

Immunocompromised people with persistent enteroviral infection may benefit from immunoglobulin.

Antiviral agents are in development. One of these, pleconaril, interferes with the viral capsid protein, altering attachment and uncoating. It reduces illness duration in adults with enteroviral meningitis.

Lymphocytic choriomeningitis virus

Lymphocytic choriomeningitis virus (LCMV) is found worldwide. It is an ssRNA virus (family *Arenaviridae*) and causes an asymptomatic infection in mice (its reservoir). Human cases are rare, and one-third of such infections are subclinical; 50% of clinical infections have neurological involvement.

Infection is by inhalation or consumption of infected excreta and it typically causes a febrile, self-limited, biphasic disease. Individuals exposed to rodents (living conditions, pet handlers, lab personnel) are at risk for the infection. Transmission of infection during organ transplantation has occurred.

Primary viremia leads to CNS infection and a nonspecific febrile illness with rash and lymphadenopathy. Secondary viremia follows a few days later and is associated with meningitis/meningoencephalitis. Clinical course is benign with <1% of cases being fatal.

It is a significant teratogen. Acquired congenitally it produces similar abnormalities to congenital CMV; 35% of congenital infections are thought to lead to fetal loss; 84% of surviving infants have neurodevelopmental sequelae (e.g., cerebral palsy, seizures, mental retardation, visual problems, hydrocephalus).

Togaviridae

This family of viruses contains two key genera: *Rubivirus* (containing just rubella, p. 335) and *Alphavirus*. The alphaviruses are considered here.

The virus

Lipid-enveloped virions contain 11–12 kB positive-stranded RNA.

Epidemiology

All medically significant alphaviruses are vector borne (they were once called the group A arboviruses). "New World" viruses predominantly cause encephalitis and circulate in North and South America. "Old World" viruses cause predominantly fever, rash, and arthropathy. Geographic spread is determined by the distribution of their vectors.

Only some of the many viruses identified are known to cause human disease or cause only a rare and mild fever-arthropathy.

Some are maintained in an animal-vector cycle (e.g., eastern equine encephalitis [EEE]: birds and mosquito), with a third party vector transmitting to other animals (e.g., horses) or humans. Animal infections may precede human ones; animal health surveillance can warn of human outbreaks.

Humans can develop a viremia significant enough to infect mosquitos with some agents (Venezuelan equine encephalitis [VEE]) but not others (EEE).

Pathogenesis

Incubation is 1–12 days. Bite of an infected mosquito deposits virus in the subcutaneous tissues. VEE has been acquired by aerosol in the lab.

Non-neurotropic agents cause viremia, skin lesions (lymphocytic perivascular cuffing and red cell leak from superficial capillaries), arthralgia, and an inflammatory frank arthritis (aspirates are inflammatory—no virus is present).

Neutrotropic viruses cause viremia and fever in early infection, indicating replication in non-neural tissues. Infection of capillary endothelial cells is thought to allow subsequent CNS invasion. Acute encephalitis follows and lesions may be seen throughout the brain and spinal cord. Transplacental spread can occur with VEE and western equine encephalitis (WEE).

Clinical features

- *Encephalitis:* headache, high fever, chills, nausea and vomiting. Respiratory symptoms may be seen with WEE. In cases with CNS involvement (<1% adults, 4% children), confusion and somnolence follow within a few days. Seizures are more common in the young. Infants may develop bulging fontanelles. CSF protein and lymphocyte counts are high. Sequelae (70% infants after EEE, 30% WEE) include mental retardation, behavior change, and paralysis. Case fatality rate is <1% overall, 20% for encephalitis cases.
- *Fever, rash, arthritis:* rapid-onset fever (up to 40°C) and chills may last several days, remit, then recur (saddle-back fever chart). Rash usually appears on day 1 (can be late). A face and neck flush evolves to maculopapular lesions on the trunk, limbs, face, palms and soles and may be pruritic. Arthralgia lasts a week to a few months, is polyarticular, and affects small joints, which may be swollen. Other features include headache, photophobia, and sore throat. Long-term joint problems may be associated with HLA B27.

Diagnosis

- History: the epidemiology of each disease is fairly specific (Table 3.22).
- Acute and convalescent serology

Treatment and prevention

There is no specific therapy. Prevention depends on vector control and mosquito avoidance. Vaccines exist for EEE, WEE, VEE, and chikungunya, in limited human use.

Table 3.22 Clinical syndromes caused by alphaviruses

Name	Location	Vector	Features
New World: cause predominantly encephalitis			
Eastern equine encephalitis (EEE)	Eastern and Gulf Coast U.S., southern Canada, and northern South America	Enzoonotic vector: *Culiseta melanura*, breeds in freshwater swamps and feeds on birds (which become infected but may be asymptomatic). Vectors to human: *Aedes* and others	Summer disease of horses, children and elderly. Rare, but case fatality over 50%
Western equine encephalitis (WEE)	North and South America	*Culex tarsalis*	Summertime disease of horses and humans. Highest incidence in infants
Venezuelan equine encephalitis	South and Central America	Many different mosquito species	Rainy season; human disease follows horse by 1–2 weeks. Severest in children
Old World: cause predominantly fever, rash, and polyarthritis			
Chikungunya	Africa and Asia	*Aedes stegomyia* and *A. aegypti.*	Sporadic outbreaks (90% population seropositive in Sub-Saharan Africa)
O'nyong-nyong	Africa	*Anopheles*	Fever and rash
Mayaro	South America, Caribbean	*Haemagogus* and others	
Sindbis	Africa, Scandinavia, CIS, Asia	*Culex* maintains a bird cycle, several species infect humans	Outbreaks occur at times of rainfall and flooding
Ross river	Australia, Oceania		Epidemic polyarthritis. Joint symptoms can last up to 3 years after infection.

Bunyaviridae

The virus
There are four genera: *Bunyavirus*, *Phlebovirus*, *Nairovirus*, and *Hantavirus*. They are spherical, lipid membrane-contained viruses containing three negative-sense RNA segments coding for around six proteins.

Epidemiology
- *California encephalitis (CE) viruses:* CE is the most common childhood CNS infection in the United States. La Crosse virus is the main cause. The virus is maintained in the mosquito vector population by transovarial transmission, and each summer the infected mosquito mass increases as they feed on viremic squirrels, foxes, etc.
- *Rift Valley fever (RVF):* maintained in Sub-Saharan Africa by transovarial transmission in some *Aedes* species. Infected eggs in the soil remain viable for years, hatching in heavy rains. Sheep and cattle amplify infection.
- *Congo–Crimean hemorrhagic fever (CCHF):* tick transmission. It may also be acquired through infection with infected animals that may be asymptomatic (cattle and sheep).
- *Hantaviruses:* each viral species has a principal rodent host. They become chronically infected and excrete virus in urine and saliva for months. Infection is acquired through animal bite or aerosols of virus-contaminated urine or feces.

Clinical features

California encephalitis
Most human infections are asymptomatic. Incubation is 3–7 days, then fever, encephalitis, or meningoencephalitis occurs. Severity ranges from mild viral meningitis to a severe disease similar to herpes encephalitis. Aphasia, ataxia, paralysis and convulsions (50% cases) can occur.

CT is usually normal, MRI may be positive, EEG is usually abnormal; 90% of La Crosse virus cases occur in those under 15 years old. Mortality in acute disease is around 1%. Sequelae include EEG abnormalities (75% at 1–5 years), epilepsy (10%), and emotional lability (10%).

Rift Valley fever
This is a febrile illness, with 10% experiencing retinitis and vasculitis that can cause a permanent loss of vision; 1% develop fulminant disease after 3–6 days of fever, with hemorrhage and hepatitis. Half of these patients die. There are rare cases of severe encephalitis.

Congo–Crimean hemorrhagic fever
There is shock, DIC, bleeding, and thrombocytopenia. Mortality is 20–50%.

Hantavirus
Hemorrhagic fever with renal syndrome occurs after incubation of 5–40 days. Patients develop fever, thrombocytopenia, and acute renal failure (interstitial nephritis).

In the severe form (Hantaan virus), a toxic phase (headache, back pain, fever, blurred vision, erythematous rash, and petechiae) may be followed by severe shock. Those surviving can have prolonged renal insufficiency (oliguria, electrolyte, and acid–base abnormalities, then polyuria), bleeding, and pneumonitis. Mortality is 5% with Hantaan infection—one-third in the shock phase, two-thirds in the renal phase.

The milder form (Puumala virus), fatal in less than 1% of clinical cases, is hantavirus pulmonary syndrome: a 4- to 5-day febrile prodrome is followed by pulmonary edema and shock. If hypoxia and shock are well managed, the vascular leak resolves in a few days. Thrombocytopenia may be seen.

Diagnosis
Diagnosis of CE and *Hantavirus* infection is serological.

CCHF and RVF viruses are detected using PCR from the blood of infected patients. Antigen detection by ELISA may be useful in severe cases, but the aerosol infection risk limits its usefulness. Culture needs to be conducted in biosafety level 4 laboratories. Antibodies can be detected at 5–14 days, coinciding with clinical improvement.

Treatment and prevention
There are no vaccines in general use, and prevention is through public health measures to reduce vector numbers, and personal avoidance.

Ribavirin has been used effectively in treating *Hantavirus* infection, and evidence suggests it has a role in the therapy of RVF and CCHF.

Supportive measures include anticonvulsants, fluids, and circulatory and renal support.

Adenovirus

Adenovirus is a cause of acute infections of the respiratory tract and conjunctivae.

The virus
This DNA virus of around 70 nm diameter has a complex outer capsid consisting of 252 subunits forming a 20-sided icosahedron.

The three different types of subunits (hexons, pentons, and fibers) differ immunologically: some antigenic sites are common to all adenoviruses, others are type specific.

There are around 50 human serotypes, some of which are associated with specific clinical syndromes. Similar viruses are found in some animals.

Epidemiology
Adenovirus infection is worldwide, with different geographic areas seeing different syndromes associated with different serotypes. Transmission is via respiratory and feco-oral routes.

Most people have experienced at least one infection by age 10 years; 75% of all infectious illnesses in U.S. infants may be attributable to adenovirus.

Infecting serotype and consequent disease are related to age. Types 1, 2, 5, and 6 are more common in young children (cause URTI); types 3, 4, and 7, in young adults (URTI and LRTI); types 8 and 19 cause adult eye infections.

Pathogenesis

The virus generally causes lytic infection of epithelial cells, resulting in cell death with the release of up to 1 million progeny (up to 5% are infective).

Latent or chronic infection can be demonstrated in lymphoid cells (e.g., tonsils), where only small numbers of virus are released.

Oncogenic transformation is demonstrated experimentally in animals and tissue culture. Viral DNA integrates with host DNA. No infectious virus is produced.

Clinical features

- *Respiratory infection:* serological surveys suggest adenovirus causes 10% of all childhood respiratory infections in the developed world. Incubation is around 4–5 days, and illness takes the form of mild pharyngitis/tracheitis (cough, fever, sore throat and rhinorrhea) or, less commonly in infants, bronchiolitis and atypical pneumonia (serotype 7). Most cases improve over 3–5 days.
- *Pharyngoconjunctival fever* (serotype 3): a syndrome occurring in outbreaks among children and characterized by the acute onset of conjunctivitis, pharyngitis, fever, and adenitis. Initially it affects one eye, the other usually becoming involved. Symptoms last 3–5 days, bacterial superinfection is uncommon, and there is no permanent eye damage. Respiratory involvement rarely progresses to the lungs. Contaminated swimming areas have been implicated in some outbreaks.
- *Epidemic keratoconjunctivitis* (serotypes 8, 19, 37): a slow-onset, usually bilateral conjunctivitis, seen in adults and acquired through such routes as contaminated hand towels and ophthalmic solutions. Incubation is 4–24 days with the subsequent development of keratitis. The cornea may be involved for several months. Secondary spread to household contacts occurs in 10% of cases.
- *Hemorrhagic cystitis* (type 7, 11, 21): seen in children (males more than females) and causes around 3 days of macroscopic hematuria. The means of infection is unclear. It is also seen in children and adults undergoing BMT.
- *Infantile diarrhea* (serotype 40, 41): a common cause of watery diarrhea and fever lasting up to 2 weeks. There are distinct causative serotypes. Certain of the common respiratory adenoviruses may be associated with intussusception.
- *Intussusception* (serotype 1, 2, 3, 5): adenovirus was isolated in over 40% of intussusception cases in one series.
- *Encephalitis/meningoencephalitis* (serotypes 7, 1, 6, 12): pneumonia is often an associated finding. Chronic meningoencephalitis occurs in patients with hypogammaglobulinemia.

- *The immunosuppressed:* those undergoing BMT or solid-organ transplant are at increased risk of adenoviral infection, both of the organ system transplanted and through disseminated disease (e.g., lung, gut, CNS). Dissemination is most common in children but occurs in adults and has a high mortality. Adenovirus may be detected in those with AIDS (particularly in the urine or GI tract), and diseases such as colitis, parotitis, and encephalitis have been attributed to it. The significance is not clear, as most patients are asymptomatic.
- *Other:* fatal dissemination in neonates, pericarditis, congenital abnormalities

Diagnosis

- *Culture:* it is easy to culture virus from respiratory specimens, stool, urine, and conjunctival scrapings. Typical cytopathic changes are seen in human epithelial monolayers at 2–7 days. Isolated virus can be grouped by hemagglutination and serotyped.
- *Antigen detection:* indirect immunofluorescence allows detection of virus quickly and cheaply and correlates well with culture.
- *Serology:* infection is demonstrated by a fourfold rise in antibodies between acute and convalescent samples, as demonstrated by complement fixation (group specific), viral neutralization (serotype specific), or ELISA.

Treatment and prevention

Most infections are self-limited.

There is no proven benefit of antiviral treatments. There are anecdotal reports suggesting a beneficial effect in severe cases from agents such as ribavirin, ganciclovir, cidofovir, or immunoglobulin.

Effective vaccines have been developed and have been used in the U.S. military but are generally not available.

Human herpesvirus type 8

HHV-8 is a herpes virus associated with several human neoplasms, most importantly Kaposi sarcoma (KS).

The virus

The virus is a gammaherpesvirus (like EBV), first identified in KS tissue from patients infected with HIV.

Epidemiology

KS was first recognized in the 1870s among those of Mediterranean and Eastern European descent. Later, a more aggressive form was recognized across black populations of eastern Africa. In the 1980s, clusters of KS among gay men contributed to the recognition of HIV. It has also been seen in solid-organ transplant recipients.

HHV-8 has since been identified in lesions from all forms of KS. Epidemiological studies suggest a sexual route of HHV-8 transmission.

More than 95% of HIV-associated KS cases are in gay men in whom it is up to 15 times more common than in those acquiring HIV nonsexually.

Serological studies are conflicting: two studies in the United States gave seropositive rates of 2% or 25% in healthy adults, 25% or 90% in gay HIV-positive men without KS, and 80% or 100% of KS patients.

HHV-8 DNA has been detected in the semen and saliva of HIV-infected patients with KS and not in healthy controls.

Pathogenesis

The sites of replication are not known, but viral DNA has been detected in leukocytes, which suggests they may be involved in viral dissemination.

It encodes cell cycle regulatory proteins and cytokine homologs, which probably contribute to the pathogenesis of KS and other malignancies.

KS lesions consist of inflammatory, endothelial, and red blood cells.

Clinical features of Kaposi sarcoma

Lesions are vascular, often nodular (0.5–2 cm diameter) and appear on skin, mucous membrane, or viscera (lung and biliary tract particularly). They are violaceous or brown/black in pigmented skin. Visceral disease may involve any organ (e.g., gastrointestinal, which can bleed, pulmonary, producing effusions). Lymphedema may follow lymph node infiltration.

Endemic KS is slow growing and has little prognostic significance.

In AIDS patients with KS, the health impact of the lesions is generally of less importance than that of opportunistic infections.

Diagnosis

Diagnosis is clinical and histological.

Treatment

Isolated lesions can be observed. Individual lesions of cosmetic impact can be irradiated or intralesional vinblastine administered. Other indications for treatment include lymphedema, bulky lesions in the oropharynx, and pulmonary disease. Extensive disease may be treated with recombinant INF-A or single cytotoxic agents (doxorubicin or vinblastine). Life-threatening disease may require combination chemotherapy.

Antiviral agents have not yet been demonstrated to be of benefit. HIV patients with KS require HAART. Taxanes (e.g., paclitaxel) have antiangiogenic properties and may be beneficial.

Other malignancies associated with HHV-8

- *Primary effusion lymphoma* is an uncommon, aggressive B-cell lymphoma seen in AIDS patients and presenting as lymphomatous effusions arising predominantly in the pleural, pericardial, or peritoneal cavities.
- *Castleman's disease* is an angiofollicular lymph node hyperplasia. Localized forms are benign and may be cured by surgical excision. Multicentric disease is associated with HIV and is aggressive and usually fatal.
- *Other:* inconclusive claims have been made of HHV-8 isolation in some skin cancers and certain cases of multiple myeloma.

Human papillomavirus

HPV is a group of viruses producing epithelial tumors of the skin and mucous membranes and associated with genital tract malignancies. Seventy percent of cervical cancers in women worldwide are associated with infection by HPV-16 and HPV-18.

The virus

These are nonenveloped dsDNA viruses of the *Papillomavirus* genus of the family *Papovaviridae*. They are identified in many vertebrates and are highly species specific.

The genome comprises a noncoding regulatory region, an early region involved in viral transcription and regulation, and a late region that codes capsid proteins. Certain viral early proteins have transforming properties and may contribute to the development of malignancy.

More than 100 HPV types have been identified by DNA sequence homology. They vary in the pathological process with which they are associated (Table 3.23).

Pathogenesis

All types of squamous epithelium may be infected by HPV. Warts develop around 3 months (range 6 weeks to 2 year) after inoculation.

Virus infects the basal cells of the stratum germinativum, with replication and viral assembly taking place as basal cells mature and move to surface. Virions are shed along with dead keratinocytes.

Warts and condylomata are associated with proliferation of epidermal layers, resulting in acanthosis and hyperkeratosis. Some infected cells may develop characteristic perinuclear vacuolation—koilocytosis.

HPV DNA may be found in normal-looking cells, accounting for recurrence after treatment for warts. Excessive proliferation of the basal layer is a premalignant feature. DNA is extrachromosomal in benign disease but usually integrated in malignancy.

Table 3.23 Clinical spectrum of HPV disease

Clinical manifestation	Most common HPV types
Cutaneous warts	1, 2, 3, 10
Warts in meat and fish handlers	7, 2
Epidermolysis verruciformis	2, 3, 10, 5, 8, 9, 12, 14, 15, 17
Condylomata acuminata	6, 11
Low-grade intraepithelial neoplasia	6, 11
High-grade intraepithelial neoplasia and cervical carcinoma	16, 18
Recurrent respiratory papillomatosis	6, 11

Disease occurs at increased frequency and severity in those with immunodeficiencies (primary, lymphoproliferative disease, HIV) and receiving immunosuppressive therapy and may be more severe in pregnancy.

Antibodies are often raised against HPV. Their significance is uncertain.

Clinical features

Cutaneous warts

Groups at risk of developing warts include butchers and fish handlers. Close personal contact may be important in transmission, with minor trauma at the infection site facilitating infection. The warts are asymptomatic but may become painful and resolve in 90% by 5 years. Very rarely do they progress to verrucous carcinoma.

Common warts (71%) occur frequently among school-aged children, with a well-defined, exophytic appearance. They are commonly found on the back of the hand, between fingers, and on palms and soles. They may coalesce.

Plantar (and palmar) warts (34%) are most common among adolescents and young adults. They appear as raised bundles of fibers and are often painful. Planar warts (4%) are irregular, slightly elevated papules seen in childhood.

Epidermodysplasia verruciformis

This rare genetic condition is characterized by the appearance of disseminated cutaneous warts in early life (under 10 years old), with a high incidence of malignant transformation (one-third of patients in young adulthood). It is associated with a relatively specific group of HPV types. The warts vary in appearance.

Anogenital warts

This is the most common viral sexually transmitted infection (STI), with highest rates in women aged 16–19 years and in men aged 20–24 years. Incidence is increased in those with many partners or not using barrier contraception. Around 66% of those having sex with an individual with warts will develop them within 3 months.

Young children may develop genital warts from hand contact with non-genital lesions. Their presence should, however, prompt consideration of abuse. Seventy-five per cent of patients with anogenital warts are asymptomatic, with the remainder experiencing itching, burning, and tenderness. Appearance is of exophytic papules, which may be sessile or pedunculated, small (<1 mm), or coalesce into large plaques.

In men, the most commonly affected area in uncircumcised men is the preputial cavity (85%); in circumcised men the penile shaft is more commonly involved. Other sites include urethral meatus, distal urethra, and perianal involvement (common in gay men, low in heterosexual men). There is an increased risk of anal cancer with a history of anal warts.

Women are mostly affected over the posterior introitus, the labia, and the clitoris. The application of 3% acetic acid may whiten vulval lesions. The presence of external genital warts should prompt the consideration of cervical HPV and cervical intraepithelial neoplasia (CIN). Genital warts may spontaneously remit (approximately 10% of cases over 4 months).

Lesions can become very large, particularly during pregnancy or when immunosuppressed. They may cause local destruction, enter the spectrum of CIN, or, rarely, transform into invasive squamous cell carcinoma. CIN has a highly variable outcome depending on the HPV type and grade of tumor (grade 1, 60% regress, 1% become invasive; grade 3, 33% regress, 12% progress).

Recurrent respiratory papillomatosis
This disease of the larynx and airways exists in two forms: juvenile and adult onset.

Juvenile infection is probably acquired intrapartum. Median age at onset is 3 years. Patients present with hoarseness or an altered cry. Disease may spread to the trachea and lungs, resulting in obstruction, stridor, infection, and respiratory compromise. It may require surgical excision.

Adult disease is associated with a high number of sexual partners and oral–genital contact. Presentation is less aggressive; malignant transformation occurs rarely.

Other
Other clinical features include conjunctival papillomas, epidermoid cysts, and coinfection with EBV in oral hairy leukoplakia in HIV-infected patients.

Diagnosis
Diagnosis is usually made from clinical examination assisted by use of colposcopy and 3% acetic acid.

Biopsy may be indicated to confirm diagnosis. HPV antigen detection and PCR-based tests are available.

Prevention
Two vaccines are FDA cleared for use in the United States. Gardasil® targets the four types of HPV that cause cervical cancer and warts (16, 18, 6, and 11). Another bivalent vaccine (Cevarix®, for types 16–18) is also available. Both vaccines have high efficacy against infection, CIN, and consequent HPV-associated cervical cancer.

Guidelines for their use have been set forth by various committees, the main differences being the target age range for immunization. For greatest efficacy, young women would need to be vaccinated prior to becoming sexually active.

Barrier contraception may reduce HPV transmission during intercourse.

Cervical smears are essential in detecting premalignant change.

Treatment
- *Cutaneous warts:* most cutaneous warts undergo spontaneous resolution. The two main treatment modalities for hand warts are daily salicylic acid–based preparations or cryotherapy every 3 weeks. Both achieve cure in up to 70% of cases. Salicylic acid cures around 80% of deep plantar warts, but only 50% of mosaic plantar warts. Other modalities exist: curettage, cryotherapy, and electrosurgery.

- *Anogenital warts:* treatments include the use of local caustic agents (e.g., podophylum or trichloroacetic acid), crytotherapy, electrosurgery, and surgical excision.
- *Epidermodysplasia verruciformis:* lesions should be carefully observed and malignant lesions treated rapidly.
- *Recurrent respiratory papillomatosis:* endoscopic crytotherapy or laser surgery. There may be a role for INF-A and cidofovir.

Polyomaviruses

These viruses cause widespread infection that is asymptomatic in the majority, but are important causes of disease in the immunosuppressed.

The virus

Polyomaviruses are members of the *Papovaviridae* family (small, nonenveloped viruses with dsDNA genomes). There are two genera: *Polyomavirus* and *Papillomavirus*. Polyomaviruses are found in humans, monkeys, and mice and are relatively species specific.

Two of the human polyomaviruses, BK and JC, are named with initials of the patient in whom each was first identified. JCV is associated with progressive multifocal leucoencephalopathy (PML), BKV with post–renal transplant urethral stenosis. They have around 75% nucleotide homology.

Epidemiology

From 60 to 80% of European adults have antibodies to JCV, BKV, or both. BKV infection probably occurs at around age 4 years and JCV infection at age 10 years. There is no evidence of perinatal infection.

Immunosuppressed patients and pregnant women can develop asymptomatic viruria. PML used to be seen only in older patients with hematological malignancy or receiving steroid therapy. Now over half the deaths associated with PML occur in those with HIV infection.

Pathogenesis

Primary viremia probably leads to the establishment of latent infection in the kidney. Immunosuppression allows viral reactivation and replication leading to viuria (and the renal clinical features described below).

JCV and BKV sequences have been identified in peripheral blood mononuclear cells in patients with leukemia, HIV infection, and PML. These cells may provide the means for JCV to reach the CNS.

It is not known whether PML follows reactivation of latent JCV in the CNS or new CNS infection occurs following reactivation of renal JCV. Virus probably directly infects oligodendrocytes, leading to demyelination. Three cases of PML occurring in patients treated with natalizumab have been described.[1]

Clinical features

Primary infection is usually asymptomatic, but children may experience mild upper respiratory tract symptoms.

BKV and JCV viruria

This is rare in those without immune impairment.
- *Pregnant women:* JCV/BKV is found in <3% of pregnant women in the last trimester, ceasing rapidly postpartum. It probably represents reactivation (due to immunosuppression or hormonal change).
- *Renal transplant recipients:* seen in 10–45% of patients after transplantation, representing both reactivation and primary infection of the recipient from a previously infected kidney. Most cases occur in the first 3 months after surgery and are asymptomatic. Some cases of BKV infection have been associated with ureteric stenosis.
- *Bone marrow transplant recipients:* BKV viruria occurs in <50% of patients, most <2 months after the procedure and probably due to reactivation. It is associated with development of hemorrhagic cystitis.
- *Other immunodeficiencies:* BKV viruria with renal complications has been reported in cases of other causes of immunodeficiency.

Progressive multifocal leucoencephalopathy (PML)

Presentation is similar in both those with HIV and those with other immunodeficiencies: rapidly progressive focal neurological deficits including hemiparesis, visual field defects, aphasia, ataxia, and cognitive impairment.

Late features include cortical blindness, quadriparesis, dementia, and coma. Abnormalities occur predominantly in cerebral white matter and less commonly in the cerebellum and brainstem. Spinal cord involvement is rare. Death usually occurs within 6 months of diagnosis, although some patients experience a 2- to 3-year fluctuating course.

Diagnosis

Serology is unhelpful given the high seroprevalence, so diagnosis relies on virus detection and pathological findings. Viral culture is difficult, as both JCV and BKV are very slow growing and require specialized cell lines.

Viruria

Cytological examination is useful for detection of viruria, although normal appearance does not exclude infection. Infected cells have large nuclei with a large basophilic intranuclear inclusion. Although relatively distinctive, these changes can be confused with those caused by other viral infections, e.g., CMV and adenovirus.

PCR detects virus, but it is also positive in a proportion of normal controls and apparently healthy elderly. BK DNA PCR is confirmatory.

PML and JCV

Brain biopsy allows definitive diagnosis, demonstrating multiple asymmetric foci of demyelination, cytopathic change apparent in oligodendrocytes, and EM revealing viral particles within their nuclei. Fluorescent antibody staining allows identification of JCV.

CT scan appearance may be less dramatic than the severity of clinical findings suggests: hypodense nonenhancing white matter lesions. MRI is more sensitive.

PCR of CSF to identify JCV DNA should only be used in combination with imaging and clinical findings. Sensitivity is variable depending on technique and may be positive in the immunosuppressed without PML.

Treatment

Most patients with BKV and JCV are asymptomatic and do not require treatment. PML patients with HIV may demonstrate marked improvement with the introduction of HAART. Treatment of other immunosuppressed patients is supportive and symptomatic.

Cytarabine has been shown to have no clinical benefit. Evidence is awaited to demonstrate a role for interferon or cidofovir.

Reference

1. Yousy TA, et al. (2006). Evaluation of patients treated with natalizumab for progressive multi-focal leucoencephalopathy. *N Engl J Med* 2006;354:924–933.

Poxviruses

Unlike most other DNA viruses, replication occurs in the infected cell's cytoplasm rather than within the nucleus.

The viruses

Large, asymmetric virions contain dsDNA, and enzymes enable cytoplasmic replication. Viruses are extremely resistant to chemical and physical inactivation and remain infective for months at room temperature or for years if frozen.

See Table 3.24 for viruses and respective hosts.

Table 3.24 Genera of the *Poxviridae* with example species

Genera	Viruses	Normal host
Orthopoxvirus	Vaccinia	Humans, derived from cowpox
	Variola	Humans (monkeys)
	Monkeypox	Monkeys (humans)
Avipoxvirus	Fowlpox	Chickens
Capripoxvirus	Sheep-pox	Sheep
Leporipoxvirus	Myxoma	Rabbit
Parapoxvirus	Bovine papular stomatitis virus	Cow (humans: "milker's nodule")
	Pseudocowpox virus	Cattle (humans)
	Orf	Sheep and goats (humans)
Suipoxvirus	Swinepox	Pigs
Molluscipoxvirus	Molluscum contagiosum	Humans
Yatapoxvirus	Tanapox	Monkeys (human form resembles monkeypox)

Vaccinia

Vaccinia was derived from cowpox in the early 19th century via person-to-person transmission. It now has no natural host. Jenner observed in 1798 that inoculating people with pustular material from cowpox gave protection from smallpox, inventing vaccination. Routine vaccination for smallpox has been discontinued.

Vaccinia continues to have a role among military personnel, as a vaccine vector for other infections, and in immunotherapy. Protection is almost 100% for 1–3 years, with disease-attenuating protection for <20 years. Complications of vaccination include fever, regional lymphadenopathy, postinfectious encephalitis (1–2 weeks later), and skin eruptions.

Variola (smallpox)

Unlike vaccinia, variola infects only humans and, occasionally, monkeys.

Two main viral strains are the virulent variola major (mortality 20–50%) and the milder variola minor (mortality <1%).

Rapid diagnosis can be made using PCR, electron microscopy, or gel diffusion techniques on vesicular fluid. It no longer exists in nature (last case: Somalia 1977).

Incubation is <12 days, then a 2-day prodrome is followed by rash (maculopapules, vesicles to pustules and scabs). Dense rash on the trunk and appearance of lesions in crops are characteristics of varicella that are not seen in smallpox. In fulminant disease, death can occur before the rash. Today only two laboratories in the world are known to have isolates of variola.

Monkeypox

This virus causes vesicular illness in monkeys, similar to smallpox. Sporadic cases of human infection occur in endemic areas (rainforests of Western and Central Africa and some imported cases have been seen in the United States).

Rash resembles smallpox and is contagious to other humans. A 1996/97 outbreak in the Congo had a fatality rate of 1.5%.

Parapoxviruses

These are found worldwide. They are native to a variety of animals, and some members are capable of infecting humans. They can persist within herds for long periods.

Orf (sheep and goats) and pseudocowpox (cattle) cause lesions in the mouth and skin, and passage to humans is acquired by direct contact with the animal or contaminated objects. Lesions in humans are milder (vesicle to pustules) with prolonged incubation and can last for weeks.

Diagnosis is from vesicular material, examined by PCR, EM, or culture.

Molluscum contagiosum

This is the only poxvirus specific for humans in the post-smallpox era. It is found worldwide and is spread by close human contact.

It causes small, firm, umbilicated papules on exposed epithelial (children) or genital areas (adults). These usually resolve spontaneously but can persist for months in the context of immunosuppression or become generalized in atopic patients.

An opportunistic pathogen in AIDS patients, it can cause generalized infection with large atypical lesions resembling basal cell carcinomas.

Diagnosis is by histology and EM. Management is by local therapy (cryotherapy, incision) and improving immunological function.

Poliovirus

The virus

Viruses are members of the *Picornaviridae* family, genus *Enterovirus* (p. 372). There are three serotypes; infection by one confers protective immunity only to that type, with little heterologous protection. Prior to widespread vaccination, paralytic disease was caused largely by type 1.

Wild-type and/or vaccine-strain virus may circulate in different populations depending on regional vaccine use and the level of endemic naturally occurring viral transmission.

Humans are the only natural host (infections can be achieved experimentally in primates). Wild-type strains vary widely in neurovirulence.

Epidemiology

Transmission is similar to that of other enteroviruses.

Polio was largely sporadic in the 19th century, affecting mostly children <5 years of age. By 1950, developing-world infections were epidemic in nature, most cases being in children aged 5–9 years (one-third in those over 15 years). Incidence in older children was attributed to rising standards of hygiene delaying inapparent infections that previously took place in childhood and conferred widespread immunity. The resulting pool of older, susceptible individuals facilitated epidemics—the higher rate of paralytic disease being due to the loss protective maternal antibody.

Rates fell dramatically after vaccine introduction. Of the 25 cases of paralytic polio notified since 1983, most were vaccine associated (see below), some were imported, and wild-type virus was not detected in the remainder.

The WHO has certified that polio transmission is interrupted in the Americas, Western Pacific, and Europe. India, Pakistan, Afghanistan, and Nigeria are the main remaining reservoirs.

Pathogenesis

Virus enters through the GI tract and replicates in the gut and adjacent lymphoid tissue. It reaches susceptible reticuloendothelial tissue via the bloodstream.

Asymptomatic cases stop at this point. Type-specific antibodies are formed. Otherwise, replication and viremia occur (the "minor illness").

The CNS is probably infected by retrograde axonal transport from muscle to nerve to cord. Neurons throughout the gray matter are affected, especially those within the anterior horn of the spinal cord and motor nuclei of medulla and pons. Distribution of lesions is similar in all cases; it is their severity that determines clinical disease.

Clinical features

Incubation is 9–12 days from acquisition to prodrome ("minor illness": 1–3 days of fever, headache, sore throat, anorexia, vomiting, abdominal pain), and 11–17 days until the onset of paralysis ("major illness").

Manifestations

Inapparent: 95% of cases are asymptomatic

Abortive: 4–8% of infections experience just the prodrome and appear as any nonspecific viral infection

Nonparalytic polio: similar to severe cases of abortive but with signs of viral meningitis

Spinal paralytic polio

Frank paralysis occurs in 0.1% of infections. Children experience the classic biphasic illness: the 2- to 3-day minor illness coincides with viremia and is followed by 2–5 asymptomatic days before the abrupt onset of the major illness.

Headache, fever, malaise, vomiting, neck stiffness, and muscle pains are followed after 1–2 days by flaccid weakness and paralysis of anything from a single muscle to quadriplegia (very rare in infants). Initially hyperactive reflexes become absent.

Paralysis is asymmetric with proximal involvement more severe than distal, and the legs more commonly involved than the arms. Bladder paralysis usually accompanies the legs. Occasional cases progress from onset of weakness to quadriplegia and bulbar involvement within hours. More commonly, progression is over 2–3 days, halting when the patient becomes afebrile.

Sensory loss is rare (consider Guillain–Barré syndrome).

Bulbar paralytic polio

Paralysis of those muscle groups innervated by the cranial nerves results in dysphagia, nasal speech, and dyspnea. This condition is seen in 5–35% of paralytic cases. Medullary circulatory and respiratory centers may become involved. Mixed bulbar and spinal involvement is common.

Polio encephalitis

This uncommon form, occurring mainly in infants, is characterized by confusion, disturbed consciousness, and seizures with spastic paralysis (upper motor neuron involvement).

Prognosis

Prior to vaccination, mortality of paralytic disease was 5–10%, rising to 20–60% with bulbar involvement. Two-thirds with paralytic disease have a degree of permanent weakness on recovery, and complete recovery is rare when acute paralysis is severe, particularly if requiring ventilation.

Those surviving bulbar disease show the best recovery, with significant improvement by 10 days and ultimately usually attaining normal function. Most reversible muscle paralysis in spinal disease will have resolved by 1 month with some improvement up to 9 months.

Post-poliomyelitis syndrome

From 20 to 30% of previously paralyzed patients experience a new onset of weakness, pain, and atrophy in previously affected muscle groups 25–3 years after acute illness. This is thought to be due to attrition of motor units in innervated muscle that is already less innervated because of the initial disease.

Risk factors for paralysis

These include prepubertal males, pregnancy, B-cell immunodeficiency (increases the risk of oral polio vaccine [OPV]-associated disease), strenuous exercise within first 3 days of major illness, intramuscular injection (paralysis localizes to the limb injected or injured within 2–4 weeks before infection), and tonsillectomy (8 times the risk of those with tonsils).

Complications

These include respiratory compromise (diaphragmatic and intercostal muscle paralysis, upper airway obstruction, respiratory center impairment), myocarditis, gastrointestinal hemorrhage, ileus, and complication of paralysis.

Diagnosis

- *CSF:* abnormalities do not distinguish poliovirus from other viral causes of aseptic meningitis. Unlike other enteroviruses, polio is rarely isolated from CSF.
- *Virus isolation:* poliovirus can be isolated from the throat in the first week of illness and from feces for several weeks. In areas of low incidence, it is important to identify the viral strain as either wild type or vaccine related. If achievable, CSF viral isolation is valuable, as recovery of vaccine-virus in feces is common and does not demonstrate conclusive etiology.
- *Serology:* acute and convalescent sera, but cannot distinguish wild type from vaccine

Treatment

There is no specific antiviral therapy. Management is supportive. Bed rest is essential in the acute phase to reduce extension of paralysis.

Avoid intramuscular injections.

Ventilatory assistance is required once vital capacity falls to <50%. Tracheal intubation is indicated in severe cases of bulbar paralysis.

Physiotherapy can start once the progression of paralysis has ceased.

Multidisciplinary management of long-term physical sequelae is required.

Vaccination

IPV (inactivated polio vaccine)

IPV was developed by Salk and introduced in the UK in 1956. The preparations now used contain all three serotypes and have seroconversion rates equal to those of OPV. Neutralizing antibodies are found in 100% of people after the third dose.

Recipients develop little or no secretory antibody and are thus capable of asymptomatic infection and shedding to unimmunized contacts.

OPV (oral polio vaccine)

OPV was developed by Sabin in 1963. It is trivalent: four doses are required to achieve seroconversion to all three serotypes. Nonimmune recipients shed virus in feces for up to 6 weeks. OPV promotes antibody formation in the gut (providing local protection against viral entry) and boosts community immunity (recently vaccinated children excrete virus that may be acquired by their contacts).

However, around 1 dose in every 2.6 million results in vaccine virus–related disease, both in receivers (usually those under 4 months of age, 7–21 days after administration) and their contacts (usually young adults, 20–29 days after administration); 22% of reported cases occur in those with humoral immunodeficiency. The syndrome is similar to naturally occurring disease but is more protracted.

Developing world

OPV is in widespread use in developing nations because of its lower cost and easy administration. Even those in tropical countries who receive all the recommended doses may fail to seroconvert for all three serotypes. This may be related to the prevalence of diarrheal disease and vaccine formulation.

Human T-cell lymphotropic virus

Human T-cell lymphotropic viruses (HTLV) 1 and 2 are retroviruses. HTLV-1 is associated with certain forms of adult T-cell leukemia/lymphoma and neurological disease. HTLV-2 has not yet been definitively linked to a specific disorder.

The virus

HTVLs are members of the primate T-cell leukemia/lymphoma viruses. Nonhuman primates are thought to constitute the natural reservoir of HTLVs.

They differ from lentiviruses (retroviruses such as HIV) in that although both are capable of prolonged asymptomatic infection, lentiviruses have a cytopathic effect, whereas HTLV transforms T cells, immortalizing them.

They are spherical virions, with 65% nucleotide homology between HTLV-1 and -2. HTLV-1 isolates show a high degree of similarity (92–97%) across the world (unlike HIV-1). Small variations seem to reflect geographic origin; it has been classified into five clades.

HTLV-2 has three subtypes: 2a (among IV drug users in North America), 2b (indigenous groups in Panama, Colombia, and Argentina), and 2c (urban Brazil).

Epidemiology

HTLV-1 is widely scattered. It is endemic in some regions (e.g., 20% of adults are seropositive in some islands of southwest Japan) and widespread in immigrants from parts of the Caribbean, Central and West Africa, Melanesia, Middle East, India, and parts of South America.

HTLV-2 is found largely among IV drug users and their sexual contacts as well as in some Native American populations.

Transmission occurs sexually (mostly male to female; risk is increased in the presence of genital ulceration); via blood products (those containing cellular components, not plasma derivatives—the infectious titer in plasma is extremely low); or from mother to child (breastfeeding being the predominant route; 15–20% of breastfed children of HTLV-positive mothers acquire it). Most infections are lifelong and asymptomatic.

Clinical features

Adult T-cell leukemia/lymphoma (ATL)

ATL is a proliferative disorder of mature CD4+ CD25+ T cells. Integration of the provirus into the cellular genome is monoclonal (T cells originate from a single transformed cell), and the virus may be latent in neoplastic cells. An HTLV-1 carrier has a 1–4% lifetime risk of developing it.

Clinical features include lymphadenopathy, hypercalcemia, lytic bone lesions, skin lesions (nodules through to erythroderma), and hepatosplenomegaly. Patients can be immunocompromised, and opportunistic infections are common (*Strongyloides stercoralis* in Japan).

ATL is classified into four types:
- Smoldering ATL (normal cell count but 5% or more abnormal T-cell morphology with skin lesions and can last for years)
- Chronic ATL (raised cell count with organomegaly, skin or pulmonary involvement but no effusions, bone, or CNS involvement; median survival is 24 months)
- Lymphomatous ATL (lymphadenopathy with histological confirmation but normal cell counts; median survival is 10 months)
- Acute ATL (presents as leukemia or high-grade non-Hodgkin's lymphoma; median survival is 6.2 months)

HTLV-1-associated myelopathy (tropical spastic paraparesis)

This chronic, progressive demyelinating disease affects the spinal cord and white matter of the CNS. There is a 5% lifetime incidence in HTLV-1 carriers, with onset typically at >30 years of age.

Clinical features include gait disturbance, leg weakness or stiffness with moderate to severe spasticity, back pain, bladder and bowel dysfunction and variable degrees of sensory loss. Progression varies: some patients have long periods of mild difficulty walking, others become bed-bound.

Unlike ATL, infected lymphocytes are polyclonal and may cause disease indirectly by activating autoimmune T cells or by infecting CNS glial cells precipitating a cytotoxic response against them.

Other disease associations
- *HTLV-1:* arthropathies, uveitis, polymyositis, infectious dermatitis, Sjögren's syndrome, and possibly mycosis fungoides
- *HTLV-2:* unconfirmed associations with rare hematological malignancies and neurodegenerative disorders

Diagnosis

- *ELISA-based tests* are used to screen for HTLV. Positives are confirmed using more sensitive techniques to distinguish HTLV-1 and -2 (e.g., PCR).
- *ATL* diagnosis is by histology (blood cell appearance, skin lesion biopsy), cytogenetics, immunophenotyping, and confirmation of the monoclonal integration of proviral DNA into malignant cells.
- *HTLV-1-associated myelopathy:* MRI may show lesions, CSF may reveal atypical lymphocytes.

Treatment

ATL

Combination chemotherapy is used. Side effects may outweigh benefits in indolent disease. Durable remissions are rare, with most relapsing within 12 months. The role of BMT or stem cell transplantation has not been established.

Zidovudine in combination with IFN-α was reported to induce remission in 26% of patients in one series.

Monoclonal antibodies (coupled to yttrium 90) against the IL-2R chain (expressed by ATL cells) are reported to be effective in some patients.

HTLV-1-associated myelopathy

There is no effective treatment.

Danazol has been reported to improve gait and bladder function. Corticosteroids, plasmapheresis, cyclophosphamide, and IFN-α may produce transient responses.

Flaviviruses

The Family *Flaviviridae* includes the genus *Flavivirus*, along with the *Pestivirus* genus and the hepatitis C–like viruses. Although genetically similar, there is no known antigenic relationship between these genera.

This group of viruses derives its name from yellow fever (the type species, *flavus* being Latin for "yellow"). The *Flavivirus* genus has around 70 members, 30 of which are known to cause human disease. Most are arthropod born or zoonotic viruses. Here we consider those members for which encephalitis is the defining clinical feature. Dengue and yellow fever itself are covered on pp. 401 and 399.

Viral structure

Virions are spheres 50 nm in diameter, with an outer lipid envelope packed with the membrane (M) and envelope (E—involved in cell attachment and containing several epitopes involved in viral neutralization) glycoproteins. Positive sense ssRNA is contained within the nucleocapsid.

Cross-neutralization assays allow flaviviruses to be classified into one of eight antigenic groups, the most important of which are the JE complex (Japanese encephalitis, St. Louis encephalitis, West Nile virus, Murray Valley encephalitis virus), dengue complex, tick-borne virus complex (central European encephalitis, Russian spring–summer encephalitis, Kyasanur Forest disease).

Pathogenesis

Incubation is 4–28 days (usually 1 week). One in 250 infections is symptomatic. Old age is the most significant risk factor for severe disease.

Virus replicates locally. Brief viremia (virus is rarely recovered from blood) is followed by CNS invasion. CNS spread is cell to cell, which causes meningeal inflammation, cerebral edema, and encephalitis (particularly temporal, thalamus, brainstem, and anterior spinal cord).

Viruses causing encephalitis

Japanese encephalitis (JE)

Epidemiology

JE is found throughout Asia (Pakistan to eastern Russia) and responsible for up to 65% of hospitalized encephalitis cases in areas of high endemicity. Outbreaks have occurred in northern Australia and Pacific islands. Widespread childhood immunization in China, Japan, and Korea has resulted in a large fall in incidence.

The virus is transmitted by *Culex* mosquitoes, with viral amplification occurring in pigs and aquatic birds. Humans are incidental hosts. Conditions for mosquito breeding are most favorable in rural areas (e.g. rice paddies) where the risk of infection is highest.

Most infections are subclinical and occur in childhood (2–10 years of age), thus 80% of young adults are immune in endemic areas. Regions with high vaccine uptake see most infections in the elderly.

Clinical features

Although infection is symptomatic in <1% of cases, these patients experience a severe encephalitis (25% fatality even with intensive care facilities). Main findings at presentation are high fever and altered consciousness (personality change to coma). Early symptoms are lethargy, fever, headache, abdominal pain, and vomiting. Over a few days, they progress to agitation, delirium, motor abnormalities (facial paralysis, dysconjugate gaze, convulsions, hemiparesis, focal weakness, flaccid and spastic paralysis, ataxia, tremor, choreoathetosis, and other extrapyramidal signs), neck stiffness, and coma (some patients needing ventilatory support).

Severe cases may be quickly fatal. Milder cases see improvement after 1 week. Neurological recovery can take weeks to years, with one-third having residual problems at 5 years, and psychological sequelae occurring in over 50% of afflicted children.

Secondary complications include infections and pressure sores. Abortion may be precipitated when infection is acquired in the first or second trimester.

Laboratory findings

These include leukocytosis, hyponatremia, raised CSF lymphocytes, and CSF protein normal or slightly raised. EEG shows diffuse delta waves (occasionally seizure activity). CT/MRI may show cerebral edema and evidence of abnormalities in the brainstem, cerebellum, and spinal cord.

Treatment and prevention

There is no specific therapy. Anecdotal reports of benefit from INF-A and immunotherapy need further validation.

JE vaccines are available: three doses of an inactivated vaccine over 4 weeks is ~90% effective. Side effects include angioedema and urticaria, and there have been reports of encephalomyelitis. Because of the low risk of acquiring JE while traveling, it is not recommended routinely. A live vaccine is available only in China.

St. Louis encephalitis

Epidemiology

Outbreaks have occurred throughout the United States and in parts of Canada and Mexico; sporadic cases occur further afield including in South America and parts of the Caribbean. Virus is transmitted in an enzootic cycle (birds) by differing *Culex* species in different geographic areas; human infection is incidental.

The eastern United States sees periodic regional outbreaks in late summer, usually in urban areas where polluted water provides mosquito-breeding areas. Vectors are most active in the evening. Incidence of infection is highest in men and the homeless.

In the western United States, infection occurs at low levels throughout the year, often associated with irrigated areas. The risk of illness is greatest in the elderly.

Clinical features

There are three broad syndromes: febrile illness, aseptic meningitis, and fatal encephalitis. Most severe and fatal cases occur in adults and elderly.

Early symptoms include malaise, fever, headache, myalgia and upper respiratory and abdominal symptoms. After several days, lethargy, confusion, tremor, ataxia and other cerebellar signs, vomiting and diarrhea, generalized weakness, meningism (children), tremor (eyelids, lips, extremities), and cranial nerve palsies can occur. Most patients do not progress to coma, and convulsions are rare, with 8% overall fatality (20% of cases in those over 60 years of age).

Children often have residual deficits but late recovery. Adults may have residual neurological and psychological disturbances for months.

Laboratory findings

These include leukocytosis, hyponatremia, proteinuria, raised CSF pressure in one-third of cases, and raised CSF protein in two-thirds. EEG shows generalized slowing with delta waves.

Treatment and prevention

There is no specific treatment. Bird and mosquito surveillance may enable outbreak prediction. The early use of insecticides in at-risk areas along with public health education can reduce mosquito exposure.

Tick-borne encephalitis

Epidemiology

Ixodes tick-borne viruses causing encephalitis include central European encephalitis (CEE, principally in Austria and surrounding countries but also Scandinavia and other parts of Europe), Russian spring–summer encephalitis (RSSE, eastern Russia, Korea, China, Japan), louping ill (Britain, an occupational disease of vets and butchers), and Powassan virus (North America). Incidence is highly variable within countries at risk (e.g., RSSE occurs primarily in sylvatic locations).

Viruses are transmitted between ticks and vertebrates and passed vertically to tick offspring. Human infections are incidental and in central Europe tend to occur from April to November.

Most cases occur in adults 20–50 years of age. Infection has been acquired by the consumption of unpasteurized milk from infected animals (CEE) and through handling infected meat (louping ill, CEE).

Clinical features

Incubation may be as long as a month; 1 in 250 of CEE infections is symptomatic, and of those, 5–30% develop neurological features. Illness is biphasic (initial phase may not be reported). Early features include fever, headache, malaise, and vomiting. Symptoms resolve at 1 week.

Those who develop the second, neurological phase do so after a 2- to 10-day remission, after which fever, headache, and vomiting return. Neurological features are aseptic meningitis, encephalitis, myelitis (particularly shoulder girdle and upper limb paralysis, which may be permanent), autonomic and bladder disturbances, and bulbar involvement; 1% of cases are fatal (mostly elderly), 40% experience sequelae (ataxia, psychological disturbance). RSSE tends to be monophasic and more severe, with seizures, coma, brainstem involvement, and serious neurological sequelae being much more common. Powassan virus produces a severe disease that may resemble herpes encephalitis.

A history of tick bite is given in only half of cases. Neuroborelliosis should be considered, both as a differential and because ticks and patients may be dually infected.

Laboratory findings include early-phase leukopenia, late-phase leukocytosis, and moderate CSF lymphocytosis.

Treatment and prevention

Passive immunization with TBE immunoglobulin has been tried, but there is a significant risk of exacerbating the disease. Corticosteroids reduce fever duration but prolong hospital stay. Inactivated vaccines are available and are widely used in areas at risk.

Local control through the use of acaricides to reduce tick numbers is effective but not practical over large areas.

Other

West Nile fever

This is related to JE but produces a febrile illness and arthropathy. Elderly people are at increased risk of more severe manifestations, including hepatitis, pancreatitis, and myocarditis. Severe neurological disease leads to death in 5% of cases. It is transmitted between *Culex* mosquitoes and birds, and is the most widespread of the arboviruses (Africa, Europe, Asia, America, Middle East).

Murray Valley encephalitis
This is related to West Nile fever and found in Australia and Papua New Guinea. It causes encephalitis with coma, limb paralysis, and respiratory depression in severe cases.

Kyasanur Forest disease and Omsk hemorrhagic fever
These two related viruses are transmitted by ticks and found only in the Kyasanur Forest of India and parts of Siberia, respectively. A 3- to 8-day incubation is followed by the abrupt onset of fever, headache, and photophobia with hepatosplenomegaly and petechiae.

Gum, GI tract, and pulmonary hemorrhage can occur with renal failure in severe cases. Symptoms then remit for up to 3 weeks before the onset of a neurological syndrome. Case fatality: Kyasanur 5–10%, Omsk 3%.

Diagnosis
Viral isolation is rarely useful with neurotropic flaviviruses, and most clinical laboratories do not have the cell lines required for growth. Isolation from blood is only likely in the first week (before the onset of neurological features). Isolation from CSF is possible in early fulminant disease, and it may be isolated from tissue samples (brain, spleen, etc.) in some cases. PCR of acute-phase serum may allow early diagnosis.

Serology of both blood and CSF is the main means of diagnosis. ELISA for IgM is positive in one or the other by day 10 in nearly all cases of flaviviral encephalitis. Tests can remain positive for months. In areas where several flaviviruses circulate, it can be difficult to distinguish acute from previous infection and between different flaviviruses.

Yellow fever

Yellow fever is the type species of the genus *Flavivirus* (p. 395).

Epidemiology
The disease originated in Africa and was probably introduced into the Americas by mosquito-infested slave-trading ships. It is now found in areas of Sub-Saharan Africa and South America but has not been documented in Asia. Two patterns of transmission occur:
- *Urban* (epidemic): occurs in Africa and represents human-to-human transmission by *Aedes aegypti* mosquitoes
- *Jungle*: infection is maintained in monkeys, transmission occurring via *Haemogogus* and *Aedes* mosquitoes. Human cases occur when susceptible individuals come into contact with infected mosquitoes (e.g., forestry workers). Viremic individuals may precipitate an urban transmission cycle on returning home.

African epidemic attack rates can be high (30 people in 1000), with death rates of 20–50%. Declining epidemics reflect changes in viral activity and human immunity (natural and vaccination related). In South America, 7100 cases are reported each year; urban outbreaks are unusual.

Person-to-person transmission is theoretically possible in any area where the vector exists (including southern United States).

Pathogenesis

Virus is inoculated by a mosquito and replicates in local lymph nodes spreading via the bloodstream to other lymphoid sites and tissues.

Viremia peaks around day 5–6, corresponding with an increase in inflammatory cytokine production and the onset of symptoms.

Widespread hemorrhages develop on mucosal surfaces, skin, and other organs. Gastric erosions may precipitate hematemesis, and there can be extensive hepatocellular damage with lobular necrosis. Renal impairment may be secondary (prerenal) or due directly to viral infection. Neurological impairment is usually due to edema and hemorrhage rather than to encephalitis. Other features may include coagulation deficiency, myocarditis, and systemic inflammatory response syndrome.

Clinical features

Incubation is 3–6 days. Mosquitoes may become infected if biting within the first 3–5 days of illness.

Symptoms range from asymptomatic to a hemorrhagic fever. Commonly they are biphasic, starting with abrupt-onset headache, fever, and myalgia lasting 3–4 days. Most people recover at this point.

After a few hours' to days' respite, severe cases go on to a second phase of high fever, back pain, nausea, vomiting, abdominal pain, and drowsiness before jaundice, hepatitis, and bleeding develop. Hematemesis, melena, epistaxis, petechial, and purpuric rashes may occur. Patients may become oliguric and uremic.

Other features are myocarditis, arrhythmias, shock, metabolic acidosis, acute tubular necrosis, confusion, seizures, and unconsciousness.

Laboratory findings include leukopenia in the early stages, thrombocytopenia, coagulation abnormalities, very high transaminases (AST may be more than ALT if myocarditis), normal or slightly raised ALP, uremia, metabolic acidosis, albuminuria (a characteristic feature of yellow fever hepatitis), and raised CSF protein.

Those who survive the critical period commonly get bacterial pneumonia or sepsis. Hepatic recovery is good; chronic hepatitis is not a feature. The death rate in severe cases of hemorrhagic fever can be as high as 50%.

Diagnosis

Severe yellow fever resembles other viral hemorrhagic fevers circulating in Africa and South America, so lab confirmation is required for conclusive diagnosis.

Viral detection

This is frequently possible, as patients present while still viremic, allowing the detection of viral antigens, or virus culture. Virus isolation is accomplished by inoculation of mosquito or mammalian cell cultures in specialized laboratories.

Serology

In primary infections, IgM detection by ELISA is over 95% sensitive on serum samples taken 7–10 days after illness onset. In secondary infections, positive assays for IgG and IgM can be 100% sensitive at 5 days.

Paired serum samples showing a fourfold rise in titer confirm the diagnosis. Cross-reactivity is problematic in those who have been exposed to several flaviviruses.

Neutralization assays are most specific but are only offered in specialized laboratories. Complement fixation assays can distinguish between the flavivirus complexes but rise at only 4–6 weeks after onset.

Treatment

Treatment is supportive: fluid balance, management of coagulopathy, and renal insufficiency, reducing risk of GI bleeding.

In some areas of the world, it may be necessary to exclude the patient from mosquitoes to prevent onward transmission.

The 17D vaccine is highly effective and a single dose produces long-term protection in 95% of people. This is a live attenuated virus vaccine. There are rare cases of encephalitis. Infants are at higher risk, and it is contraindicated in those under 4 months of age.

Travelers to at-risk countries should receive the vaccine every 10 years. It is recommended for routine use in 35 African countries but uptake is low. The 17D vaccine should not be administered to immunocompromised individuals or pregnant women.

Vector reduction is difficult and expensive but has been achieved in some areas.

In South America, surveys to identify dead monkeys can warn of an increased risk of to humans.

Dengue

A flavivirus (p. 395) and arbovirus are transmitted by *Aedes* mosquitoes, causing fever (dengue fever [DF]), which may be complicated by fluid leak, shock, and hemorrhage (dengue hemorrhagic fever [DHF]).

Epidemiology

The virus exists in four distinct serotypes. Infection with one serotype provides brief (around 6 months) cross-protection to all four upon recovery, after which immunity remains to the infecting serotype only. Later secondary infection with one of the other three is then associated with an increased risk of severe disease, DHF.

Worldwide outbreaks of dengue began at the start of the 20th century. "Breakbone fever" was recorded in Greece (1928), Australia (1897), Florida (1934), and the tropics. After World War II, transmission of multiple serotypes greatly increased in Southeast Asia, with a consequent increase in cases of DHF.

Today, dengue occurs in regions of the tropics in which its vector is found (*Aedes aegypti* and, to a lesser extent, *A. albopictus* and *A. polynesiensis*), particularly in Southeast Asia, parts of South and Central America, and certain parts of Sub-Saharan Africa. DHF can be endemic where more than one viral type circulates.

It takes around 2 weeks for a mosquito to become infective after feeding on a viremic individual. *Aedes* are day biting and are easily disturbed while feeding. A single mosquito can infect an entire household. They breed in any source of open water (domestic containers, puddles, tires); thus transmission can be very intense in tropical cities.

Tropical transmission occurs throughout the year, increasing in the rainy season. Epidemic attack rates can be as high as 70%. Around 3 billion people live in areas at risk of dengue, with 100 million cases per year of dengue fever, and 500,000 cases of dengue shock.

Pathogenesis

Virus disseminates in the blood within 2–3 days of an infected bite. Patients are viremic for 4–5 days. Malaise reflects the cytokine response.

Most people infected with virus experience a significant but self-limited febrile illness. Some patients, usually those who have experienced previous infection, develop a severe immunopathological response (DHF), thought to be due to antibody-dependent enhancement: heterologous antibody is non-neutralizing and enhances viral uptake and increases the infected cell mass. The consequently exaggerated inflammatory response includes vasoactive cytokines (e.g., TNF-A), which contribute to fluid leak. Unlike viral hemorrhagic fevers such as Ebola, structural damage to blood vessels is not a feature.

It is rare for individuals to have more than two episodes of dengue.

Clinical features

Dengue fever

Dengue fever is asymptomatic in up to 80% of infants and children (it is often difficult to distinguish from other causes of fever).

DF tends to be more severe in adults; 4–7 days' incubation is followed by abrupt fever, headache, retro-orbital pain, marked muscle and joint pain, as well as rash (macular erythema with petechiae on extensor surfaces), with rapid progression to prostration and back and abdominal pain. The joint and muscle pains evoked the term "break-bone fever."

Defervescence occurs after 2–7 days—it may settle and recur (saddleback fever pattern). Recovery may be followed by prolonged fatigue and, occasionally, depression.

Other features include minor mucosal bleeding (severe in some cases, e.g., pre-existing peptic ulcer), subcapsular splenic bleeds, hepatitis, and neurological features (may represent the effects of cerebral edema or viral encephalitis).

DHF (dengue shock syndrome)

The early features are identical to mild disease. Severe symptoms tend to occur at defervescence (when, notably, viral load is falling rapidly) with reduced perfusion, central cyanosis, sweating, and other signs of shock. Platelets fall and petechiae develop, with spontaneous bruising and bleeding from mucosal surfaces.

Hemorrhagic tendency is demonstrated by a positive tourniquet test or spontaneous bleeding. Fluid leak occurs (increased hematocrit, pleural effusions, and ascites). The duration of illness is 7–10 days. With support in the critical period (fluid therapy, etc.), mortality is under 1%. Without support, death rates can reach 50%.

Complications include encephalopathy, hepatic failure, renal failure, and dual infections (Gram-negative sepsis, parasitic disease).

Diagnosis

- *Clinical:* DF is not easily distinguished from other causes of childhood febrile disease, even in cases of shock. DHF may resemble yellow fever. Leukopenia, low platelets, and abnormal LFTs are common.
- *Viral detection:* culture is definitive but impractical and rarely achieved if samples are taken more than 1–2 days after defervescence. Detection of viral RNA by RT-PCR is used in some centers.
- *Serology:* serological techniques are less specific than culture because of cross-reactivity between different flaviviruses. Neutralization assays allow different dengue serotypes to be distinguished in primary infection. Acute infection (as opposed to recent infection) can only be confirmed by demonstrating a rise in anti-dengue immunoglobulin in paired sera, e.g., IgM antibody capture (MAC)-ELISA for IgM (which tends to be specific to dengue complex).

Treatment and prevention

Supportive treatment includes antipyretics, oral rehydration, and close observation of fluid status with appropriate interventions (IV fluids, circulatory support). Avoid invasive procedures.

The WHO algorithm for classifying, monitoring, and identifying severe disease (e.g., 20% increase in hematocrit, narrowed pulse pressure, etc.), and guiding fluid replacement has been responsible for large falls in mortality.[1]

For prevention, there are several experimental vaccines, but none in widespread use. Vector control is effective but expensive and rarely practical in the regions that most need it.

Reference

1. World Health Organization (1997). *Dengue hemorrhagic fever: diagnosis, treatment, prevention and control*, 2nd edition. Geneva: World Health Organization.

Viral hemorrhagic fevers

Viral hemorrhagic fevers (VHF) are severe, potentially life-threatening illnesses caused by members of several viral families (Table 3.25). Most patients are not severely unwell when they present, and VHF should be considered as a cause of fever, rash, and sore throat in patients who have visited at-risk areas (e.g., rural West or Central Africa) within the last 3 weeks. *But* remember malaria is a much more likely diagnosis.

Here we consider the filoviruses and arenaviruses. Certain bunyaviruses (p. 378) and flaviviruses (p. 395) may cause similar presentations.

Table 3.25 Viral families

Virus	Source or vector	Distribution
Arenaviridae		
Junin (Argentine hemorrhagic fever)	Rodent	Agricultural areas of northern Buenos Aries province
Machupo (Bolivian haemorrhagic fever)	Rodent	Northeastern Bolivian savannah
Guanarito (Venezuelan haemorrhagic fever)	Rodent	Cleared forest areas of Venezuela
Lassa	Rodent	West Africa
Bunyaviridae		
Congo–Crimean haemorrhagic fever	Tick, or contact with infected animals	CIS, Middle East, Africa
Hantavirus (haemorrhagic fever with renal syndrome)	Rodent	Parts of China, Asia, Russia, Europe
Rift valley fever	Mosquito	Sub-Saharan Africa
Filoviridae		
Ebola	Unknown	DRC, Sudan, and Côte d'Ivoire
Marburg	Unknown	Uganda, Western Kenya
Flaviviridae		
Yellow fever	Human or monkey, via mosquito	South America, Sub-Saharan Africa
Dengue	Human via mosquito	Asia, Sub-Saharan Africa, South America
Omsk haemorrhagic fever	Tick	Siberia
Kyansanur forest disease	Tick	Kyansanur forest, India
Togaviridae		
Chikungunya	Mosquito	Africa and Asia

Management of suspected viral hemorrhagic fever
Presentation
Consider VHF in a patient with a febrile illness who has returned from a tropical African or VHF endemic country within 3 weeks and discuss with a local expert. Patients are infectious only after they develop symptoms. Early clinical features are mild and are not particularly characteristic: fever, cough, headache, sore throat, nausea, vomiting, weakness, and abdominal and chest pains. Severe features present later: hemorrhage, encephalopathy, hepatitis, and shock.

Differential diagnosis
Malaria should be excluded as soon as possible. Also consider typhoid fever, dengue, and rickettsial infection.

Infection control
Strict infection control precautions aim to prevent secondary infection of other patients and hospital and laboratory staff. Onward transmission to other people requires contact with the patient or infected secretions; aerosol transmission is not thought to be a significant means of infection.

Medical and lab staff should be meticulous in taking blood, handling fluids, disposing of excreta, and performing invasive procedures. Gloves, water-repellant aprons, face visors, and masks should be used. Sharps and other contaminated equipment should be disposed of carefully.

Risk assessment
- *Minimum:* the patient has not been in an endemic area or left more than 3 weeks before symptom onset.
- *Moderate:* the patient was in a known endemic area within 3 weeks of onset in the absence of any other features listed below or was in an adjacent area within 3 weeks and has severe illness that could be due to VHF.
- *High:* if (a) the patient was in a known endemic area within 3 weeks of onset and stayed in a house with a VHF case or suspected case, nursed a case or suspected case, had contact with fluids or the body of a case or suspected case (e.g., lab worker), or was moderate risk but has gone on to develop severe illness (organ failure, hemorrhage) or (b) was not in an endemic area within the 3-week window but has cared for a case or suspected case, or handled fluids or the body of a case or suspected case

Sample processing
If samples have already been sent to the lab, then it should be informed immediately so that they may be stored. Defer further samples, with the exception of malaria screening, until a detailed risk assessment has been performed. If patients are considered moderate to high risk, call the Special Pathogens Branch at the CDC (404-639-1115) for advice before sending samples.

Subsequent management
The following documents provide guidance on managing patients with VHF (1), isolation precautions (2), and decontamination procedures (3):
1) www.cdc.gov/ncidod/hip/BLOOD/vhf interimGuidance.htm
2) www.cdc.gov/ncidod/hip/ISOLAT/Isolat.htm
3) www.cdc.gov/ncidod/hip/enviro/guide.htm

Care is supportive
Minimum-risk patients are usually managed in a standard side room with specimens transported and processed as for other blood-borne viruses.

Moderate-risk patients should be isolated and full special precautions taken in acquiring and transporting samples. Only malaria films should be performed (at a minimum of category 3 containment). If positive with a good response to malaria therapy, most moderate-risk patients are recategorized as minimum risk.

High-risk patients (especially those with a negative malaria film) should be managed in accordance with CDC directives. Recovering patients may excrete virus in the urine for weeks.

Filoviruses

Named after their characteristic filament-like morphology, filoviruses are elongated structures 80 nm across and 800–1000 nm long. Genetic material is negative sense ssRNA. The two agents identified to date (Ebola and Marburg) show no serological cross-reactivity. Details of their natural history remain elusive. Viral particles are stable and highly infective.

Epidemiology

Outbreaks emerge abruptly. The source may be traced to a single human or primate index case but no further. No conclusive animal reservoir has been identified; however, prolonged infection has been demonstrated in bats.

Exact routes of transmission are unknown. Infection acquired parenterally has a high mortality, but most infections probably occur through skin or mucous membrane contact. Aerosol transmission may occur in monkeys but is not thought to be important in human-to-human spread.

Marburg virus was identified in 1967 when African green monkeys brought from Uganda to Germany developed a hemorrhagic illness subsequently transmitted to humans (7 deaths among 31 cases). Primary cases were associated with close contact with monkey blood or cell culture, and secondary cases with human blood exposure. Cases have occurred in western Kenya and once in Zimbabwe. Mortality is ~25%.

Ebola was identified in 1976. Four subtypes are identified: Zaire, Sudan, and Côte d'Ivoire in Africa, and Reston, which was first identified in the United States in monkeys imported from the Philippines. Early Ebola outbreaks were exacerbated through use of infected needles. Without precautions, rates of infection of household contacts can reach 17%. Case fatality rates range from 50% (Sudan) to over 80% (Zaire subtype).

Clinical features

Incubation is 5–10 days. There is abrupt onset of fever, myalgia, and headache. Nausea, vomiting, abdominal pain, diarrhea, and chest pain follow. Petechiae, hemorrhages, and spontaneous bruising occur as disease progresses. A maculopapular rash can develop around the fifth day.

In week 2, patients either become afebrile and improve or develop shock and multi-organ dysfunction with DIC and renal and liver failure.

Convalescence is prolonged. Virus is detectable in semen and urine for weeks.

Diagnosis

Clinical clues include travel to at-risk areas or contact with monkeys, maculopapular rash (not seen with other VHF).

Viral detection is by culture, which is usually positive acutely and viral particles may be seen on EM of histological specimens. Viral antigen detection and PCR-based tests are also available.

Seroconversion occurs at around day 10.

Treatment and prevention

There are no specific treatments; management is supportive.

Prevention is by early recognition of outbreaks and barrier nursing. Experimental vaccines show promise.

Arenaviruses (Lassa fever)

Arenaviruses are a family of ssRNA viruses. All are parasites of rodents, each virus showing specificity for a single rodent species. Here we consider Lassa fever. Other members include lymphocytic choriomeningitis virus (a cause of fever and meningitis) and the *Tacaribe* complex of viruses (causes of VHF in South America).

Epidemiology

The virus is found in West Africa. The *Mastomys* rodent hosts are chronically infected and show no evidence of disease. Humans are infected through contact with excreta.

Unlike other arenaviruses, person-to-person transmission of Lassa can occur. Endemic transmission occurs throughout the year with nosocomial outbreaks (where aerosol and parenteral transmission have been implicated) in the dry season.

Clinical features

Incubation is 7–12 days. Most infections in Africa are mild, with severe disease in <10% of cases. Mortality in this group can be as high as 25%.

Symptoms include fever, chest pain, back and abdominal pain, cough, vomiting, diarrhea, sore throat, conjunctivitis, facial edema, and CNS features (encephalitis, meningism).

Severe cases develop in the second week, with shock, fluid leak (facial and pulmonary edema, ascites, pleural effusions), and mild hemorrhages from mucosal surfaces. Pregnancies in maternal infections frequently abort; there is a high maternal mortality.

Late complications in less severe cases include cranial nerve deafness (up to one-third of hospitalized cases), pericarditis, uveitis, and orchitis.

Diagnosis

- *Viral detection:* culture from blood, throat swabs, and urine is possible within first 7–10 days.
- *Serology:* IgM detection is rapid and sensitive; around 75% of patients are positive on admission in Sierra Leone in one study.

Treatment and prevention

No vaccine is available.

Ribavirin therapy initiated before day 7 reduces mortality significantly (55% to 5% in one study) but improves survival at all stages of illness.

Contacts should be monitored for development of illness, with early presumptive use of ribavirin if fever develops.

Nosocomial transmission can be reduced through barrier nursing and isolation wherever possible (person-to-person spread by aerosol appears to occur).

Rodent control is rarely practical in the countries affected.

Rabies virus

Present throughout history, rabies (Latin for "madness") virus produces near-uniformly fatal encephalitis.

The virus

This negative-sense ssRNA virus is a member of the family *Rhabdoviridae*, genus *Lyssavirus*. Virions are bullet shaped (180 nm long by 75 nm wide).

The genus has six members—classic rabies is serotype 1. The other five rarely cause human disease.

Epidemiology

Rabies is worldwide, with the exception of Antarctica and certain islands. From 40,000 to 70,000 deaths occur each year, most in Asia. In 1999, 100 countries reported cases of rabies; 45 had none.[1]

Many mammals maintain and transmit rabies—foxes, skunks, raccoons, and bats are the primary reservoirs in the United States; dogs rarely transmit the infection. Other animal species are susceptible but, like humans, develop disease and do not participate in onward transmission (camels, horses).

Epidemiology of human disease reflects the pattern of animal infection. In developing regions, most human cases are acquired through dog bites. Developed nations have largely eliminated disease from domestic animals; most human infections follow exposure to rabid wild animals. Cases have followed corneal and solid-organ transplantation.

Animal rabies has been increasing in the United States, generally arising in raccoon populations. In 2003, there were two cases of human rabies reported in the United States.

Pathogenesis

Virus enters through a break in the skin or across mucosal surfaces, attaching to muscle and nerve cells. Internalization is followed by local replication within muscle cells.

Rapid administration of antirabies immunoglobulin and immunization are able to prevent spread of the virus at this stage. Once virus has entered peripheral nerves, it is not possible to prevent replication and spread.

Nerve innervating the muscle spindle is infected first, replication continuing in peripheral neurons as viral particles migrate along the axon. Virions travel by retrograde axoplasmic flow, unlike herpes simplex virus, which uses microtubular transport systems and therefore infects faster.

On reaching the cord, the rabies virus spreads throughout the CNS, reaching the rest of the body (e.g., saliva) via peripheral nerves.

The mechanism of CNS damage is uncertain. It may interfere with neurotransmission, with endogenous opioid systems, or act in an excitotoxic manner. Pathological examination of the brain in furious rabies reveals findings characteristic of encephalitis with Negri bodies (round eosinophilic cytoplasmic inclusions up to 7 micrometer across and containing viral nucleocapsids). These are concentrated in hippocampal pyramidal cells but may be found in cortical neurons. Paralytic rabies affects the spinal cord (inflammation and necrosis) and may cause segmental demyelination. Myocarditis can occur, and Negri bodies may be identified in the myocardium, suggesting a direct viral pathology.

Clinical features

Risk of acquiring rabies is related to the size of the inoculum (e.g., multiple bites, bite directly on skin vs. through clothing) and the location of the bite (greater risk is with the face than with extremities).

Incubation is days to years; most patients develop symptoms within 3 months.

Initial symptoms include fever, headache, malaise, vomiting with altered sensation at the bite site, and subtle personality changes. There may be myoedema (localized contraction of the muscle when struck with a tendon hammer, disappearing over a few seconds).

Acute neurological disease develops 4–10 days later and lasts 2–14 days, before coma intervenes. Patients die an average of 18 days after symptom onset. There are two main clinical presentations:

- *Furious (encephalitic) rabies* (80% of cases): anxiety, biting, hydrophobia (an exaggerated respiratory tract irritant reflex), delirium, agitation, seizures, hyperventilation, pituitary dysfunction (e.g., diabetes insipidus), cardiac arrhythmias, and autonomic dysfunction (papillary dilatation, salivation, priapism). Patients eventually enter a coma.
- *Paralytic rabies* (20% of cases): the spinal cord and brainstem are predominantly affected, and patients develop an ascending paralysis that may resemble Guillain–Barré syndrome or a symmetrical quadriparesis. Meningeal signs may develop. Disease progression is marked by confusion and a decline into coma.

Diagnosis

- *Incubation:* no tests are useful during incubation, and history is paramount in determining exposure to a potentially rabid animal and prompting the initiation of prophylactic treatment.
- *Symptomatic:* collection of samples should be performed after consulting with the local state health department or the Rabies Program at the CDC (www.cdc.gov/rabies). The diagnostic standard is direct fluorescent antibody staining of a skin biopsy taken from the nape of the neck. Virus localizes in hair follicles; 50% of samples are positive in the first week of illness, increasing thereafter. RT-PCR of tissue, CSF, or saliva is in increasing use. Other standard tests do not distinguish other causes of encephalitis.

Treatment and prevention

Prevention
Reducing disease in animal populations is central to the control of human disease. Vaccination of cats and dogs is a legal requirement in many countries, and vaccination of wild animals is effective in regions that can maintain it.

Pre-exposure vaccination
This is generally offered to those in high-risk occupations or traveling to at-risk countries with limited access to medical facilities. It is given as three intramuscular (IM) or intradermal injections on days 0, 7, and 21. Booster doses are recommended every 2–3 years.

Post-exposure treatment (PET)
Wound care by thorough washing with 20% soap solution and irrigation with a virucidal agent (e.g., iodine) may reduce the risk of rabies by as much as 90%. Local advice should be sought regarding the risk of rabies from the species involved.

Observe the responsible animal for 10 days if apparently healthy. It should undergo pathological examination if its behavior changes. If PET is considered necessary, it should be started immediately. It has a good record and appears safe in pregnancy. Immunocompromised patients may not respond sufficiently to vaccination and should have antibody titers checked at 2–4 weeks.

- If not previously vaccinated, rabies immunoglobulin (20 IU/kg body weight) should be infiltrated around the wound with any remaining dose given IM at an anatomical site distant from that of vaccine administration. Vaccine should then be given IM deltoid on days 0, 3, 7, 14, and 28.
- If previously vaccinated, immunoglobulin should not be given, and vaccine should be given IM deltoid on days 0 and 3.

Treatment after symptom onset
Generally, treatment initiated after symptom onset is of no benefit. In October 2004, a 15-year-old girl developing symptoms after a bat bite survived despite no history of vaccination or post-exposure treatment. Her treatment involved early induction of coma, ventilatory support, ribavirin, and amantadine.[2] However, ribavirin had been used before without success, and it is not clear what elements of this case or treatment regime contributed to recovery.

References

1. World Health Organization. Rabies: epidemiology. Retrieved August 6, 2008, at http://www.who.int/rabies/epidemiology/en/.

2. Willoughby RE, et al. (2005). Survival after treatment of rabies with induction of coma. *N Engl J Med* 352:2508–2514.

Creutzfeldt–Jakob disease (CJD)

CJD is one of the transmissible neurodegenerative, or prion (proteinaceous infectious particle), diseases. A *prion* has been defined as a small infectious pathogen containing protein and is resistant to procedures that modify or hydrolyze nucleic acid, including UV radiation. This raises issues regarding infection control; see Box 3.15. Prions are, however, fairly sensitive to procedures that digest or denature protein.

Human prion diseases have certain properties in common:
- Pathological manifestations confined largely to the CNS
- Long incubation times (kuru up to 30 years)
- Progressive and fatal
- Similar neuropathological features (astrocytosis with little inflammatory response and usually small vacuoles—the spongiform change)
- All result in the accumulation of an abnormal prion protein (PrP), a protease-resistant protein.

Other prion diseases include the following:
- Scrapie, a spongiform-encephalopathy of sheep and goats
- Bovine spongiform encephalopathy (BSE)
- Kuru (p. 414)
- Gerstmann–Sträussler–Scheinker syndrome (GSS) (p. 414)
- Familial fatal insomnia (FFI) (p. 414)

Box 3.15 Transmission of prion diseases

Kuru, CJD, and BSE have been transmitted to primates via the oral route. Repeated oral inoculations are more effective than single doses. There is no evidence that ingestion is a means of transmission for sCJD, GSS, or FFI. The highest concentrations of infectious material are to be found in brain, spinal cord, and eye, with material also present in CSF, lymphoreticular organs, lung, and kidney.

There have been four cases of probable blood transfusion–transmitted CJD. Iatrogenic transmission appears to require direct inoculation, implantation, or transplantation of infectious material. In terms of health care workers' protection, universal precautions are adequate and care should be taken to identify and safely dispose of material that may carry an infection risk.

There are specific guidelines for the performing of autopsies in suspected cases of CJD. Controversy continues on the best means of sterilizing instruments or other materials known to contain prions.

For guidance, see "Transmissible spongiform encephalopathy agents: Safe working and prevention of infection. Guidance from the Advisory Committee on Dangerous Pathogens TSE Working Group" at http:// www.advisorybodies.doh.gov.uk/acdp/tseguidance/index.htm.

Epidemiology

Familial cases are inherited in an autosomal dominant fashion; penetrance varies. Mean age of onset is around 65 years and these patients have the longest clinical course.

Sporadic cases (sCJD, around 90% instances) are rare, with an incidence of around 1 per million worldwide. Age of onset is 57–62 years. Cases have occurred in older teenagers. Early onset should prompt the consideration of iatrogenic sources of infection, as cases have occurred in association with cadaveric growth hormone and gonadotropin, dural grafts, corneal transplants, liver transplant, and contaminated neurosurgical instruments.

Blood can be demonstrated to have low-level infectivity, but there have been no recorded cases of CJD transmission by blood or blood products, nor do epidemiological studies identify previous transfusions as a risk factor for the development of CJD. The illness duration is around 4–8 months.

New-variant CJD (vCJD) is an entity distinct from sCJD, affecting younger patients (mean age 29 years, compared with 65 years for sCJD) with a longer illness duration (14 months) and a distinct clinical presentation. vCJD is attributed to consumption of cattle infected with BSE.

A large outbreak of BSE in the UK, thought to be due to cattle feed made from scrapie-infected sheep carcasses, peaked in 1992, 4 years after the introduction of a ban on ruminant feed. Five million animals were slaughtered in the effort to halt the epidemic.

By October 2008, 167 human cases of definite or probable vCJD had been reported in the UK, of which 164 had died. The number of reported cases has remained relatively stable. Only five cases were confirmed each year between 2005 and 2007.

Pathogenesis

Much of our current understanding of prion disease comes from studies of scrapie. A protein similar to PrP^{sc}, PrP^{C} is present in the brains of uninfected animals and is expressed constitutively. It is thought to have a role in neuronal development.

The proteins have very different biological properties (PrP^{C} is sensitive to protease degradation and exists predominantly on the cell surface in an A-helix form, PrP^{sc} is resistant to protease degradation and is found predominantly intracellularly with a B-sheet secondary structure). It is thought that PrP^{sc} is formed by post-translational modification of PrP^{C}. This conformational change may be induced by the interaction of PrP^{sc} with normal PrP protein, resulting in an exponential increase in abnormal forms.

Several mutations in the gene encoding prion protein have been identified in familial CJD, and some have associations with particular disease phenotypes (e.g., age of onset, rate of progression, associated symptoms). Prion gene mutations are very rarely found in cases of sporadic CJD.

Clinical features

sCJD

sCJD presents as a rapidly progressive dementia with myoclonus. The early clinical picture of around one-third of patients may be dominated by visual or cerebellar features. Myoclonus can be aggravated if the patient is startled. Two-thirds of patients eventually develop extrapyramidal signs; 40–80% develop corticospinal tract signs such as hyperreflexia and spasticity; visual features include cortical blindness and agnosia.

Seizures, sensory signs, cranial nerve lesions, and autonomic dysfunction may occur but are uncommon. Average duration from symptom onset to death is 7–9 months. There are rare cases of long duration.

vCJD

These cases are dominated by sensory (pain and parasthesia of face, hands, feet, and legs) and early psychiatric features such as depression and delusions that persist until obscured by dementia. They show the spongiform changes and neuronal loss of sCJD but differ in having prominent cerebellar involvement and widespread PrP^{sc}-positive amyloid plaques throughout the cerebellum and cerebrum.

Diagnosis

Routine tests, including standard CSF examination, are rarely helpful. Other causes of dementia and encephalopathy should be excluded (e.g., syphilis, HIV, nutritional, metabolic).

- *Imaging:* MRI is more sensitive than CT imaging in picking up abnormalities associated with CJD and certain findings specific to vCJD, but a normal brain scan does not significantly decrease the diagnostic probability of CJD.
- *EEG:* between 70% and 95% of patients ultimately develop a typical EEG pattern of slow background waves interrupted by generalized bilaterally synchronous biphasic or triphasic periodic sharp wave complexes. They are said to be 86% specific for CJD. Lack of this pattern after 4 months of symptoms should challenge the diagnosis. These abnormalities may not be seen in familial or variant CJD.
- *Certain specific CSF proteins* have been noted to have an association with CJD: protein 14-3-3 (sensitivity and specificity around 96% in sporadic cases, but only 50% and 91%, respectively in vCJD), tauprotein (the best sensitivity and specificity for vCJD at 80% and 94%, respectively). Elevations may be seen in herpes encephalitis, metabolic encephalopathies, and cerebral metastases.
- *Tonsil biopsy:* patients with vCJD (but not sporadic) may have detectable PrP^{sc} in follicular dendritic cells within lymphoid germinal centers. This may be detected by immunocytochemistry, and this is highly sensitive and specific for vCJD.

The gold standard remains examination of brain material: spongiform change, neuronal loss, reactive gliosis, and little inflammatory response. PrP^{sc} can be identified by Western blot of material obtained at autopsy or biopsy.

Treatment

All prion diseases seem to be invariably fatal, and there is no effective therapy. Symptom progression has apparently slowed in individual patients treated with pentosan polysulfate. Trials are in progress assessing the efficacy of pentosan polysulfate and quinacrine.

Kuru

Originally endemic within a specific tribal group of Papua New Guinea, epidemiological studies suggested it was transmitted through ritual cannibalism, and there have been no further cases since the practice was abandoned. A prodromal phase of headache and arthralgia is followed by progressive neurological decline (ataxia, tremor, choreoathetosis, myoclonus) and dementia.

Cranial nerve abnormalities, weakness, and sensory loss occur late in the disease, if at all. Laboratory tests are unhelpful, and EEG does not share the characteristic features of those seen in some cases of CJD.

The pathologically distinct feature of kuru is the presence of PrP^{sc} plaques, predominantly in the cerebellum (similar but not identical to those seen in vCJD).

Gerstmann–Sträussler–Scheinker syndrome

This rare prion disease (incidence <10 cases per 100 million people per year) is predominantly familial in nature. It is inherited in an autosomal dominant fashion with nearly complete penetrance. The key feature is spinocerebellar degeneration with dementia developing at a mean age of around 43–48 years.

The average illness duration is 5 years. It is associated with several prion protein gene mutations, which may contribute to the clinical heterogeneity; some families have prominent dementia, others have extrapyramidal signs for example. Even within a family the same mutation can produce a varied phenotype.

Laboratory tests including EEG are helpful only insofar as they may allow the exclusion of other diagnoses. Definitive diagnosis requires the examination of brain, which shows the finding typical of prion disease together with plaques similar to those of kuru and vCJD.

These plaques may have an atypical distribution resembling that of Alzheimer's disease. In the past, some cases may have been diagnosed as Alzheimer's disease.

Fatal familial insomnia

Fatal familial insomnia (FFI) is a prion disease showing autosomal dominant inheritance and presenting in middle age or above (range 35–61 years) with insomnia, autonomic dysfunction (hyperthermia, hypertension etc), and motor abnormalities (ataxia, myoclonus, etc.).

Patients can experience hallucinations, confusion, and memory problems, but dementia is rare. Some patients develop endocrine disturbance (increased cortisol, loss of circadian pattern of growth hormone secretion). Average disease duration is 13 months.

Neuropathology (neuronal loss, gliosis) is focused in thalamic nuclei, with changes seen occasionally in the cerebellar and cerebral cortices. Spongiform change is rare. PrP^{sc} can be identified on immunostaining, but concentrations are the lowest of the prion diseases.

Changes may be seen in EEG and sleep studies.

Overview of fungi

Fungi are aerobic eukaryotes with limited anaerobic capabilities. They have chitinous cell walls and ergosterol-containing plasma membranes (human cell walls contain cholesterol). They may grow as yeasts (single-celled, reproduce by budding), molds (form multicellular hyphae which grow by branching and extension), or both—dimorphic, growing as yeasts in vivo and at 37°C in vitro but as molds at 25°C.

Fungal infection is the seventh most common cause of infection-related death in the United States, with HIV being the most common predisposing factor.

Reproduction

Fungal reproduction may be sexual or asexual. Virtually all fungi can produce asexual spores by mitosis. Sexual spores are formed by the fusion of two haploid nuclei followed by meiotic division of the diploid nucleus (thus they carry half the chromosome number).

Certain fungi can only sexually reproduce with other colonies of a different, compatible mating type (e.g., *Histoplasma* spp.).

Pathogenesis

Fungal infections may be cutaneous (e.g., dermatophyte infection, pityriasis versicolor), subcutaneous (e.g., following traumatic inoculation: sporotrichosis), or systemic (see Table 3.26).

Systemic mycoses usually follow inhalation-acquired primary lung infection but may be caused by normal flora in an immunocompromised host (e.g., *Candida albicans* infection may be part of the normal flora, yet cause systemic disease in the immunosuppressed). Disease may be a consequence of toxin production (e.g., aflatoxin) or the host immune response to an infecting agent.

Organism characteristics facilitating infection include good growth at 37°C, production of substances such as keratinases by dermatophytes (digests keratin in skin, hair, and nails), the ability to change form (exist in nature as molds but take on yeast forms in a host, allowing them to spread and become pathogenic), the ability to adhere to surfaces (e.g., *Candida albicans*), antiphagocytic capsules (*Cryptococcus neoformans*), and persistence following phagocytosis, allowing dissemination with macrophages.

Generally, hosts have a high level of innate immunity to fungi; most infections are mild and self-limiting. This resistance derives from the fatty acid content of the skin, pH of the skin, mucosal surfaces and body fluids, epithelial turnover, competition with the normal bacterial flora, transferrin, and cilia of respiratory tract.

Table 3.26 Overview of common fungi causing human disease

Phylum	Organism	D	O	SC	SU	Comment
Basidiomycota	**Yeasts**					
	Cryptococcus neoformans	-	-			Mild lung granuloma in healthy persons
	Trichosporon beigelii	-			-	May disseminate
	Rhodotorula spp.		-			
	Malassezia furfur		-			Pityriasis versicolor
Ascomycota	*Candida* spp.	-	-			
	Pneumocystis jiroveci (was *carinii*)		-			
	Dimorphic fungi					
	Histoplasma capsulatum	-				Histoplasmosis
	Blastomyces dermatidis	-				Blastomycosis
	Sporothrix schenkii	-		-	-	Acquired by local trauma. Rare dissemination
	Coccidioides immitis, Paracoccidioides brasilensis	-				In the Americas
	Penicillium spp.		-			Disseminate in immunosuppressed
	Molds					
	Aspergillus spp.	-	-		-	Allergic, localized and invasive disease
	Epidermophyton spp.; *Trichophyton* spp.; *Microsporum* spp.				-	Dermatophytes – infect skin, hair, and nails
	Fusarium spp.		-			Disseminate in immunosuppressed
	Pseudallescheria boydii	-		-		Mycetoma. May infect any organ or disseminate
	Madurella spp.; *Acremonium* spp.; *Exophilia* spp., etc.			-		Mycetoma
Zygomycota	*Mucor* spp.; *Rhizopus* spp.	-				Rare invasion, e.g., mucormycosis

D, disseminated infection; O, opportunistic infection; SC, subcutaneous infection; SU, superficial infections.

Cell-mediated immunity (CMI) is important in controlling fungal infection. Humoral responses play a part, but patients with defects in CMI experience more severe fungal infections than those with humoral defects.

Epidemiology

Host factors play an important part in the epidemiology of fungal infection. Immunocompromise leads to a general increase in opportunistic fungal infection, but certain conditions predispose to specific organisms, e.g., rhinocerebral mucormycosis in patients with diabetic ketoacidosis, histoplasmosis in AIDS patients. Less dramatically, the use of antibiotics may increase the rate of candidal vaginitis.

Environment affects the pattern of fungal disease. Some are found worldwide but are seen mostly in individuals whose lifestyles place them at risk of exposure and inoculation (e.g., a gardener with subcutaneous inoculation of *Sporothrix schenckii* through minor trauma). Others are more likely to be seen in people living in or visiting specific regions (e.g., *Coccidioides immitis* in the desert of southwestern United States).

Candida species

Candida, a yeast, is the most common cause of fungal infection: candidemia is the fourth-most commonly reported bloodstream infection in the United States. *C. albicans* is responsible for 90% of cases of infection and for 40–50% of cases of fungemia. Non-*albicans* species are increasingly associated with invasive candidiasis and tend to be more resistant to certain antifungal drugs.

Mycology and epidemiology

Small, ovoid cells reproduce by budding. Both sexual and asexual forms exist. Of the over 150 *Candida* species, only nine are frequent human pathogens: *C. glabrata* and *C albicans* account for approximately 70–80% of cases of invasive candidiasis. The others are *C. guilliermondii, C. krusei, C. parapsilosis, C. tropicalis, C. pseudotropicalis, C. lusitaniae,* and *C. dubliniensis.*

C. albicans is ubiquitous and may be found in soil, food, and hospital environments. They are normal commensals of humans (skin, sputum, GI tract, female genital tract, etc.). The vast majority of human infections are of endogenous origin.

C. krusei is found in many environmental sites. It is fluconazole resistant and often found colonizing patients receiving fluconazole prophylaxis.

C. parapsilosis (adheres well to synthetic materials) and *C. tropicalis* are now more common causes of IV catheter infections and endocarditis than *C. albicans.*

C. glabrata infections of ICU patients are associated with a low survival rate. *Candida* spp. are uncommon laboratory contaminants.

Pathogenesis

The rise of *Candida* spp. infection relates to the increase in medical interventions: the use of antibiotics (suppressing normal bacterial flora and permitting the proliferation of *Candida* organisms), intravenous catheters (providing a route of entry), and GI tract surgery. Immune suppression mediated by disease (e.g., HIV) or therapies such as steroids are also associated with increased rates of infection.

The immune response to *Candida* infection is mediated by humoral and cellular mechanisms. *Candida* spp. virulence factors include surface molecules that permit organism adherence to other structures (human cells, extracellular matrix, prosthetic devices), acid proteases, and the ability to convert to a hyphal form.

General points on diagnosis

Many patients will require early treatment in the absence of a conclusive microbiological diagnosis. Those at risk (e.g., the neutropenic) who remain febrile despite broad-spectrum antibiotic therapy should be suspected of having systemic candidiasis.

Therapy should be started early and empirically in such patients. Always consider positive culture results from sterile sites to be significant. *Candida* may contaminate blood cultures, but treatment is usually indicated, as distinguishing contamination from infection is very difficult. Blood cultures are positive in 50–60% of cases of disseminated disease. Serology is rarely useful.

Culture

Strict aerobes grow well in routine blood cultures (usually positive in 48–96 hours in cases of candidemia) and on agar plates (smooth white colonies). Yeast forms (Gram-positive) and hyphae may be found on microscopy of clinical specimens (facilitated by 10% KOH).

Presumptive identification of *C. albicans*/*C. dubliniensis* is possible by inoculating organisms from a colony into a small tube of serum. Germ tubes should form within 90 minutes, which tend not to be seen with the other species. There are relatively high rates of false-positive and false-negative germ tube tests.

Accurate speciation relies on physiological characterisitics (e.g., fermentation, nitrate utilization) and can be demonstrated on commercial indicator agar preparations (ChromAgar) and with multiparameter kits.

Fungal antigen detection assays

The following assays are useful adjuncts in the diagnosis and monitoring of invasive fungal infection:

- *1-3 beta-d-glucan:* a cell wall component in a wide variety of fungi except cryptococcus and the zygomycetes. It is a broad-spectrum assay that detects *Aspergillus, Candida, Fusarium, Acremonium,* and *Saccharomyces* species The commercial blood assay (Fungitell®) has a sensitivity of 75–100% and a specificity of 88–100%. Its negative predictive value is useful, but the positive predictive value is limited by the ubiquitous nature of glucan—for example, positive tests may follow exposure to the cellulose in certain hemodialysis membranes or surgical gauze.

- *Candida mannan assay:* sensitivity ranges from 31% to 90% (less for non-*albicans* species).

Sensitivity testing

In vitro susceptibility testing can help guide the treatment of candidiasis to a greater extent than for the other fungi. Testing is not always available locally. Knowledge of the infecting species is highly predictive of likely susceptibility and can be used to guide therapy.

Susceptibility testing is important in managing deep infections of non-*albicans* species, particularly if the patient has been previously treated with an azole. *C. albicans* is rarely resistant to azoles, whereas certain non-

Table 3.27 Treatment of *Candida* infections

Presentation	First-line treatment	Duration	Comment
Candidemia in non-neutropenic adults	AmB or Flucon IV or Caspo (alternative AmB and Flucon for 7days then Flucon)	14 days after last positive blood culture and resolution of symptoms	Remove intravascular catheters.
Candidemia in children	AmB or Flucon IV (alternative Caspo)		
Candidemia in neutropenic adults	AmB or LPAmB IV or Caspo (alternative Flucon IV or PO)	14–21 days after last positive culture and resolution of symptoms and resolved neutropenia	Gastrointestinal sources of infection are common.
Chronic disseminated candidiasis	AmB or LPAmB IV	3–6 months and resolution or calcification of radiological lesions	Flucon may be given after 1–2 weeks of AmB therapy if stable or improved.
Chronic disseminated neonatal candidiasis	AmB IV (alternative Flucon)	14–21 days after clinical improvement	
Urinary candidiasis	AmB IV or Flucon (FC may be useful in cases due to non-*albicans* species)	7–14 days	Remove or replace stents or catheters.
Endocarditis	AmB IV or LPAmB IV and FC PO (alternative caspo)	At least 6 weeks after valve replacement	Valve replacement is nearly always necessary. Long-term suppression with Flucon may help if this is not possible.

Table 3.21 (Contd.)

Presentation	First-line treatment	Duration	Comment
Meningitis	AmB IV and FC IV	At least 4 weeks after resolution of symptoms and normalized CSF findings	Remove shunts if possible. Flucon has been used as a long-term suppressive therapy.
Endophthalmitis	AmB IV or Flucon IV or PO	6–12 weeks after surgery	Vitrectomy is usually necessary if vitreitis is present.
Oropharyngeal candidiasis	Clo or nystatin or Flucon PO (alternative AmB IV or PO or Caspo IV or Itracon PO)	7–14 days after clinical improvement	Long-term suppression with Flucon in patients with AIDS does not appear to lead to resistance.
Oesophageal candidiasis	Flucon PO or IV or Itracon or keto (alternative Voricon IV or PO or AmB IV or Caspo)		IV therapy maybe required in severe cases.
Genital candidiasis	Topical nystatin or Clo or short-course Flucon PO	1–7 days	10% with complicated vaginal candidiasis (severe or recurrent or caused by non-*albicans* species or in an abnormal host) may need 7–10 days of therapy with a non-azole

AmB, conventional amphotericin B; LPAmB, liposomal amphotericin B; Flucon, fluconazole; Clo, clotrimazole; Caspo, caspofungin; FC, 5-flucytosine; Itracon, itraconazole; Keto, ketoconazole.

*. Pappas PE, et al. (2009). Guidelines for the treatment of candidiasis. *Clin Infect Dis* 48:503–535.

albicans species may show intrinsic resistance to these and certain other antifungal agents (see Table 3.27, p. 419).

Superficial *Candida* infections

See p. 685 for details of the cutaneous manifestations of candidal infection.

Mucous membrane infection

Thrush

Thrush is a form of oral candidiasis characterized by white, creamy patches on the tongue and oral mucosa. Scraping removes the lesions, leaving a sore, bleeding surface. Diagnosis can be confirmed using a KOH smear or Gram stain to demonstrate pseudohyphae and yeast forms.

Other manifestations include acute atrophic candidiasis (affecting the tongue), chronic atrophic candidiasis (associated with denture use), angular cheilitis (not caused solely by *Candida*), and *Candida* leukoplakia (white plaques affecting cheek, lips and tongue; may be precancerous).

Oral thrush is associated with the use of inhaled steroids (often resolves spontaneously even without reduction in steroid use or with topical therapy), malignancy, and AIDS. Treatment is usually topical (systemic where this fails).

Prophylaxis with fluconazole has been effective in the prevention of oral *Candida* infections in cancer and AIDS patients but remains controversial. It is no longer routinely recommended in AIDS patients because of the development of resistance. It does reduce the rate of clinical candidiasis in patients undergoing immunosuppressive therapy.

Candida esophagitis

Most cases are associated with HIV or the treatment of malignant disease of the hematopoietic or lymphatic systems. It may occur in the absence of oral disease. Symptoms include dysphagia, retrosternal chest pain, nausea, and vomiting. Symptoms may be mild even in extensive disease. Diagnosis is made by endoscopy and biopsy.

In practice, diagnosis is often made presumptively in those with AIDS or malignancy on the basis of oral thrush and symptoms of esophagitis.

Extensive disease may result in intraluminal protrusions and partial obstruction. Perforation is rare. Severely immunocompromised patients may be coinfected with CMV or HSV.

Gastrointestinal candidiasis

This is usually associated with malignant disease, the most common manifestation being focal invasion of benign stomach ulcers. Diffuse gastric mucosal involvement is rare. Small and large bowel infection also occurs with white plaques, erosions, pseudomembrane, and ulceration visible on endoscopy.

Vulvovaginitis

Candida is the most common cause of vaginitis, and 75% of women have at least one episode in their lives. Predisposing factors include diabetes, antibiotic therapy, and pregnancy. Edema and vulval pruritis may be accompanied by discharge, which may be scanty or thick. Secondary infection of perineal skin and the urethra can occur.

Invasive *Candida* infections

Candidemia

Candida bloodstream infection is becoming more common, with a rise in the number of susceptible patients and the increased use of indwelling catheters. Venous and arterial vessels may be affected, as well as prosthetic vascular materials.

Complications include obstruction (e.g., of the superior vena cava [SVC]), endocarditis, and pulmonary venous thrombosis. Disease may be more extensive than symptoms suggest. Patients should always be checked for endocarditis and eye involvement. Management always involves removal of any lines or other prosthetic material.

CNS candidiasis

Candida may infect both brain substance and meninges. Around 50% of *Candida* meningitis cases (most common in premature neonates) occur in the context of disseminated disease. Meningitis may present non-specifically or with features typical of meningism.

Parenchymal infection takes the form of scattered multiple microabscesses and can have extremely variable clinical presentations. Infection may follow trauma, neurosurgery, or colonization of a ventricular shunt. CSF may show lymphocytosis with low glucose, but these findings are not consistent. Organisms are visible on Gram stain in 40% of cases.

The mortality rate is very high without therapy. Hydrocephalus is a common complication.

Cardiac candidiasis

Candida endocarditis usually affects the aortic and mitral valves. Associations include valve disease, chemotherapy, implantation of prosthetic heart valves, prolonged use of IV catheters, heroin addiction (*C. parapsilosis* is the most common cause), and pre-existing bacterial endocarditis.

Around 50% of cases follow cardiac surgery (associated with the length of the postoperative course, reflecting use of IV lines and antibiotics). Most cases present within the first 2 months postoperatively; <40% of cases are caused by non-*albicans* species; >70% of patients have positive blood cultures. Prior to antifungal therapy, mortality was 90%. Combined prolonged (6–10 weeks) medical and early surgical treatment has brought this to around 45%.

There is a high risk of relapse. Patients should be followed up for at least 2 years postoperatively. It may be appropriate to use long-term suppressive therapy, e.g., fluconazole.

Other cardiac manifestations include myocardial microabscesses, which may be a relatively frequent occurrence in cases of disseminated candidiasis. *Candida* is emerging as a cause of pericarditis.

Urinary tract infection

UTI probably follows extension of vaginitis in women, or in men is acquired by sexual contact with a woman with candidal vaginitis. There is frequently a history of recent antibiotic use. Candiduria is a common finding (particularly in those with urinary catheters) and does not equal renal tract infection.

Candida cystitis is associated with prolonged catheterization. Bladder perforation occurs in severe cases. Renal infection may occur hematogenously or less commonly by retrograde spread (particularly in association with renal tract obstruction or diabetes), causing papillary necrosis, fungal balls, and perinephric abscesses. Surgery may be required to remove fungal balls. Prosthetic material within the tract should be removed.

Asymptomatic candiduria should be treated in renal transplant patients, the neutropenic, low-birth-weight infants, and those undergoing urinary tract interventions (e.g., nephrostomy).

Bone and joint infection

Candida osteomyelitis may affect the vertebrae and discs, wrist, femur, scapula, humerus, and the costochondral junctions. Blood cultures are usually negative. Diagnosis is by aspiration of the affected area. Most cases follow hematogenous spread but may occur secondary to spread from the skin. Surgery may be required.

Septic arthritis due to *Candida* occurs in the context of dissemination, trauma, surgery, and intra-articular injection of steroids. It may be a complication of AIDS and rheumatoid arthritis. *C. albicans* is the most common cause in the context of disseminated infection.

Non-*albicans* species are more common when infection is local.

Intra-abdominal infection

Peritonitis may complicate peritonial dialysis (PD), GI perforation, and surgery. Infection tends to remain localized; dissemination is extremely rare in cases associated with PD and around 25% in cases secondary to GI perforation. Other GI organs that can be affected include the gall bladder, spleen, liver, and pancreas. Hepatosplenic infection occurs in the severely immunocompromised.

Candida peritonitis due to PD can be treated by local instillation of amphotericin B (can be painful) or fluconazole. Catheter removal may be indicated. *Candida* from postoperative drains need not always prompt antifungal treatment. Therapy is required for treatment of *Candida* identified in ascites from an undrained abdomen.

The failure rate for treatment of liver and spleen infection is high, even with combination therapy. Results may be better with liposomal amphotericin. Candidiasis of the biliary tract may require drainage.

Disseminated candidiasis

Patients at risk of dissemination include those with malignancy (particularly acute leukemia), burn patients, and those with complicated postoperative courses (e.g., organ transplants, GI tract surgery). Multiple organs tend to be affected, most frequently the kidney, brain, myocardium, and eye.

The pathological features are small abscesses and diffuse microabscesses with a granulomatous reaction. Many patients have negative blood cultures, and diagnosis is often made very late or at postmortem.

Tests for *Candida* antigen and serum antibodies have a high rate of false-negative results; diagnosis is largely clinical. A positive blood culture should be considered abnormal.

The consensus is that all patients should be treated with antifungals and examined carefully for evidence of ocular involvement or other manifestations of disseminated disease. Cultures should be repeated several times and catheters removed or replaced (but not by passing the new one over a wire at the site of the old one). Speciation and isolate sensitivity should be confirmed. Therapy should be continued for 2 weeks after the last positive blood culture.

Other

- *Respiratory tract candidiasis:* definitive diagnosis depends on biopsy: recovery of *Candida* from sputum or bronchoalveolar lavage (BAL) alone is not sufficient (high levels of colonization).
- *Ocular infection:* see Uveitis (p. 672).

Treatment

The treatment of *Candidia* infections is summarized in Table 3.27. Updated 2009 guidelines for the treatment of candidiasis have been published by the IDSA[1] and are available online (www.idsociety.org).

Points to remember in treatment

- Remove infected IV lines, replace infected valves, if possible.
- Amphotericin B is the first-line agent for treatment of disseminated and deep-organ infection; most strains are sensitive. It may be combined with flucytosine in systemic neonatal infection.
- Knowledge of the infecting species is highly predictive of likely susceptibility and can be used to guide therapy. The new azoles (e.g., voriconazole) and candins (caspofungin) are useful against non-*albicans* species, which are commonly fluconazole resistant:
  - *C.glabrata* is less susceptible to azoles.
  - *C. krusei* is intrinsically resistant to ketoconazole and fluconazole and less susceptible to other antifungals, including intraconazole, voriconazole, and amphotericin B. It remains sensitive to the candins.
- *C. lusitaniae* is susceptible to azoles but frequently resistant to amphotericin B. Susceptibility testing is important in managing deep infections of non-*albicans* species, particularly if the patient has been previously treated with an azole when resistance must be considered.
- Azoles are a useful continuation therapy for *C. albicans* infections initially controlled with IV amphotericin B.

Reference

1. Pappas PE, et al. (2009). Guidelines for the treatment of candidiasis. *Clin Infect Dis* 48:503–535.

Malessezia infections

These lipophilic yeasts (grow in the presence of certain fatty acids) are oval or round in shape and normal commensals of the skin, which they colonize in late childhood. They are a cause of skin infections and have been known to cause catheter-acquired sepsis.

Pityriasis versicolor

Superficial skin infection is characterized by hypopigmented lesions usually confined to the trunk and proximal limbs. It is usually caused by *M. globosa* or *M. furfur*.

Pathogenesis

Clinical infection is usually associated with yeasts transforming to hyphal forms from their round/oval appearance. Although seen at greater frequency in those with Cushing's syndrome, there is no clear association with T-cell suppression.

Infection is more common in the tropics and may be precipitated by sun exposure. A carboxylic acid produced by the yeast may lead to the depigmentation.

Clinical features

Non-itchy macules develop on the trunk and proximal limbs and may be hypo- or hyperpigmented. They can coalesce, forming scaly plaques.

Diagnosis

Direct microscopy of the lesions will reveal yeasts and hyphae, often described as "spaghetti and meatballs." They may fluoresce under UV light. Organisms are best seen in skin scrapings after ink and potassium hydroxide staining.

Treatment

Some lesions resolve spontaneously. Otherwise, topical treatment for 2 weeks with an azole, terbinafine cream, selenium lotion, or 20% sodium thiosulphate is usually effective.

Severe cases may require a course of oral azole.

Malassezia folliculitis

Topical therapy may be effective. Systemic treatment is often necessary. There are three clinical presentations:
- Itchy papules and pustules on the back and upper chest, sometimes appearing after sun exposure
- Multiple small papules across the back and chest in patients with seborrheic dermatitis. Lesions may display erythema and scaling.
- Multiple pustules across the trunk and face in patients with HIV.

Seborrheic dermatitis

Once thought simply to colonize a pre-existing area of hyperproliferative skin, *Malassezia* is now implicated in the pathogenesis.

Pathogenesis

Although it is unlikely that direct invasion precipitates the appearance of seborrheic dermatitis, an indirect mechanism such as sensitization may exist. Most cases resolve with a course of azole, and improvement in clinical appearance follows eradication of the organism.

Clinical features
Erythema and itching and scaling of chest and upper back occur. Facial lesions have a greasy appearance and appear around the eyebrows, ears, and nose. Scalp lesions are scaly, and pustules may develop. Patients with AIDS may develop abrupt and widespread lesions.

Diagnosis
Diagnosis is clinical, and topical treatment is usually sufficient.

Other yeasts

Trichosporon species
Trichosporon beigelii can be part of the commensal flora of humans. It can cause invasive infections in the immunocompromised and has also been identified in prosthetic valve infections. Trichosporonosis is an acute, febrile infection with dissemination to multiple organs. The means of acquisition is not clear.

Diagnosis is by biopsy and culture. Blood cultures tend to be positive late in the course of illness. Amphotericin B has been used in treatment.

Rhodotorula species
This is a cause of disseminated infections in immunocompromised patients, usually acquired through IV catheter infection following bone marrow transplant.

Cryptococcus neoformans

Cryptococcosis is a systemic fungal disease caused by the yeast-like organism *Cryptococcus neoformans*.

The organism
C. neoformans is an encapsulated yeast-like organism that reproduces by budding. The cell is round or ovoid (4–6 micrometer in diameter) and surrounded by a capsule of variable size. There are five capsular serotypes (A, B, C, D and AD). Types A and D were previously classified as *C. neoformans* var. *neoformans* and B and C as *C. neoformans* var. *gattii*.

Genotypic evidence has led to a recent reclassification. Serotype A is considered var *grubii*, serotypes D and AD var. *neoformans,* and B and C are now considered a separate species: *Crypotococcus gattii. C. gattii* tends to cause infections in immunocompetent individuals, whereas *C. grubii* and *neoformans* (the majority of clinical isolates) infect the immunocompromised.

Epidemiology
C. neoformans is a ubiquitous environmental saprophyte. Serotype A (most common) and serotype D are found worldwide and have been isolated

from pigeon droppings and nesting places, from contaminated soil and decaying woodchips, or, occasionally, from fruit.

Infections caused by serotypes B and C are largely restricted to tropical and subtropical areas. The organism has been cultured from eucalyptus trees.

Transmission

Circumstantial evidence suggests that infection occurs by inhalation of aerosolized organisms, but there is no evidence of person-to-person transmission or laboratory-acquired infection. Rare routes of transmission include organ transplantation from infected donors or cutaneous inoculation. Cryptococcosis also occurs in animals, but there is no evidence of zoonotic transmission.

Risk factors

Cryptococcosis occurs more commonly in patients with defects in T-cell-mediated immunity. Predisposing factors include the following:

- AIDS (80–90% of cryptococcal infections, AIDS-defining illness in 5–88% of patients, associated with CD4 count <100 cells/mm^3)
- Post-transplantation (peak period 4–6 weeks)
- Others: corticosteroid therapy, lymphoreticular malignancies (especially Hodgkin's disease), sarcoidosis

Pathogenesis

A number of potential virulence factors have been identified:

- Capsular polysaccharide
- Melanin production
- Mannitol production
- Lack of soluble anticryptococcal factors in CSF

The inflammatory response to infection is variable. The characteristic lesion consists of cystic clusters of fungi with no inflammatory response that are spread throughout the brain.

Less commonly, focal inflammatory lesions (cryptococcomas) are found. In severe infections, the leptomeninges are thickened with distension of the subarachnoid by a white gelatinous material (attributed to capsular polysaccharide).

Clinical features

- *Cryptococcal meningitis:* onset may be acute or chronic, and symptoms may be mild and nonspecific. On examination, fever may be absent; there may be minimal or no nuchal rigidity, papilloedema (30%), cranial nerve palsies (20%), and blindness. Seizures occur late. Differential diagnosis is other mycoses, TB meningitis, viral meningoencephalitides, and meningeal metastases.
- *Pulmonary cryptococcosis:* may be asymptomatic or present with dyspnea, cough, and chest pain. Physical signs are unusual. May be rapidly progressive in AIDS. Differential diagnosis includes tumor (HIV-negatives), *Pneumocystis* pneumonia, pulmonary TB, histoplasmosis.
- *Other sites:* C. neoformans may cause skin lesions, bone lesions, oral lesions, vulvar lesions, post-transplant pyelonephritis, and prostatic cryptococcosis.

Laboratory diagnosis

CSF examination

CSF findings include elevated opening pressure (may be >500 mm CSF), low glucose, high protein, and high white cell count (>20/mm³, lymphocyte predominance). CSF abnormalities may be minimal or absent in AIDS. A cryptococcal antigen test should be performed.

India ink smear

India ink or nigrosin staining of the CSF deposit shows a capsule, double cell wall, and refractile inclusions in the cytoplasm in 20–50% of HIV-negative cases and around 75% of AIDS patients.

Fungal culture

Appropriate samples include CSF deposit, sputum, and urine, which are cultured on Sabouraud agar. Positive blood cultures may occur in extensive infections. *C. neoformans* colonies are smooth, convex, and yellow or tan on solid media. It produces brown colonies on birdseed agar (melanin production). Unlike other yeasts, it does not produce pseudomycelia on cornmeal or Tween agar.

It can be identified by biochemical tests, e.g., API or biotyping agars. There are commercially available DNA hybridization probes.

Cryptococcal antigen test

A variety of latex agglutination tests and EIAs are available with reported sensitivities of ≥90%. They can be performed on both CSF and serum.

False-positive tests may occur, but titers are usually ≤1:8 and can result from infection with *Trichosporan beigelii* and certain bacterial genera (e.g., capnocytophaga).

Histopathology

Methenamine silver or periodic acid–Schiff staining shows a yeast-like organism with narrow-based buds. Mayer's mucicarmine stain stains the capsule rose red.

Treatment

Meningitis

Multiple studies have compared various treatment regimes. All consist of an induction phase (usually 2 weeks), a consolidation phase (around 6 weeks), and for those patients with long-term immunosuppression (e.g., HIV with low CD4 counts), a long-term maintenance phase, as relapse is common.

Aggressive management of raised intracranial pressure (ICP) by repeated lumbar puncture (LP) has been associated with significantly better outcomes. Those with raised ICP at diagnosis or who develop symptoms suggestive of it should have daily LP to reduce the pressure to <20 cm CSF or 50% of the opening pressure. Those requiring LP after 4 weeks will probably need a permanent ventricular shunt.

- *Induction* should be with amphotericin and flucytosine. This has been shown to be the most rapidly fungicidal and should be continued for 2 weeks or until the patient is asymptomatic.

- *Consolidation* follows with high-dose fluconazole (400 mg daily) for 6–10 weeks.
- *Maintenance therapy* with lower-dose fluconazole (200 mg daily) is required for at least a year in patients with HIV. Cessation may then be considered in those who have responded to HAART.
- Selected AIDS patients with mild, asymptomatic CNS cryptococcosis have been treated successfully with a long course of very high dose oral fluconazole (<1 g/day) and flucytosine; however, many have significant problems with drug side effects (GI and bone marrow toxicity).

Pulmonary disease

Mild to moderate infections in the immunocompetent can be treated with oral fluconazole alone. Those with severe disease or multi-organ involvement should be treated as for meningitis. Surgical excision may be curative.

Prognosis

Prognosis depends on the severity of the illness at presentation and the nature of any underlying disease. Relapse is rare in those HIV patients who respond to treatment, continue suppressive therapy, and experience improved immune function on HAART.

Reference

Perfect JR, et al. (2010). IDSA Practice guidelines for the management of cryptococcal disease. Infectious Diseases Society of America. *Clin Infect Dis* 50:291–322.

Pneumocystis jiroveci

For many years, *Pneumocystis carinii* was thought to be a protozoan, but rRNA analysis suggests that it is more closely related to fungi. The human-derived organism was recently renamed *Pneumocystis jiroveci*, whereas the rat-derived organism remains *Pneumocystis carinii*.

Microbiology

P. jiroveci is an unusual fungus that lacks ergosterol in its cell wall and is therefore not susceptible to certain antifungals. It has proved extremely difficult to culture in vitro, so biochemical and metabolic studies of the organism have been limited. Three developmental stages exist: the trophic form, the sporocyte, and the spores.

Epidemiology

P. jiroveci is ubiquitous in the environment and has a worldwide distribution. Primary infection occurs in childhood and is probably asymptomatic. The principal mode of transmission is by the airborne route.

Once infection is acquired, there is some debate about how long the organism resides in the host. One view is that *P. jiroveci* remains quiescent and reactivates when immune deficiency develops. The other school of thought is that infection is transient but people are frequently exposed to the organism.

Risk factors include the following:
• Premature, debilitated infants
• Severe protein malnutrition
• Primary immunodeficiency, e.g., severe combined immunodeficiency disease (SCID)
• Immunosuppressive drugs, e.g., corticosteroids, cytotoxics
• Organ transplantation.

Pathogenesis

Once inhaled, the trophic form attaches to the alveolar type I cell and undergoes proliferation. The host immune defects that contribute to the uncontrolled proliferation of *P. jiroveci* and the development of disease are incompletely understood, but impaired humoral and T-cell-mediated immunity both appear to be important.

The host immune response results in the production of inflammatory cytokines (e.g., TNF-A and interleukin-1 [IL-1]), which may contribute to lung damage. The principal histological finding is a foamy eosinophilic alveolar exudate. There may be hyaline membrane formation, interstitial fibrosis, and edema.

Clinical features

Pneumonia (P. jiroveci pneumonia, or PJP)

There is insidious onset of fever, dyspnea, a nonproductive cough, and reduced exercise tolerance. Occasionally, there may be sputum production, hemoptysis, or chest pain. Examination reveals tachypnea, tachycardia, exercise-induced hypoxia, and crackles (in <30% adults).

Infants may be cyanosed with respiratory distress.

Extrapulmonary disease

This occurs mainly in the context of advanced HIV infection and is rare. The most commonly affected sites are the lymph nodes, spleen, liver, bone marrow, GI tract, eyes, thyroid, adrenal glands, and kidneys.

Clinical findings may vary from incidental findings at autopsy to severe progressive disease, with or without pulmonary involvement.

Laboratory diagnosis

• *Specimens:* *P. jiroveci* is rarely found in expectorated sputum but can be found in induced sputum (50–90% sensitivity). Bronchoalveolar lavage (BAL) increases the diagnostic rate to >90%, especially if multiple lobes are sampled or the procedure is directed to the site(s) of radiographic involvement. Transbronchial biopsy may provide further information but is associated with risk of complications, e.g., bleeding, pneumothorax. Open lung biopsy may be helpful if BAL is non-diagnostic.
• *Histopathology:* a variety of stains have been used to identify *P. jiroveci*, e.g., methenamine silver, Wright Giemsa, calcofluor white. Commercial immunofluorescence tests are more sensitive than histological stains but more expensive. Immunohistochemistry has also been used.
• *Molecular diagnostics:* PCR amplification and detection of *P. jiroveci* DNA has proved highly sensitive and reasonably specific. However,

the detection of a PCR product in a clinical specimen may represent subclinical infection or result from antibiotic pretreatment.

* *1,3-beta-D glucan (Fungitell):* glucan is a cell wall component of most fungi, including *Pneumocystis*. This assay appears to have utility for diagnosing PJP.

Treatment

The treatment of choice is high-dose trimethoprim/sulfamethoxazole (15–20 mg/kg/day trimethoprim, 75–100 mg/kg/day sulfamethoxazole) for 14–21 days. Side effects are common in HIV patients and include skin rash, fever, cytopenias, nausea, vomiting, hepatitis, pancreatitis, nephritis, hyperkalemia, metabolic acidosis, and CNS symptoms.

Alternative regimens include the following:

* Trimethoprim and dapsone
* Clindamycin and primaquine
* Atovaquone
* Intravenous pentamidine

Adjunctive corticosteroids are recommended in patients with hypoxia. Patients should be tested for glucose-6-phosphate deficiency before taking dapsone or primaquine.

Prognosis

Untreated PJP in immunocompromised patients is fatal. Poor prognostic factors include hypoxia (partial pressure of arterial oxygen [PaO_2] <7 kPa), high alveolar–arterial oxygen gradient (>45 mmHg), and extensive pulmonary infiltrates.

The short-term mortality (1–3 months) in HIV-infected patients has fallen to 10–20%, whereas the mortality in HIV-negative patients remains 30–50%. Patients who recover are at risk of developing recurrent episodes or pneumothoraces.

Prevention

HIV-infected patients

Primary prophylaxis with trimethoprim/sulfamethoxazole is recommended in HIV-infected patients with a CD4 count <200 cells/mm^3. Secondary prophylaxis is recommended for life but may be discontinued in patients with CD4 count consistently >200 cells/mm^3.

Alternative regimens are atovaquone; dapsone pyrimethamine + folinic acid; aerosolized or IV pentamidine; pyrimethamine + sulfadoxine; or clindamycin + primaquine.

HIV-negative patients

Although no formal guidelines exist, chemoprophylaxis should probably be considered in all patients with predisposing conditions (see above). Trimethoprim/sulfamethoxazole is the agent of choice, as there is more limited clinical experience in HIV-negative individuals with other regimens.

Reference

Briel M, Bucher HE, et al. (2006). Adjunctive corticosteroids for pneumocystis pneumonia in patients with HIV infection. *Cochrane database* 2006, article No.CD006150

Aspergillus

Aspergillus is a mold capable of causing a wide range of disease in both healthy and immunocompromised individuals.

Mycology

Many species cause invasive disease in humans. The most frequently identified include *A. fumigatus* (around 90%), *A. flavus*, and *A. niger*.

Pathogenic species grow better on routine mycological media at 37°C than nonpathogenic, most of which cannot grow at this temperature. Colonies become apparent at 36–90 hours. Sporulation occurs up to 2 days later but may take longer with less common species.

Identification of common species is possible by microscopic and colonial appearance, although more detailed identification requires specialized media and molecular methods.

Microscopy of pathological specimens may reveal hyphae (best seen on silver stains), but sporulation is not often seen (save in specimens taken from air-containing areas such as the lung), thus the organism cannot be distinguished from other pathogenic molds by this means.

Epidemiology

The organism is found worldwide, favoring decomposing vegetable material (e.g., potted plants, spices, and particularly around farms). Molecular techniques have demonstrated that colonized individuals and those with aspergilloma tend to pick up several different genotypes over time. Most invasive infections, however, are caused by a single genotype.

Pathogenesis

Disease spectrum is wide, from superficial infection, to allergic, to disseminated. Time from exposure to disease in invasive aspergillosis ranges from 36 hours to 3 months. Disease may follow infection by organisms that have already colonized an individual (e.g., in neutropenia).

Many factors influence disease form and severity: organism growth rate (*A. fumigatus* being the fastest), spore size (*A. fumigatus'* small spores allow them to pass deep into the lung), the hydrophobic coat of conidia (protection from host defense), the ability to adhere to epithelial surfaces (achieved by *A. fumigatus* much more effectively than other species), and enzyme/toxin production (e.g., aflatoxin produced by *A. flavus*).

Host defenses include lung macrophages (capable of ingesting and killing conidia), T lymphocytes (appear to be important in chronic and allergic disease), complement proteins, and neutrophils (damage hyphae). Corticosteroids impair macrophage and neutrophil killing.

Pathological appearances include vascular invasion (with consequent infarction of distal tissue) with acute invasive disease in the immunosuppressed; alveolar consolidation, necrotizing granulomatous pneumonia, and bronchiectatic cavities in chronic invasive aspergillosis; and exudative bronchiolitis and eosinophilic pneumonia with allergic bronchopulmonary aspergillosis.

Clinical features of noninvasive *Aspergillus* disease

Superficial

Cutaneous infections are rare, usually occurring in neutropenic patients at the site of IV catheter insertion or in burn wounds. More common s otomycosis, a growth of *A. niger* in those with chronic otitis externa which may cause itch and discomfort. Appearance may be of nonspecific inflammation.

Cleaning and topical therapy with an agent such as amphotericin B 3% or clotrimazole is curative.

Allergic disease: allergic bronchopulmonary aspergillosis (ABPA)

ABPA occurs in those with asthma or cystic fibrosis and hypersensitivity to airway colonization by *Aspergillus*. It presents with worsening asthma or lung function. Patients may have an eosinophilic pneumonia or airway sputum impaction. Blood tests may reveal eosinophilia early in disease.

Oral corticosteroids can help exacerbations, and inhaled steroids may prevent episodes from occurring. Oral itraconazole may help those requiring long-term steroids. *Aspergillus* may also cause allergic sinusitis; this is best managed by aeration of the affected sinus.

Aspergilloma: pulmonary aspergilloma

This follows *Aspergillus* colonization of pre-existing cavities or cysts left from TB, sarcoidosis, or *Pneumocystis* pneumonia. TB cavities 2 cm or larger have a 15–25% risk of developing an aspergilloma. Some patients are asymptomatic; most have productive cough, hemoptysis, weight loss, wheeze, and clubbing.

Culture of sputum may reveal the organism, and precipitating IgG may be detected in serum. Radiological imaging demonstrates the hyphal mass as a cavity surrounded by a rim of air.

Complications include massive hemoptysis (may be fatal; embolization may help those in whom surgery is not possible), contiguous spread of infection to pleura or vertebrae, and dissemination. Aspergilloma must be distinguished from chronic invasive disease requiring systemic therapy.

In terms of treatment, 10% of cases resolve spontaneously. Surgical resection has a role in the treatment of isolated lesions in those with good lung function. Amphotericin B has been injected into cavities with some effect. Oral itraconazole or voriconazole may provide symptomatic relief. Sinus aspergilloma may develop in the ethmoid or maxillary cavities. Surgical drainage is usually sufficient in those with no evidence of mucosal involvement.

Medical therapy should be used in combination with surgery in those with invasive disease or involvement of the frontal or sphenoid sinus.

Eye

Aspergillus keratitis (and less commonly endophthalmitis) may occur following ocular trauma or hematogenously (e.g., IV drug users, endocarditis). Early recognition and treatment is essential for a good outcome. Corneal smears may reveal hyphae, and cultures are usually positive.

Keratitis may be treated with topical amphotericin B (27% response when given hourly). Superficial infections may be treated with topical clotrimazole. Oral itraconazole is effective in up to 75% of cases.

Surgery is required when medical therapy fails or when there is the threat of ocular perforation or the formation of a descemetocele (a herniation of the posterior limiting layer of the cornea). Vitrectomy may be required to establish the diagnosis and, where possible, intraoperative examination of the specimen for hyphae is useful, as it allows immediate administration of intravitreal amphotericin B or voriconazole. Systemic therapy is also recommended.

Clinical features of invasive *Aspergillus* disease

Invasive pulmonary disease

Over 80% of patients with invasive disease have pulmonary infection. The immunocompromised tend to experience few symptoms but progress rapidly, whereas the less immune impaired have more symptoms with a slowly progressive, chronic course.

Acute invasive pulmonary aspergillosis

Around 25% have no symptoms in the early stages, with the remainder experiencing dry cough and a mild fever. Pleuritic chest pain and hemoptysis may occur, as may breathlessness in those with bilateral disease who can become hypoxic. Signs resemble pulmonary embolism (PE) or mucormycosis.

CXR changes can be nonspecific (consolidation, cavities, wedge-shaped lesions, lower lobe shadowing) and may appear normal in 10% of cases. High-resolution CT images are useful in aiding early diagnosis. Early in disease, radiological imaging may demonstrate nodules with the halo sign (a zone of ground-glass attenuation surrounding a nodule or mass).

In later disease, with neutrophil recovery, nodules may cavitate, producing the air-crescent sign. Focal or nodular disease has a better prognosis than diffuse or bilateral infection. In focal disease, the danger is of massive hemoptysis, which may occur with no warning.

Chronic invasive pulmonary aspergillosis

This occurs less frequently than the acute form. Predisposing conditions include AIDS, alcoholism, diabetes mellitus, chronic granulomatous diseases, and corticosteroid therapy for chronic pulmonary diseases. Some patients have no identifiable predisposing factors.

Presentation is with weeks of chronic productive cough. Other symptoms include hemoptysis, fever, and weight loss. Infection may extend to the chest wall, spine, or brachial plexus.

CXR shows cavitation and consolidation, and in the absence of previous images to demonstrate the presence or absence of a pre-existing cavity, it can be difficult to distinguish from aspergilloma. Definitive diagnosis can be made through positive culture of a biopsy specimen.

Airways

More common in lung transplant recipients and AIDS patients, *Aspergillus* tracheobronchitis varies from mild inflammation to severe ulcerative disease; 80% experience symptoms (cough, fever, breathlessness, chest pain, hemoptysis) that become more severe with progression. Complications include wheeze or stridor, tracheal perforation, dissemination, airway occlusion, and death.

Bronchoscopy allows definitive diagnosis. CXR is usually normal in early disease.

Sinus

Invasive *Aspergillus* sinusitis can be acute or chronic:

Acute

Early symptoms include fever, cough, nose-bleeding, headaches, discharge, and sinus discomfort. Ulceration is preceded by decreased blood flow to the affected nasal areas; these may be identified by careful examination for loss of sensitivity. Infection may extend to the palate, orbit, or brain.

CT or MRI allows identification of the extent of disease, and culture or hyphal identification tissue confirms diagnosis

Chronic

Most cases have no identifiable immunocompromise. Early symptoms include nasal congestion and discharge, loss of smell, and headache. It is clinically indistinguishable from other causes of sinusitis. As disease extends, proptosis, loss of vision, ocular pain, and even features of stroke may develop.

Radiological features are similar to those of acute disease. Obtaining a positive culture may require multiple samples.

Brain

From 10 to 20% of cases of disseminated disease develop cerebral aspergillosis. It is rare in the immunocompetent, when it is usually secondary to neurosurgery. Severely immunocompromised individuals have a nonspecific presentation with confusion and seizures, and death following a few days later. Less severely immune impaired patients tend to have headache and focal neurological features. Fever may occur. Meningitis is rare.

Contrast CT appearances are of infarction or of a ring-enhancing abscess with edema. Lesions may be deep and surgically inaccessible.

Diagnosis rests on culture and microscopy of a biopsy or aspiration sample. This may not be possible, and diagnosis can be made presumptively in those with invasive disease elsewhere and typical radiological appearances.

Other

Aspergillus endocarditis can occur in isolation or as part of disseminated disease. Blood cultures are usually negative, and valve replacement is necessary to achieve cure. Other sites of infection include pericardial, intestinal, esophageal, renal, vascular graft, and bone.

Diagnosis

Radiology

Once clinical suspicion of invasive disease has been raised, CT or MRI assessment of the lungs, sinuses, and brain should be performed within 24 hours.

Airway disease

Bronchoscopy is useful, but biopsy is rarely positive in focal lung disease. A needle biopsy or surgical resection (superior to open biopsy) is appropriate for peripheral pulmonary lesions. Focal lesions near the great vessels should prompt urgent resection given the high risk of massive hemoptysis.

Respiratory samples should be examined by microscopy (rapid but does not distinguish species) and cultured. Antigen testing (galactomannan) of BAL may be useful.

Culture in invasive disease

Positive cultures from any site should prompt a thorough evaluation, particularly in the immunocompromised. Definitive diagnosis of invasion requires culture of the organism from a sterile site. Combinations of other positive findings have less certainty, as other molds can give the same appearance.

The most common *Aspergillus* species are *A. fumigatus*, *A. flavus*, *A. terreus*, and *A. niger*.

Antibody testing

Aspergillus antibody tests are useful in the diagnosis of ABPA, aspergilloma, and chronic invasive disease. They are not sensitive in the severely immunocompromised.

Serum antigen tests

The galactomannan (a fungal exoantigen released by all pathogenic *Aspergillus* species during growth) assay has moderate accuracy for diagnosis of invasive aspergillosis in immunocompromised patients. The test is most useful in patients who have hematological malignancy or who have undergone hematopoietic cell transplantation.

It can become positive a week before clinical disease is manifest, and the titer corresponds to the tissue burden, with a high level having prognostic significance. It is of low sensitivity in pediatric patients with primary immunodeficiencies. False positives may follow absorption of galactomannan from the diet in those with mucositis, or the administration of Piperacillin/tazobactam®.

The 1–3 beta-D-glucan test has a high negative predictive value, which may help exclude invasive disease in adults (see *Candida* species, p. 417).

Treatment[1]

Invasive aspergillosis is fatal in virtually all cases if untreated. Good outcomes require aggressive diagnosis in those groups at risk, early presumptive treatment, early changes in treatment where the response is poor, early surgical resection of focal lung lesions located near the hilum and great vessels, and reduction or reversal of immunosuppression when possible. Evaluating the response takes longer in those with less immunocompromise.

For invasive aspergillosis, voriconazole is the drug of choice. A lipid preparation of amphotericin B, echinocandin, or posaconazole is an alternative. Primary combination therapy is not routinely recommended, based on lack of clinical data.

Treatment is often prolonged and should be continued at least until the disease has stopped progressing. It may be appropriate to continue therapy with voriconazole or posaconazole while the patient remains immunocompromised. Itraconazole was previously used but is limited by its variable bioavailability (e.g., in those with intestinal problems such as that resulting from graft-versus-host disease [GVHD]) and drug interactions (e.g., agents activating P-450, cyclosporine, protease inhibitors).

For invasive sinusitis, treatment is similar to that for invasive pulmonary aspergillosis. Relapse is common.

For cerebral disease, surgery is useful only for diagnosis unless the lesion is superficial and isolated. Otherwise, treatment rests on antifungal therapy.

Surgery is indicated for focal invasive pulmonary diseases, significant hemoptysis, lesions near great vessels and pericardium, or invasion of the chest wall. Also consider it for localized skin or soft tissue infection, infected catheter or device, endocarditis, osteomyelitis, or sinusitis.

No significant clinical benefit has been seen with G-CSF, GM-CSF, granulocyte infusions, or IFN-γ.

See IDSA guidelines for treatment of aspergillosis.[2]

References

1. The Aspergillus Web site: www.aspergillus.man.ac.uk (accessed 6 August 2008).

2. Walsh TJ, Anaissie EJ, Denning DW, et al. (2008). Treatment of aspergillosis: clinical practice guidelines of the Infectious Diseases Society of America. *Clin Infect Dis* 46:327–360.

Mucormycosis

Mucormycosis is a clinical syndrome caused by a number of fungal species belonging to the order *Mucorales* (class *Zygomycetes*).

Mycology

Fungi are spore forming and grow rapidly in the mold form in both tissues and the environment. Common species causing mucormycosis include *Rhizopus*, *Rhizomucor*, and *Mucor*. Microscopy allows a degree of speciation (e.g., appearance of the columellae and rhizoids if present).

Epidemiology

All members of the order are widespread in decaying matter. As testament to their ubiquitous nature, they have been isolated from wooden tongue depressors and infection has resulted from their use as splints in neonates.

Clinical disease is limited largely to the immunocompromised, transplant patients, those with diabetes mellitus, and trauma patients. Infection may be rhinocerebral, respiratory, cutaneous, disseminated, or localized to specific organs.

Pathogenesis

Infection is acquired via the respiratory tract or in primary cutaneous infection, via the inoculation of spores into skin abrasions. Spore germination follows in hosts whose immune response is deficient. Macrophages and neutrophils are important in preventing growth, and normal human serum is fungistatic.

Invasive disease is favored by hyperglycemia, acidosis, and in patients receiving desferrioxamine (an agent that enhances fungal growth experimentally). Cases are not as significantly raised in those with AIDS as might otherwise be expected. Hyphae invade tissues, penetrate blood vessel walls, and may grow along the vessel, contributing to thrombosis and necrosis.

Clinical features

Rhinocerebral disease

This is a disease of the immunosuppressed, seen in diabetic patients (particularly if acidotic) and neutropenic leukemia patients on antibiotics, and is almost invariably fatal. Fungal infection causes septic necrosis and infarction of the tissues of the nasopharynx and orbit.

Patients develop facial pain or headache with fever and may have orbital cellulitis, with proptosis and conjunctival swelling, evolving cranial nerve defects, and black crusty material apparent in the nasopharynx. Fungal invasion of vessels may lead to retinal artery thrombosis and visual impairment. Other complications include ptosis/pupil dilatation (secondary to cranial nerve lesions), cerebral abscess, and cavernous sinus/internal carotid artery thrombosis.

X-ray of the sinuses may show mucosal thickening, and fluid and bone destruction may be apparent on CT. Features may recur after apparently successful therapy; patients should be monitored.

Pulmonary disease

This is usually secondary to neutropenia and seen in BMT or leukemia patients receiving chemotherapy. Symptoms are initially mild: fever, mild shortness of breath, and cough. With progression, hemoptysis may develop and erosion of a blood vessel can cause severe pulmonary hemorrhage.

CXR may show infiltration, consolidation, and cavities. Infection may start in one lung segment but often disseminates in the late stages (e.g., multiple lung area, spleen, kidney).

Diabetics may develop a milder chronic form of pulmonary infection.

Cutaneous disease

Outbreaks have been associated with colonized bandages. The appearance is of cellulitis but if unrecognized, the organism penetrates deeper into the skin, and necrosis may follow vascular invasion. Dissemination may follow. It may take the appearance of a chronic ulcer.

Cases have occurred with minor trauma (e.g., gardeners), major trauma, burns, and insect bites. Skin lesions may also develop following dissemination from a distant site.

Gastrointestinal disease

This is seen in those suffering from malnutrition, although cases have occurred in patients with inflammatory bowel disease and in renal transplant recipients. Any part of the tract may be infected; and it is rapidly fatal. Symptoms include abdominal pain, fever, nausea, and vomiting.

CNS disease

This is rare and usually due to direct invasion from infected sinuses. Cases have occurred in leukemia patients with no obvious route of acquisition and as a result of open head trauma. Presentation is with decreasing levels of consciousness and multiple focal neurological deficits.

Other features include endocarditis, osteomyelitis, renal infection, and allergic sinusitis.

Diagnosis

Clinical suspicion should be raised by the presence of vascular invasion and tissue necrosis, which may manifest as black eschars and discharges. These are markers of advanced disease, and the earlier the diagnosis the better the outcome. Lesions may be apparent only on the nasal mucosa and palate.

Diagnosis rests on identifying the organism in tissue biopsy. Swabs are insufficient. Broad, nonseptate fungal hyphae with right-angle branching can be seen on routine hematoxylin and eosin (H&E) stains and help distinguish it from *Aspergillus*. There is usually an associated neutrophilic infiltrate, and tissue necrosis may follow blood vessel invasion with an inflammatory vasculitis. Organisms rarely appear in blood cultures.

The differential includes *Aspergillus* infection, rapidly progressive orbital tumor, cavernous sinus thrombosis, pulmonary embolism, and acute leukemia.

Treatment

Good outcomes rest on early diagnosis and correction of any predisposing factors, e.g., acidiosis, hyperglycemia, and immunosuppression. Overall mortality is around 50%.

For invasive disease, most clinicians use a lipid amphotericin preparation (less nephro- and infusion related toxicities) in combination with aggressive surgical debridement of necrotic tissue. Reconstructive surgery may be necessary once recovered. Posaconazole has activity in vitro and has been used as salvage therapy.

Other therapies suggested but unproven include colony-stimulating factors, oxygen therapy, the iron chelating agent deferasirox, and combination therapy including a polyene and an echinocandin.

For primary cutaneous disease use local debridement and topical amphotericin B. Treatment duration should be guided by response.

Eumycetoma

Mycetoma is a chronic, slow-growing, destructive infection usually involving hands or feet and characterized by the spread of the infecting organism from its subcutaneous site of implantation to adjacent structures. Serous discharges contain small grains of organism colonies.

- Actinomycetoma is caused by filamentous branching bacteria.
- Eumycetoma is caused by fungi.

Epidemiology

It is found worldwide in tropical regions, most commonly in India, Mexico, parts of Sub-Saharan Africa, and Yemen, among others. It is rare in temperate areas but may be seen in the southwestern United States.

The causative organism varies with geography: *Madurella mycetomatis* accounts for most cases worldwide; *Madurella grisea* is a common cause in South America; *Pseudallescheria boydii* in the United States; *Leptosphaeria senegalensis* and *Leptosphaeria tompkinsii* are common causes in West Africa. Geographic distribution of the causative agents is related to local climate (e.g., rainfall).

Pathogenesis

Soil fungi enter tissues of the foot or hand after local trauma. Infection spreads along tissue planes, destroying connective tissue and bone. Multiple sinuses and tracts form between the surface, each other, and deep abscesses. Inflammation and scarring lead to enlargement and disfiguring of the infected area.

Histologically, the appearance is of a suppurative granuloma with grains embedded in abscesses. Grain appearance is often characteristic of the specific organism.

Clinical features

Mycetoma is seen most frequently in men aged 20–40 years, often farmers and rural laborers. The foot is the most commonly affected area; other regions include the hand, leg, arm, head, thigh, and even back (carrying contaminated sacks). Early manifestation is a small, painless nodule. This quickly increases in size (faster in actinomycetoma) and ruptures forming a sinus. Additional nodules appear in adjacent areas as some areas heal.

The cycle of swelling, discharge, and scarring leads to a swollen mass of deformed tissue with multiple discharging fistulas. Lymphatic spread to regional nodes may occur. Cortex of bone may be invaded. Osteolytic lesions can be seen on X-ray.

Pathological fractures are less common than would be expected. Constitutional symptoms are rare. Fever implies secondary bacterial infection.

Diagnosis

The appearance is fairly typical: indurated swelling, and deformity with multiple sinus tracts draining grainy pus. Grains may be black, white, yellow, red, or pink, depending on the causative organism, e.g., white to yellow grains with *Acremonium* species, *Aspergillus nidulans*, *Aspergillus flavus*,

Cylindrocarpon cyanescens, *P. boydii*, and *Fusarium* species; black grains with *Corynespora cassicola*, *Curvularia* species, and *M. mycetomatis*. They can be difficult to spot in tissue sections.

Tissue Gram stain can detect the fine branching hyphae of actinomyc-etoma, but other stains are better for the detection of eumycetoma grains (e.g., periodic acid–Schiff stain). A good idea of the causative organism can be drawn from grain characteristics. They can be cultured for more-exact diagnosis; biopsy specimens are best to avoid contamination.

Serological diagnosis is possible in some centers.

Treatment

Mycetoma at all stages is usually amenable to prolonged medical therapy. Surgery usually leads to recurrence or mutilation that is more severe than that pre-existing.

Treatment success depends on identification of the causative organism and continues in all cases for at least 10 months. There is a role for surgery in combination with effective medical treatment, e.g., for bulk reduction.

Dermatophytes

This group of fungi is capable of invading the dead keratin of skin, hair, and nails, causing dermatophytosis (tinea). Also known as "ringworm," several species infect humans and belong to the *Epidermophyton*, *Microsporum*, and *Trichophyton* genera.

Clinical classification is by the body area involved: tinea capitis (scalp hair, most common in children); corporis (trunk and limbs); pedis (soles, most common overall worldwide); cruris (groin); barbae (beard area and neck), faciale (face); and unguium (nail, also known as onychomycosis).

Mycology

Dermatophytes may be anthrophilic, zoophilic (causing incidental human infection), or geophilic (found primarily in soil and infrequent causes of human infection outside certain specific tropical regions). All favor humid or moist skin. Cases occur worldwide, but incidence is highest in hot, humid regions where they may be the most common skin infections.

The most common anthrophilic species is *Tricophyton rubrum*, a common cause of tinea pedis or tinea cruris in temperate regions, and tinea corporis in the tropics. Spread is through contact with infected desquamated skin scales, primarily through sharing common washing facilities.

Epidermophyton floccosum may cause tinea cruris and foot infections either sporadically or in outbreaks in institutions.

T. concentricum is a cause of tinea corporis in remote parts of the humid tropics, often affecting infants shortly after birth.

Some other species have fairly specific geographic distributions. *T. tonsurans* is the predominant cause of tinea capitis in the UK, United States, and Mexico, whereas it is *T. violaceum* in India, East Africa, and the Middle East.

Pathogenesis

Infection is transmitted by hardy arthrospores, formed by dermatophyte hyphae. Direct contact between individual people is not necessary. Fungal cells adhere to keratinocytes, where they germinate and invade. Host susceptibility to infection appears to be influenced by genetic factors, local moisture, and cell-mediated immunity.

Risk factors include moist conditions, communal baths, athletic activities leading to abrasions (e.g., wrestling), atopy, genetic predisposition, and impaired cell-mediated immunity (e.g., Cushing's disease, AIDS, which may lead to severe infection, e.g., extensive skin involvement, abscess, and dissemination).

Clinical features

The key feature is an annular scaling patch with a raised margin showing a degree of inflammation; the center is usually less inflamed than the edge. The precise appearance varies with the affected site, the fungal species involved, and the host immune response.

Inappropriate application of topical steroids may lead to an infection showing none of the classical signs. Interdigital fungal infection may cause cracks in the skin and lead to bacterial cellulitis. Differential diagnosis includes seborrheic dermatitis, psoriasis, eczema, erysipelas, impetigo.

Tinea capitis

This is a disease of childhood (perhaps due to the presence of medium chain-length fatty acids in sebum that inhibit growth in postpubertal adults). It is found worldwide.

Endemic infections affecting a large number of children tend to be caused by anthrophilic organisms and sporadic cases by zoophilic fungi. Those infections in which the arthrospores are found on the hair surface are termed *ectothrix* infections, and those in which the spores develop within the hair, *endothrix* infections.

The main clinical findings are scalp scaling and hair loss. It may resemble dandruff. In ectothrix infections, hair tends to break a few millimeters above the skin, in contrast to endothrix infections, where the hair breaks at the skin surface. Inflammation is variable and may be severe with pustules and exudative crust.

Untreated scalp ringworm usually remits spontaneously after puberty.

Tinea corporis

This is commonly known as ringworm and is due to infection with one of a number of species. Anthrophilic species produce only mild inflammation and a consequently less well-defined skin lesion (e.g., *T. rubrum*), whereas zoophilic species produce more inflamed lesions that may contain pustules (e.g., *M. canis*).

Tinea barbae affects only the beard area with scaly plaques, pustules and vesicles. Tinea imbricata is a variant caused by *T. concentricum*, characterized by rash with concentric rings of scales. It is endemic in Southeast Asia, the South Pacific, Central America, and South America.

Tinea pedis

This is seen in children and young adults and is usually due to infection with *T. rubrum* or *T. mentagrophytes*. It causes toe-web fissures, maceration caling of soles, erythema, vesicles and pustules, and bullae. Scaling between the toes is often called "athelete's foot," but infection with other organisms (including bacteria) can produce an identical appearance.

Tinea cruris

This is usually due to infection with *T. rubrum* or *E. floccosum*. Erythematous lesions with central clearing and raised borders occur in the groin and, less commonly, the scrotum. It is usually seen in young men.

Tinea unguium (onychomycosis)

This usually occurs in association with infection of the adjacent skin. In the most common form, the nail is invaded from the distal and lateral aspects with onycholysis (separation of nail from nail bed) and thick, discolored (white, yellow, brown, black), dystrophic nails. It can occur at any age but is more common with increasing age.

A number of other fungi may cause onychomycosis, including *Scopulariopsis brevicaulis*, *Acremonium* spp., and *Fusarium* spp.

Diagnosis

Skin scrapings, nail specimens, or plucked hairs are treated with KOH and examined by direct microscopy. Samples should be taken from the edge of the lesion. Look for hyphae and arthrospores around the hair shaft.

Fungal cultures may be performed (culture on Sabaroud's agar containing antibiotics and antifungal agents to selectively suppress the growth of environmental fungi; growth may take at least 2 weeks). Examination of the lesions under UV light may help in the diagnosis of tinea capitis. Hairs infected with *Microsporum audouinii* and *M canis* fluoresce yellow-green, those infected with *Trichophyton schoenleinii*, dull green.

It is important to identify the organism causing scalp infection, as the presence of an anthrophilic species should prompt screening of classmates and the family of affected children. Zoophilic infections rarely spread from child to child.

Treatment

Treatment is generally topical, although oral therapy may be considered in extensive or unresponsive disease. Hair and nail disease usually requires oral therapy.

For infections confined to heavily keratinized areas (palms and soles), keratolytic agents such as Whitfield's ointment (salicyclic and benzoic acid compound) may be effective.

For tinea corporis, tinea cruris, and tinea pedis, use topical ketoconazole 2%, miconazole 2%, or clotrimazole 1% rubbed into the affected area daily for 2–6 weeks. Extensive or unresponsive disease may need systemic therapy with one of the agents below.

Nail infections rarely respond to topical therapy; terbinafine, itraconazole, or fluconazole are suitable. Treatment may need to last 3–4 months. Drugs are well tolerated—there is a low risk of hepatic injury (1 in 70,000). Terbinafine tends to show the best response rates (70–80% cure for fingernails after 6 weeks' and toenails after 12 weeks' treatment).

Other molds

Pseudallescheria boydii

This fungus is found in soil and fresh water throughout the world. The asexual form (anamorph) is called *Scedosporium apiospermum*. It causes two distinct diseases: mycetoma (see Eumycetoma, p. 440) and pseudallescheriasis (all other infections).

Pseudallescheriasis may affect lung, bone, joints, and the CNS, as well as causing skin and soft tissue infections. Infection may be acquired by inhalation or through skin trauma. Invasive pulmonary disease reminiscent of pulmonary aspergillosis may be seen in the immunocompromised (e.g., those undergoing BMT).

Infections in the immunocompetent have subacute or chronic courses. Those in the immunocompromised tend to be acute and severe.

Osteoarticular infection manifests as a painful swollen joint with overlying erythema. Weeks or months may pass between local fungal inoculation and the development of symptoms.

Cerebral abscesses may develop in association with lung infection in the immunocompromised. Abscesses are usually multiple. In immunocompetent individuals they may be associated with instances of near-drowning in polluted water.

CNS infection can also occur as a result of contiguous spread from infected paranasal sinuses. There have been cases of indolent meningitis caused by *P. boydii*. Isolation of the organism from sterile sites is diagnostic. It is rarely cultured from blood.

Effective antifungal therapy has not been established. Resistance to amphotericin B has been reported. Successful treatment regimes have used both surgical debridement and voriconazole.

Scedosporium prolificans

This is an uncommon cause of human infection, with several dozen cases reported worldwide. Immunocompetent patients experience focal, usually osteoarticular, disease. Immunocompromised patients frequently develop disseminated infection, e.g., those undergoing BMT. Fungemia, skin lesions, myalgia, pulmonary infiltrates, and cerebral lesions have all been reported.

Diagnosis is made by culture. The organism is intrinsically resistant to most antifungals.

Most therapy successes have involved debridement. Disseminated disease carries a high mortality.

Fusarium **species**

This is found commonly in soil, and in healthy individuals causes disease only rarely, usually through traumatic inoculation. *Fusarium* species may cause endophthalmitis, skin infection, musculoskeletal infections, mycetoma, and, particularly in the immunocompromised, disseminated infections. Systemic fusariosis occurs most commonly in patients with acute leukemia and prolonged neutropenia and those undergoing BMT.

Presentation is with fever and myalgia unresponsive to antibiotics. Skin lesions are seen in up to 80% of cases, often starting as macules and progressing to necrotic papules. In the severely neutropenic, infection progresses rapidly to death. In those whose neutrophils recover, infection is more subacute and progresses slowly or is controlled and cured.

Diagnosis is by culture. Unlike aspergillosis, blood cultures are often positive (50% cases). The optimal treatment has not been established. Lipid formulations of amphotericin B have been used successfully in some patients. Voriconazole and posaconazole may also have in vitro activity against certain isolates.

Overall mortality ranges from 50% to 80%, and survival is nearly always associated with recovery from neutropenia.

Dark-walled fungi

Phaeohyphomycosis is a loose term designating infection with molds with dark walls in culture, but not always in tissue. These organisms are a cause of brain abscess (e.g., *Cladophialophora bantiana*), allergic fungal sinusitis (e.g., *Bipolaris, Exserohilum*), and cutaneous disease.

Sporothrix schenckii

This is a dimorphic fungus and the cause of sporotrichosis, which may take the form of cutaneous infection, granulomatous pneumonitis, or disseminated disease.

Mycology

The fungus is dimorphic. Demonstrating the temperature-dependent conversion is a useful means of identification. Hyphal colonies are initially white and later turn brown/black as they produce pigment.

Epidemiology

It is found across the world; most human infections occur in tropical and subtropical parts of the Americas.

Animal-to-human transmission has occurred. Human-to-human is rare.

It is identified in soil, plants, straw, and wood, and outbreaks have occurred in association with exposure to mine timbers, hay, and thorned plants.

Clinical features

Cutaneous sporotrichosis

Fungus is inoculated into skin at sites of minor trauma, with disease usually arising in cooler body areas such as distal extremities. There are no systemic symptoms. Lesions take one of two forms, both of which wax and wane over years:

- Painless smooth or verrucous erythematous papulonodular lesions (0.5–4 cm diameter) that often ulcerate and can be followed by secondary lesions along the line of proximal lymphatics
- A fixed (plaque) form that does not spread locally. Spontaneous resolution has been described.

Extracutaneous sporotrichosis

Osteoarticular

This is the most common extracutaneous form. Infections involve the extremities, e.g., elbow, knee, hand, foot, not the hip, shoulder, or spine. Most present with primary involvement of a single joint that is swollen and painful, with an effusion and possibly a sinus tract. Other joints may become involved without therapy. There are few systemic features.

Repeated joint aspiration and culture or synovial biopsy may be necessary to make a diagnosis.

Pulmonary sporotrichosis

One-third of patients are alcoholic, one-third have pre-existing illness (e.g. diabetes, sarcoid), and one-third are healthy. They may be asymptomatic, but productive cough, fever, and weight loss are common, as are raised inflammatory markers.

Chest X-ray reveals cavitation with or without hilar lymphadenopathy and effusions. Sputum Gram stain and culture is usually diagnostic, but long-term follow-up with repeated cultures may be necessary for diagnosis. Untreated disease leads to progressive respiratory decline.

Other sites of infection

Meningitis is rare. In cases of CNS disease, the CSF shows high lymphocytes, high protein, and low glucose. Endophthalmitis, involvement of sinuses, kidney, or testes are also uncommon sites of *Sporothrix* infection.

Multifocal extracutaneous sporotrichosis

In healthy people, lesions tend to be single site. Multifocal disease with systemic features is usually seen in those with immunosuppression. Untreated infection is fatal.

Patients with HIV

Those with low CD4 counts are at greater risk of widespread ulcerative skin lesions and systemic dissemination. Presentation may be with arthritis and resemble seronegative arthropathies such as Reiter's syndrome. Visceral involvement occurs: meningitis, lung abscess, liver and spleen, endophthalmitis, bone marrow, and sinus invasion.

Diagnosis

- *Culture:* success may require multiple samples taken from affected sites at different times. A positive blood culture indicates multifocal disease. Although culture of skin lesion fluid may be positive, biopsy is best.
- *Histology:* a pyogranulomatous response is usually apparent, and in the presence of yeast, forms can be diagnostic. Again, multiple samples may be necessary. Yeast may be cigar or oval in shape.

Differential diagnosis

- *Cutaneous disease:* fixed lesions: bacterial pyoderma, foreign body granuloma, dermatophyte infections, cutaneous tuberculosis, and other granulomatous conditions; lymphocutaneous lesions: nocardiosis, leishmaniasis, mycobacterial infections (e.g., *M. chelonae, M. marinum*)
- *Osteoarticular disease:* TB, gout, rheumatoid arthritis

- *Pulmonary disease:* TB and other mycobacteria, histoplasmosis, coccidioidomycosis

Treatment

- *Cutaneous disease:* itraconazole or saturated potassium iodide (5–10 drops PO three times a day, increased slowly to 40 drops per dose. Side effects include anorexia, diarrhea, and parotid gland enlargement). Treatment course is usually 6–12 weeks. Prognosis is good. There have been cases described in which simply warming the lesion has been curative, reflecting the organism's temperature sensitivity.
- *Osteoarticular disease:* itraconazole is used as initial therapy. Amphotericin B deoxycholate (or lipid formulation) is used for extensive disease or in those who do not respond to itraconazole. Courses are long, and relapse is common. The role of surgery is not known.
- *Pulmonary disease:* prior to cavitation amphotericin B may be effective. Advanced disease requires surgical resection of cavities and a course of amphotericin B.
- *Meningitis:* varying response to amphotericin and some advocate combination therapy with 5-flucytosine

Immunocompromised patients may require lifelong itraconazole therapy for multifocal extracutaneous disease.

Chromomycosis

This is a localized chronic fungal infection of cutaneous and subcutaneous tissue caused by several species and producing verrucous lesions.

Mycology

Several different species cause chromomycosis—all take the appearance of dark brown cells occurring singly or in small clusters. Culture colonies are dark with a gray/green or brown/black surface. Agents grow slowly, and culture may take 6 weeks.

Organisms include *Fonsecaea pedrosoi* (the most commonly isolated agent), *Fonsecaea compacta*, *Phialophora verrucosa*, and *Cladosporium carrionii* (common in Australia, South Africa, and Venezuela).

Epidemiology

It occurs worldwide but is most common in tropical or subtropical areas, among barefoot workers.

Fungus is found in soil and decaying vegetation and is inoculated into skin by minor trauma. Thus feet and legs are most commonly affected.

Clinical features

Lesions can appear a long time after inoculation. The primary lesion is usually a small, pink papule that may itch and is followed (possibly many months later) by crops of either warty, violaceous nodules or firm tumors. These tend to enlarge and form groups with ulceration and dark hemopurulent material on the surface. Satellite lesions may occur.

Some people develop annular, papular lesions with active edges and healing in the center, which can become scarred or form keloid. Fibrosis and edema of the affected limb may occur in severe cases.

Complications include secondary infection, lymphedema (elephantiasis), fistula formation, hematogenous spread (rare), squamous carcinoma in longstanding lesions, and late recurrence (years later sometimes).

Differential diagnosis includes blastomycosis, yaws, tertiary syphilis, leishmaniasis, mycetoma, sporotrichosis, *M. marinum*, and leprosy.

Diagnosis

All forms of disease produce characteristic sclerotic bodies that may be identified on biopsy along with pyogranulomata and microabscesses. Microscopy of exudates may reveal hyphal strands.

Culture is necessary to confirm identity and may take 6 weeks.

Treatment

- *Early small lesions:* surgical excision or cryotherapy is effective.
- *Late disease:* most cases present late with large lesions. Local heat and several antifungals have been reported as effective, e.g., itraconazole. Treatment duration may last well over a year. It has been used in combination with flucytosine in cases of relapse.

Histoplasma capsulatum

This is a dimorphic fungus causing opportunistic infection in parts of the United States and elsewhere.

The organism

It is a member of the class *Ascomycetes*. It was first identified in 1905 and mistaken for a protozoan. Its characterization as a fungus in the 1930s led to the re-evaluation of many tuberculosis cases in the United States whose diagnosis had been made on chest X-ray alone.

H. capsulatum contains between four and seven chromosomes. Restriction fragment length polymorphism (RFLP) of certain genes permits strains to be placed in one of six groups that correlate with virulence and geographic location.

Mating types exist: (+) and (−). These are found in equal ratio in soil, but the (−) predominates in clinical isolates.

It is dimorphic: the mycelial phase grows at ambient temperatures, the yeast phase at 37°C. These differ in their growth requirements (e.g., mycelial needs calcium, yeast does not).

The mycelial phase exists in two forms: macroconidia (<15 micrometer) and microconidia (<5 micrometer, and thought to be the infective form being small enough to reach terminal bronchioles).

Epidemiology

It is found throughout the world but is most common in warm, humid environments, e.g., southern United States. It is associated with the presence of bat and bird guano. Birds do not carry the organism; bats can, and shed it in their droppings.

Infection tends to occur when soil disruption (e.g., excavation) releases fungal elements that are then inhaled.

Disease develops in men more often than women (4:1), which may reflect the association of chronic pulmonary disease with smoking (previously more common in men).

Pathogenesis

The key pathological determinant is the transition from mycelial to yeast form. Artificially blocking the transition blocks infection in experimental systems. Mycelial forms are rarely seen in established infection.

Microconidia settle in the terminal airways where they are phagocytosed by neutrophils and macrophages. Transition to the yeast phase takes hours to days, after which they migrate (probably intracellularly) from the pulmonary parenchyma to the local lymph nodes and beyond.

The resulting inflammatory response produces caseating or non-caseating granulomas. These consist of fungal elements, mononuclear cells, T lymphocytes, and calcium deposits. Excessive granuloma formation may be followed by fibrosis.

Macrophages are the key mediator of resistance to *H. capsulatum*. Macrophages from HIV-infected individuals are impaired in their ability to kill and inhibit fungal growth.

T cells (CD4+ in particular) are important in acquired immune defense; B cells and antibodies have little role in host resistance. CD4 cells seem to be vital for the activation of mononuclear phagocytes through cytokine release.

Cell-mediated immunity limits but does not eliminate infection. Infected people contain dormant organisms for years. These pose risk only if the individual subsequently becomes immunosuppressed.

Clinical features

Pulmonary histoplasmosis

Acute primary infection

Most patients are asymptomatic or experience mild flu-like symptoms. Around 10% become very unwell. Severity is affected by: inoculum size, age (the young and the old), underlying disease, and the presence of immunodeficiency. Incubation is 1–3 weeks.

Symptoms include high fever, headache, dry cough, substernal chest pain, malaise, weakness and fatigue, arthralgias, erythema nodosum, and erythema multiforme.

Examination reveals some added respiratory sounds, hepatosplenomegaly rarely. CXR shows hilar lymphadenopathy and patchy pneumonitis, which may calcify with time. Consider sarcoidosis and hematological malignancy in those presenting with isolated hilar lymphadenopathy.

Most symptoms settle by day 10 but may persist in those with a large initial inoculum. Lab tests are nonspecific: transient rises in ALP and rises or falls in white cell count.

Around 6% of patients infected with histoplasmosis develop pericarditis, probably representing the granulomatous inflammatory response of nearby lymph nodes.

Acute reinfection

Those in endemic areas who experience repeated infection develop mild flu-like symptoms within 3 days of re-exposure. The illness is shorter than with primary infection.

Cavitary pulmonary histoplasmosis

This is a distinct presentation of acute infection generally seen in men over age 50 with existing lung disease (e.g., COPD). Symptoms include low grade fever, cough, weight loss, night sweats, and chest pain. Any existing pulmonary impairment may be exacerbated.

CXR shows cavitating lesions, mostly in the upper lobes (90%) near a bulla. Lymphadenopathy is not a feature.

Spontaneous resolution is seen in up to 60%. Healing leads to fibrosis of the affected area with consequent respiratory impairment. Recurrence is seen in 20%. Death is rare.

Histoplasmoma

This is a mass lesion resembling a fibroma and a rare complication of primary infection. It is usually located in the lung. It enlarges slowly over years, forming a calcified mass. On CXR, it may appear to have a core of calcium or as a collection of calcified clusters.

Mediastinal granuloma and fibrosis

Granulomatous inflammation in response to infection leads to massive enlargement of the mediastinal lymph nodes (up to 10 cm). They may be asymptomatic or cause airway impingement. Fibrotic tissue formed during healing may distort airways (leading to pneumonias and bronchiectasis), the esophagus, or the superior vena cava. Large nodes can penetrate the airways, creating sinuses or fistulas to the pericardium or esophagus.

Rarely, mediastinal fibrosis can develop, affecting all structures within the mediastinum.

African histoplasmosis

H. capsulatum var. *duboisii* is found in Africa along with classical var. *capsulatum*. Infection is associated with a distinct clinical presentation, skin and bone being the most frequently affected organs, perhaps reflecting an increased incidence of cutaneous inoculation.

Patients develop ulcers, nodules, and rashes that may resemble psoriasis. Osteolytic lesions affecting the skull, ribs, and verterbrae may become cystic with time. Infection can become disseminated and affect multiple organs with a pathology that resembles infection with *Coccidioides immitis* more than it does classic disseminated histoplasmosis. This may reflect the larger size of var. *duboisii* yeast form than that of var. *capsulatum*.

Ocular histoplasmosis

Uveitis or panophthalmitis occurs rarely as part of histoplasmosis.

Presumed ocular histoplasmosis syndrome (POHS) involves visual impairment secondary to macular choroidal neovascularization. Although incidence is epidemiologically associated with areas where histoplasmosis occurs in the United States, there is no proven pathological link.

Progressive disseminated histoplasmosis (PDH)

There is continued growth of histoplasma in multiple organs. PDH occurred in 78% of infections in some outbreaks. Risk factors include age and immunosuppression. Most cases probably represent reactivation of quiescent fungi, although PDH may result from primary infection or reinfection with a large inoculum.

Acute PDH

This is associated with a fulminant course and seen in children and immunosuppressed patients (HIV and hematological malignancies). Symptoms are abrupt onset of fever, cough, weight loss, and diarrhea.

Children

Chest features predominate. Findings include hepatosplenomegaly, cervical lymphadenopathy, mouth ulcers, jaundice (a few), and pancytopenia. LFTs may be raised. CXR may show enlarged hilar lymph nodes and patchy pneumonitis.

Untreated mortality is 100%, and prior to antifungal therapy, children died around 6 weeks after symptom onset as a result of DIC, hemorrhage, or secondary bacterial infections.

Adults with HIV infection

CD4 is usually <200 cells/mm^3 with positive histoplasma serology prior to illness. Before HAART, up to 25% of AIDS patients in an endemic area could develop infection.

Findings include pancytopenia (may predate PDH), hepatosplenomegaly, lymphadenopathy, and cutaneous signs (maculopapular rash, bruising, petechiae). Rarer manifestations are colonic masses, perianal ulcers, meningitis, and encephalitis. CXR may be normal or show diffuse reticulonodular shadowing.

Untreated fatality is 100%; with therapy, acute survival is 80%. The rare severe form, reactive hemophagocytic syndrome, is nearly always fatal despite therapy.

Subacute PDH

Symptoms are prolonged. Hepatosplenomegaly is common, but fever, weight loss, and lab abnormalities are less pronounced.

Infective lesions may occur in the GI tract (ulceration), CNS (chronic meningitis, cerebritis, and mass lesions), adrenal glands (affected in 80% but overt Addison's seen in only 10%), and vascular structures (endocarditis and infection of aortic aneurysms).

CSF in chronic meningitis shows lymphocytosis, elevated protein, and low glucose. Basilar meninges are badly affected; hydrocephalus may develop.

Chronic PDH

This is seen exclusively in adults. It is distinguished from subacute disease by the mild chronic nature of the symptoms. Malaise and lethargy are the key complaints. Fever is less common. The most common physical finding is painless mouth ulceration (which may have the appearance of malignancy).

Yeasts and macrophages can be identified on biopsy from the center of the lesion. Disease usually remains undiagnosed for some years until features associated with a single organ become apparent.

Diagnosis

Culture

Isolation of *H. capsulatum* is the only sure way to confirm a diagnosis of histoplasmosis. Blood cultures using the lysis-centrifugation technique or BACTEC myco/F lytic system should be performed in all suspected cases. Specimens are cultured for up to 6 weeks at 30°C in brain-heart infusion agar with blood, antibiotics, and cycloheximide; 90% of positives will exhibit fungus by day 7. Isolates' identification is confirmed using a probe for ribosomal DNA.

Recovery rates depend on the source of the specimen and burden of infection: 10–15% for sputa from patients with acute pulmonary histoplasmosis, up to 60% from patients with cavitary disease, up to 90% for bronchoscopic specimens taken from AIDS patients with pulmonary disease, and 25–65% for CSF from patients with *H. capsulatum* meningitis (best if large volumes are taken, >20 mL).

In endocarditis, blood cultures are often negative, heart valves are frequently positive. The organism is rarely found in pleural or pericardial fluid and is better grown from pleura or pericardium.

Organism detection

Tests are available that can detect polysaccharide antigen in urine or serum. They are positive in 90% of patients with progressive disseminated disease and 20% of those with acute pulmonary histoplasmosis.

It can be performed on BAL from patients with pulmonary disease. It is useful for detecting relapses in those with PDH, particularly in the immunosuppressed, and is more sensitive than serology. It is sensitive and fairly specific in the diagnosis of meningitis from CSF samples.

Cross-reactivity with *Blastomyces* and *Coccidioides* species causes false-positive results. PCR tests are available and are rapid and specific.

Serology

Tests are negative in up to 50% of immunosuppressed patients. The detection of complement-fixing antibodies has been widely used in diagnosis. Around 10% of healthy people living in endemic regions have low-level responses. A titer of 1:8 is considered positive. A fourfold rise, or a titer of 1:32, is indicative of active infection and is seen in 75% of patients by 6 weeks of infection.

Rising titers in those who have been treated hints at relapse. There is a false-positive rate of around 15%, seen often in those with coccidiomycosis or blastomycosis due to antibody cross-reactivity.

The precipitin bands test detects antibodies to the H and M glycoproteins in patient sera. These are released by yeast and mycelial forms.

The presence of anti-H antigen indicates active infection but is seen in <10% of patients. Anti-M antigen is detected in 80% of cases but does not distinguish active disease from previous infection.

Histochemical stains

These can enable rapid identification of fungus from tissues and body fluids. It may be detected in blood smears from up to 40% of patients with acute PDH.

Skin test

The histoplasmin skin test is useful only for epidemiological studies. It is positive in up to 90% of those in endemic areas and can be negative in cases of PDH.

Treatment

- *Drugs:* the major choices of therapy are amphotericin B deoxycholate (or one of its lipid formulations) or an azole drug (particularly itraconazole). The choice depends on the severity of disease.
- *Acute pulmonary histoplasmosis:* most cases do not require treatment; bed rest and antipyretics are sufficient. Those who have had a high level of exposure, experience respiratory compromise and malaise, and continue to have fevers after 1 week should receive therapy. Itraconazole for 4–6 weeks is usually sufficient. An alternative if this is not tolerated is amphotericin B
- *Mediastinal granuloma:* enlarged mediastinal lymph nodes can impinge on major airways and may require treatment as above. Amphotericin B may be preferable if rapid resolution of symptoms is required. Surgical excision may rarely be necessary.
- *Mediastinal fibrosis:* surgery, steroid, and antifungal therapy have all been tried with little success. Surgery is often difficult and fibrosis may recur.
- *Histoplasmoma* require surgical excision only if enlarging. 2–3 months' therapy with an azole may be beneficial afterward. Fluconazole is the only azole that penetrates the CNS.
- *Cavitary pulmonary histoplasmosis:* cavities with thin walls usually resolve spontaneously. Treatment should be given to those with progressive infiltrates, thick-walled cavities, or persistent cavities impairing respiratory function. Itraconazole 400 mg daily for 6 months leads to improvement in up to 85% of patients. Amphotericin B should be used in the immunosuppressed or if disease progresses on therapy. Relapse is seen in up to 20%. Surgical resection may be necessary in such cases.
- *Acute PDH:* acute life-threatening PDH should be treated with early amphotericin B. Most patients show significant improvement in the first week. Mild acute PDH can be treated with a 6-month course of itraconazole. Patients with AIDS and those on long-term immunosuppressive therapy should receive lifelong itraconazole.
- *Subacute and chronic PDH:* itraconazole 400 mg daily gives a 90% success rate. An alternative is amphotericin B.
- *Meningitis:* treatment is with amphotericin B, with weekly lumbar punctures to assess efficacy. Relapses are common, with overall cure seen in around 50% (more in the immunocompetent, less in the immunocompromised).
- *Endocarditis:* amphotericin B and surgical removal of infected valve

- *Pericarditis* may be seen after acute PDH. The pericardium is rarely infected, and pericarditis does not require antifungal therapy in its own right. Bed rest, NSAIDs, and possibly steroids (beware of exacerbating active histoplasmosis lesions) usually suffice. Cardiac tamponade is uncommon. In the rare cases where the pericardium is itself infected, antifungal therapy is indicated.
- *Presumed ocular histoplasmosis:* antifungal therapy is not required. Laser therapy can prevent neovascularization.

See the IDSA guidelines for further details on the treatment of histoplasmosis.[1]

Prevention

There is no vaccine available. Prevention rests on educating those who work in areas where there is a risk of acquiring infection, e.g., workers in buildings and other environments that have served as bat habitation. In HIV-infected patients who have had histoplamosis, secondary prophylaxis is given until the CD4 count is consistently above 200 cells/mm³.

Reference

1. Wheat LJ, Freifeld AG, Kleiman MB et al. (2007). Clinical practice guidelines for the management of patients with histoplasmosis: 2007 update by the Infectious Diseases society of America. *Clin Infect Dis* 45:807–825.

Blastomyces dermatitidis

This is a dimorphic fungus and the cause of blastomycosis, a systemic pyo-granulomatous disease.

Mycology

It grows in the mycelial form at room temperature and as a yeast at 37°C. The mycelial form grows on plates by 3 weeks and produces the infectious conidia (2–10 micrometer in diameter).

Yeast cells are multinucleate with thick cell walls and have a similar appearance in vitro as in clinical specimens. *B. dermatitidis* is the asexual stage of *Ajellomyces dermatitidis*, the sexual form which requires opposite mating types for reproduction.

Epidemiology

Information is limited because of the lack of a sensitive skin test. Endemic areas include southeastern United States, parts of South America, the Middle East, and India. African strains are serologically distinct from American isolates. It is probably a saprobe of soil, favoring decaying wood material in moist areas.

Symptomatic disease occurs in less than 50% of infected people.

Pathogenesis

Infection is acquired via the lungs. Conidia are inhaled and convert to the yeast phase. A non-caseating granulomatous response usually follows.

although respiratory disease may not be apparent. The organism may disseminate to other sites.

The histology of cutaneous disease is distinct, producing pseudoepitheliomatous hyperplasia with microabscesses. In appearance it may resemble other skin lesions (e.g., squamous cell carcinoma). Mucosal involvement of the mouth and larynx may take a similar appearance.

Protection from infection is mediated primarily by natural resistance (e.g., alveolar macrophages—rates are not greatly increased in those with immunocompromise) and cellular immunity (antibodies confer no protection).

Clinical features

Almost any organ can become infected. Some patients present with an acute pneumonic-type illness. Most experience a more chronic course; symptoms may be systemic or purely pulmonary.

Acute infection

Following exposure, there is an incubation period of 4–6 weeks before the development of nonspecific flu-like symptoms: fever, arthralgia, and cough (initially nonproductive but may later producing purulent sputum). CXR may demonstrate an area of consolidation.

There have been reports of spontaneous resolution of such acute pneumonias.

Chronic infection

Pulmonary
There is chronic pneumonia with productive cough, pleuritic chest pain, hemoptysis, weight loss, and low-grade fever. CXR may show infiltrates, mass lesions (which may resemble malignancy), and cavities, but effusions are rare. Miliary disease or diffuse pneumonitis is unusual; both have a high mortality.

Skin
Infection of skin is the most common extrapulmonary manifestation, seen in up to 80% of cases and may occur in the absence of respiratory features. Lesions may be verrucous or ulcerative; both may occur in the same patient. Verrucous lesions resemble squamous cell carcinoma with a crusted gray to violet appearance. Where there is discharge, microscopy may reveal yeast forms.

Subcutaneous nodules represent cold abscesses and are usually seen in acutely ill patients with severe pulmonary or extrapulmonary disease at another site.

Bone and joint
Long bones, vertebrae, and ribs are common sites, and extension may lead to arthritis. Organisms are seen easily in synovial aspirates.

Genitourinary tract
Around 25% of men have GU involvement, usually of the prostate.

CNS

CNS involvement is uncommon in the normal host but seen at increased frequency (e.g., as abscess or meningitis) in patients with AIDS who develop blastomycosis.

Other

The liver, spleen, gut, thyroid, or pericardium may be involved.

The immunocompromised

This is an unusual opportunistic pathogen in HIV patients. Disease is more severe and more likely to be fatal in those with late-stage AIDS. CNS infection is seen in 40% of cases. Similar severity is seen in patients with immunocompromise due to steroid therapy and chemotherapy. Up to 40% of cases are fatal.

Treat suspected cases early, as most deaths occur within a few weeks. Relapse is common if immunodeficiency remains, and long-term suppression should be considered.

Diagnosis

Microscopy of secretions

The characteristic broad-based budding yeast cell may be seen in a wet preparation of sputum or pus. Body fluids such as urine or pleural fluid should be centrifuged and the sediment examined. BAL may be useful in patients who are not producing sputum. When organisms are sparse, they may be more easily identified on Papanicolaou preparations.

Histology

Gomori's methenamine silver and PAS stains readily visualize the fungus.

Culture

Material should be inoculated onto Sabouraud's or more enriched agar and incubated at 30°C. The mycelial form is not diagnostic, and ideally conversion to yeast at 37°C should be demonstrated.

This is not always possible, and mycelial identification can be achieved by nucleic acid probes for *Blastomyces* RNA.

Serology

Complement fixation, immunodiffusion, and ELISA-based tests are available, but sensitivity and specificity vary widely. A negative test does not rule out disease, and a positive one does not on its own warrant therapy; rather, it should fuel the hunt for the organism.

Treatment

All patients should receive therapy. A small number of cases do resolve spontaneously, but these cannot be predicted at presentation. Surgery has a role in the drainage of large abscesses and the resection of necrotic bone tissue in combination with medical therapy.
- Mild-to-moderate disease in the immunocompetent: itraconazole. Therapy should be continued for at least 6 months.
- Relapses do occur (around 10% with ketoconazole), and patients should be followed up for 2 years.

- Severe, including CNS disease: amphotericin B (or lipid formulation). Relapse is more common in those with immunocompromise, and long-term azole therapy should be considered.
- The role of the newer azole antifungal agents has not been established.

See the IDSA guidelines for further details on the management of blastomycosis.[1]

Reference

1. Chapman SW, Dismukes WE, Proia LA, et al. (2008). Clinical practice guidelines for the management of blastomycosis: 2008 update by the Infectious Diseases Society of America. *Clin Infect Dis* 46:1801–1812.

Coccidioides immitis

Dimorphic fungi of the genus *Coccidioides* (*C. immits,* and *C. posadasii*) are found in certain regions of the western hemisphere and a cause of respiratory illness.

Mycology

These fungi may exist as a mycelium or a spherule (a structure unique to this organism seen only in tissue). The mycelial form is present on routine laboratory agar and in soil. Some mature cells develop a hydrophobic outer layer that renders them capable of prolonged survival in the environment (arthroconidia).

Once airborne, arthroconidia may be inhaled and deposited in the lungs, where they begin to multiply. The resultant tissue spherule consists of a thin wall containing many endospores. This wall eventually ruptures, allowing the spread of endospores.

Epidemiology

Endemic to certain lower deserts of the western hemisphere with an arid climate, hot summers, and alkaline soil, *Coccidioides* spp. are found in parts of western Texas, southern Utah, Arizona, southwestern New Mexico, and central California in the United States. Arthroconidia transport (e.g., in dust storms) has resulted in infections in nonendemic areas.

Infections tend to occur when the soil is dry toward the end of the summer. The organism is most easily isolated after the winter rains.

The number of new infections varies greatly from year to year; 30% of people living in the endemic regions of the United States show evidence of prior exposure.

Pathogenesis

Most infections follow inhalation of arthroconidia. There are rare cases of cutaneous infection (which tend to resolve without treatment). Inflammation follows its conversion to a spherule. The resulting pulmonary lesion consists of neutrophils and eosinophils and, if infection becomes chronic, granulomas with lymphocytes and multinucleated giant cells. Both acute and chronic lesions may be found at different sites in the same individual.

Control of infection relies on the T-cell response, and those with deficient T-cell immunity are at risk of severe disease. The innate immune response appears to be important against arthroconidia and endospores.

Clinical features

Up to two-thirds of infections produce only mild or subclinical disease, and of those producing respiratory symptoms most follow a self-limited course. Complications may occur up to 2 years later and do not correlate with the severity of the original infection.

Early respiratory infection

Symptoms develop 1–3 weeks after exposure: cough, pleuritic chest pain, breathlessness, and fever. Onset is usually slow but can be abrupt. Inhalation of a large number of arthroconidia may result in early symptoms. Weight loss and migratory arthritis can occur, and some patients develop skin rashes ranging from a fine papular rash early in illness to erythema multiforme and nodosum (particularly in women).

Laboratory tests may reveal peripheral blood eosinophilia and raised inflammatory markers. Around 50% of patients have CXR changes: effusions, infiltrates, hilar lymphadenopathy, and cavities.

Most infections resolve without complications over several weeks. There are rare cases of severe diffuse coccidioidal pneumonia (due either to massive exposure or hematogenous seeding), leading to respiratory failure and septic shock with a high mortality. One-third of coccidioidal infections in HIV-positive patients (typically those with CD4 <100 cells/mm^3) presents in this manner.

Pulmonary nodules and cavities

Four percent of lung infections result in a nodule that may reach up to 5 cm in diameter. Although usually asymptomatic, a biopsy may be necessary to distinguish it from a neoplastic lesion.

Nodules may liquefy and drain via a bronchus to form a cavity. Cavities are usually peripheral, and although half close within 2 years, some may cause pain, cough, and hemoptysis as well as providing a focus for the development of mycetoma. Peripheral cavities can rupture, causing a pyopneumothorax.

Chronic fibrocavity pneumonia

This is associated with diabetes or pre-existing lung fibrosis; some people develop a chronic fibrotic pneumonia with widespread pulmonary infiltrates and cavities involving more than one lobe. As well as local symptoms, people may experience night sweats and weight loss.

Dissemination

Of the general population, 0.5% develops disseminated infection. Those with immunodeficiency (solid organ transplants, late-stage HIV infection, those on high-dose steroids, Hodgkin's disease) are at greater risk. Many with disseminated disease do not develop respiratory features and have normal CXRs.

Sites of dissemination include skin (causing maculopapular lesions, verrucous ulcers, and abscesses with a predilection for the nasolabial fold), joints (knee, hand, wrist, feet), bone (particularly the vertebrae, which may progress to develop a paraspinous abscess), and meningitis, the most serious manifestation. Meningitis develops a few weeks to a few months after initial infection and is usually fatal within 2 years of diagnosis.

CSF findings include elevated pressure, raised protein, low glucose, and raised eosinophils. The basilar meninges are usually involved, and hydrocephalus is a common complication in children.

Diagnosis

Clinical features of coccidioidal infection are not specific and lab tests are required to establish diagnosis. Travel history is vital. Remember that exposure can be subtle (e.g., changing planes within an endemic area).

Complications are usually apparent within 2 years of exposure, but infection may have occurred many years previously in the immunodeficient.

Isolation of the organism

Definitive diagnosis is by culture of, or identifying fungal elements within, clinical specimens (e.g., biopsy, sputum). These can be collected without risk to personnel, as infection is not transmitted from primary specimens.

Stains such as silver, periodic acid–Schiff, or H&E will reveal spherules. *C. immitis* grows on standard microbiological media in aerobic conditions and typically takes the form of a white mold at around 5–7 days. At this point it is highly infectious.

Unlike the spherule, the mycelial form is not unique, and identification is made by reference laboratories either antigenically or by the detection of specific ribosomal RNA.

Serology

Most patients are not very symptomatic, and diagnosis is by serology. Serology is important in the diagnosis of coccidioidal meningitis, as CSF is usually culture-negative. Tests are highly specific, and even borderline positive results should be treated seriously. Negative tests do not exclude infection.

The tube precipitin (TP) antibody (IgM) test detects a fungal cell wall polysaccharide, and 90% of patients will have a positive test in the first 3 weeks of illness. Complement-fixing antibodies (predominantly IgG) are detected later and for longer than TP antibodies, and their presence in CSF is important in the diagnosis of coccidioidal meningitis. ELISA for IgG and/or IgM is sensitive and in increasing use.

Skin testing

Skin-testing for delayed-type hypersensitivity to coccidioidal antigens is useful epidemiologically but limited as a diagnostic tool.

Treatment

Newly diagnosed patients should be assessed for the extent of disease and factors that increase the risk of future complications. Amphotericin B (or lipid formulation) is the preferred agent in cases of severe pulmonary disease or those who are deteriorating. Azoles are used in cases of chronic infection (itraconazole or fluconazole).

Surgery may be required in some patients. Debridement and drainage of infected sites is essential in the management of extensive bone infection, and in cases of vertebral infection, stabilization may be required.

Uncomplicated pulmonary disease

This may not require therapy in healthy individuals. Those at risk of dissemination (e.g., the immunosuppressed, pregnant women) should usually receive antifungal therapy. Those at risk of severe pulmonary disease (e.g., diabetics and those with pre-existing lung fibrosis) should also be considered for treatment.

More severe pulmonary infection

This infection is associated with weight loss of over 10%, night sweats for 3 or more weeks, infiltrates that are either bilateral or involve more than half of a lung, persistent hilar lymphadenopathy, or symptoms persisting for over 2 months. Treatment is with azole antifungals for 3–6 months.

Diffuse pneumonia

Treat with an amphotericin product for a few weeks, with azole therapy following for at least 1 year.

Pulmonary cavity

Cavities that do not resolve spontaneously should be resected if it is safe to do so to avoid future complications.

Persistent fibrocavitary pneumonia

Treatment is usually started with oral azoles. Up to 60% respond with improved symptoms and CXR. Those who do not, may respond to amphotericin.

Dissemination

Coccidioidal meningitis is treated initially with fluconazole, which achieves a response rate of 70%. Those who do not respond may benefit from intrathecal amphotericin B. Hydrocephalus may require shunting. Occasionally, cerebral abscesses develop, which may need draining.

Other forms of disseminated disease can usually be treated with oral azoles except in those who are showing rapid deterioration or have infection in critical places (e.g., vertebrae) when amphotericin B tends to be preferred. Treatment is continued for at least a year, and for 6 months beyond the end of recovery. Relapses occur in one-third of patients, and lifelong suppressive therapy may be required.

See IDSA guidelines for further details on the management of cocciodioidomycosis.[1]

Reference

1. Galgiani JN, Ampel NM, Blair JE, et al. (2005). Coccidioidomycosis. *Clin Infect Dis* 41:1217–1223.

Paracoccidioides brasiliensis

This is a cause of chronic progressive systemic mycosis in South America.

Mycology

Paracoccidioides brasiliensis is a dimorphic fungus (at 37°C an oval or round mold of variable size reproducing by budding; below 28°C, a slow-growing mold). At 37°C, colonies take around 10 days to appear and have a creamy, soft appearance. Mold-form colonies take up to a month to develop.

Epidemiology

Geographic distribution is very limited: it has been found in South America from Argentina as far north as Mexico. Within these regions, it tends to cause infections in forest areas with high year-round humidity and mild temperatures. Brazil has the highest number of reported cases. It has been isolated from soil but is not widespread, and the organism's ecological niche is not clear.

Human infection is probably acquired by inhalation. Most cases occur in men over 30 years of age, yet skin testing demonstrates that men and women are equally exposed. The rare prepubescent cases have an equal sex distribution.

Agricultural workers, smokers, and alcoholics are at greater risk.

Clinical features

Most primary cases are subclinical. The organism can remain dormant for prolonged periods, disease becoming apparent only in states of debilitation or immunosuppression. Paracoccidiomycosis tends to cause subacute severe disease in the young and chronic disease in adults, in whom it has a better prognosis with therapy. Infection is acquired via the lungs.

- *Lung:* patients complain of breathlessness, and CXR may reveal nodular infiltrates that are often bilateral. Lesions are concentrated in the mid and lower zones, apices are usually clear. Cavities, fibrosis, areas of emphysema, and right ventricular hypertrophy become more likely as disease becomes chronic.
- *Mouth and upper respiratory mucosa:* ulcerated lesions of the mouth, lip, gums, tongue, and palate are common. Other features are tooth loss, dysphonia, and nasal lesions.
- *Cutaneous lesions:* warty ulcerated lesions infiltrate the subcutaneous tissue. They appear over legs and orifices.
- *Other:* lymphadenopathy (sometimes with fistulas), bone marrow dysfunction (e.g., aplastic anemia), diminished adrenal function, spleen, liver, gut, vascular system, bone, and CNS involvement

Diagnosis

- *Microscopy with KOH* reveals the organism in over 90% of cases where sputum or exudates is available. The typical appearance is that of a large mother cell surrounded by multiple budding daughter cells of varying sizes, often called a "pilot's wheel" or "Mickey mouse head" when only two budding cells are present.
- *Biopsy* is often diagnostic. Histology shows granuloma with multinucleated giant cells that may contain fungi. Ulcerated lesions may show a pyogenic reaction, and skin lesions may have intraepithelial microabscesses.
- *Culture* on Sabouraud-dextrose agar confirms diagnosis. Cultures should be kept for 6 weeks.
- *Serology:* immunodiffusion test is useful for diagnosis but remains positive after successful treatment. Complement fixation tests allow

an assessment of response to treatment but cross-react with *H. capsulatum*. Tests that are more specific have been developed.

- *Skin testing* is not useful for diagnosis.

Treatment

It is important that specific therapy be combined with measures to improve general health. *P. brasiliensis* is sensitive to most antifungal agents and sulfonamides.

Imidazoles

Itraconazole has been used extensively and appears to be more effective than ketoconazole, requiring shorter treatment courses with fewer side effects and lower relapse (3–5%).

Sulfadiazine and amphotericin B

Paracoccidiomycosis is the only mycosis sensitive to sulfa drugs. Treatment takes months and can be reduced only when improvement is apparent. Courses often last as long as 5 years to avoid relapse (up to 25% of cases). Mortality can be as high as 25%.

In severe cases, it is used in combination with amphotericin B, which may also be added to imidazole-based regimes in patients unresponsive to a single agent.

Penicillium marneffei

This thermally dimorphic fungus (exists in a yeast or mold form depending on the temperature) causes life-threatening disseminated infection.

Epidemiology

Its distribution is limited to Southeast Asia and southern China. Humans and bamboo rats are the only known hosts. The exact route of transmission is unknown but is thought to be inhalation or, rarely, inoculation.

Infection is commonly seen in young adults with HIV, but cases are seen in immunocompetent children and adults.

Occupational exposure to soil is a risk factor.

Clinical features

Patients present with around a 1-month history of illness with low-grade fever, weight loss, and skin lesions (pustules, papules, ulcers, or abscesses of the face, upper trunk, or extremities). Pharyngeal and palatal lesions are common in those with HIV. Most have anemia and weight loss, with around half presenting with fungemia or lymphadenopathy. Hepatomegaly, splenomegaly, hemoptysis (secondary to cavitating lung lesions), joint infections, and pericarditis may occur.

The diagnosis should be considered in those with immunocompromise and history of travel to an affected area. Infection may present many years after travel.

Diagnosis

Diagnosis may be made on smear (skin lesion, sputum), biopsy (lymph node, bone marrow), or culture. Microscopic examination may reveal yeast forms both extracellularly and within phagocytes. Histology may demonstrate either a granulomatous (commonly seen in immunocompetent individuals), suppurative, or necrotizing (commonly seen in the immunocompromised) response.

Culture at 30°C produces a mold with sporulating structures that may be converted to yeast form by culture at 37°C. This dimorphism is not seen in other members of the genus *Penicillium*. In vitro *P. marneffei* is highly sensitive to itraconazole, voriconazole, terbinafine, and flucytosine. It is intermediately sensitive to amphotericin. There are no randomized controlled trials on the acute treatment of penicilliosis.

Treatment[1]

Disseminated infection is most successfully treated with 2 weeks IV amphotericin B followed by 10 weeks PO itraconazole. Patients with mild disease can be treated with oral itraconazole 400 mg/day for 8 weeks.

All HIV-infected patients who complete treatment for penicilliosis should be given secondary prophylaxis with oral itraconazole 200 mg/day. Secondary prophylaxis may be found in patients on antiretroviral therapy who have a CD4 count of >100 cells/mm^3 for at least 6 months.

Reference

1. Guidelines for the prevention and treatment of opportunistic infection in HIV infected adults and adolescents (2008). Available from http://AIDSinfo.nih.gov

overview of parasitology

Plasmodium species (malaria)

Malaria, an infection caused by *Plasmodium* species, has affected humankind for millennia. The word *malaria* means "bad air" and refers to the association between the illness and the marshes where *Anopheles* mosquitoes breed.

Although malaria has virtually disappeared from Europe and the United States (apart from imported cases), it remains a major problem in tropical countries, where it causes 3–500 million cases and 2–3 million deaths per year.

Plasmodium species

Five *Plasmodium* species cause human infection:

- P. falciparum can invade red blood cells of all ages, may be drug resistant, and is responsible for most severe, life-threatening infections. It does not produce dormant liver stages (hypnozoites) or cause relapse.
- P. vivax and P. ovale cause clinically similar, milder infections. They produce hypnozoites and may cause relapse months after the initial infection.
- P. malariae rarely causes acute illness in normal hosts, does not produce hypnozoites, but may persist in the bloodstream for years.
- Plasmodium knowlesi causes malaria in macaques and has recently been recognized as a cause of human malaria in Southeast Asia. Microscopically, it resembles P. malariae but can cause fatal disease (like P. falciporum).

Mixed infections may occur in 5–7% of patients.

Life cycle

Humans acquire malaria from sporozoites transmitted by the bite of the female *Anopheles* mosquito. Sporozoites travel through the bloodstream and enter hepatocytes. Here they mature into tissue schizonts, which rupture and release merozoites into the bloodstream. These invade red blood cells and mature into ring forms, then trophozoites, and finally schizonts, before rupturing to release merozoites.

Alternatively, some erythrocytic parasites develop into gametocytes (sexual forms), which are ingested by the mosquito and complete the sexual life cycle. In *P. vivax* and *P. ovale* infections, some parasites remain dormant in the liver as hypnozoites for months before they mature into tissue schizonts.

Epidemiology

The epidemiology of malaria varies and depends on a number of factors: climate, *Plasmodium* species and life cycle, efficiency of transmission by vectors, and drug resistance. Thus, in Sub-Saharan Africa, *P. falciparum* can survive as a result of the year-round presence and efficient transmission by its mosquito vectors (*A. gambiae* and *A. funestus*).

In contrast, *P. vivax*, which is found in more temperate zones, requires hypnozoites to sustain its transmission.

Pathogenesis

The following mechanisms contribute to the pathogenesis of severe falciparum malaria:

- *Cytoadherence:* adherence of parasitized red blood cells to the vascular endothelium is mediated by *P. falciparum*–infected erythrocyte membrane protein 1 (PfEMP1), which binds to specific endothelial receptors, e.g., thrombospondin, CD36, ICAM-1, VCAM1, and ELAM1. This results in peripheral sequestration of parasites, which protects them from removal from the circulation as they pass through the spleen, and oxidant damage as they pass through the lungs.
- *Rosetting:* PfEMP1 also binds to complement receptor-1, resulting in clustering of unparasitized red cells around parasitized red cells.
- *Hyperparasitemia* (>5%) is associated with a greater risk of death, particularly in nonimmune patients. Reasons for this include more severe metabolic effects, e.g., hypoglycemia and lactic acidosis.

Clinical features

- Fevers (cyclical or continuous with intermittent spikes)
- Malarial paroxysm: chills, high fever, sweats
- Complications include cerebral malaria, pulmonary edema, severe anemia, hyperparasitaemia, hypoglycemia, uremia, and lactic acidosis.

Laboratory diagnosis

- Thick and thin blood smears, stained with Field's stain or Giemsa stain, examined under light microscopy. Giemsa is better for species identification.

- *Rapid diagnostic tests:* most employ immunochromatographic lateral flow technology for antigen detection. There are numerous tests available worldwide. The BinaxNOW® Malaria Test Kit is FDA cleared in the United States and is based on detection of malarial HRP-2 and aldolase antigens. The assay differentiates *P. falciporum* from non-*falciporum* infection.
- *Laboratory findings:* hemolytic anemia, thrombocytopenia (common), uremia, hyperbilirubinemia, abnormal LFTs, coagulopathy

Treatment

Antimalarials (p. 96)

These remain the mainstay of therapy, but successful treatment is threatened by increasing drug resistance. The main classes of drugs are as follows:

- Quinoline derivatives (chloroquine, quinine, mefloquine, halofantrine)
- Antifolates (pyrimethamine, sulfonamides)
- Ribosomal inhibitors (tetracycline, doxycycline, clindamycin)
- Artemisinin derivates (artemisinin, artemether, arteether, artesunate)

Combination therapy with artemisinin derivatives shows rapid parasite clearance, low toxicity, and no clinical reports of resistance. Despite superior efficacy to quinine, most artemisinin derivatives are not available in the United States.

Supportive therapy

Good supportive therapy with careful management of seizures, pulmonary edema, acute renal failure, and lactic acidosis is essential in severe malaria. Exchange transfusion may be helpful in hyperparasitemia.

Adjunctive therapies

Adjunctive therapies for severe malaria have proved disappointing. Monoclonal antibodies directed against TNF-A reduced fever but showed no effect on mortality and may have increased morbidity. Dexamethasone has been shown to increase the duration of coma and was associated with poorer outcome in cerebral malaria.

Prevention (see Box 3.16)

- *Insecticide-treated bed nets* have been shown to reduce intradomilcilary vector populations and protect against infection.
- *Insect repellents* such as diethyltoluamide (DEET) reduce the risk of transmission in areas where mosquitoes are active before bedtime.
- *Chemoprophylaxis*, taken rigorously, is efficacious in reducing the incidence of malaria in travelers.
- *Vaccines:* a number of candidate vaccines using various antigens have been developed. Intense efforts to produce a vaccine have so far failed to yield a good candidate, but studies are ongoing.

Reference

Warell DA, Hooareeoyran S, Warrell MJ, et al. (1981). Dexamethasone proves deleterious in cerebral malaria. A double-blind trial in 100 comatose patients. *N Engl J Med* 306:313–319.

Box 3.16 Malaria treatment and prevention guidelines

Treatment

- U.S. guidelines: CDC. Treatment of Malaria (Guidelines for Clinicians). http://www.cdc.gov/malaria/diagnosis_treatment/tx_clinicians.htm
- WHO guidelines: *Management of Severe Malaria: A Practical Handbook*, 2nd ed. Geneva: WHO, 2000. http://www.who.int

Prophylaxis

- U.S. guidelines: National Center for Infectious Diseases Travellers' Health; The Yellow Book – Health Information for International Travel 2008. Atlanta: Centers for Disease Control, 2008. http://wwwn.cdc.gov/travel/ybToc.aspx
- WHO guidelines: World Health Organization. International Travel and Health: Vaccination Requirements and Health Advice. Geneva: WHO, 2004. http://www.who.int/ith

---

Babesia

Babesiosis is a zoonotic infection caused by *Babesia* spp., a malaria-like parasite that parasitizes erythrocytes of animals and causes fever, hemolysis, and hemoglobinuria. It typically causes mild illness in humans, but fulminant disease may occur in asplenic or immunosuppressed patients.

The parasite

There are more than 70 *Babesia* species worldwide that infect a wide range of mammals and birds. The rodent strain *B. microti* (United States) and the cattle strains *B. divergens* and *B. bovis* (Europe) are the main causes of human disease. *Babesia* spp. vary in length from 1 to 5 micrometer and are pear-shaped, oval, or round; their ring conformation and peripheral location in erythrocytes may lead to their misidentification as *P. falciparum*.

Babesia spp. are transmitted from their animal reservoir to humans via a tick vector *Ixodes scapularis* (United States) or *Ixodes ricinus* (Europe). The tick has three developmental stages (larva, nymph, and adult) and requires a blood meal, often from different mammalian species (e.g., deer, rodent) to mature to the next stage.

Epidemiology

The first fatal human case of babesiosis was reported in 1996. Since then, more than 100 cases have been reported worldwide, most from the northeastern coastal regions of the United States. Based on seroprevalence data, most infections appear to be subclinical. Transfusion-associated, transplacental, and perinatal transmission may occur.

The clinical features of babesiosis vary markedly between regions. Virtually all of the European cases have been caused by *B. bovis* or *B. divergens*, have occurred in splenectomized patients, and have had a fulminant and usually fatal course. In contrast, epidemiological data from the United States suggest that most infections are caused by *B. microti* and are mild or subclinical; clinical infections are more likely in the asplenic, immunosuppressed, or elderly, or in patients with concomitant Lyme disease.

Clinical features

Clinical features include fever, chills, malaise, fatigue, anorexia, headache, myalgia, arthralgia, nausea, vomiting, abdominal pain, dark urine, depression, and emotional lability. Photophobia, conjunctival injection, sore throat, cough, and adult respiratory distress syndrome have also been described.

Laboratory abnormalities include hemolytic anemia, reticulocytosis, normal or low WBC, thrombocytopenia, raised erythrocyte sedimentation rate (ESR), positive direct Coombs' test, mild elevations in LFTs, renal impairment, and reduced serum haptoglobin levels.

Urinalysis reveals hemoglobinuria and proteinuria.

Laboratory diagnosis

- *Microscopy:* examination of thin blood smears stained with Giemsa or Wright stains show parasitized erythrocytes, sometimes with diagnostic tetrads, referred to "Maltese Cross," of merozoites. *Babesia* spp. can be distinguished from *P. falciparum* by its lack of hemozoin and absence of schizonts and gametocytes.
- *Serology:* indirect immunofluorescent antibody titer for *B. microti* is available from the CDC, Atlanta. A titer of ≥1:256 is considered diagnostic for acute *B. microti* infection.
- *Molecular methods:* a PCR-based assay may be used for the detection of low levels of parasitemia.

Treatment

Most patients with *B. microti* infection have mild, self-limited illness that does not require specific treatment.

In patients with severe infections, a combination of quinine and clindamycin for 7–10 days appears to be effective.

Atovaquone and azithromycin is an alternative regimen—less rapidly effective but with fewer adverse effects.

Exchange transfusion is used in critically ill patients to reduce parasitemia.

Prevention

Avoid exposure to ticks in endemic areas between May and September. Wear light-colored, long-sleeved clothing, and tuck trousers into socks or boots.

Use insect repellent (e.g., diethyltoluanide) on skin and clothes. Carefully remove any ticks.

Discourage blood donations from donors in endemic areas between May and September, from donors with fevers 2 months prior to donation, and from donors with a history of tick bite.

Toxoplasma gondii

Toxoplasmosis is a zoonotic infection caused by *Toxoplasma gondii*, a coccidian parasite of cats that affects humans and other mammals as intermediate hosts. Although infection with *T. gondii* is common, it rarely causes disease apart from in congenitally acquired infection and in patients with cell-mediated immunodeficiency, especially AIDS.

Classification

T. gondii belongs to subphylum *Apicomplexa*, class *Sporozoa* and exists in three forms: the oocyst (which releases sporozoites), the tissue cyst (which contains bradyzoites), and the tachyzoite.

Life cycle

Oocysts are produced in the cat's intestine and shed in its feces. Once outside the cat, the oocysts sporulate and develop sporozoites. Oocysts are ingested by other animals and release sporozoites, which develop into tachyzoites.

These infect a wide variety of cells, multiply rapidly to form rosettes, lyse the cells, and spread to other cells or parts of the body. In the tissues, formation of tissue cysts may occur, with slowly replicating bradyzoites inside them.

Epidemiology

Toxoplasmosis is a worldwide zoonosis infecting a wide variety of mammals. Human infection occurs through the following means:

- Ingestions of tissue cysts in raw or undercooked meat
- Ingestion of food or water contaminated with oocysts
- Transplacental transmission from mother to fetus
- Rarely, through organ transplantation from a seropositive donor, contaminated blood transfusion, or needle stick injury

In HIV-infected patients, cerebral toxoplasmosis is usually due to reactivation of latent infection from advanced immunosuppression (CD4 count <100 cells/mm^3.) The incidence of toxoplasmosis among HIV-infected individuals is directly related to the seroprevalence of *T. gondii* antibodies in the general HIV population.

Thus rates are higher in Western Europe and Africa than in the United States. However, the introduction of HAART and use of trimethoprim/sulfamethoxazole prophylaxis for PCP have resulted in a dramatic fall in the incidence of toxoplasmosis in the developed world.

Pathogenesis

T. gondii penetrates intestinal epithelial cells and multiplies intracellularly. Organisms spread to the regional lymph nodes before being carried to distant organs in the lymphatics and blood. Infection with *T. gondii* induces both humoral and cellular immune responses, which are important for the early clearance of organisms from the blood and limit the parasite burden in other organs.

Cyst formation is responsible for persistent or latent infection; the main sites are the brain, skeletal and cardiac muscle, and the eye. In immunocompetent individuals, initial infection is often asymptomatic, chronic or latent infection is not clinically significant, and immunity is lifelong.

In immunosuppressed patients, toxoplasmosis may be caused by primary infection but is usually due to reactivation of latent infection and uncontrolled proliferation of organisms. The histological features of cerebral toxoplasmosis include focal (or diffuse) necrotizing encephalitis, microglial nodules, multiple brain abscesses, and hydrocephalus.

Clinical features

Immunocompetent patients

From 10% to 20% of infections are symptomatic. Clinical features include lymphadenopathy and/or an infectious mononucleosis–like syndrome. Rarely, severe, disseminated disease (myocarditis, pneumonitis, hepatitis, encephalitis) may occur.

Immunodeficient patients

Toxoplasmosis in HIV-negative patients is associated with organ transplants and lymphoma and presents with CNS, myocardial, or pulmonary involvement.

In patients with AIDS, cerebral toxoplasmosis is the most common diagnosis and presents subacutely with focal neurological symptoms. Other manifestations include spinal cord involvement, pneumonitis, chorioretinitis, pituitary abnormalities, orchitis, and GI involvement.

Ocular toxoplasmosis

T. gondii is an important cause of chorioretinitis. Congenitally acquired infection usually presents in the second or third decade of life, with bilateral disease, macular involvement, and old retinal scars.

Postnatal infection usually presents in the fourth to sixth decade of life with unilateral involvement and macular sparing.

Ocular toxoplasmosis has also been reported in HIV-infected patients, especially from Brazil.

Congenital toxoplasmosis

The incidence of fetal infection varies with trimester: 10–25% in the first trimester, 30–54% in the second trimester, and 60–65% in the third trimester. The risk of severe congenital infection is highest in the first and second trimesters (weeks 10–24). Clinical features include chorioretinitis, strabismus, blindness, seizures, microcephaly, intracranial calcification, hydrocephalus, anemia, jaundice, rash, encephalitis, pneumonitis, diarrhea, and hypothermia.

In contrast, infants who acquire infection in the third trimester may be born with subclinical infection but, if untreated, go on to develop disease, e.g., chorioretinitis, developmental delay.

Laboratory diagnosis

Serology

This remains the mainstay of diagnosis. The main problem with serological tests is that antibodies are present in many healthy individuals and persist at high levels for years. Different tests measure different antibodies, and there is no single test that can be used to differentiate acute from chronic infection. A combination of tests is often used:

- IgG antibodies usually appear within 1–2 weeks, peak at 1–2 months, and persist for life. The most widely used tests are: ELISA, indirect fluorescent antibody (IFA) test, modified direct agglutination test, IgG avidity test, and Sabin–Feldman dye test (gold standard).
- IgM antibodies may appear and decline more rapidly than IgG antibodies. However, high IgM levels may persist for years, limiting its use as the sole marker of acute infection. Various tests exist: ELISA (false positives with antinuclear antibody [ANA] and rheumatoid factor); IFA; and IgM immunosorbent agglutination assay (ISAGA).
- IgA antibodies have higher sensitivity than the IgM assays for the diagnosis of congenital toxoplasmosis
- IgE antibodies are present for a shorter duration than that of IgM or IgA and may be useful for diagnosing recently acquired infection.

PCR

The detection of *T. gondii* DNA in body fluids and tissues has been used to diagnose all forms of *Toxoplasma* infection. It has been used for the diagnosis of intrauterine infection and disseminated disease. Sensitivity is 15–85% in blood/buffy coat, and 11–77% in CSF.

Isolation

Isolation of *T. gondii* from blood, body fluids, placenta, or fetal tissues is diagnostic of acute infection. Isolation is not routinely performed but may be considered in neonates. The organism can be grown in tissue culture (3–6 days) or by mouse inoculation.

Histology

Demonstration of tachyzoites in tissues or body fluids is also diagnostic of acute infection. Various methods may be used to demonstrate organisms: fluorescent antibody staining, immunoperoxidase, ELISA, fluorescein-labeled monoclonal antibodies, electron microscopy, and Wright–Giemsa staining of centrifuged deposit or smear.

Antigen-specific lymphocyte transformation and typing

Lymphocyte proliferation in response to *T. gondii* antigens is a sensitive and specific indicator of previous infection in adults and has been used to diagnose congenital infection. An increase in CD8+ T cells may occur with acute infection in immunocompetent adults.

Radiological features

Radiological imaging is helpful in patients with CNS disease. In neonates with congenital toxoplasmosis, ultrasound or CT may demonstrate intracranial calcification and ventricular dilatation. In immunodeficient adults with cerebral toxoplasmosis, CT typically shows multiple ring-enhancing lesions. However, scans may be normal or show solitary lesions or cortical atrophy.

MRI appears to be more sensitive than CT and is the imaging modality of choice.

Treatment[1]

Recommended drugs act primarily against the tachyzoite form and do not eradicate the encysted form. Pyrimethamine is the most effective agent and should be given with folinic acid to prevent bone marrow suppression. A second drug, sulfadiazine or clindamycin, is also given.

Alternative agents include trimethoprim/sulfamethoxazole or pyrimethamine plus one of azithromycin, clarithromycin, atovaquone, or dapsone.

- *Immunocompetent adults* do not usually require treatment unless symptoms are severe and persistent, visceral disease is overt, or infection is parenterally acquired.
- *Immunodeficient patients:* acute/primary therapy is recommended for 3–6 weeks followed by lifelong maintenance therapy/secondary prophylaxis. AIDS patients with cerebral toxoplasmosis usually respond clinically within 2 weeks; those who do not should be investigated for other alternative diagnoses, e.g., CNS lymphoma.
- *Ocular toxoplasmosis:* treatment may not be required for small peripheral retinal lesions in immunocompetent adults but is generally indicated for lesions that threaten or cause visual loss.
- *Toxoplasmosis in pregnancy:* patients with suspected acute toxoplasmosis in pregnancy should be referred to a specialist unit for further investigation and management. Treatment with spiramycin, a macrolide antibiotic similar to erythromycin, reduces the risk of transmission to the fetus. As spiramycin does not cross the placenta, if fetal infection occurs, treatment should be changed to pyrimethamine (not in the first trimester) and sulfadiazine.
- *Congenital toxoplasmosis:* infants with congenital toxoplasmosis should be referred to a specialist unit. Treatment is with pyrimethamine and sulfadiazine for up to 12 months.

Prevention[1]

Prevention of primary infection in susceptible individuals, e.g., pregnant women and immunosuppressed patients, is by education:

- Avoid contact with cat feces in gardens and cat litters.
- Avoid ingestion of undercooked meat.

For HIV-infected patients with CD4 count <200 cells/mm^3, primary prophylaxis with trimethoprim/sulfamethoxazole has been shown to reduce the incidence of cerebral toxoplasmosis. Prophylaxis may be discontinued when the CD4 count remains persistently >200 cells/mm^3.

Some countries, e.g., France and Austria, advocate monthly screening of seronegative pregnant women during pregnancy.

Reference

1. Guidelines for prevention and treatment of opportunistic infections in HIV-infected adults and adolescents (2008). Available from http://AIDSinfo.nih.gov.

Cryptosporidium

Cryptosporidium is an intracellular protozoan, first described in 1907 in mice, and thought to be rare and clinically insignificant for 50 years.

It has since been recognized as a common enteric pathogen and is associated with waterborne outbreaks and diarrhea in patients with AIDS. It infects and replicates in epithelial cells of the digestive and respiratory tracts of most vertebrates.

Twenty species are recognized; *Cryptosporidium parvum* is the most important species.

Life cycle

Ingestion of oocysts is followed by encystation, usually after exposure to digestive enzymes or bile acids, then release of four sporozoites, which attach to the epithelial cell wall. Sporozoites mature asexually into meronts and release merozoites intraluminally.

Some of these re-invade the host cells (autoinfection), while others mature sexually into oocysts, which are excreted in the feces.

Epidemiology

Cryptosporidium is a ubiquitous enteric pathogen of all age groups. Transmission occurs by person-to-person, animal-to-person, water-borne or, less commonly, food-borne spread.

The prevalence of fecal oocyst excretion varies from 1–3% in industrialized countries to 5–10% in Asia and Africa. Seroprevalence data indicate that cryptosporidiosis is more common than surveys of fecal oocyst excretion demonstrate, e.g., 25–35% seroprevalence in Europe and North America.

Cryptosporidiosis has been recognized as an important cause of diarrhea in patients with HIV/AIDS. Other risk factors include malnutrition, immunoglobulin deficiencies, intercurrent viral infections, diabetes mellitus, organ transplantation, and hematological malignancies.

Clinical features

Symptoms usually develop 7–10 days after ingestion of oocysts.
- *GI symptoms:* diarrhea (may be copious), cramping abdominal pains, anorexia, nausea, vomiting, toxic megacolon (rare)
- *Other symptoms:* low-grade fever, weakness, malaise, fatigue, cholecystitis (especially HIV patients), hepatitis, pancreatitis, reactive arthritis, respiratory symptoms, disseminated disease. Recovery depends on the immune status of the patient: immunocompetent individuals have self-limited disease

Diagnosis

- *Stool microscopy:* examination of several specimens may be required (intermittent shedding). Most laboratories use a fecal concentration method followed by microscopy using a modified acid-fast stain: oocysts stain red/pink (carbol fuschin) against a blue (methylene blue) or green (malachite green) counterstain. Other stains include safranin-methylene blue, methenamine silver-nigrosin acridine orange, auramine-rhodamine, and auramine-carbolfuschin.

- *Antigen detection:* immunofluorescent antibody or ELISA tests may be used to detect cryptosporidial antigens in clinical or water specimens.
- Serology is primarily used as an epidemiological tool rather than for acute diagnosis.
- PCR-based assays have been developed but are not in routine use.
- Histology has low sensitivity and is now rarely used.

Treatment

Disease is usually self-limited in immunocompetent patients, and supportive therapy (hydration, parenteral nutrition) is key. Nitazoxanide has been used in immunocompetent patients. Antiretroviral therapy has been associated with improvement in patients with HIV/AIDS.

Prevention

Good hygiene is important, such as handwashing and proper disposal of contaminated material. Children with cryptosporidial diarrhea should avoid public swimming pools for at least 2 weeks after symptoms have resolved because of the continued shedding of oocysts and the resistance of these infectious particles to chlorination.

Prevent exposure in at-risk individuals, e.g., use water filters; avoid exposure to human and animal feces; and boil water during outbreaks.

Isospora

Isospora belli, a coccidian parasite first described in 1915, is the only species that infects humans. It is found predominantly in tropical and subtropical climates. It causes a self-limited diarrheal illness in immunocompetent patients. It has been recognized as an important cause of chronic or severe diarrhea in immunocompromised individuals especially patients with HIV/AIDS. Rare presentations include disseminated disease, cholecystitis, and reactive arthritis.

Diagnosis is by identification of oocysts in stool in wet mounts or acid-fast smears of fecal concentrates. Ultraviolet autofluorescence microscopy is a rapid, simple, and sensitive diagnostic test based on detection of oocyst autofluorescence when a 330–380 nm UV filter is used.

Treatment is with trimethoprim/sulfamethoxazole.

Cyclospora

Cyclospora cayetanensis was first described in humans in Papua New Guinea in 1977. Since then, it has emerged as a worldwide cause of diarrhea in travelers, children, and HIV-infected patients. Transmission is by contaminated food and water. Most of the early cases were described in Nepal, Peru, and Haiti.

The epidemiology of the disease varies according to the type of patient. In endemic areas, the duration of illness is short, and there are many asymptomatic carriers. In travelers, diarrhea may last for over a month. In immunocompromised patients, symptoms may be severe and last longer.

Diagnosis is by microscopic detection of oocysts in stool using modified acid-fast or safranin stains. Ultraviolet autofluorescence of oocyst is both rapid and sensitive but not specific.

Treatment is with trimethoprim/sulfamethoxazole (160 mg bid for 7 days for immunocompetent patients, 160 mg qid for 10 days followed by lifelong suppressive therapy in HIV patients, until the CD4 count is consistently >200 cells/mm^3.

Trypanosoma

The genus *Trypanosoma* consists of approximately 20 species of protozoa. They are common animal pathogens causing severe disease in domestic animals. Three species infect humans:

- *Trypanosoma cruzi*, which causes Chagas' disease
- *Trypanosoma brucei gambiense, which* causes West African sleeping sickness
- *Trypanosoma brucei rhodesiense*, which causes East African sleeping sickness

Trypanosoma cruzi

Chagas disease is a zoonosis caused by *T. cruzi*. The disease is endemic in wild and domestic animals in Central and South America. It is transmitted by blood-sucking insects called *triatome* or "kissing" bugs, which transmit the parasite between and among many mammalian species. Humans are considered accidental hosts.

Transmission of *T. cruzi* may also occur through blood transfusions, organ transplantation, or vertically from mother to child.

Life cycle

The parasites multiply in the mid-gut of the insects as promastigotes. In the hindgut they transform into trypomastigotes, which are passed out in the feces during blood meals.

Transmission to a second mammalian host occurs when breaks in the skin, mucous membranes, or conjunctivae are contaminated with bug feces. The parasites enter host cells, transform into amastigotes, and multiply and differentiate into trypomastigotes. The cell ruptures, releasing the parasites, which invade local tissue and spread hematogenously.

Pathogenesis

In acute Chagas disease, the inflammatory lesion that develops at the site of entry is called the *chagoma*. Trypomastigotes released by cell rupture may be detected my microscopic examination of the blood. Muscles are the most heavily parasitized tissues.

The heart is the most commonly affected organ in chronic Chagas disease; clinical features include myocarditis and conduction defects. The gastrointestinal tract is also affected, with dilatation and muscular hypertrophy of the esophagus and the colon.

Clinical features

There are four main clinical syndromes.

Acute Chagas disease

This is usually an illness of children. An inflammatory lesion, a chagoma, develops at the site of entry. Romaña's sign (painless perioribital edema) may be seen if the site of entry is the conjunctivae. Localized signs may be followed by fever, malaise, anorexia, edema, lymphadenopathy, and hepatosplenomegaly.

CNS involvement is rare but carries a poor prognosis. Severe myocarditis with congestive cardiac failure may also occur. The acute illness is usually resolved and the patient enters the asymptomatic phase.

Cardiac disease

Chronic disease becomes symptomatic many years after the primary infection. The heart is the most common site and clinical features are dizziness, syncope, arrhythmias, seizures, congestive cardiac failure, and thromboembolism. Death occurs within months of developing cardiac failure.

Gastrointestinal disease

Patients with megaesophagus present with symptoms of achalasia, e.g., dysphagia, odynophagia, cough, chest pain, and regurgitation. Aspiration pneumonitis is common and may be fatal. An increased incidence of esophageal cancer has been reported.

Patients with megacolon present with constipation, abdominal pain, intestinal obstruction, or bowel perforation.

Disease in immunosuppressed patients

Reactivation of *T. cruzi* may occur in immunosuppressed patients, e.g., with solid-organ transplantation or HIV. The clinical presentation is similar to that of acute Chagas disease but may be more severe, with CNS involvement.

Diagnosis

Diagnosis of Chagas disease is based on the following:

- History of exposure to *T. cruzi*, e.g., residence or travel to an endemic area, blood transfusion in an endemic area
- *Acute Chagas disease:* wet prep or Giemsa smear for detection of circulating parasites. In immunocompromised patients, other specimens may need to be examined, e.g., lymph node, bone marrow aspirates, pericardial fluid, CSF. If the smear is negative, culture of blood or specimens in liquid media or xenodiagnosis may be attempted.
- *Chronic Chagas disease* is diagnosed by detection of IgG antibodies to the parasite. Many serological assays are available, but their performance is variable.
- PCR assays have been developed over the past 20 years. Sensitivity is usually >90% (range 47–100%).

Treatment

The current treatment of Chagas disease is far from ideal.

Nifurtimox, a nitrofuran derivative, has been used to treat acute and congenital Chagas disease. Although it reduces the duration and severity of symptoms, parasitological cure rates are only ~70%. Side effects include nausea, vomiting, abdominal pain, weight loss, and neurological symptoms.

Benznidazole, a nitroimidazole derivative, is the alternative agent. Its efficacy is similar to that of nitrofurimox. Side effects include rash, peripheral neuropathy, and neutropenia.

For chronic infection, treatment is supportive. Patients have an ECG every 6 months. Pacemakers are helpful in patients with bradyarrhythmias. Megaesophagus may be treated with balloon dilatation/myomectomy of the lower esophageal sphincter. Megacolon is managed with high-fiber diet and laxatives and enemas. Surgery may be required for complications.

Trypanosoma brucei complex

The organisms that cause African sleeping sickness are morphologically indistinguishable and belong to the *T. brucei* complex:

- *T. brucei brucei* (animal pathogen)
- *T. brucei rhodesiense* (East African trypanosomiasis)
- *T. brucei gambiense* (West African trypanosomiasis)

They are transmitted by the blood-sucking tsetse flies in Africa.

Life cycle

Tsetse flies ingest trypomastigotes during a blood meal from an infected mammalian host. Once in the mid-gut, the short, stumpy trypomastigotes transform into long, slender, procyclic trypomastigotes. After several cycles of replication, they migrate to the salivary glands, where they differentiate into epimastigotes and continue to multiply. The epimastigotes transform into infective trypomastigotes, which are inoculated into a second mammalian host at the next blood meal.

African trypanosomes differ from *T. cruzi* in that they exhibit antigenic variation and are thus able to evade the host immune response.

Pathogenesis

The pathogenesis of African sleeping sickness is complex and incompletely understood. An acute inflammatory lesion (trypanosomal chancre) develops at the site of the tsetse fly bite. Multiplication of the parasite occurs in this lesion, resulting in inflammation, edema, and local tissue destruction. The parasites spread to the local lymph nodes and then disseminate in the bloodstream.

In stage 1 disease (hemolymphatic), there is widespread lymphadenopathy and histiocytic infiltration followed by fibrosis. The heart may be involved. Stage 2 disease (meningoencephalitic) is characterized by CNS invasion.

Clinical features

West African trypanosomiasis is caused by *T. brucei gambiense*. Infected humans are the main reservoir of infection. A trypanosomal chancre develops 1–2 weeks after the tsetse fly bite and resolves within several weeks.

Stage 1 disease is marked by the onset of intermittent high fevers, posterior cervical lymphadenopathy (Winterbottom's sign), hepatosplenomegaly, transient edema, pruritis, and rash.

Stage 2 disease is characterized by the insidious onset of neurological symptoms (headache, somnolence, listless gaze, extrapyramidal signs), accompanied by CSF abnormalities.

East African trypanosomiasis is caused by *T. brucei rhodesiense*. Infected wild animals are the main reservoir of infection. The illness is more acute than the West African disease, with onset of symptoms a few days after the insect bite. Intermittent fever and rash are common features; lymphadenopathy is less prominent than in West African disease.

Cardiac manifestations such as arrhythmias and congestive cardiac failure may result in death prior to the onset of CNS disease. Untreated, this condition is fatal in weeks to months.

Diagnosis

The diagnosis of African trypanosomiasis is based on the following:
• History of exposure e.g., residence in or travel to an endemic area
• Compatible clinical features
• Examination of chancre fluid or lymph nodes for trypanosomes (wet prep and Giemsa stain)
• Examination of blood for trypanosomes (wet prep and Giemsa stain). This is more likely to be positive in the hemolymphatic stage and in East African trypanosomiasis (higher parasitemia). Serial specimens should be examined.
• Examination of Buffy coat for trypanosomes (if blood film is non-diagnostic)
• CSF examination shows increased cell count, increased CSF pressure, elevated IgM, and total protein concentrations. A patient with any CSF abnormalities should be regarded as having CNS disease.
• Bone marrow aspiration may be helpful in patients whose other tests are negative.
• Serology: assays are available but limited by variable performance.

Treatment

A number of drugs are available to treat African trypanosomiasis (Table 3.28):
• Melarsoprol (p. 103)
• Pentamidine (p. 104)
• Suramin (p. 105)
• Eflornithine.

The treatment of African trypanosomiasis depends on the infecting species, drug resistance patterns, and stage of disease.

Table 3.28 Treatment of African trypanosomiasis

	Stage 1 disease	Stage 2 disease
T. brucei gambiense	Pentamidine or eflornithine	Eflornithine or melarsoprol
T. brucei rhodesiense	Suramin or pentamidine	Melarsoprol

Prevention

Control programs involving vector eradication and drug treatment of animals and humans have had limited success. Chemoprophylaxis is not recommended because of drug toxicity.

Leishmania

Leishmaniasis is caused by various *Leishmania* spp. that vary in their geographic distribution and clinical features. There are three clinical syndromes, each of which may be caused by several species:
- Visceral leishmaniasis (kala-azar)
- Cutaneous leishmaniasis
- Mucosal leishmaniasis (espundia)
- Post kala-azar dermal leishmaniasis

The parasite

Leishmania spp. have a dimorphic life cycle and live in macrophages as intracellular amastigotes in mammalian hosts and extracellular promastigotes in the gut of their sand fly vectors.

Leishmania spp. cannot be differentiated on the basis of morphology. Speciation was initially based on epidemiological and clinical features; several molecular assays are now used.

Pathogenesis

Cell-mediated immune responses are responsible for controlling leishmanial infections. The clinical manifestations depend on complex interactions between the parasite's invasiveness, tropism, and pathogenicity and the host's genetically determined immune response e.g., NRAMP-1 polymorphisms.

The resolution of leishmanial infections is associated with expansion of leishmania-specific CD4+ T cells of the TH1 type, which secrete IFN-γ and interleukin-2 (IL-2) in response to leishmanial antigens. Macrophages and their products are also important in controlling infection.

Leishmania spp. may also elicit disease-enhancing immune responses, e.g., expansion of CD4+ T cells of the TH2 type, which produce IL-4, IL-5, and IL-10.

Epidemiology

Visceral leishmaniasis has a wide geographic distribution. It is caused by *L. donovani* spp. (India, Pakistan, Nepal, East Africa, eastern China), *L. infantum* (Middle East, Mediterranean, the Balkans, central and southwest Asia, northern and western China, northern and Sub-Saharan Africa) or *L. chagasi* (Latin America). Rarely, *L. amazonensis* or *L. tropica* may cause visceral leishmaniasis.

Cutaneous leishmaniasis is also widely distributed. The classic form of Old World cutaneous leishmaniasis, the oriental sore, is found in the Middle East, Mediterranean, Africa, India, and Asia. It is usually caused by *L. major*, *L. tropica*, *L. aethiopica*, and, occasionally, *L. donovani* and *L. infantum*. New World cutaneous leishmaniasis is endemic in Latin America. It is caused by *L. brazilensis*, *L. mexicana*, *L. panamensis*, and, occasionally, *L. chagasi*.

Mucosal leishmaniasis (espundia) mainly occurs in Latin America and is usually caused by *L. braziliensis*.

Clinical features

Visceral leishmaniasis

The incubation period is 3–8 months. Onset may be acute or gradual. Symptoms include abdominal enlargement, fever, weakness, anorexia, and weight loss.

Examination shows pallor, hepatosplenomegaly ± lymphadenopathy (Sudan). The skin becomes dry, thin, scaly and discolored (kala-azar = black fever). Hemorrhage may occur at various sites. Secondary infections are common in advanced disease and may lead to death.

Laboratory findings include anemia, leukopenia, and hypergammaglobulinemia. Visceral leishmaniasis may be the presenting feature of HIV infection.

Cutaneous leishmaniasis

The incubation period is 2 weeks to several months. A wide variety of skin lesions may occur, from small, dry crusted lesions (usually *L. tropica*) to large, deep ulcers with a granulating base and overlying exudate (usually *L. braziliensis*).

Lesions may be single or multiple and tend to occur on exposed areas. Secondary bacterial infections and lymphadenopathy may occur.

Mucosal leishmaniasis

A small proportion of patients with cutaneous leishmaniasis develop mucous membrane involvement of the nose, oral cavity, pharynx, and larynx months to years after their skin lesions have healed. Symptoms include nasal stuffiness, discharge, or epistaxis.

The nasal septum may be destroyed, resulting in nasal collapse. Perforation may occur through the nose or soft palate. Occasionally, patients may be unable to eat or develop aspiration pneumonia.

Diagnosis

Visceral leishmaniasis

Splenic (most sensitive), bone marrow, lymph node, or liver biopsy may confirm the diagnosis. Amastigotes may be seen in Wright- or Giemsa-stained smears. Specimens should be inoculated into special media (e.g., Novy, McNeal and Nicoll medium, Schneider insect medium) and cultured at 22–26°C. Motile promastigotes develop after days to weeks.

Anti-leishmanial antibodies may be present at high titer in immunocompetent patients but may be absent or low titer in HIV-infected patients. False-positive reactions occur with leprosy, Chagas disease, malaria, schistosomiasis, toxoplasmosis, or cutaneous leishmaniasis.

An antigen test has been developed.

Cutaneous leishmaniasis

Skin biopsies taken from the edge of a lesion may show on amastigotes on Wright or Giemsa staining. Lesions may also be injected and aspirated with saline and examined for amastigotes. Samples may be cultured using special media (see above). Anti-leishmanial antibodies may be present in some patients. The leishmanin (Montenegro) skin test becomes positive during the course of the disease but is no longer used.

A *Leishmania* PCR test has recently been developed and evaluated.

Mucosal leishmaniasis

A definitive diagnosis is made by identification of amastigotes in tissue biopsies or isolation of promastigotes in culture. However, the diagnosis is often presumptive and based on the presence of a characteristic scar and positive leishmanin skin test or anti-leishmanial antibodies.

Treatment

Pentavalent antimony compounds (sodium stiboglutamate or meglumine antimoniate) have been used for decades, but drug resistance, treatment failures, and relapses are becoming more common. The recommended dose is 20 mg/kg/day pentavalent antimony for 20–28 days, depending on clinical syndrome.

Side effects include abdominal pain, anorexia, nausea, vomiting, myalgia, arthralgia, headache, malaise, raised amylase and lipase, renal failure, ECG abnormalities, cardiac arrhythmias, and sudden death (high doses).

Liposomal amphotericin B is licensed for the treatment of visceral leishmaniasis. It is as effective as, but less toxic than, pentavalent antimony. Conventional amphotericin B deoxycholate and pentamidine isetionate are effective but more toxic alternatives.

Fluconazole and itraconazole have been shown to be effective in cutaneous leishmaniasis.

Miltefosine has been used to treat both cutaneous and visceral leishmaniasis in the developing world.

Topical therapy with paromycin and methylbenzethonium has been used in cutaneous leishmaniasis.

Local heat therapy or cryotherapy has been used in cutaneous leishmaniasis.

Prevention

Prevention strategies include the following:
- Controlling sand fly vectors (insecticides, bed nets)
- Controlling animal reservoirs (difficult)
- Treating infected humans.

Although there is no effective form of immunoprophylaxis, there are ongoing efforts to produce a vaccine.

Giardia lamblia

Giardia lamblia, a flagellated intestinal protozoan, is a common cause of diarrhea throughout the world.

The pathogen

G. lamblia is the only *Giardia* species that infects humans. The life cycle consists of two stages: trophozoite and cyst.

Epidemiology

G. lamblia has a worldwide distribution and is the most commonly identified intestinal parasite. It is usually acquired by ingestion of contaminated water but may also be spread by person-to person (children in daycare centers, institutionalized people, sexual) or food-borne transmission.

Natural or experimental infections with *Giardia* spp. have been documented for many mammalian species; whether these act as reservoirs for transmission to humans is less clear.

Pathogenesis

Infection occurs after ingestion of as few as 10–25 cysts. After encystation, trophozoites colonize and multiply in the small bowel. Several pathogenic mechanisms have been postulated: disruption of the brush border, mucosal invasion (rare), stimulation of inflammatory infiltration leading to fluid and electrolyte secretion, and villous changes.

The production of gastrointestinal secretory IgA antibodies appears to be key in preventing and clearing infection. The cellular immune response is also important in clearing infection, by coordinating IgA secretion and cellular cytotoxicity.

Susceptibility to giardiasis has been seen in patients with common variable immune deficiency, X-linked agammaglobulinemia, previous gastric surgery, or reduced gastric acidity.

Clinical features

- Incubation period: symptoms develop 1–2 week after ingestion of cysts; detection of cysts in the stool may take longer.
- Clinical features include asymptomatic cyst passers (5–15%), diarrheal syndrome (25–50%), and subclinical infection (35–70%).
- Symptomatic giardiasis is characterized by diarrhea, abdominal cramps, bloating, flatulence, malaise, nausea, anorexia, and weight loss. Initially, stools may be profuse and watery but later may become greasy and foul-smelling and may float. Vomiting, fever, and tenesmus are less common.
- Unusual features include urticaria, reactive arthritis, biliary disease, and gastric infection (if achlorhydria).
- Severe volume depletion may occur in young children and pregnant women, necessitating hospital admission.

Diagnosis

The diagnosis should be considered in all patients with chronic diarrhea, particularly if associated with malabsorption or weight loss.

- Stool examination: a wet mount of fresh liquid stool may show motile trophozoites; iodine staining may reveal cysts. Formol-ether concentration techniques may increase the yield.
- Antigen detection assays that detect *G. lamblia* by immunofluorescence or ELISA are significantly more sensitive than stool microscopy.
- Duodenal string test (Entero-Test) may be helpful in difficult cases.
- Duodenal aspirate and biopsy is more invasive but may help to exclude other diagnoses.

- Antibody tests are not widely available but are useful in distinguishing acute from past infection and in epidemiological surveys.
- In vitro culture and molecular assays are available in research settings.

Treatment

Metronidazole is the drug of choice and has an efficacy of 80–95%. Drug resistance can be induced in vitro and may occur in vivo. Side effects include metallic taste, nausea, dizziness, headache disulfiram reaction (with alcohol), and neutropenia (rare). Concerns about teratogenicity mean that it is contraindicated in pregnancy (first trimester) and not recommended in children.

Tinidazole (p. 106), another nitroimidazole, is given in a single dose and has an efficacy of approximately 90%.

Furazolidone (see Nitrofurans, p. 61), a nitrofuran, has a lower efficacy rate (80%) but is available as a liquid suspension. Side effects include GI symptoms, brown discoloration of urine, and mild hemolysis (in G6PD deficiency).

From the benzimidazoles (see Anthelmintic drugs 1, p. 107), mebendazole has proved disappointing, but albendazole looks promising in several pediatric studies.

Paromomycin (see Aminoglycosides, p. 39), an oral aminoglycoside, has been used in pregnancy but has a lower efficacy rate (60–70%) than that of other drugs.

Prevention

Good sanitation with proper treatment of public water supplies is important. Boiling or purification of water with chlorine- or iodine-based preparations should be carried out in endemic areas.

Prevention of person-to-person spread consists of good personal hygiene, handwashing, and avoidance of orogenital or oroanal sex.

Trichomonas vaginalis

T. vaginalis, a flagellated protozoan, was initially thought to be a harmless commensal but has since become recognized as an important cause of genital infection.

The pathogen

On microscopic examination of genital specimens, *T. vaginalis* is a pear-shaped organism (10 × 7 micrometer) with twitching motility. There are four anterior flagella that arise from a single stalk and a fifth flagellum that is embedded in the undulating membrane.

The organism only exists as a vegetative cell, reproduces by binary fission, and generates energy with unique organelles called *hydrogenosomes*.

Epidemiology

The incidence appears to be declining in Western Europe and the United States. Trichomoniasis is usually sexually transmitted and its incidence is highest in women with multiple partners, in patients with other STIs, and in HIV-infected patients.

Trichomoniasis is occasionally acquired nonvenereally (e.g., in institutionalized patients) or by vertical transmission during delivery.

Pathogenesis

All areas of the cell surface are capable of phagocytosis and can ingest bacteria, leucocytes, erythrocytes, and epithelial cells. Trichomonads appear to damage genital epithelium by direct contact, which is mediated by surface proteins, and cause microulceration.

Specific virulence factors have not been defined, and the immune response is incompletely understood. T. vaginalis activates the alternative complement pathway and attracts neutrophils that may kill the protozoan.

Clinical features

The incubation period is 5–28 days.

Symptoms often begin or worsen during periods and include vaginal discharge (may be smelly or itchy), dyspareunia, dysuria, and lower abdominal discomfort. Signs include vulvar erythema, yellow/green or frothy vaginal discharge, vaginal inflammation, and punctuate hemorrhages on the cervix ("strawberry cervix").

Most infected men are asymptomatic, but those that are symptomatic may have urethritis that is clinically indistinguishable from other causes of nongonococcal urethritis.

Complications of vaginal trichomoniasis include vaginitis emphysematosa (gas-filled blebs in the vaginal wall), vaginal cuff cellulitis after hysterectomy, premature labor, and low-birth-weight infants.

Diagnosis

Diagnosis relies on identification of the organism in genital specimens.

The wet mount will identify organisms in 48–80% of infected women and 50–90% of infected men. The organisms remain motile for 10–20 minutes after sample collection. Other findings, while not diagnostic, are an elevated vaginal pH (>4.5) and increased PMNs on saline microscopy.

Various staining methods (e.g., Gram, Giemsa, Pappenheim, and acridine orange) are less sensitive than the wet mount.

Other methods (e.g., direct fluorescent antibody staining, latex agglutination, ELISA, DNA probe, and PCR-based assays) are more sensitive than wet prep but less sensitive than culture.

Culture remains the most sensitive technique, and trichomonads can be cultured on a variety of media; modified Diamond's media is best.

Serological diagnosis is hampered by low sensitivity and poor specificity, particularly in high-risk populations.

Treatment[1]

Metronidazole (p. 59) is the treatment of choice and can be given as a single 2 g dose or in divided doses for 7 days. The main disadvantage of a single dose is the risk of reinfection if the partner is not treated simultaneously.

Alternative drugs, for metronidazole intolerance or resistance (which appears to be increasing), include tinidazole. Although cross-resistance to tinidazole is frequent, it is not inevitable.

The most common causes of treatment failure are nonadherence and reinfection.

Prevention

- General advice about prevention of STIs
- Use of barrier contraceptive methods if sexually active

Reference

1.2006 CDC treatment guidelines for sexually transmitted infections. www.cdc.gov/std/treatment/

Entamoeba histolytica

E. histolytica is a common cause of diarrhea worldwide, particularly in the tropics. It can also cause extraintestinal disease sites, e.g., abscessses in the liver, lung, brain, or genitourinary tract.

The parasite

E. histolytica is one of several *Entamoeba* species that infect humans. Other species are nonpathogenic and include *E. dispar* (morphologically identical), *E. hartmanii,* and *E. coli.* The organism exists in two forms: the trophozoite (10–60 micrometer with single nucleus ± ingested erythrocytes) and the cyst (5–20 micrometer with four nuclei). Ingestion of the cyst results in excystation in the small bowel and trophozoite infection of the colon, resulting in symptoms.

When conditions are no longer favorable, the trophozoite encysts and is passed out in the feces. Cysts remain viable for weeks or months in moist environments.

Epidemiology

It is estimated that 10% of the world's population is infected with *E. histolytica.* There is a wide geographic variation in prevalence, ranging from ≤5% in developed countries to 20–30% in the tropics. Risk factors for amebiasis in endemic areas include low socioeconomic status, poor sanitation, and overcrowding.

In low-prevalence countries, certain groups are at higher risk: immigrants or travelers from endemic regions, institutionalized individuals, and promiscuous gay men.

Factors associated with severe disease include neonates, pregnancy, corticosteroid therapy, and malnutrition.

Pathogenesis

The pathogenesis of invasive amebiasis requires adherence of trophozoites by galactose-inhibitable lectin, direct cytolytic and proteolytic effects that damage tissue, and resistance of the parasite to the host immune response.

Clinical features

The clinical features of amebiasis can be divided into intestinal and extraintestinal syndromes:

- *Intestinal manifestations* include asymptomatic infection, symptomatic noninvasive infection, amebic dysentery (gradual onset, abdominal pain/tenderness, bloody diarrhea), fulminant colitis (rare but carries a high mortality), toxic megacolon, chronic colitis, ameboma (annular lesion of the colon), and perianal ulceration
- *Extraintestinal manifestations* include amebic liver abscess (complications: empyema, pericarditis, peritonitis), lung abscess, brain abscess, and genitourinary disease; 50% of liver abscess patients have no history of dysentery.

Diagnosis

Stool microscopy (ova and parasite examination [O&P]) remains the cornerstone of diagnosis, but sensitivity is poor and multiple specimens may need to be examined. A fresh liquid stool should be examined by wet mount for motile trophozoites. A formol-ether concentrate with examination of iodine-stained deposit increases the likelihood of seeing cysts.

Antigen detection in stool using ELISA, radioimmunoassay, or immunofluorescence is commercially available and more sensitive than stool O&P. These assays also distinguish *E. histolytica* from *E. dispar* infections

Stool culture is also more sensitive than microscopy but not routinely available.

Colonoscopy and biopsy may be helpful in confirming the diagnosis in patients with colitis. Endoscopic features range from nonspecific mucosal thickening to punctuate hemorrhages and/or the classic "flask-shaped" ulcers, but may appear normal in early disease.

Serological tests, e.g., indirect hemagglutination assays, are helpful in the diagnosis of invasive intestinal amebiasis, but titers may be negative in early disease and remain high for years. Other less sensitive assays (e.g., counterimmunoelectrophoresis or gel diffusion precipitation) wane more rapidly and may be helpful in diagnosing acute disease.

PCR-based assays are not currently widely available.

Imaging studies, e.g., ultrasound, CT, or MRI scans, are useful in assessing patients with suspected amebic liver abscess. Aspiration of the abscess yields a brown, odorless, sterile liquid, which may show trophozoites. The main risk of aspiration is peritoneal spillage or peritonitis. Many cases may be diagnosed and treated with aspiration.

Treatment

The treatment of amebiasis is complicated by a number of factors, including a variety of clinical syndromes, varying sites of action of different drugs, and the availability of different drugs in different countries.

Intraluminal carriage (e.g., asymptomatic cyst passers) should be treated because of the risk of invasive disease. Possible regimens include diloxanide furoate, paromomycin, tetracycline + iodoquinol.

Invasive disease (e.g., dysentery, colitis) should be treated with metronidazole or tinidazole followed by an intraluminal agent (see above).

Extraintestinal amebiasis (e.g., liver abscess) should be treated by metronidazole followed by an intraluminal agent (see above). In severely ill patients, emetine or dehydroemetine (less toxic) may be added for the first few days. Aspiration or percutaneous drainage is usually only required for large cysts or to confirm the diagnosis. Surgical attempts to correct amebic bowel perforation or peritonitis should be avoided.

Prevention

Avoid ingestion of contaminated water and food. In endemic areas, vegetables should be treated with a detergent and soaked in acetic acid or vinegar. In endemic areas, water should be boiled, as purification with chlorine or iodine may not be sufficient to kill cysts.

Sexual practices that involve feco-oral contact should be avoided.

Free-living amoebae

Human infection with free-living amoebae is infrequent but may be severe and life threatening. Three clinical syndromes occur:
- Primary amebic meningoencephalitis, caused by *Naegleria fowleri*
- Granulomatous amebic encephalitis, caused by *Acanthamoeba* spp. and *Ballamuthia mandrillaris*
- Amebic keratitis, caused by *Acanthamoeba* spp.

Naegleria fowleri

Epidemiology

This is found throughout the world in soil, rivers, lakes, and thermally polluted water. It grows well in temperatures up to 45°C. It causes primary amebic encephalitis in children and young adults who have recently swum in warm freshwater lakes or ponds.

Pathogenesis

Amoebae penetrate the olfactory mucosa and enter the CNS through the cribriform plate, resulting in a diffuse meningoencephalitis, purulent leptomeningitis, and cortical hemorrhages.

Clinical features

Symptoms occur 2–5 days after exposure. Patients may initially report changes in smell or taste followed by an abrupt onset of fever, anorexia, nausea, vomiting, headache, meningismus, and altered mental status. Patients rapidly progress to coma and death within a week.

Myocarditis is found in 7–16% of patients at autopsy, but patients do not appear to develop arrhythmias or heart failure.

Diagnosis

Diagnosis is based on clinical suspicion and confirmed by the demonstration of trophozoites in the CSF. A variety of molecular assays have been developed but are not widely available.

Serological tests are not helpful, as the majority of adults tested in endemic areas, e.g., Florida, have antibody.

Treatment

Few patients are known to have survived primary amebic encephalitis. Most were treated with systemic and intrathecal amphotericin B. One patient was treated with miconazole, rifampin, and sulfisoxazole.

Various other agents have been tried in animal models, including passive immunotherapy.

Acanthamoeba spp.

Epidemiology

Acanthamoeba spp. have been isolated from soil, water, and air. Serological surveys indicate that exposure is common and the organism may be isolated in pharyngeal swabs from healthy people. Encephalitis tends to occur in debilitated or immunosuppressed patients, e.g., HIV, liver disease, diabetes mellitus, organ transplantation, corticosteroid therapy, and chemotherapy. In contrast, keratitis occurs in healthy patients.

Pathogenesis

Granulomatous amebic encephalitis is characterized by necrotizing granulomatous lesions containing perivascular trophozoites and cysts located in the cerebellum, midbrain, and brainstem. Keratitis is characterized by cysts and trophozoites in the cornea, with an acute or mixed inflammatory infiltrate.

Granulomatous amebic encephalitis

This has an insidious onset and presents with focal neurological deficits. Clinical features include altered mental status, seizures, fever, headache, hemiparesis, meningismus, visual disturbance, and ataxia. The duration of CNS illness until death is 7–120 days.

Other clinical syndromes include skin lesions, pneumonitis, adrenalitis, leucocytoclastic vasculitis, and osteomyelitis.

Amebic keratitis

This is associated with minor corneal trauma or the use of soft contact lenses. Clinical features include a foreign-body sensation followed by severe pain, photophobia, tearing, blepharospasm, conjunctivitis, and blurred vision. The diagnosis is often delayed because of initial misdiagnosis or periods of temporary remission.

Diagnosis

Granulomatous amebic encephalitis is usually diagnosed postmortem. CT brain scans have shown multiple lucent nonenhancing lesions. Lumbar puncture is contraindicated because of the risk of herniation. When performed, CSF examination has been nondiagnostic, with elevated white cell counts and protein and decreased glucose levels.

Organisms may be found in brain biopsy material or by skin biopsy in those with skin lesions. The diagnosis of amebic keratitis depends on the demonstration of *Acanthamoeba* in corneal scrapings, contact lenses, or contact lens fluid by histology or culture.

Corneal scrapings may be examined by wet mount for motile trophozoites or fixed and stained using a variety of stains. A non-nutrient agar overlaid with *E. coli* is most commonly used for culture. Molecular techniques include PCR and DNA probes.

Treatment

Little is known about the treatment of granulomatous amebic encephalitis. Drugs that are active in vitro include propamidine, pentamidine, ketoconazole, miconazole, paromomycin, neomycin, 5-flucytosine, and, to a lesser extent, amphotericin B.

One case has been successfully treated with trimethoprim- sulfamethoxazole. The treatment of amebic keratitis involves aggressive surgical debridement and topical therapy for 2–3 months.

In clinical practice, topical propamidine 0.1% and polyhexamethylene biguanide 0.02% or biguanide chlorhexadine 0.02% drops are often selected as initial choices. When medical therapy is unsuccessful, cornea transplantation must be considered.

Ballamuthia mandrillaris

Epidemiology

B. mandrillaris is a soil inhabitant that contaminates fresh water. It causes granulomatous amebic encephalitis in both immunocompetent and immunocompromised hosts.

Pathogenesis

CNS lesions are characterized by a chronic inflammatory infiltrate with or without granulomas. Cysts and trophozoites occur in perivascular pattern and are associated with angiitis and hemorrhagic necrosis of the meninges and underlying brain tissue.

Clinical features

A subacute or chronic meningoencephalitis involves fever, headache, nausea, vomiting, seizures, and focal neurological signs. Death occurs 1 week to several months after onset of symptoms.

Diagnosis

CT brain scan shows multiple hypodense lesions with mass effect. CSF abnormalities include a mononuclear pleocytosis (10–500 cells), raised protein, and low glucose. Brain biopsy specimens may demonstrate the cyst and trophozoite.

Previously, *B. mandrillaris* was difficult to distinguish from *Acanthamoeba* spp., but an immunofluorescence assay and a cell-free growth medium have been developed, mainly as a research tool.

Treatment

There is no known effective treatment for *B. mandrillaris* encephalitis. In vitro, pentamidine isetionate, azithromycin, and amphotericin B have amebastatic activity. Pentamidine has shown some clinical efficacy.

Microsporidia

First identified in 1857, the microsporidia are a diverse group of obligate intracellular, spore-forming protozoa that belong to phylum *Microspora*, order *Microsporida*. Although eukaryotic, they are unusual in having 70S ribosomes, no mitochondria, and simple vesicular Golgi membranes.

The microsporidial spore is a highly specialized structure that varies in size and shape according to species.

Over 1200 species exist and they infect a wide range of vertebrate and invertebrate hosts. At least 14 species have been implicated in human disease, e.g., *Enterocytozoon bieneusi* and *Encephalitozoon* spp., being the most common.

Epidemiology

Human infection has been identified worldwide (except in Antarctica). Most severe infections are associated with immunocompromise, e.g., HIV infection, organ transplantation, and corticosteroid therapy. However, infections are becoming increasingly recognized in immunocompetent patients, e.g., residents of or travelers from tropical countries.

Routes of transmission include water-borne, person-to person spread, inhalation/aerosol, or by zoonotic spread.

Pathology

Microsporidia can infect many different organs:
- *Eye:* punctuate epithelial keratopathy
- *Respiratory tract:* rhinitis, sinusitis, nasal polyposis, tracheitis, bronchitis, bronchiolitis ± pneumonia
- *Genitourinary tract:* chronic and granulomatous interstitial nephritis, acute tubular necrosis, microabscesses, granulomas, necrotizing ureteritis and cystitis, prostatic abscess
- *Gastrointestinal and hepatobiliary tract:* enteritis, ulceration, mucosal invasion, granulomatous hepatitis, and cholecystitis
- *Central nervous system:* ring-enhancing lesion with central areas of necrosis filled with spores and macrophages, surrounded by microsporidia-filled astrocytes
- *Musculoskeletal system:* myositis, muscle fibrosis

Clinical features

The clinical manifestations of microsporidiosis can be divided into two groups, according to the host's immune status.

Immunocompetent patients

Intestinal infections are the most common manifestation. It is caused by *Ent. bieneusi* or *Enc. intestinalis*. It presents with watery diarrhea, nausea, abdominal pain, and fever and is usually self-limited.

Ocular infections are rare and may present with corneal stromal infection or keratoconjunctivitis.

Cerebral or disseminated infections are extremely rare.

HIV-infected patients

Ent. bieneusi typically causes intestinal infections with chronic diarrhea, anorexia, weight loss, and malabsorption. CD4 counts are typically <100 cells/mm^3. Patients may also develop cholecystitis or cholangitis with fever, nausea, vomiting, and abdominal pain.

Enc. intestinalis causes intestinal and systemic infections that appear similar to those caused by *Ent. bieneusi*. Disseminated disease, particularly to the kidneys, may occur.

Enc. hellem and *Enc. cuniculi* can both cause keratoconjunctivitis sicca. Patients often have laboratory evidence of disseminated infection and may present with bronchiolitis, sinusitis, nephritis, cystitis, urethritis, prostatitis, hepatitis, peritonitis, cerebral infection, or nodular skin infections.

Myositis may be caused by various microsporidial species, e.g., *Pleistophora* spp., *Trachipleistophora hominis*, *Brachiola vesicularum*.

Systemic infections due to other microsporidial species have been described in case reports.

Diagnosis

The clinical laboratory should be alerted of the potential diagnosis and specific stains requested, since routine ova and parasite examination will not detect the microsporidia spores.

Stool examination is the easiest and most practical method for diagnosing intestinal infections. The modified trichrome stain that stains the microsporidial wall bright pink is most commonly used. Chemiluminescent stains may also be applied.

Cytology is used for diagnosis of microsporidiosis in other organs. Various stains may be used, e.g., Weber, Gram, Giemsa, Steiner silver, trichrome blue, chemiluminescent stains.

Histology remains important in the diagnosis of microsporidiosis; however, infection of the bowel may be patchy. Various stains may be used, e.g., modified Gram, Giemsa, periodic acid–Schiff and Steiner silver stains.

Electron microscopy may be useful to identify microsporidia to genus or species level.

Nucleic acid amplification assays: several PCR-based assay have been developed for species-specific diagnosis. They are usually restricted to a few research laboratories.

Immunofluorescent detection methods using polyclonal antisera can detect microsporidia (except *Ent. bieneusi*) in most clinical specimens. Sensitivity is poor in stool specimens.

Serology is unhelpful in the diagnosis of microsporidiosis. Tissue culture is only available in a few specialist laboratories.

Treatment

There are limited data on the therapy of human microsporidiosis:
- Albendazole is effective against most species (except *Ent. bieneusi*) and improves symptoms in HIV-associated *Enc. intestinalis* infections.
- Topical fumagillin has been used for ocular infections, while systemic therapy has been tried with some success for *Ent. bieneusi*.[1]
- HAART appears to improve symptoms, normalize intestinal architecture, and clear parasites from the stool. However, recurrent diarrhea and parasitological relapse can occur.

Prevention

Prevention strategies for environmental or zoonotic exposure have not been established, but meticulous handwashing and adherence to existing guidelines for the general prevention of opportunistic infections in HIV-infected patients may be pertinent.

As yet there are no clinical trial data to support antimicrobial prophylaxis. HAART may be important in preventing microsporidiosis.

Reference

1 Molina JM, Toumeur M, Sarfati C, Cherret S, et al. (2002). Fumagillin treatment of intestinal microspondiosis. *N Engl J Med* 346:1963–1969.

Nematodes

There are more than 60 species of nematodes or roundworms that infect humans, some of which are shown in Table 3.29. They are the most common human parasites and are estimated to infect 3–4 billion people worldwide. Helminth infections are a major public health burden in the developing world.

All nematodes are elongated, cylindrical, nonsegmented organisms with a smooth cuticle and body cavity containing a digestive tract and reproductive organs.

Intestinal nematodes

Intestinal nematodes are the largest group of human helminths. The most common intestinal nematodes (*Ascaris lumbricoides*, *Ancylostoma duodenale*, *Necator americanus*, and *Trichuris trichuria*) cannot reproduce in humans and are referred to as *geohelminths*, as their eggs have to develop in the soil.

The exceptions are *Stronglyoides stercoralis* and *Enterobius vermicularis*, which can be transmitted from person to person.

Tissue nematodes

The tissue-dwelling roundworms are also a major public health problem, particularly in the tropics. Some affect humans only, while others have an animal reservoir. All of the parasites have a complex life cycle involving intermediate hosts, except *Trichinella* spp.

Adult worms do not multiply in humans, so the worm load and severity of disease depend on intensity of exposure.

Table 3.29 Medically important nematodes

Type	Disease	Species
Intestinal	Ascariasis	*Ascaris lumbricoides*
	Trichuriasis	*Trichuris trichiura*
	Hookworm	*Ancylostoma duodemale, Necator americanus*
	Strongyloidiasis	*Strongyloides stercoralis*
	Pin worm	*Enterobius vermicularis*
Tissue	Trichinosis	*Trichinella spiralis*
	Dracunculiasis	*Dracunculus medinensis*
	Filariasis	*Wuchereria bancrofti, Brugia malaya, Brugia timori*
	Onchocerciasis	*Onchocerca volvulus*

Ascaris lumbricoides

Ascariasis is the most common helminthic infection of humans, with an estimated prevalence of >1 billion. It is caused by *Ascaris lumbricoides* (roundworm) and is found worldwide, most commonly in the tropics.

The parasite

The adult worms (white or reddish yellow, 15–35 cm in length) live in the small intestine and have a lifespan of 10–24 months. Each female produces up to 200,000 ova per day, which pass out in the feces.

When ingested, the eggs hatch in the small intestine, penetrate the intestinal wall, migrate through the venous system to the lungs where they break into the alveoli, migrate up the bronchial tree before they are swallowed, and develop into mature worms in the intestine.

Epidemiology

Ascaris infection is most common in young children but can occur at any age. Transmission is by feco-oral route and is enhanced by the high output of ova and their ability to survive unfavorable environmental conditions. In endemic areas, most people have light to moderate worm burdens.

Clinical features

Most infected patients are asymptomatic. Clinical features depend on the site and intensity of infection:

- Pulmonary manifestations occur during larval migration through the lungs. Patients may present with Löffler's syndrome (respiratory symptoms, pulmonary infiltration, and peripheral eosinophilia).
- Gastointestinal manifestations include malnutrition, malabsorption, steatorrhea, and intestinal obstruction.
- Biliary obstruction may cause abdominal pain, cholangitis, pancreatitis, and obstructive jaundice.
- Ectopic infections occur rarely, e.g., umbilical or hernial fistulae, fallopian tubes, bladder, lungs, and heart.

Diagnosis

Stool examination by wet prep usually confirms the diagnosis. The eggs are oval with a thick mamillated shell and measure 45–70 micrometers (length) by 35–50 micrometers (breadth) (Fig 3.3).

Treatment

Mebendazole (see Anthelmintic drugs 1, p. 107) and albendazole are the mainstays of treatment. Pyrantel pamoate is also used and is the drug of choice in pregnancy.

Nitazoxanide is very effective in patients with light infections (i.e., <10,000 eggs/gram of stool).

Ivermectin causes paralysis of adult worms but is not routinely used.

Piperazine citrate syrup via nasogastric tube has been used for intestinal or biliary obstruction; piperazine narcotizes the worms and helps to relieve symptoms. This agent is being withdrawn from the market in many developed countries because other options are less toxic.

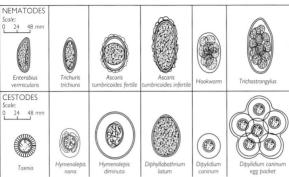

Fig. 3.3 Identification of helminth ova (nematodes and cestodes).

Trichuris trichiuria

Trichuriasis is one of the most prevalent helminthic infections, with an estimated 800 million cases worldwide. Infection is mainly asymptomatic, but heavy infection may cause anemia, bloody diarrhea, growth retardation, or rectal prolapse.

The parasite

T. trichiura (a.k.a. whip worm) principally infects humans, residing in the cecum and ascending colon. The mean life span of adult worms is 1 year, and each female worm produces 5–20,000 eggs per day.

After excretion, embryonic development occurs over 2–4 weeks. The embryonated egg is ingested and the larva escapes its shell, penetrating the small intestinal mucosa before migrating down into the cecum or colon. The anterior whip-like portion remains embedded in the mucosa, while the shorter posterior end is free in the lumen.

Epidemiology

T. trichiura has a worldwide prevalence but is more common in most tropical environments, particularly in rural communities with poor sanitation. Infection results from ingestion of embryonated eggs by direct contamination of hands, food, or drink, or indirectly through flies or other insects.

The intensity of infections is usually light; heavy infection is more common in children.

Clinical features

Infection is mainly asymptomatic, but heavy infection may present with a variety of symptoms:
• Iron-deficiency anemia
• Abdominal symptoms and signs
• Acute bloody diarrhea
• Chronic colitis with growth retardation
• Rectal prolapse

Diagnosis
Stool examination is required. The diagnosis is confirmed by detection of characteristic lemon-shaped ova (52 × 22 micrometer) in the stool (see Fig 3.3).

Treatment
Albendazole is the treatment of choice. Alternatives are mebendazole or ivermectin.

Prevention
Improved sanitation and meticulous handwashing may help to prevent infection.

Ancylostoma duodenale and *Necator americanus*

Human hookworm infection is estimated to affect 25% of the world's population and is caused by two species, *Ancylostoma duodenale* and *Necator americanus*.

The parasite
Adult hookworms are small, cylindrical (1 cm long), and grayish-white in color. They live in the upper small intestine, attached to the mucosa. Adult worms produce about 7000 eggs per day. They pass out in the stool and, under suitable conditions, hatch into larvae that molt once to become infective to humans.

Skin penetration requires contact-contaminated soil for 5–10 minutes. The larvae are carried by the venous circulation to the lungs, where they migrate up the respiratory tree to be swallowed and carried to the small intestine.

Epidemiology
The distribution and prevalence of hookworm infections are limited by environmental conditions: ova fail to develop at temperatures below 13°C; larvae are destroyed by drying or direct sunlight.

Transmission requires walking barefoot through fecally contaminated topsoil. Transmission is also thought to occur from mother to child, either transplacentally or during breastfeeding.

Clinical features
- *Skin rash:* patients may present early in the disease with "ground itch," intense pruritis, erythema, and a papular/vesicular rash at the site of larval penetration.
- *Pulmonary manifestations:* patients may present with Löffler's syndrome (respiratory symptoms, pulmonary infiltration, and eosinophilia) caused by migration of larvae through the lungs.
- *Iron deficiency anemia* is the most common manifestation. The average daily blood loss is 0.2 mL for *A. duodenale*, and 0.03 mL for *N. americanus*.

- *Protein malnutrition* is a common complication. Patients may also have abdominal pain, diarrhea, weight loss, and malabsorption.

Diagnosis

Stool examination by wet mount readily identifies the ova in clinically significant hookworm infections but is not useful early in infection. The ova are ovoid and thin-shelled and measure 58 × 36 micrometers. Eggs of *N. americanus* or *N. duodenale* are morphologically indistinguishable.

Treatment

Mebendazole is the treatment of choice. Albendazole or pyrantel pamoate are alternatives.

Iron-deficiency anemia should be treated.

Strongyloides stercoralis

Strongyloidiasis, although uncommon compared with other intestinal nematode infections, is important because of its potential to cause overwhelming infection in immunocompromised hosts.

The parasite

S. stercoralis worms can survive as parasitic forms in humans or free-living forms in the soil. The female worm is 2.2 mm, whereas the male is 0.7 mm. Adult worms inhabit the small intestine, where the females deposit ova. Eggs hatch in the mucosa, releasing larvae, and enter intestinal lumen where they pass out in the feces.

The usual route of infection is through skin contact with contaminated soil. Humans can also be infected via the feco-oral route. The larvae migrate through the bloodstream to the lungs, where they migrate up the respiratory tree to be swallowed to the small intestine.

Epidemiology

S. stercoralis infection is most common in the tropics where transmission depends on climatic conditions, soil conditions, and sanitation. In the United States, the highest rates of infection are among residents of southeastern states and individuals who have been in endemic areas.

The patient's worm burden depends on the size of the inoculum and the degree of autoinfection.

Clinical features

Asymptomatic infection occurs in about one-third of infected people.
- *Skin rash*: patients may present with a pruritic papulovesicular rash at the site of larval penetration; 5–22% of patients develop an urticarial rash that starts perianally and extends to the buttocks, thighs, and abdomen.
- *Pulmonary manifestations*: patients may present with Löffler's syndrome (respiratory symptoms, pulmonary infiltration, and eosinophilia) caused by migration of larvae through the lungs.
- *Abdominal symptoms* are common and include colicky abdominal pain, diarrhea, passage of mucus, nausea, vomiting, weight loss, malabsorption, and protein-losing entropathy. Eosinophilia is common.

- *Hyperinfection syndrome:* massive larval invasion may occur with autoinfection, particularly in immunocompromised hosts, e.g., patients with leukemia, lymphoma, lepromatous leprosy, receiving corticosteroids, or HIV infection. Clinical features include shock, severe abdominal pain, ileus, pulmonary infiltrates, and Gram-negative bacillary meningitis or septicemia. Mortality is high.

Diagnosis

Diagnosis depends on demonstration of the larvae in stool or duodenal aspirates. Larvas are excreted intermittently. As a result, three or more concetrated stool examinations may fail to detect strongyloidiasis, especially if the parasite burden is low.

Serological or molecular assays may be used to support the diagnosis.

Treatment

Ivermectin is the treatment of choice, usually administered as two single 200 mcg/kg doses on one or two consecutive days. Albendazole (see Anthelmintic drugs 1, p. 106) is an alternative.

The optimal treatment of disseminated disease and hyperinfection is not certain. In Immunocompromised patients it may be necessary to prolong or repeat ivermectin therapy.

Enterobius vermicularis

Infection with *Enterobius vermicularis*, or pinworm, is highly prevalent, particularly in temperate climates. Pinworm infection is most common in young children and institutionalized populations.

The parasite

E. vermicularis is a small, white, thread-like worm that inhabits the cecum and ascending colon. Female worms contain about 11,000 ova and live for 11–35 days. The gravid females migrate at night to the perianal/perineal region where they deposit their eggs. The eggs embryonate within hours and are transferred from the perianal region to pajamas, bedding, dust, and air.

The most common route of transmission is via the patient's hands.

Epidemiology

The prevalence of pinworm is highest in children aged 5 to 14 years. Pinworm is primarily a family or institutional infection, with no particular socioeconomic associations.

As the lifespan of the worm is relatively brief and eggs can only survive out of the body for 20 days, longstanding infections must be due to continuous reinfection.

Clinical features

Most infected patients are asymptomatic.

Perianal/perineal pruritis and disturbed sleep are the most common symptoms. Occasionally, migration of the worms may cause ectopic disease, e.g., appendicitis, salpingitis, ulcerative bowel lesions.

Serum eosinophilia or raised IgE are uncommon.

Diagnosis

The "Scotch Tape test" is performed by sticking clear cellophane tape to a slide or plastic stick to enable collection of worms from the perianal region. The ova are oval but flattened on one side and measure 56 × 27 micrometers.

The number of examinations is correlated with rate of detection, e.g., 50% for a single examination, 90% for three examinations.

All family members of an affected individual should be screened for infection.

Treatment

Mebendazole (see Anthelmintic drugs 1, p. 107) should be given to all family members. Albendazole is an alternative drug.

Pyrantel pamoate is recommended for pregnant women.

Prevention

Although good personal hygiene is a useful general principle, its role in the management of enterobiasis is debatable.

Cutaneous larva migrans

Cutaneous larva migrans is characterized by an erythematous, pruritic, serpinginous skin lesion. It is usually caused by *Ancylostoma braziliense*, the dog and cat hookworm.

Other animal and human hookworms may cause similar findings, e.g., *Ancylostoma caninum, Unicinaria stenocephala, Bunostomum phlebotomum, Strongyloides stercoralis,* and *Gnathostoma spinigerum*.

The parasite

The larvae infect dogs or cats by burrowing through the skin. The adults live in the host's intestine and shed eggs in the feces, which develop into larvae in the sandy soil.

Epidemiology

Infections are most common in warmer climates, especially tropical sandy beaches. Infection is more common in children than in adults.

Clinical features

The larvae penetrate the skin of humans (an accidental host), causing tingling, itching, and vesicle formation. They then migrate through the skin, causing a characteristic raised, erythematous, pruritic serpinginous track. In severe infections many tracks may be seen.

Systemic symptoms are rare, although pulmonary symptoms and lung infiltrates have been reported.

Diagnosis

The diagnosis is usually made clinically Skin biopsy may show an eosinophilic inflammatory infiltrate, but the migrating parasite is rarely found.

Treatment

Without treatment, the skin lesions will gradually disappear.

Topical thiabendazole is effective but may be difficult to obtain in the United States. Oral albendazole (for 3 to 7 days) or ivermectin (one dose) is also highly effective.

Visceral larva migrans

Visceral larva migrans is characterized by fever, hepatomegaly, and eosinophilia. It is usually caused by *Toxocara canis* but may be caused by *Toxocara cati* or other helminths.

The parasite

T. canis infects dogs and other animals by a variety of mechanisms. Usually, ingested eggs hatch in the small intestine and migrate to the liver, lung, and trachea. They are then swallowed and mature in the lumen of the small intestine where eggs are shed.

Other larvae migrate to the muscles and remain dormant but remain capable of development months or years after infection, particularly in pregnancy. During or post-pregnancy, pups may become infected transplacentally or by breast milk and shed larvae in their feces.

Epidemiology

Toxocariasis has a worldwide distribution. The prevalence of infection is unknown, but seroepidemiological surveys show prevalence rates ranging from 3% to 54%, depending on the community selected. Most seropositive people are asymptomatic.

Visceral larva migrans occurs most commonly in children <6 years.

Clinical features

Most infections are asymptomatic. Disease manifestations vary from mild symptoms to fulminant disease and death.

Clinical features include fever, cough, wheeze, hepatomegaly, splenomegaly, lymphadenopathy, urticaria, skin nodules, seizures, and eye involvement (ocular larva migrans).

Laboratory abnormalities include eosinophilia, leukocytosis, hypergammaglobulinemia, and elevated isohemagglutinin titers to blood group A and B antigens (due to host immune response to cross-reacting antigens on *T. canis*).

Diagnosis

The diagnosis is usually made clinically in a young child with typical clinical features and a history of exposure to puppies. A definitive diagnosis is made by finding larvae in the tissues by histological examination.

Serological tests, e.g., ELISA, may help to confirm the diagnosis (but may also be positive in asymptomatic patients).

Treatment

There is no proven effective therapy, and most patients recover without specific treatment.

Anthelmintic drugs (e.g., albendazole or mebendazole may be helpful in patients with severe disease affecting the lungs, heart, or brain. However, treatment may provoke a severe inflammatory response and worsen the clinical condition.

Corticosteroids have been used, with or without anthelmintics, with some reports of success.

Prevention

Prevention measures include preventing dogs from contaminating the environment, and preventing children from ingesting the eggs.

Trichinella species

Trichinosis occurs after ingestion of *Trichinella* larvae. Most infections are asymptomatic, but heavy exposure may cause fever, diarrhea, periorbital edema, and myositis.

The parasite

The genus *Trichinella* comprises five species: *T. spiralis* (the most common cause of human infection), *T. nativa*, *T. brotovi*, *T. pseudospiralis*, and *T. nelsoni*. The cysts are ingested in undercooked meat and the larvae liberated by acid-pepsin digestion of the cysts in the stomach.

The larvae invade enterocytes, where they develop into adult worms. The adult worms may disseminate in the bloodstream and seed the skeletal muscles, where they encyst.

Epidemiology

Trichinella spp. have a worldwide distribution, infecting a wide range of animals, e.g., pigs, rats, horses, bears, foxes, wild boar, and big cats. Humans are incidental hosts.

Clinical features

Most infections are subclinical.

Clinical features include fever, myalgia, malaise, periorbital edema, headache, rash, edema, diarrhea, nausea, subconjunctival hemorrhages, splinter hemorrhages, cough, and vomiting.

Diagnosis

The diagnosis should be suspected in any patient who presents with fever, periorbital edema, and myositis, particularly if there is a history of ingestion of undercooked meat.

Routine laboratory tests show eosinophilia, raised ESR, and elevated creatine phosphokinase (CPK) and lactate dehydrogenase (LDH) levels.

Antibodies are detectable 3 weeks after infection. Various assays may be used, e.g., ELISA, immunofluorescence, indirect hemagglutination, precipitin, and bentonite flocculation assays.

Molecular DNA detection assays have been developed.

The definitive diagnosis is made by finding larvae in biopsied muscle. Biopsy is usually limited to patients in whom the diagnosis is in doubt.

Treatment

There is no satisfactory treatment; patients are treated symptomatically with bed rest and salicylates. Corticosteroids have been given for severe disease, but the evidence to support this is equivocal.

When a patient is known to have recently ingested trichinous meat, oral mebendazole or albendazole may be given. This is active against intestinal worms but not tissue larvae and does not alter the course of established disease.

Prevention

The most effective way to prevent trichinosis is to cook meat properly.

Dracunculus medinensis

Dracuculiasis (guinea worm infection) occurs after drinking water containing crustaceans infected with *Dracunculus medinensis*. It is characterized by a chronic ulcer from which the worm protrudes.

The parasite

After ingestion of crustaceans containing *D. medinensis*, the larvae are released in the stomach, pass into the small intestine, penetrate the mucosa, and reach the retroperitoneum, where they mature and mate.

About a year later, the female worm migrates to the subcutaneous tissues of the legs. The overlying skin ulcerates, and a portion of the worm protrudes. On contact with water, large numbers of larvae are released. These are ingested by crustaceans, where they undergo further development before the cycle is repeated.

Epidemiology

D. medinensis is found predominantly in Africa where water supplies are used both for drinking water and for bathing.

Clinical features

There are often no clinical signs until the worm reaches the skin surface. Initially, a stinging papule develops on the lower leg.

Some patients may develop generalized symptoms such as urticaria, nausea, vomiting, diarrhea, and dyspnea. Over the next few days, the lesion vesiculates and ruptures and forms a painful ulcer. If the area is rinsed with water, a milky fluid containing larvae wells up.

Discharge continues intermittently over weeks and the worm is slowly absorbed or extruded, after which the ulcer heals.

Multiple ulcers may occur and secondary infection is common.

Diagnosis

The diagnosis is mainly clinical, but larvae may be seen on examination of the discharge fluid.

Treatment

There is no specific therapy besides slow extraction of the worm.

Thiabendazole (see Anthelmintic drugs 2, p. 108), mebendazole, or metronidazole (see Nitroimidazoles, p. 59) have no effect on the worms but produce resolution of the inflammation within days. This permits gradual removal of the worm by rolling it around a small stick.

Corticosteroid ointments shorten the time to healing, and topical antibiotics may reduce the risk of secondary infection.

Unerupted worms may be removed by minor surgery under local anesthesia. Secondary bacterial infections should be treated with antibiotics.

Prevention

Boiling, chlorinating, or sieving drinking water prevents guinea worm infection. In West Africa, major advances in prevention have dramatically reduced infection rates.

Filariasis

Filariasis is caused by three species: *Wuchereria bancrofti, Brugia malayi,* and *Brugia timori.*

The parasites

After the bite of an infected mosquito, larvae enter the lymphatics and lymph nodes, where they mature into white, thread-like adult worms. The adults live for 5 years, and females discharge microfilariae into the bloodstream, usually around midnight. In the South Pacific, the peak is less pronounced and occurs during the day.

Epidemiology

It is estimated that 120 million people are infected with these parasites.

- *W. bancrofti* occurs throughout the tropics and subtropics.
- *B. malayi* occurs in South and Southeast Asia.
- *B. timori* is restricted to eastern Indonesia.

Humans are the only host for *W. bancrofti,* but *B. malaya* has been found in felines and primates. Only a small proportion of people who are bitten by infected mosquitoes develop clinical disease.

Clinical features

Most patients are asymptomatic despite microfiliaremia.

Acute infection may present with lymphangitis, lymphadenitis, fever, headache, backache, nausea, epididymitis, or orchitis.

Chronic hydrocele is the most common manifestation. Chronic lymphadenopathy is common and may progress to lymphedema or elephantiasis of the lower limb. Ulceration and secondary infection may occur.

Chyluria may occur if lymphatics burst into the urinary tract.

Diagnosis

Definitive diagnosis depends on demonstrating microfilariae in the peripheral blood smear. Bancroftian and Brugian filariasis show nocturnal periodicity. Ideally, specimens should be collected between 10 PM and 2 AM.

Micofilariae are occasionally seen in hydrocele fluid, chylous urine, or lymph node aspirates.

Serological tests may be positive but do not distinguish the different species or current from past infection. Immunoassays and PCR-based assays have been developed.

Ultrasonography of the lymphatic vessels in the spermatic cord may show motile adult worms.

Treatment

The drug of choice has traditionally been diethylcarbamazine (DEC), which is not distributed for use on the United States but can be obtained from the CDC under an Investigational New Drug (IND) protocol. Albendazole or ivermectin are alternatives. Doxycycline has been shown to be effective in reducing microfilaraemia and adverse effects.

Prevention

Avoid mosquito bites (wear protective clothing, use insect repellent).

Loa loa

Loiasis is caused by *Loa loa* and characterized by transient subcutaneous swellings. Occasionally, worms can migrate through the subconjunctiva, causing conjunctivitis.

The parasite

The white, thread-like worms measure 30 to 70 × 0.3 mm and migrate through the connective tissues. The microfilariae measure 300 × 8 micrometers and appear in the blood during the day.

Epidemiology

Loa loa is endemic in West and Central Africa. It is transmitted to humans by tabanid flies (*Chrysops* spp).

Clinical features

Many patients are asymptomatic but may have eosinophilia.

The characteristic feature is transient edematous swellings (Calabar swellings), which are caused by worms migrating through the subcutaneous tissues. They are usually preceded by localized pain and itching, solitary, commonly found around joints, and may last for days to weeks. Occasionally, a worm may migrate across the subconjunctiva causing conjunctivitis.

Complications include worms in the penis or breast tissue, endomyocardial fibrosis, retinopathy, encephalopathy, peripheral neuropathy, arthritis, and pleural effusion.

Diagnosis

The diagnosis is often clinical, based on finding typical clinical features in a patient from West or Central Africa.

The diagnosis is confirmed by demonstrating microfilariae in a peripheral blood smear taken during the daytime.

A PCR-based assay has been developed but is not widely available.

Occasionally, an adult worm may be extracted from the eye.

Treatment

Diethylcarbamazine (see Anthelmintic drugs 1, p. 106) eliminates microfilariae from the blood but does not kill adult worms. Treatment may precipitate encephalopathy in patients with high microfilarial loads.

Ivermectin decreases microfilarial loads in the peripheral blood. Side effects include fever, pruritis, headache, and arthralgia.

Albendazole slowly reduces microfilarial loads.

Prevention

Avoid insect bites (protective clothing, insect repellent) in endemic areas.

Mass treatment with diethylcarbamazine or ivermectin interrupts transmission in endemic areas.

Temporary visitors to endemic areas may take prophylactic diethylcarbamazine.

Onchocerca volvulus

Onchocerciasis (river blindness) is caused by *Onchocerca volvulus* and is characterized by dermatitis, subcutaneous nodules, keratitis, and choroidoretinitis.

The parasite

O. volvulus is transmitted to humans by the *Simulium* black fly. After a bite, the larvae penetrate the skin and migrate into the connective tissues, where they develop into filiform adults. The worms are often found tangled in nodules of subcutaneous tissue.

Each female produces large numbers of microfilariae that migrate through the skin and connective tissues.

Epidemiology

O. volvulus occurs in West, Central, and East Africa, with scattered foci in Central and South America. There is no known animal reservoir.

Clinical features

- *Skin lesions:* initially there is an itchy, erythematous, papular rash. In severe infections, thickening of the skin, depigmentation, lymphedema, and lymphadenopathy occur. Fibrous nodules containing adult worms may develop over bony prominences. Systemic features include fever, weight loss, and musculoskeletal pains.

- *Eye manifestations* include punctuate keratitis, pannus formation, and corneal fibrosis. Iridocyclitis, glaucoma, choroiditis, and optic atrophy may occur.

Diagnosis

The diagnosis is confirmed by detecting microfilariae in skin snips or in the cornea or anterior chamber of the eye on slit-lamp examination. Microfilariae are sometimes found in the urine.

Reliable immunodiagnostic tests are not generally available, but molecular tests are being developed.

If the diagnosis is strongly suspected but the parasite cannot be found, a test dose of diethylcarbamazine may exacerbate the rash (see Treatment).

Treatment

Diethylcarbamazine (see Anthelmintic drugs 1, p. 106) kills microfilariae but not the adult worms. Severe Mazotti reactions may occur, e.g., fever, rash, generalized body pains, keratitis, and iritis.

Ivermectin has been shown to be safer and more effective. It also kills microfilariae but not adult worms. Side effects include fever, pruritis, headache, and arthralgia.

Other active drugs include suramin (not recommended), albendazole, and amocarzine.

Prevention

Avoid insect bites (wear protective clothing, use insect repellents). Vector control with larvicides is being used in West Africa.

Cestodes

Human cestode infections occur in one of two forms: mature tapeworms residing in the gut, or larval cysts in the tissues. The form that the infection takes depends on the species. The medically important cestodes are summarized in Table 3.30.

Table 3.30 Medically important cestodes

Type of cestode	Disease	Species
Intestinal	Tapeworm	*Taenia saginata*
		Taenia solium
		Diphyllobothrium latum
		Hymenolepis nana
Invasive	Cysticercosis, echinococcosis	*Taenia solium*
		Echinococcus granulosus
		Echinococcus vogeli
		Echinococcus multilocularis

Parasite structure

The parasitic cestodes are flatworms (platyhelminths). The worms consist of several parts: a head (scolex, which has suckers and sometimes hooks), a short neck, and a strobila (a segmented tail made of proglottids). The proglottid has both male and female sexual organs and is responsible for egg production. They become gravid and eventually break free of the tapeworm, releasing eggs in the stool or outside the body.

Parasite life cycle

Cestodes divide their life cycle between two animal hosts: the definitive carnivorous host and the intermediate herbivorous/omnivorous host. Mature tapeworms reside in the intestinal tract of the definitive host and shed eggs into the stool.

The eggs may be embryonated (can immediately infect the intermediate host) or nonembryonated (require development outside the body). The intermediate host is infected by the ingestion of eggs that hatch in the intestine, releasing an oncosphere. This penetrates the gut mucosa and spreads through the circulation to the tissues, where it forms a larval cyst. The life cycle is completed when the carnivorous host ingests the cyst-infected tissues of the intermediate host.

Taenia saginata (beef tapeworm)

- *The parasite:* adult worms are long (up to 10 m in length) and contain >1000 proglottids, each capable of producing thousands of eggs.
- *Epidemiology:* transmitted to humans by ingestion of larval cysts in rare or undercooked meat from infected cattle. Common in cattle breeding areas of the world such as central Asia, the Near East, and central and eastern Africa where prevalence of infection may be >10%. Areas of lower prevalence (<1%) include Europe, Southeast Asia, and Central America,
- *Clinical features:* patients are usually asymptomatic but a minority complain of abdominal cramps and malaise. The proglottids are motile and may be seen on the perineum or clothing.
- *Diagnosis* is confirmed by examination of proglottids (with 15–20 lateral uterine branches). The eggs are morphologically indistinguishable from those of *T. solium*.
- *Treatment* is with praziquantel (5–10 mg/kg) or niclosamide (2 g) PO. Praziquantel kills adult worms, but not eggs. Precautions must be taken to prevent autoinfection and transmission to others.

Taenia solium (pork tapeworm)

- *The parasite:* *T. solium* tapeworms may live for 10–20 years and grow up to 8 m in length.
- *Epidemiology:* humans can be definitive or intermediate hosts for *T. solium*. Individuals who ingest larval cysts in raw or undercooked pork acquire pork tapeworm; those who ingest eggs develop tissue infection with cysts (cysticercosis, p. 506). *T. solium* infection is endemic in Mexico, Central and South America, Southeast Asia, India, the Philippines, and southern Europe.
- *Clinical features:* most patients are asymptomatic unless autoinfection with parasite eggs occurs.

- *Diagnosis:* infection is readily diagnosed by detection of eggs in the stool (morphologically indistinguishable from those of *T. saginata*). Definitive diagnosis is by examination of the proglottids (with 7–13 lateral uterine branches).
- *Treatment* is with praziquantel (5–10 mg/kg) or niclosamide (2 g) PO stat.

Diphyllobothrium latum (fish tapeworm)

- *The parasite:* D. latum tapeworms may grow up to 25 m in length. The tapeworm takes 3–6 weeks to mature and may survive for more than 30 years.
- *Epidemiology:* human infection is acquired by uncooked freshwater fish containing cysts. Areas of endemic infection (>2% prevalence) include Siberia, Scandinavia, and other Baltic countries, North America, Japan, and Chile where there is stable zoonotic transmission through other animal hosts, e.g., seals, cats, bears, foxes, and wolves.
- *Clinical features:* infection is usually asymptomatic but patients may report weakness, dizziness, salt cravings, diarrhea, or intermittent abdominal discomfort. Prolonged/heavy infection may lead to megaloblastic anemia caused by vitamin B_{12} deficiency ± folate deficiency.
- *Diagnosis:* stool examination shows operculated eggs (45–65 micrometers). Recovery of proglottids (with a characteristic central uterus) also confirms the diagnosis.
- *Treatment* is with praziquantel (5–10 mg/kg) or niclosamide (2 g) PO. Mild vitamin B_{12} deficiency resolves with eradication of the tapeworm; severe deficiency requires parenteral treatment.

Hymenolepis nana (dwarf tapeworm)

- *The parasite:* H. nana is the only tapeworm that can be transmitted directly from human to human. Adult tapeworms measure 15–50 mm.
- *Epidemiology:* areas of endemic infection (up to 26%) include Asia, southern and eastern Europe, Central and South America, and Africa. Infection is more common in children and institutionalized patients.
- *Clinical features:* heavy infection may be associated with abdominal cramps, nausea, diarrhea, and dizziness.
- *Diagnosis* is made by identification of eggs (30–47 micrometers, with a characteristic double membrane) in the stool.
- *Treatment* is with praziquantel (25 mg/kg PO stat, repeated after 1 week) or niclosamide (2 g PO daily for 1 week).

Cysticercosis

The parasite

Cysticercosis is an infection with larval cysts of the cestode *Taenia solium* (see above).

Epidemiology

Infection is acquired by consumption of *T. solium* eggs. The cumulative risk of infection increases with age, frequency of pork consumption, and poor household hygiene.

Clinical features

Infected individuals may harbor multiple cysts throughout the body but are often asymptomatic. Symptoms may develop because of local inflammation at the site of infection.

Serious disease is rare but occurs with cardiac or CNS involvement (neurocysticercosis). The latter may present with focal symptoms, seizures, chronic meningitis, or spinal cord compression.

Neurocysticercosis is the most common cause of seizures in Central America. Racemose cysticercosis is an aggressive form of basilar neurocysticercosis, resulting in coma and death.

Diagnosis

Asymptomatic patients may be diagnosed incidentally by detection of calcified cysts on plain radiographs. Neurocysticercosis may be diagnosed by CT or MRI scan, which show multiple enhancing and nonenhancing unilocular cysts.

The diagnosis may be supported by a positive ELISA indicating prior exposure to *T. solium* antigens. However, patients infected with other helminths may have cross-reactive antibodies.

Stool examination is insensitive, since most patients with cysticercosis do not have viable tapeworms at the time of diagnosis.

Treatment

Treatment depends on the characteristics (calcified vs. viable), location, and number of cysts. For complicated neurocysticercosis, treatment may be given with high-dose praziquantel (50 mg/kg/day for 1–21 days) or albendazole (10–15 mg/kg/day for 7–30 days). Evidence favors albendazole over praziquantel and suggests that longer courses may be needed in patients with multiple lesions.

CNS inflammation may be reduced by concurrent administration of dexamethasone, but this may reduce the efficacy of praziquantel.

Seizures should be treated with antiepileptic medication, and hydrocephalus with shunting.

Echinococcosis

The parasite

The canine tapeworms *Echinococcus* spp. inadvertently infect humans, causing visceral cysts. Hydatid cyst disease is caused by *Echinococcus granulosus* or *Echinococcus vogeli*, whereas alveolar cyst disease is caused by *Echinococcus granulosus*.

Epidemiology

Infection is acquired by ingestion of parasite eggs excreted by tapeworm-infected animals. *E. granulosus* is prevalent worldwide and transmitted by sheep, goats, horses, camels, and domestic dogs (livestock-rearing areas). *E. multilocularis* is transmitted by wild canines and found in northern forest areas of Europe, Asia, North America, and the Arctic. *E. vogeli* is found in South America.

Clinical features

The hydatid cysts of *E. granulosus* usually affect the liver (50–70%) or lungs (20–30%) but may affect any organ of the body. They are often asymptomatic and found incidentally on radiological imaging. Symptoms may occur as a result of expansion or rupture into adjacent organs.

Cyst rupture may cause a severe allergic reaction or seeding to distant organs. Alveolar cyst disease caused by *E. multilocularis* is more aggressive, with invasion of adjacent tissue and metastasis to distant organs.

Complications include biliary disease, portal hypertension, and Budd–Chiari syndrome.

Diagnosis

Infection detected by radiological imaging (ultrasound, CT or MRI scan) may be confirmed serologically by ELISA or Western blot assay. This confirms exposure to the parasite and is most sensitive for liver cysts.

Treatment

Asymptomatic cysts may be monitored, whereas symptomatic cysts should be treated. The optimal treatment is by surgical resection of the whole cyst 30 minutes after instillation of a cysticidal agent, e.g., 30% saline, iodophor, or 95% ethanol. Perioperative anthelmintic agents (e.g., albendazole 400 mg bid or mebendazole 40–50 mg/kg/day in 3 divided doses) may be given, and care must be taken to prevent cyst rupture or spillage during surgery.

For inoperable cysts, medical therapy improves symptoms (55–79%), although cure rates are low (29%). In patients treated surgically, an antiparasitic agent, preferably albendazole, is continued for at least 2 years.

In inoperable patients, treatment is considered for years, and possibly for life. The PAIR procedure (puncture, aspiration, injection, and re-aspiration) is becoming more popular, as it is less invasive than surgery.

Trematodes (flukes)

Flukes are parasitic worms of the class *Trematoda*. They are usually oval shaped and vary in length (1 mm to several cm). Structurally, they have an oral sucker, a ventral sucker (usually), a blind bifurcate intestinal tract, and prominent reproductive organs.

The human flukes belong to the digenetic group in which sexual reproduction is followed by asexual multiplication. Most human parasites are hermaphrodites.

Schistosoma **spp.**

Humans are the principal host of the five *Schistosoma* species (see Table 3.29). Adult worms live in the venous plexus of the urinary bladder (*S. haematobium*) or the portal venous system (*S. mansoni*, *S. japonicum*), where they mate and shed their eggs.

Eggs are passed out in the urine or feces and hatch in fresh water, releasing miracidia that enter the snail (intermediate host). The miracidia multiply asexually in the snail and eventually release cercariae. These infective forms penetrate human skin and migrate through the lungs and the liver, before passing to their final habitat.

Table 3.31 Medically important trematodes

Type of fluke	Disease	Species
Blood	Schistosomiasis	*Schistosoma haematobium*
		Schistosoma japonicum
		Schistosoma mansoni
		Schistosoma mekongi
		Schistosoma intercalatum
Liver	Clonorchiasis	*Clonorchis sinensis*
	Opisthorchiasis	*Opisthorcis felineus*
		Opisthorcis viverrini
	Fascioliasis	*Fasciola hepatica*
Intestinal	Fasciolopsiasis	*Fasciolopsis buski*
	Heterophyiasis	*Heterophyes heterphyes*
Lung	Paragonimiasis	*Paragonimus westermani*

Epidemiology
200 million people worldwide are estimated to be infected with *Schistosoma* spp. Each species has a specific geographic location: *S. haematobium* (Africa, Middle East), *S. mansoni* (Arabia, Africa, South America, Caribbean), *S. japonicum* (Far East), *S. mekongi* (southeast Asia), *S. intercalatum* (West and Central Africa).

Two factors are responsible for endemicity: the presence of the snail vector, and contamination of fresh water by human waste.

Pathogenesis
The disease syndromes that characterize schistosomiasis coincide with the three stages of parasite development:
- Cercariae penetrate the skin to cause a rash.
- Some weeks after infection, the mature worms deposit their eggs; this may be accompanied by acute schistosomiasis (Katayama fever).
- Production of large numbers of eggs results in chronic granulomatous inflammation and fibrosis of the urinary tract or portal venous system.

Clinical features of schistosomiasis
- *Swimmer's itch:* a papular, pruritic dermatitis that occasionally occurs 24 hours after penetration of the skin by cercariae. It is appears to be a sensitization phenomenon, as it rarely occurs on primary exposure.
- *Acute schistosomiasis or Katayama fever* occurs 4–8 weeks after infection and is characterized by fever, chills, sweating, headache, cough, hepatosplenomegaly, and lymphadenopathy. Peripheral eosinophilia is common. Symptoms usually resolve within a few weeks but, rarely, death may occur.
- *Chronic schistosomiasis* occurs in patients with heavy infestation.
- *Intestinal schistosomiasis,* caused by *S. mansoni, S. japonicum,* or *S. mekongi,* may present with fatigue, colicky abdominal pain, diarrhea,

dysentery, chronic granulomatous bowel lesions, mucosal ulceration, or anemia. *S. intercalatum* infection may also present with symptoms.
- *Hepatic schistosomiasis*, also caused by *S. mansoni*, *S. japonicum*, or *S. mekongi*, may present with hepatomegaly, portal hypertension, splenomegaly, esophageal varices, or decompensated liver disease. *S. mekongi* infection may also present with hepatomegaly.
- *Urinary schistosomiasis*, caused by *S. haematobium*, produces granulomatous inflammation in the bladder and ureters. Patients may complain of dysuria and terminal hematuria. Hematospermia is common. Progression of disease may cause urinary obstruction with hydronephrosis and hydroureter.
- *Central nervous system schistosomiasis* is rare, but complicates 3% of *S. japonicum* infections. It may present with a space-occupying lesion, encephalopathy, or seizures. *S. haematobium* and *S. mansoni* may cause spinal cord lesions and present with a transverse myelitis.

Diagnosis
The diagnosis should be suspected in patients with compatible symptoms and an appropriate travel history. The diagnosis is confirmed by detection of eggs in a concentrated urine sample collected between 10 A.M. and 2 P.M. (*S. haematobium*) or in concentrated stool specimens. Serodiagnostic tests may be useful in returning travelers.

Management
Praziquantel is the treatment of choice for all species. The dose is 40 mg/kg in 1 or 2 divided doses (*S. haematobium* and *S. mansoni*) or 60 mg/kg in 2 or 3 divided doses (*S. japonicum* and *S. mekongi*). Side effects are mild: abdominal discomfort, fever, and headache. Drug resistance may become a problem in endemic areas with mass treatment.

Glucocorticoids are considered for Katayama fever and schistosomiasis involving the CNS.

Clonorchiasis
Clonorchis sinensis (Chinese or oriental liver fluke) is a parasite of fish-eating mammals in the Far East. The adult flukes are flat, elongated worms (15 × 3 mm) that inhabit the distal biliary capillaries, where they deposit small, yellow, operculated eggs (30 × 14 micrometer).

The eggs pass out in the stool and are ingested by snails, inside which they hatch into miracidia. Miracidia multiply into cercariae that pass into the water and penetrate freshwater, where they encyst as metacercariae.

Humans are infected by ingestion of raw or undercooked fish. Once ingested, the metacercariae excyst in the duodenum and migrate to the bile ducts.
- *Epidemiology:* millions of humans are estimated to be incidentally infected, mainly in China, Hong Kong, Korea, and Vietnam.
- *Clinical features:* most infected people are asymptomatic. Heavy infection may result in cholangitis and cholangiohepatitis. Infection has been associated with an increased risk of cholangiocarcinoma.
- *Diagnosis:* infection is confirmed by demonstration of characteristic operculated, embryonated eggs in the stool (see Fig 3.4).

- *Management:* praziquantel (see Anthelmintic drugs 2, p. 107) 75 mg/kg in 3 divided doses, or albendazole (see Anthelmintic drugs 1, p. 106) 10 mg/kg/day for 7 days. Surgery is needed, rarely, to relieve biliary obstruction.

Opisthorciasis

Opisthorcis felineus and *Opisthorcis viverrini* are common liver flukes of cats and dogs that are occasionally transmitted to humans. (see Fig 3.4) The life cycle is similar to that of *Clonorchis sinensis* (see above).

- *Epidemiology:* O. felineus is endemic in Southeast Asia and eastern Europe, whereas O. viverrini is found in Thailand.
- *Clinical features:* mild or moderate infection is usually asymptomatic. Biliary tract symptoms and ultrasonographic signs are more common in patients aged 20–40 years with heavy infection. An association between O. viverrini infection and cholangiocarcinoma has been reported in Thailand.
- *Diagnosis* is confirmed by the detection of eggs in the stool (Fig 3.4).
- *Management:* praziquantel is the drug of choice.

Fascioliasis

Fasciola hepatica is a liver fluke of sheep and cattle that can infect humans. The adult worms are large, flat, brown, and leaf-shaped, (2.5 × 1 cm) and live in the biliary tract of their mammalian host. The large, oval, yellow-brown, operculated eggs (140 × 75 micrometers) pass out in the feces and complete their development in water.

The miracidia hatch and enter the snail intermediate host, where they multiply into unforked-tail cercariae. These emerge and undergo encystment into metacercariae on aquatic plants, grasses, and sometimes soil. After ingestion, the metacercariae excyst, releasing larvae that penetrate the intestinal wall, peritoneum, and liver capsule to migrate to the biliary tract.

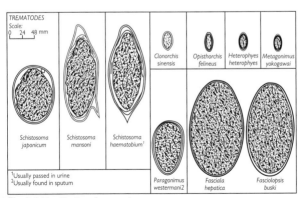

TREMATODES
Scale:
0   24   48 mm

Schistosoma japonicum

Schistosoma mansoni

Schistosoma haematobium[1]

Clonorchis sinensis

Opisthorchis felineus

Heterophyes heterophyes

Metagonimus yokogawai

Paragonimus westermani[2]

Fasciala hepatica

Fasciolopsis buski

[1] Usually passed in urine
[2] Usually found in sputum

Fig. 3.4 Identification of trematode eggs.

- *Epidemiology*: infection is more common in sheep- and cattle-rearing areas, e.g., South America, Europe, Africa, China, and Australia.
- *Clinical features*: F. hepatica infection has two distinct clinical phases:
  - Acute hepatic migratory phase, characterized by fever, right upper quadrant pain, hepatomegaly, and peripheral eosinophilia. Nodules or linear tracks may be seen on ultrasound, CT, or MRI scan.
  - Chronic biliary phase, which may be asymptomatic or present with biliary obstruction or cirrhosis
- *Diagnosis* is confirmed by detection of characteristic ova in the stool or bile (see Fig 3.4). Serological tests may also be helpful.
- *Management*: triclabendazole 10 mg/kg PO 1 dose is the treatment of choice, available on a compassionate-use basis in the United States from the manufacturer. Alternatives are nitazoxanide (500 mg bid for 7 days) or bithionol.

Fasciolopsiasis

Fasciolopsis buski is a large intestinal fluke (2–7.5 cm in length) that is endemic in Southeast Asia and the Far East. It inhabits the duodenum and jejunum, producing large, operculated eggs (135 × 80 micrometers), which are excreted and hatch into miracidia in fresh water. These enter the snail intermediate host, where they multiply and develop into cercariae that encyst into metacercariae on aquatic plants.

Humans are infected by ingestion of contaminated plants. The metacercariae excyst in the intestine and develop into adult worms.
- *Clinical features*: fasciolopsiasis is usually asymptomatic, but heavy infection may present with diarrhea, abdominal pain, or malabsorption.
- *Diagnosis* is confirmed by detection of eggs in the stool (Fig 3.4).
- *Management*: praziquantel 75 mg/kg in 3 divided doses

Heterophyiasis

Heterophyes heterophyes is a tiny intestinal fluke (<2 mm in length) that is endemic in the Nile Delta, Southeast Asia, and the Far East. The life cycle is similar to that of *Fasciolopsis buski* (see above), except that the metacercariae encyst in fish. Humans are infected by consumption of undercooked fish.
- *Clinical features*: infection may present with abdominal pain and diarrhea.
- *Diagnosis*: adult worms produce small operculated eggs (30 × 15 micrometers), which may be detected in the stool (Fig 3.4).
- *Management*: praziquantel 75 mg/kg in 3 divided doses

Paragonimiasis

Paragonimus westermani is a lung fluke that is widely distributed (West Africa, Indian subcontinent, Far East, and Central, and South America).

Life cycle

Adult worms inhabit the lungs and produce golden brown operculated eggs that pass into the bronchioles and are coughed up or swallowed and pass out into the feces. In fresh water, the eggs mature and release miracidia that infect the snail intermediate host. After 3–5 months, cercariae are released and infect freshwater crustaceans (crayfish and crabs) where they encyst in the muscles.

Humans are infected by ingestion of raw or pickled crustaceans. The metacercariae excyst in the intestine, penetrate the intestinal wall, enter the peritoneal cavity, and migrate through the diaphragm and pleural cavities to the lungs. Worms may lodge in the peritoneal cavity or brain.

Clinical features
Infection may be asymptomatic or present with cough, brown sputum, intermittent hemoptysis, pleuritic chest pain, and peripheral eosinophilia. Complications include lung abscess and pleural effusion.

Ectopic infection is rare and may present with abdominal masses, epilepsy, or focal neurological signs.

Diagnosis is confirmed by detection of characteristic eggs in the sputum or feces (see Fig. 3.4). Serology may be helpful in ectopic infections.

Management
Give praziquantel 75 mg/kg in 3 divides doses for 2 days. In areas where it is available, triclabendazole has started to replace praziquantel as first-line therapy, given its superior tolerability. Biothionol 30–50 mg/kg PO every other day for 10 days or niclosamide 2 mg/kg as a single dose were used commonly but have been supplanted because of side effects.

Abdominal angiostrongyliasis

The parasite
Angiostrongylus cantonensis, a rodent parasite, may cause abdominal symptoms or eosinophilic meningitis (see Chronic meningitis, p. 650). The definitive host is the rat, where the parasite lives in the arteries and arterioles of the ileocecum. Eggs hatch in the intestinal tissue and are excreted in the feces before being ingested by a slug intermediate, where a similar cycle occurs.

Humans may be infected by accidental ingestion of foods contaminated by larvae or slugs.

Epidemiology
Infection usually affects children in Central and South America and, rarely, Africa.

Clinical features
Patients usually complain of abdominal pain, fever, and vomiting. Physical findings include fever, abdominal tenderness, and a right lower quadrant mass (50%).

Diagnosis
The syndrome resembles appendicitis, apart from the presence of eosinophilia. Radiological features are nonspecific. Serology and PCR detection of DNA exist but are not routinely available.

Treatment

Most patients undergo laparatomy and removal of infected tissue. Some patients have been successfully treated with diethycarbamazine and thiabendazole. An alternative is mebendazole.

Anisakiasis

Anisakis and *Phocanema* are parasites of marine mammals, e.g., dolphins, seals, and whales. The eggs are excreted in the feces and hatch as free-swimming larvae, which are ingested by crustaceans and then by fish and squid. Humans are accidentally infected following ingestion of raw or poorly cooked seafood.

Epidemiology

Infection occurs most frequently in countries where raw fish is consumed, e.g., Japan and the Netherlands.

Clinical features

Symptoms usually occur 48 hours after ingestion and are caused by penetration of the worms into the gastrointestinal tract. Gastric anisakiasis is usually caused by *Phocanema* and characterized by abdominal pain, nausea, and vomiting. Small intestinal involvement is usually caused by *Anisakis* and characterized by lower abdominal pain and signs of obstruction.

Symptoms may become chronic with development of abdominal masses. Occasionally, acute allergic symptoms, e.g., urticaria and anaphylaxis, may also occur with *Anisakis*.

Diagnosis

The diagnosis should be suspected in any patient with a history of ingestion of raw fish and suggestive abdominal symptoms. Leukocytosis commonly occurs with intestinal involvement, but eosinophilia is rare.

Gastric anisakiasis may be confirmed by radiological features, endoscopy, and histological examination of biopsy specimens. Intestinal anisakiasis is confirmed by radiological features and detection of eosinophils in aspirated ascites. Serological tests are not routinely available.

Treatment

Symptoms usually improve without specific therapy but may resolve more quickly if gastric worms are removed by endoscopy. Occasionally, removal of an intestinal mass may be required.

Prevention

Infection may be prevented by cooking or freezing fish for 24 hours prior to ingestion.

Capilliariasis

Although the life cycle of *Capillaria philippinensis* is incompletely understood, its larvae have been found in freshwater fish and are known to be infectious for human and birds.

After ingestion of raw fish, the larvae invade the jejunum and ileum and produce both eggs and larvae. The parasite multiplies in the gut and may cause autoinfection and overwhelming infection (similar to that of *Strongyloides stercoralis*, p. 495).

Epidemiology

Infections usually occur in the Philippines and Thailand, but two cases have been reported in the Middle East.

Clinical features

These are consistent with malabsorption and protein-losing enteropathy and include abdominal pain, vomiting, diarrhea, abdominal distension, borborygmi, malaise, weight loss, and peripheral edema.

Diagnosis

This is confirmed by detecting ova or larvae in the stool. There are no serological tests.

Treatment

Treatment with mebendazole or albendazole is therapeutic and lifesaving and has superseded thiabendazole (25 mg/kg/day for 30 days). Mortality rates of up to 30% have been reported in untreated patients.

Ectoparasites

An *ectoparasite* is an organism that survives through interaction with the cutaneous surface of the host (e.g., obtaining a blood meal or living in the skin). Most ectoparasites belong to the phylum *Arthropoda*.

Two classes are important in human disease: *Hexapoda* (six-legged insects, e.g., lice, bugs, flies, mosquitoes) and *Arachnida* (eight-legged mites, spiders, and ticks). Ectoparasitic diseases are a common health problem in nonindustrialized tropical countries.

Lice (pediculosis)
Etiology

Three species of sucking lice affect humans: *Pediculus humanus* var. *capitis* (head louse), *Pediculus humanus* var. *corporis* (body louse), and *Phthirus pubis* (pubic or crab louse). The first two species are morphologically similar, with small, flat, elongated bodies and pointed heads. The pubic louse is shorter and wider and resembles a crab.

Small, ovoid eggs (nits) are laid by the adult female and adhere to hair and clothing; 7–10 days later, the nymphs emerge and, after three successive molts, the adult lice develop and mate. The females produce up to 300 eggs per day for 3–4 weeks until they die. Lice pierce the skin, inject saliva, and defecate while feeding.

Epidemiology
Lice infestations occur worldwide, are transmitted by direct contact, and are associated with poor hygiene and overcrowding. Lice cause skin disease and can also act as vectors for other infectious diseases, e.g., epidemic typhus (*Rickettsia prowazekii*), trench fever (*Bartonella quintana*), and relapsing fever (*Borrelia recurrentis*).

Clinical features
Pediculus capitis affects the scalp and causes pruritis. Complications include secondary bacterial infection and regional adenopathy.

Pediculus corporis is usually found in the seams of clothing. Symptoms include pruritis, erythematous macules, papules, and excoriations, usually on the trunk. Complications include impetigo, hyperpigmentation, and hyperkeratosis

Phthirus pubis resides in the pubic hair but may also be found in eyebrows, eyelashes, and axillary and chest hair. Symptoms include pruritis, erythematous macules, papules, and excoriations but are usually less severe than with other species. Small grayish-blue macules (maculae cerulae), caused by injection of an anticoagulant, may be seen. Eyelash infestation may be associated with nits at the base of the eyelashes and crusting of the eyelids.

Diagnosis
Diagnosis is usually clinical but may be confirmed by microscopic examination of the organism.

Management
- *Pediculus capitis:* 0.5% malathion lotion has been shown to be the most effective treatment but requires prolonged application (8–10 hours) and has an unpleasant odor. Other pediculicides are comparable in efficacy and require only a 10-minute application. These include 1% lindane, gamma benzene hexachloride shampoo, pyrethrins, and 1% permethrin cream rinse. Nits can be removed by combing the hair with a fine-toothed comb. Permethrin-resistant organisms have been reported.
- *Pediculus corporis:* body lice can be eradicated by discarding the clothing, washing clothes in a hot cycle, and ironing the seams or dusting clothing with 1% malathion powder or 10% DDT powder.
- *Phthirus pubis* may be treated with the same agents as those used for head lice (see above). Eyelid infestation may be treated by applying a thick layer of petrolatum bid for 8 days, or 1% yellow oxide of mercury daily for 2 weeks.

Pruritis is treated symptomatically with antihistamines and topical corticosteroids. Secondary bacterial infection should be treated with an oral antistaphylococcal agent.

Scabies
Etiology
Sarcoptes scabiei var. *hominis* is an eight-legged mite that resides in human skin. The adult female lays 2–3 eggs per day that burrow into the skin. After 72–84 hours, the larvae emerge and, after several molts, develop

into adults and mate. The males die shortly afterward but the gravid female lives for 4–6 weeks.

Epidemiology
Scabies occurs worldwide and epidemics are associated with poverty, malnutrition, overcrowding, and poor hygiene. Scabies is transmitted by direct contact (often sexual) or by fomites.

Clinical features
- *Human scabies:* symptoms include intense pruritis (more severe at night). Signs include linear burrows, erythematous papules, excoriations and, occasionally, vesicles. Complications include secondary bacterial infection and hypersensitivity reactions, e.g., eczematous eruption, nodular scabies.
- *Norwegian scabies* is a severe variant that may occur in institutionalized, debilitated, or immunosuppressed patients. Cutaneous lesions are hyperkeratotic, crusted nodules, or plaques, and nail involvement may occur. Complications include secondary bacterial infection, septicemia, and even death.
- *Animal scabies:* humans may occasionally be infected by *Sarcoptes scabiei* var. *canis* from their pet dog. Skin lesions are pruritic, papular, or urticarial.

Diagnosis
Diagnosis is usually clinical but may be confirmed by microscopic examination of skin scrapings for the organism, egg, or feces.

Management
Permethrin 5% cream applied for 8–10 hours is the most effective treatment. Lindane 1% lotion is also effective but is absorbed through the skin and may cause toxicity, e.g., irritability and seizures in infants.

Pregnant women and children may be treated with 6–10% precipitated sulfur in petrolatum daily for 3 days.

Ivermectin (see Anthelmintic drugs 1, p. 107) 200–250 microgram/kg single dose has been used experimentally in HIV-infected patients and institutional outbreaks.

Secondary bacterial infection should be treated.

Household members and close contacts should be treated simultaneously. Infected clothing and bed linen should be washed and dried on a hot cycle.

Myiasis

Epidemiology
Myiasis is an infestation caused by the larvae (maggots) of dipterous (two-winged) flies. It occurs more commonly in tropical climates and is an important veterinary problem. Human disease occurs as a result of travel to an endemic area or exposure to infected animals.

Etiology
A number of species may cause myiasis:
- *Dermatobia hominis* (human or tropical botfly)
- *Cordylobia anthrophaga* (tumbu fly)
- *Cordylobia rodhaini*

- *Oestrus ovis* (sheep botfly)
- *Gasterophilus* spp. (horse botfly)
- *Hypoderma bovis* (cattle botfly)
- *Cuterebra* spp. (North American botfly)
- *Cochliomyia hominivorax* (New World screwworm)
- *Chrysomyia bezziania* (Old World screwworm).

Clinical features

Furunculoid myiasis is usually caused by *D. hominis, C. anthrophaga,* or *C. rhodhaini* and occurs in travelers returning from Latin America or Africa. It is characterized by single or multiple cutaneous nodules, each containing a larva. A central punctum develops and may exude serosanguinous or purulent fluid. *D. hominis* infestations occur in the scalp, face, and extremities and may be associated with local pain.

C. anthrophaga usually affects the trunk, buttocks, and thighs. *C. rodhaini* is similar, but lesions are larger and more painful.

Subcutaneous infestation is caused by *Gastrophilus* spp. and characterized by migratory integumomiasis (creeping eruption), which is due to migration of larvae through the skin. *H. bovis* may cause similar lesions, which become furunculoid as the larvae mature.

Wound myiasis may be caused by *C. hominovorax* or *C. bezziana* and is characterized by local tissue destruction and secondary bacterial infection.

Ophthalmomyiasis is caused by *O. ovis* and may be superficial (ophthalmomyiasis externa), with conjunctivitis, lid edema, and punctuate keratopathy, or deep (ophthalmomyiasis interna), with invasion of the globe.

Management

- *Cutaneous myiasis:* removal of larvae from the affected tissue may be achieved by occlusion of the punctum, e.g., with Vaseline or clingfilm that encourages the larva to partially emerge from the punctum to avoid asphyxiation. It can then be removed with forceps. Surgical excision may be required.
- *Wound myiasis:* treatment requires removal of larvae and wound debridement.
- *Ophthalmomyiasis:* external infection is managed by removal of larvae under local anesthetic using forceps and slit-lamp examination. With internal infection, dead larvae (without associated inflammation) may be left in situ. Inflammation requires topical corticosteroids and mydratics. Surgical intervention is indicated for live larvae or involvement of critical structures.

Mites

Etiology

Mites belong to the class *Arachnida.* They occur worldwide and may be free living or parasitize plants, insects, animals, and humans. The mites that infect humans include the following:

- Chiggers (harvest mite or red bug)
- Animal mites, e.g., *Sarcoptes scabiei* var. *canis, Cheyletiella* spp., *Liponyssoides sanguineus, Ornithonysus bacoti*
- Bird mites, e.g., *Dermanyssus gallinae*

- Food, grain, and straw mites
- Follicle mites, e.g., *Demodex folliculorum*, *Demodex brevis*
- House dust mites, e.g., *Dermatophagoides pteronyssinus*, *Dermatophagoides farinae*
- Scabies (see above)

Clinical features

Mites may cause cutaneous disease in humans or act as vectors for infectious diseases, e.g., rickettsial diseases (p. 296) Q fever (p. 298), tularemia (p. 266), and plague (p. 263).

Management

Treatment of mite bites is symptomatic, with oral antihistamines or topical corticosteroids. Most lesions resolve within a week. Secondary bacterial infection should be treated with an antistaphylococcal antibiotic.

Ticks

Ticks are bloodsucking arthropods of the class *Arachnida*. There are three classes: *Ixodidiae* (hard ticks), *Argasidae* (soft ticks), and *Nuttalliellidae* (with characteristics of both).

Epidemiology

Ticks occur worldwide and are important vectors of infectious diseases, e.g., Lyme disease (p. 290), babesiosis (p. 466), ehrlichiosis, rickettsial diseases (p. 269), Q fever (p. 298), tularemia (p. 266), and relapsing fever (p. 288).

Clinical features and management

Most tick bites are asymptomatic. Attached ticks should be removed with forceps to prevent disease transmission. After removal, a pruritic, erythematous papule or plaque may persist for 1–2 weeks. Sometimes a tick bite granuloma may develop.

Tick paralysis is rare complication of prolonged attachment of certain tick species. Clinical features are of an ascending paralysis caused by a neurotoxin in the tick salivary gland. Symptoms usually resolve with removal of the tick. A hyperimmune globulin against *Ixodes holocyclus* is effective against tick paralysis caused by this species.

Clinical syndromes

Fever: introduction

Fever has been recognized as a clinical syndrome since the sixth century BCE. Several centuries later, Hippocratic physicians proposed that body temperature was a balance between the four corporal humors: blood, phlegm, black bile, and yellow bile.

Devices to measure body temperature have been around since the first century BCE. Measurement of body temperature became a part of clinical practice in 1868 when Wunderlich declared 37.4°C (98.6°F) to be normal body temperature and described the diurnal variation of body temperature.

Definitions

Different terminologies exist for separate but overlapping conditions.

- *Fever* is defined as a state of elevated core temperature which is often, but not necessarily, part of the defensive responses of a multicellular organism (the host) to the invasion of live (microorganisms) or inanimate matter recognized as pathogenic or alien to the host.
- *Infection* is the presence of organisms in a normally sterile site, usually accompanied by a host inflammatory response.
- *Bacteremia* is the presence of bacteria in the blood; it may be transient.
- *Septicemia* is similar to emiabacteremia but more severe.
- *Systemic inflammatory response syndrome (SIRS)* is a response to a wide variety of clinical insults that include infectious and noninfectious causes.
- *Sepsis* is clinical evidence of infection plus evidence of systemic response to infection, e.g., hypoxia, lactic acidosis, oliguria, altered mentation.
- *Sepsis syndrome* is sepsis plus evidence of altered organ perfusion.
- *Severe sepsis* is sepsis associated with organ dysfunction, hypoperfusion, or hypotension.
- *Septic shock* is sepsis with hypotension despite adequate fluid resuscitation along with the presence of perfusion abnormalities.
- *Refractory septic shock* is septic shock that lasts for >1 hour and does not respond to interventions.

Sepsis syndrome

Sepsis and *sepsis syndrome* are clinical definitions and are not directly related to microbiological data. However, information on bloodstream infections is available from passive surveillance systems, e.g., National Nosocomial Infection Survey (NNIS). These show that the rate of bloodstream infections has increased over the past two decades, with a dramatic increase in staphylococcal bacteremias, notably methicillin-resistant *Staphylococcus aureus* (MRSA).

Pathophysiology

The usual setting for the sepsis syndrome is bacterial invasion of the host or toxin production. The best studied example is systemic disease caused by gram-negative bacteria that have bacterial endotoxin or lipopolysaccharide (LPS). LPS triggers humoral enzymatic mechanisms, including complement, clotting fibrinolytic, and kinin pathways.

Fever and inflammation are mediated by cytokines, e.g., tumor necrosis factor (TNF)-A, interleukin (IL)-1, IL-6, and IL-8, and interferon (IFN)-G. Disseminated intravascular coagulation (DIC) may occur, also mediated by cytokines. Systemic activation of coagulation results in the deposition of fibrin and microvascular thrombosis in critical target organs. Conversely, consumption of clotting factors may lead to bleeding.

Infection or shock may trigger injury to the pulmonary vascular endothelium, leading to acute respiratory distress syndrome (ARDS). In models of acute lung injury, various stimuli, e.g., LPS, thrombin, complement, platelet-activating factor, or arachidonate metabolites, may trigger this.

Clinical features

The symptoms and signs suggestive of severe bacterial infection as a cause of sepsis syndrome include the following:
- Fever, chills, hypothermia
- Hypotension, cardiac failure
- Hyperventilation, respiratory failure, cyanosis
- Jaundice, liver failure
- Oliguria, anuria, renal failure
- Skin lesions
- Bleeding
- Altered mental status.

Laboratory diagnosis

Routine investigations may show leukopenia, thrombocytopenia, and lactic acidosis.

At least two sets of blood cultures should be taken from different sites. Cultures of potential sources of infection should also be taken.

Lumbar puncture (LP) and cerebrospinal fluid (CSF) examination should be performed for all patients with altered mental status.

Management

- *Antimicrobials:* combination antimicrobial therapy is usually given empirically until the results of cultures are available. The choice of agents depends on the clinical presentation, i.e., community or hospital acquired, neutropenic sepsis, colonization with MRSA or other drug-resistant pathogens
- *Volume replacement:* careful management of fluid and electrolyte balance is crucial. Hemodynamic monitoring may help to guide therapy. Depending on the clinical situation, crystalloids, colloids, or blood products may be used.
- *Inotropes:* sympathomimetic agents, e.g., epinephrine (adrenaline) and norepinephrine (noradrenaline), have been widely used to treat shock, but there are no controlled trials of comparative efficacy. Alternative

agents, e.g., dopamine, dobutamine, vasopressin, and isoprenaline (isoproterenol), are being increasingly used of instead norepinephrine.
- *Corticosteroids:* the use of corticosteroids for the treatment of septic shock, in the absence of adrenal sufficiency, remains controversial. Early small studies suggested benefit, but this was not confirmed in larger controlled trials.
- *Anticoagulation:* routine use of anticoagulation to treat septic shock associated with DIC has not been shown to be beneficial. If there is bleeding secondary to coagulopathy, this should be corrected with appropriate replacement therapy, e.g., platelets, cryoprecipitate, or fresh-frozen plasma. For patients with refractory shock and coagulopathy despite therapeutic measures, heparin may be beneficial in terminating DIC. Activated protein C is sometimes given in severe sepsis.
- *Diuretics:* despite lack of evidence, diuretics are commonly used in the early oliguric or anuric phases of septic shock with a view to preventing acute renal failure.
- *Cytokine inhibition:* the use of antibodies directed against LPS have failed to show benefit in clinical trials of gram-negative sepsis syndrome. Similarly, results from trials using recombinant IL-receptor (IL-1Ra) antagonists, and monoclonal antibodies to TNF-A and TNF-A receptors have proved disappointing.

Prevention

A number of measures may be implemented to try to prevent sepsis:
- Infection control measures in hospitals
- Prophylactic antimicrobials, e.g., polymixin sprays, nebulized colistin, selective digestive decontamination
- Management of high-risk patients, e.g., bone marrow transplant (BMT) patients in a protective environment
- Active or passive immunoprophylaxis with type-specific or cross-reactive antibodies
- Use of granulocyte transfusions or colony-stimulating factors.

However, these approaches are controversial, as no consistent benefit has been demonstrated and concern remains about selection of drug-resistant organisms.

Fever of unknown origin

Definition

The first definition of *fever of unknown origin* (FUO) was proposed by Petersdorf and Beeson in 1961: "fever of >38.3°C (101°F) on several occasions persisting without diagnosis for at least 3 weeks despite at least 1 week's investigation in hospital.[1]"

Since then, the definition has been modified to reflect changes in medical practice and there are now four different subtypes:
- Classic FUO (>38°C for >3 weeks, >2 visits or 3 days in hospital)
- Nosocomial FUO (>38°C for 3 days, not present or incubating on admission)

- Immune-deficient FUO (>38°C for >3 days, negative cultures after 48 hours)
- HIV-related FUO (>38°C for >3 weeks for outpatients or >3 days for inpatients)

Causes of FUO

Classic FUO

Although a wide variety of conditions can cause classic FUO, most fall into five categories:

- Infections (27–50%), e.g., abscesses, endocarditis, tuberculosis, complicated urinary tract infections (UTIs). Some causes show distinct geographic variation, e.g., visceral leishmaniasis (Spain), melioidosis (Southeast Asia).
- Neoplasms (13–25%), e.g., lymphoma
- Connective tissue disorders (9–17%), e.g., Still's disease, systemic lupus erythematosus (SLE), rheumatoid arthritis (RA), temporal arteritis, polymyalgia rheumatica
- Miscellaneous disorders (15–21%)
- Undiagnosed conditions (5–23%)

The relative frequency of disorders within these five categories varies according to the era in which the study was conducted, geographic region, age of patient, and type of hospital.

Nosocomial FUO

This presents as fever after hospitalization for at least 24 hours. Risk factors include intravascular devices, urinary or respiratory tract instrumentation, surgical procedures, immobility, and drug therapy. However, knowledge is limited due to lack of published data.

Immune-deficient FUO

This occurs in patients receiving cytotoxic therapy, those with solid-organ or hematopoietic stem cell transplant, or those with hematological malignancies. Because of impaired immune function, signs of inflammation may be modest, leading to atypical presentations.

During episodes of neutropenia, infections caused by pyogenic bacteria are most common. In patients with impaired cell-mediated immunity, viral infections are more common.

HIV-related FUO

This may occur with primary infection or in advanced disease, where it is due to opportunistic infections (e.g., mycobacteria, visceral leishmaniasis, *Pneumocystis jiroveci*, bacterial infections, cytomegalovirus [CMV], toxoplasmosis, cryptococcosis) or malignancies.

Evaluation of FUO

History and examination

A comprehensive history should include details of recent travel, contact with persons who have a similar illness, exposure to animals, work environment, past medical history, drug history, and family history for hereditary causes of fever. A careful physical examination may reveal clues as to the etiology, e.g., stigmata of endocarditis.

The presence of fever should be verified, although fever patterns are neither sensitive nor specific enough to be diagnostically reliable.

Laboratory investigations

These include simple blood tests (e.g., full blood count, erythrocyte sedimentation rate [ESR], biochemistry) and urinalysis. Blood cultures (at least three separate specimens) should be taken prior to initiation of antimicrobial therapy).

Serology may be helpful for viral infections (e.g., Monospot, CMV IgM, HIV test) and autoimmune disorders (e.g., antinuclear antibody [ANA], antineutrophil cytoplasmic antibody [ANCA], rheumatoid factor).

Imaging studies

All patients should have a chest radiograph. Further radiological imaging should be guided by the clinical presentation, e.g., abdominal computerized tomography (CT) or radiolabeled leukocyte scans for suspected abscesses. Venous duplex scans of the lower extremities may reveal deep vein thromboses.

Invasive procedures

Diagnostic biopsies (e.g., needle biopsy, excision biopsy, open biopsy) may be helpful. With the exception of temporal artery biopsies, the diagnostic yield of bedside biopsies is low compared with that of CT-guided or operative biopsies.

Therapeutic trials

There are a number of limitations and risks associated with empirical therapy. The underlying condition may remit spontaneously. Empirical treatment may not be specific, e.g., rifampin is active against a range of pyogenic bacteria as well as M. tuberculosis.

Therapeutic trials may confound or delay the diagnosis of FUO. Thus therapeutic trials should be reserved for those few patients in whom all other approaches have failed, or the occasional patient who is too ill for therapy to be withheld.

Management

A fundamental principle of management of classic FUO is that therapy should be delayed until the cause has been identified so that it can be targeted appropriately. However, this ideal is frequently ignored in clinical practice and may confound or delay the diagnosis of FUO.

In contrast, for neutropenic sepsis, which carries a high risk of serious bacterial infections, empiric broad-spectrum antibiotic therapy should be started immediately after appropriate cultures are taken.

Prognosis

The prognosis of FUO depends on the cause of the fever and the underlying disease. Elderly patients and those with malignant disease have the poorest prognosis.

Diagnostic delay adversely affects outcome in intra-abdominal infections, disseminated tuberculosis and fungal infections, and recurrent pulmonary emboli.

Patients who have undiagnosed FUO after extensive evaluation generally have a favorable outcome (3.2% 5-year mortality rate).

Reference

1. Fever of unexplained origin: report on 100 cases. PETERSDORF RG, BEESON PB. Medicine (Baltimore). 1961 Feb;40:1–30.

Fever in the returned traveler

Fever in returning travelers is estimated to affect 20–70% of the 50 million people who travel from industrialized countries to the developing world each year. Although most illnesses are mild, 1–5% of people are ill enough to seek medical attention, 0.1% require medical evacuation, and 1 in 100,000 dies.

An increased risk of travel-associated infections is seen in people who visit family and friends abroad and adventure travelers, often because they underestimate the risks of illness. Potential problems include exposure to "new" pathogens (via contaminated water and food, poor hygiene, or sanitation), inexperience of clinician in diagnosis, and possible transmission of common resistant organisms between countries.

For an excellent review, see Ryan et al.[1]

Clinical features

Patients may present with a wide spectrum of disease, ranging from asymptomatic carriage to fulminant disease (see Table 4.1).

Three main syndromes are seen: fever, diarrhea, and skin conditions. Fever can be differentiated into diagnostic groups according to
- Duration of symptoms (<14 days, 14 days to 6 weeks, and >6 weeks)
- Symptoms, e.g., undifferentiated fever, respiratory symptoms, central nervous system (CNS) symptoms, or hemorrhage.

Diarrhea may be acute (<2 weeks) or chronic (2 to 4 weeks).

Skin lesions may be divided into four categories, e.g., papules, subcutaneous swellings/nodules, ulcers, or linear/migratory lesions.

Don't forget to consider non–travel-related infections or conditions.

History and examination

The following are essential in the assessment of a returning traveler:
- Travel history—where, how long, urban or rural
- Exposure history—animals and insects
- Incubation period
- Duration of illness
- Symptoms and physical findings
- Immunization status
- Antimalarial chemoprophylaxis—regimen, compliance.

Laboratory investigations (as indicated by travel history)
- Full blood count (FBC), white cell count (WCC) and differential, thick and thin films
- Blood urea nitrogen (BUN), creatinine, electrolytes, liver function tests (LFTs), C-reactive protein (CRP)

Table 4.1 Causes of fever in the returned traveler

Incubation	Syndrome	Causes
<14 days	Undifferentiated fever	Malaria, dengue, rickettsial spotted fevers, scrub typhus, leptospirosis, bacterial gastroenteritis, typhoid, acute HIV
	Fever with respiratory symptoms	Influenza, legionellosis, Q fever, acute histoplasmosis, acute coccidioidomycosis
	Fever with CNS symptoms	Bacterial meningitis, viral meningitis, encephalitis, cerebral malaria, typhoid, typhus, rabies, arboviral encephalitis, *Angiostrongylus cantonensis* eosinophilic meningitis, polio, East African trypansomiasis
	Fever with hemorrhage	Meningococcemia, leptospirosis, *Streptococcus suis*, malaria, viral hemorrhagic fevers
14 days to 6 weeks		Malaria, typhoid, hepatitis A, hepatitis E, acute schistosomiasis, amebic liver abscess, leptospirosis, acute HIV infection, East African trypanosomiasis, viral hemorrhagic fevers, Q fever
>6 weeks		Malaria, tuberculosis, hepatitis B, hepatitis E, visceral leishmaniasis, lymphatic filiariasis, schistosomiasis, amebic liver abscess, chronic mycosis, rabies, African trypanosomiasis, HIV

- Urinalysis, urine microscopy and culture
- Stool microscopy for microscopy, ova, cysts, parasites, and culture
- Skin scrapings or biopsy of lesions
- Sputum microscopy and culture
- Blood cultures
- Serology: arboviruses, rickettsia, schistosomiasis, leptospirosis, viral hepatitis, HIV
- Imaging, e.g., chest X-ray (CXR), abdominal ultrasound
- Bone marrow examination may be helpful in certain conditions, e.g., typhoid, leishmaniasis.

Treatment
- Supportive treatment (mild infections or those with no treatment)
- Specific treatment according to the causative organism

Prevention
- Pre-travel vaccination, e.g., hepatitis A (HAV), tetanus, typhoid, diphtheria, meningitis, rabies, Japanese B encephalitis, cholera, yellow fever

- Chemoprophylaxis, e.g., antimalarials
- Advice regarding risk avoidance, e.g., water purification, avoid uncooked food, barrier contraception

Reference

1. Ryan ET, Wilson ME, Kain KC (2002). Illness after international travel. *N Engl J Med* 347(7): 505–516.

Common cold

The term *common cold* is applied to the acute minor coryzal illness caused by viruses belonging to a number of different families.

Etiology

Common causes are members of the myxovirus, paramyxovirus, adenovirus, picornavirus, and coronavirus families—mostly the rhinoviruses (40%) and the coronaviruses (10%). Some of these have several different antigenic types (e.g., over 100 in the case of rhinovirus).

Other causes include parainfluenza, respiratory syncytial virus (RSV), adenovirus, certain enteroviruses, streptococcal pharyngitis (cannot be differentiated on clinical grounds alone and is considered a cause of colds).

Reinfections may occur with the same virus; ~25% of cases are attributed to agents as yet unidentified. Influenza can produce a cold-like syndrome but generally produces more severe lower respiratory tract infection (LRTI).

Epidemiology

Epidemics occur in the winter months in temperate areas and during the rainy season in tropical regions, reflecting the seasonal nature of viral circulation (perhaps due to the effects of humidity on viral survival).

In developed countries, adults experience on average 2–4 and children 6–8 colds a year. Smokers tend to experience more significant symptoms.

The prime reservoir for cold viruses is the upper airway of young children and spread occurs in schools and the home. Mothers have higher secondary attack rates than those of fathers. Spread is probably by a mix of aerosol and contact with contaminated skin and surfaces.

Pathogenesis

The pathological mechanisms of different viruses vary. All invade the mucosa of the upper respiratory tract, and sloughed nasal columnar epithelial cells may be identified in the nasal secretions.

Chemical mediators (cytokines, histamine, prostaglandin) and activation of parasympathetic nervous pathways cause inflammation and engorging of blood vessels of the nasal turbinates with congestion and discharge.

The peak of rhinovirus cold symptoms coincides with maximal viral shedding. Cold viruses may affect the bacterial flora of the respiratory tract and facilitate secondary bacterial infections.

Clinical features

Incubation is 12 hours to 3 days. Symptoms include nasal discharge, congestion, sneezing, cough, sore throat. Fever is mild and more common in children.

Symptoms reach peak severity by day 3. Most resolve by 1 week, some last up to 2 weeks. Conjunctivitis may be seen in adenovirus and enterovirus infection.

Diagnosis

Identification of the causative agent is unhelpful in uncomplicated cold.

It is important to recognize secondary bacterial sinusitis (2% of cases) and otitis media (2% of cases). Marked pharyngeal inflammation or exudates raises the possibility of streptococcal, adenovirus, herpes simplex virus (HSV) or Epstein–Barr virus (EBV) infection.

Rapid antigen detection for group A streptococci (GAS) may be useful in those with prominent pharyngeal symptoms.

Treatment

Patients should be encouraged to wash their hands and take measures to avoid contamination of others at the peak of symptoms.

Antihistamines provide relief from sneezing, discharge, and cough. Nonsteroidal anti-inflammatory drugs (NSAIDs) such as naproxen reduce cough.

Decongestants may be given topically or orally. Rebound nasal congestion may follow withdrawal of topical agents after prolonged use. Topical anesthetic-containing lozenges may relieve sore throat.

Large doses of vitamin C may have a modest therapeutic effect but have no demonstrable preventative effect in controlled trials.

There is no role for antibiotics in uncomplicated cold.

Pharyngitis

Pharyngitis is an infection or irritation of the pharynx and/or tonsils.

Etiology

- 40–60% viral (mostly rhinovirus and adenovirus)
- 5–40% bacterial (up to ≤15% caused by group A *Streptococcus*)
- Other causes include allergy, trauma, toxins, and malignancy.

It is important to distinguish pharyngitis from more serious conditions such as epiglottitis and para- or retropharyngeal abscess.

Pathogenesis

Bacteria or viruses invade the pharyngeal mucosa, causing a local inflammatory response. Certain viruses (rhinovirus) promote nasal secretions that cause secondary pharyngeal irritation.

Streptococcal protein and toxins facilitate local invasion and may lead to complications such as rheumatic fever and poststreptococcal glomerulonephritis.

Epidemiology

Pharyngitis is most common in children. Cases of both viral and bacterial etiology peak among school-aged children (4–7 years).

Group A streptococci account for 30% of childhood pharyngitis and 15% of adult cases. *Mycoplasma pneumoniae* and *Chlamydia pneumoniae* are common causes among teenagers and young adults. Consider gonococcal pharyngitis if there is a history of orogenital contact.

Clinical features

Viral and bacterial causes are not easily distinguished clinically.

General features include fever, malaise, sore throat, and myalgia. On examination there are erythema and edema of the tonsils and pharyngeal mucosa. Purulent tonsillar exudate suggests streptococcal infection or EBV. Conjunctivitis suggests adenovirus, vesicles suggest HSV stomatitis or Coxsackie A infection.

Document murmurs to monitor for potential rheumatic fever. Chest signs may indicate LRTIs by *M. pneumoniae* or *C. pneumoniae*.

Hepatosplenomegaly may be seen in EBV infection.

Specific bacterial infections

- *Group A streptococcal infection:* 15% of cases. Occur winter to early spring. Consider if there is abrupt onset, recent contact with others diagnosed with GAS, headache, vomiting, no cough, swollen tender cervical lymphadenopathy, or high WCC. Scarlet fever is also caused by GAS infection (see Group A *Streptococcus*, p. 197). Complications include rheumatic fever (1 in 400 untreated GAS infections), glomerulonephritis, abscess, toxic shock syndrome, and airway obstruction.
- *Group C, G, and F streptococci:* 10% of cases. These resemble GAS but without the immunological sequelae.
- *Other:* Arcanobacterium haemolyticum (5%, common in young adults, causing outbreaks of a scarlet fever–like rash); *M. pneumoniae* (young adults with headache, pharyngitis, chest symptoms, cough); *C. pneumoniae* (similar to *M. pneumoniae,* pharyngitis may precede pulmonary infection); *N. gonorrhoeae* (rare, usually follows orogenital contact); *Corynebacterium diphtheriae* (rare in the developed world, risk of airway obstruction), *Borrelia* species

Viral infections

Pharyngitis following several days of coughing or rhinorrhea:
- *Adenovirus:* 5% of cases and the most common cause in children under 3 years. It causes an associated conjunctivitis.
- *HSV:* vesicular lesions are common in children but may be absent in older patients (may be indistinguishable from GAS infection).
- *Other:* Coxsackie viruses A and B (similar presentation to HSV), rhinovirus, coronavirus, EBV (difficult to distinguish from GAS, see p. 197), CMV, HIV (pharyngeal edema and erythema, mouth ulcers)

Other causes

These include candidal infection (particularly in immunocompromised patients) and irritation (dry air, postnasal drip, allergy, esophageal reflux, smoking). Differential includes diphtheria, mycoplasmal pneumonia, para-pharyngeal abscess, and malignancy.

Investigations

- *Serology:* a rise in ASO titer confirms GAS infection retrospectively.
- *Throat swab:* antigen tests and culture are sensitive for the presence of GAS and are widely used in the United States. High rates of asymptomatic carriage and positivity do not indicate causality. Antigen tests do not detect group C or G streptococci or other bacterial pathogens. Culture for *N. gonorrhoea* if indicated.

Consider specific tests for other causes: EBV, *C. pneumoniae, M. pneumoniae*, etc, and viral culture. Viral serology may be useful in retrospect.

Management

For general management, consider airway and sepsis, exclude abscess, and assess hydration. Most cases are viral and do not need antibiotic treatment and resolve spontaneously within 10 days.

Early treatment of GAS infection reduces the incidence of immunological sequelae. Antibiotic therapy may prevent suppurative complications. Although antibiotics' value might be questioned, most people would treat suspected GAS infection and all patients who appear unwell, e.g., penicillin V for 10 days. Avoid ampicillin or amoxicillin in those in whom EBV infection has not been excluded because of severe rash side effect. Rates of recurrence are higher in those not completing the 10-day course.

For recurrent tonsillitis, treat with β-lactamase stable agents such as clindamycin. Consider ear, nose and throat (ENT) referral. Tonsillectomy may be appropriate.

Complications

These include LRTI, suppurative complications (abscess, sinusitis, otitis media, epiglottitis, mastoiditis), and nonsuppurative sequelae of GAS infection. Scarlet fever (see Bacterial causes of childhood illness, p. 704) may be seen in association with a streptococcal infection at any site.

Retropharyngeal abscess

This infection causes abscess in one of the deep spaces of the neck. It is potentially life threatening given the risk of airway compromise but is rare in developed countries, where antibiotic usage in the treatment of upper respiratory tract infection (URTI) is widespread. This is generally a pediatric diagnosis. Other pharyngeal abscesses (lateral pharyngeal, peritonsillar) are more common in older children and adults.

Pathogenesis

The retropharyngeal space is located posterior to the pharynx, anterior to the cervical vertebrae, and extends from the base of the skull to the level of the tracheal bifurcation.

It may become infected by contiguous spread (e.g., an URTI that has spread to the retropharyngeal lymph nodes) or through direct inoculation by penetrating trauma or instrumentation (feeding tube insertion, head and neck surgery, fish bone).

Clinical features
Patients may have experienced previous URTI (perhaps weeks previously) and may not recall the specific trauma (e.g., running and falling with a lollipop in the mouth).

Symptoms include fever, chills, malaise, voice change (classically a duck quack: "cri du canard"), sore throat, dysphagia, neck stiffness, sensation of a lump in the throat, and pain in back and shoulders on swallowing. Difficulty breathing is a serious sign that may herald airway obstruction.

On examination there is fever, septic, unilateral lymphadenopathy, neck mass, mass in the posterior pharyngeal wall on oral examination (30% cases), or signs of vascular complications (jugular vein thrombophlebitis, carotid rupture—bleeding from the ear, nose, or mouth and ecchymosis in the neck).

Consider the diagnosis in those with fever, neck stiffness, and normal lumbar puncture.

Complications include mass effect (e.g., expansion against the trachea causing airway compression), abscess rupture (pus aspiration may lead to pneumonia), and spread of infection (inflammation and destruction of adjacent tissues—mediastinitis, pericarditis, empyema, jugular vein thrombosis, carotid artery rupture, osteomyelitis of the cervical vertebrae leading to subluxation and spinal cord damage). The infection itself may rarely develop into necrotizing fasciitis and sepsis.

Diagnosis
- *Imaging:* lateral soft tissue X-ray of the neck (inspiration with the neck in normal extension) may show widening of the prevertebral tissue and gas. Contrast CT is more useful. MRI produces more detailed images, but these are usually unnecessary and children often require sedation.
- *Microbiology:* usually polymicrobial members of the oropharyngeal flora: gram-positives (group A streptococci, *S. aureus*) and anaerobes (*Bacteroides* species) predominate. Gram-negatives may also be found.
- Consider tuberculosis (TB) and coccidiosis in patients with risk factors who fail to respond to standard antibiotic therapy.
- *Differential:* foreign body, epiglottitis, cystic hygroma, other forms of pharyngeal collection

Management
- Urgent ENT referral for incision and drainage
- Intravenous (IV) antibiotic therapy with benzylpenicillin and clindamycin, or cephalosporin and metronidazole
- 30% may require a surgical airway.

Quinsy (peritonsillar abscess)

This relatively common infection of the peritonsillar space (between the capsule of the palatine tonsil and the pharyngeal muscles) usually follows bacterial pharyngitis but may arise de novo. One-third of cases occur in children. Peak incidence is at age 20–30 years.

Usually it is polymicrobial in origin (GAS, aerobes such as *S. milleri* and anaerobes such as *Peptostreptococcus*, *Streptococcus sanguis*, and *Fusobacterium* species).

Symptoms are drooling, fever, an abrupt increase in pain and dysphagia.

Examination reveals asymmetrical tonsillar enlargement and neck swelling; there may be a palpable fluctuant mass and bad breath. Trismus may render examination impossible. Ultrasound scan or CT may be useful in such patients.

Management includes ENT referral for consideration of surgical drainage and IV benzyl-penicillin or amoxicillin-clavulanateamoxicillin-clavulanate. Perimucosal needle aspiration may be appropriate in patients who can tolerate it with no evidence of deep neck tissue extension, septicemia, or toxicity. Material can also be obtained for culture.

Complications are airway obstruction.

Treatment success is 90–95% for appropriately treated uncomplicated abscesses, with a 10–15% recurrence rate (the majority very shortly after the initial episode, suggesting ongoing infection). Such patients may benefit from interval tonsillectomy.

Lemierre's disease

This oropharyngeal infection ("anaerobic tonsillitis") spreads to cause internal jugular thrombosis. Usually it is seen in young, healthy adults.

It is caused by *Fusobacterium necrophorum*. Severe sore throat progresses to sepsis with secondary abscesses (liver, lungs, pleura, bones, joints, brain) and local spread (Quinsy and vascular thrombosis).

Ultrasound, CT, and MRI confirm the diagnosis. The organism may be grown from blood or pus; some cases are mixed infections (oropharyngeal flora, e.g., *S. milleri*). Prolonged antibiotic therapy is required (e.g., 6 weeks' amoxicillin-clavulanateamoxicillin-clavulanate).

Croup

Croup is an acute laryngotracheitis or laryngotracheobronchitis of viral etiology occurring in young children and resulting in breathlessness with stridor-like inspiration and a barking, seal-like cough.

Epidemiology

It is a common illness in young children (around 10% of LRTI), peaking during the second year of life, although it can occur in children as old as 15 years.

Autumn cases tend to be due to parainfluenza types 1 and 2, winter cases to influenza and RSV, sporadic cases to parainfluenza type 3 and several less frequently identified agents, e.g., adenovirus, rhinovirus.

Measles is a cause of severe croup and remains so in areas of poor vaccination coverage. *M. pneumoniae* can cause a croup-like syndrome.

Pathophysiology

Viral infection of the upper airway spreads down and may involve the entire respiratory tract. Inflammation of the larynx and trachea causes stridor, hoarseness, and cough and is greatest at the subglottic level near the cricoid. The compliant airways of young children further restrict airflow on inspiration at this narrow point.

Decreased tidal volume leads to an increase in respiratory rate, and if the obstruction is severe, exhaustion, hypercapnia, and hypoxia may follow. Hypoxia is exacerbated by parenchymal inflammation.

The predilection of croup for young children is probably a combination of their anatomy (small compliant airways) and the fact that many children are experiencing primary infections. Immune mechanisms may play a part; not every child experiencing a parainfluenza infection gets croup, and immune defects similar to those found in atopic patients may contribute to the mechanics of disease in certain cases.

Clinical features

It is vital to distinguish croup from epiglottitis (see p. 536).

Children usually have a short history of URTI with sore throat, mild cough, and fever. The onset of croup often occurs at night with barking, seal-like cough, and hoarseness. Stridor and dyspnea may develop. The child may sit forward to aid breathing. Ausculation can reveal rhonchi and wheeze in severely affected children. Some develop pneumonia. Respiratory rates of 40/minute are not unusual. Symptoms fluctuate, improving or worsening within an hour, tending to be more severe in the evening.

In severe cases, exhaustion or severe obstruction may necessitate respiratory support or intubation.

Indicators of impending respiratory failure are stridor at rest (may be quiet), sternal wall retractions, lethargy, or decreased level of consciousness, paradoxical breathing, and quiet breath sounds.

Some children experience repeated episodes of croup (spasmodic croup), perhaps related to airway hyperreactivity and allergic disease.

Diagnosis

Diagnosis is clinical, and croup must be differentiated from other causes of stridor (e.g., foreign body) and bacterial epiglottitis. Epiglottitis has a more rapid course and children tend to be more toxic with dysphagia and drooling. Croup's distinctive cough is also absent.

- *General laboratory features:* WBC count may be normal or raised, hypoxia is seen in most hospitalized children and hypercapnia in half.
- *Viral identification:* immunofluorescence and reverse transcription polymerase chain reaction (RT-PCR) may allow rapid identification of a causative agent.

Serology is not useful in the diagnosis of croup.

Management

Steam inhalation providing humidification of the upper airways is a mainstay of home therapy. There is no evidence to demonstrate its efficacy.

Patients unwell enough to require hospitalization require close observation to identify signs of airway obstruction, exhaustion, and respiratory failure requiring intubation and ventilation. Interventions such as blood sampling should be kept to a minimum to avoid exacerbating anxiety and breathlessness.

Respiratory rate is the best indicator of hypoxia. Cyanosis may not be present, and the severity of stridor indicates the degree of subglottic obstruction and does not necessarily relate to oxygenation.

Pulse oximetry is sufficient a measure of oxygenation in most patients, but the more severely ill patient should have arterial CO_2 measured. Children who are hypoxic with normal CO_2 should respond to low concentrations of supplemental oxygen. Humidification has not been shown to have any benefit; in fact, dry air may be preferable.

Pharmacological interventions

Nebulized budesonide is associated with faster clinical improvement compared to placebo in moderate to severe cases.

- *Corticosteroid therapy:* a single dose of dexamethasone (oral or intramuscular [IM] 0.15–0.6 mg/kg) reduces the proportion of those with mild disease requiring further medical attention. It is beneficial in cases of moderate and severe croup, equal to or more efficacious than nebulized steroids, easier to give, and less distressing to the anxious child when given orally.
- *Nebulized racemic adrenaline* (epinephrine) 2.25% diminishes subglottic swelling and produces clinical improvement in those children with severe stridor. It is fast acting, but improvement is transitory, around 2 hours. It does not improve oxygenation but results in less frequent need for intubation due to exhaustion

There is no role for antibiotics in the management of croup in the absence of concomitant bacterial infection.

Epiglottitis

This is a potentially life-threatening condition of inflammation, edema, and obstruction of the epiglottis and surrounding structures. Classically, it is a disease of children (aged 3–7 years) due to infection by *Haemophilus influenzae* type B. Since the introduction of *H. influenzae* type B (Hib) vaccination, recent epidemiology suggests that it is now more common in adults, and no one organism is predominant.

Other causes include group A, B, and C *Streptococcus*, *S. pneumoniae*, *K. pneumoniae*, *Candida albicans*, *S. aureus*, *Haemophilus parainfluenzae*, *N. meningitides*, and certain viruses. Hib epiglottitis has occurred in vaccinated children.

Clinical features

There is abrupt onset of severe sore throat and fever with stridor, drooling, anxiety, and refusal to eat. Children may adopt the typical posture: sitting up, leaning forward, and generally looking seriously unwell.

Attempting to examine the throat (e.g., use of a tongue depressor) may result in total airway obstruction, as may IV cannulation. These procedures should be deferred until anesthetic support is present.

Complications include emiabacteremia, pneumonia, meningitis, arthritis and cellulitus.

Management

Securing the airway is the absolute priority. Once the airway is secured mortality is less than 1%. Outcome is significantly better with elective intubation than with emergency intubation.

- *Antibiotics:* IV cephalosporin usually for 7–10 days. However, consider *C. albicans* if there are white patches on examination.
- *Prophylaxis (Hib):* rifampin should be given to the patient and all household and daycare contacts, including adults, if there are other susceptible (unvaccinated or immunocompromised) children in the family.
- *Mortality:* around 0% with a quick diagnosis in specialist centers, 9–18% where diagnosis is delayed, and 6% where patients are managed without intubation.

Investigations

All investigations should follow securing the airway.
- WBC count and inflammatory markers are raised.
- *Cultures:* blood and epiglottic swabs
- *Radiology:* lateral neck X-ray may show an enlarged epiglottis protruding from the anterior wall of the hypopharynx ("thumb sign").
- *Differential:* croup, diphtheria, inhaled foreign body

Bacterial tracheitis

This is an atypical form of croup, its clinical picture having more in common with that of epiglottitis. It is uncommon, tending to affect older children. Those with a history of either recent intubation or viral illness are at greater risk.

Presentation is with an abrupt onset of fever, stridor, and breathlessness with large amounts of purulent sputum. Progression can be rapid, necessitating intubation. Obstruction is subglottic, the epiglottis itself being only minimally inflamed.

Organisms that may be recovered include *S. aureus*, group A, β-hemolytic streptococci, and (prior to vaccination) *H. influenzae* type B.

Antibiotics should be given promptly, and direct laryngscopy can confirm the diagnosis and provide local secretions for culture.

Laryngitis

Etiology

This is an inflammation of the larynx that may be caused by any of the major respiratory viruses, including rhinovirus, influenza, parainfluenza, adenovirus, and coronavirus. It can be a feature of streptococcal sore throat.

Other common bacterial agents associated with laryngitis include *M. catarrhalis*, *H. influenzae*, *Mycoplasma pneumoniae*, and *Chlamydia pneumoniae*. Worldwide, diphtheria continues to be an important cause.

Uncommon causes include *Candida*, *Coccidioides immitis*, *Cryptococcus neoformans*, TB, and blastomycosis.

Clinical features

Most cases occur in adults between 18 and 40 years of age. It is a feature in 38% of cases of pneumonia, 24% of cases of children with sore throat, and 75% of toddlers with croup. It presents as a hoarse or harsh voice with lowered pitch, episodes of aphonia, and sore throat.

Duration is 3–8 days.

Treatment

Management is symptomatic (analgesia and voice rest). Routine antibiotics are not recommended. Treatment should be directed at the underlying cause.

Sinusitis

Sinusitis is inflammation of the paranasal sinuses, usually due to viral, bacterial, or fungal infection to or noninfectious causes (allergy). Acute sinusitis lasts <4 weeks, and chronic sinusitis lasts >4 weeks.

Etiology

Bacterial sinusitis
- *Community acquired: Streptococcus pneumoniae, Haemophilus influenzae,* α-hemolytic streptococci, *Moraxella catarrhalis*
- *Nosocomial:* anaerobes, S. aureus, P. aeruginosa, other enterobacteria

Viral sinusitis
- Rhinovirus, influenza, parainfluenza, adenovirus

Fungal sinusitis
- *Community acquired:* generally allergic and not
- *Immunocompromised patients:* invasive *Aspergillus* spp., *Rhizopus* spp. *Mucor* spp., *Sporothrix schenkii, Scedosporium apiospermum*
- *Noninfectious causes:* chemical irritants, tumors, foreign bodies, Wegener's granulomatosis

Epidemiology

Acute sinusitis is a common diagnosis in the primary care setting.

Viral sinusitis is seen as part of the common cold from autumn to spring. Cases of acute community-acquired bacterial sinusitis peak in association with viral cases (occur in around 0.5% of colds).

Nonviral cases occur throughout the year in association with allergy, swimming, nasal polyps, foreign bodies, tumor, immunodeficiency, and cystic fibrosis.

Nosocomial cases (often polymicrobial) may occur secondary to head trauma, prolonged nasotracheal or nasogastric intubation, neutropenia, diabetic ketoacidosis, corticosteroids, or broad-spectrum antibiotic use.

Pathogenesis

- *Viral:* 90% of patients with a cold develop viscous discharge and reduced clearance of secretions from sinuses, which may be due to local viral infection or the effect of inflammatory mediators.
- *Bacterial:* most cases probably occur by spread of nasopharyngeal organisms to the usually sterile sinuses. Sinus obstruction prevents effective clearance, and bacterial growth leads to destruction of epithelial cells, inflammatory infiltration, and the formation of mucus and pus.
- *Fungal* sinusitis may be noninvasive (two forms: allergic fungal sinusitis or sinus mycetoma) or invasive (occurs in hospitalized or immunocompromised patients). There are three forms of invasive sinusitis: acute fulminant (high mortality rate), chronic, and granulomatous.

Clinical features

- *Viral infections:* cough, sneeze, nasal discharge (clear or purulent) and obstruction, headache, and facial pressure may occur in viral infections.
- *Bacterial infections:* high fever and facial pain are characteristic. Sphenoid sinus infection may cause severe headache and sensory changes. Advanced frontal sinusitis may cause swelling and edema of the forehead as pus collects under the periosteum.
- *Nosocomial cases:* infection may not be apparent if the patient is unwell or unconscious (on intensive care unit [ICU]).
- *Allergic fungal sinusitis:* consider this in patients with intractable sinusitis, and a history of allergic rhinitis and nasal polyposis.
- *Sinus mycetoma:* symptoms of sinusitis plus gravel-like material from the nose. It is often found incidentally on CT scan.
- *Acute invasive fungal sinusitis:* fever, cough, nasal discharge, headache, confusion, dark ulcers on the septum, turbinates, and palate
- *Chronic invasive fungal sinusitis:* long history; may have reduced vision or ocular mobility (mass in the superior orbit)
- *Granulomatous invasive fungal sinusitis:* chronic sinusitis and proptosis, bone erosion. It is often rapidly progressive.

Complications

These include meningitis, brain abscess, subdural empyema, cavernous sinus and cortical vein thrombosis, orbital cellulitus and abscess, and Pott's puffy tumor (osteomyelitis, usually staphylococcal, of frontal bone).

Diagnosis

Most cases are diagnosed clinically. Consider a bacterial etiology in those whose symptoms fail to improve or worsen after 1 week.

Nosocomial cases present during the second week of hospitalization.

- *Radiology:* an air–fluid level on skull X-ray correlates well with a positive bacterial aspirate culture, but sensitivity is low.
- *Microbiology:* sinus cavity specimens must be collected by sinus puncture and aspiration via the antrum below the inferior turbinate; 60% of aspirates are positive in suspected bacterial sinusitis.

Treatment

Two-thirds of cases resolve spontaneously, reflecting the fact that many of these have a viral etiology. Decongestants may relieve symptoms of obstruction but have no effect on sinus drainage.

Patients who do not respond to antimicrobial therapy should be considered for sinus puncture and lavage to avoid progression.

For bacterial disease, treatment is usually given empirically. Amoxicillin-clavulanate cefuroxime, and quinolones such as levofloxacin have been shown to be effective, and treatment should be continued for 10 days. Those with severe infection or complications such as intracranial extension should receive intravenous therapy with broad-spectrum agents until culture results are available. These groups require CT or MRI imaging and may need diagnostic lumbar puncture or surgical interventions. Nosocomial cases may require broader therapy than that for community-acquired disease.

Fungal infection (community acquired) is effectively treated by surgical debridement. Complicated cases and immunocompromised patients are likely to need a combination of surgical and antifungal therapy.

Mastoiditis

Pathogenesis

The mastoid bone is penetrated by airspaces that are lined with modified respiratory mucosa and are connected via the antrum to the middle ear. It is clinically important, as it is adjacent to many important structures: the posterior and middle cranial fossae, the sigmoid and lateral sinuses, the facial nerve canal, and the semicircular canals.

The advent of antibiotics has brought the incidence of clinically significant mastoiditis to very low levels. Infection of the mastoid leads to the collection of purulent exudates within the air cells. The thin bony septa necrose, and pus coalesces into cavities.

Clinical features

Acute mastoiditis is accompanied by acute middle ear infection. Shortly after the onset of the signs of acute otitis media, pain, swelling, and erythema develop over the mastoid. The pinna may be displaced downward and tympanic perforation is followed by a purulent discharge.

Chronic disease may lead to erosion through the roof of the antrum (causing a temporal lobe abscess) or extend posteriorly (where it may cause thrombosis of the lateral sinus).

Diagnosis

Plain X-ray may show something of the destruction of bony septa and inflammation of the air cells. CT demonstrates the extent of the disease. It is useful to obtain fresh pus as it exudes from the tympanic membrane to enable culture of material from the middle ear.

Treatment

Treatment is with systemic antibiotics providing cover for *S. pneumoniae* and *H. influenzae*, as well as *S. aureus* and gram-negative organisms in cases that have had a prolonged course. Therapy can be modified once culture results are available.

Mastoidectomy is indicated in those cases where a mastoid abscess has formed and should be performed once sepsis has been adequately controlled

Otitis externa

Otitis externa is bacterial and, less commonly, fungal infection of the external auditory canal.

Pathogenesis

The external auditory canal is ~2.5 cm long. The lateral half is cartilaginous and the medial half runs through the temporal bone with a narrowing at the junction between the two. The bacterial flora is that of skin elsewhere: *S. epidermidis*, *S. aureus*, and some anaerobes. In situations in which the skin becomes damaged, these organisms may proliferate, resulting in infection and inflammation of the skin itself.

In addition to native organisms, invasive disease may be caused by gram-negative species such as *Pseudomonas aeruginosa*. Fungal species such as *Aspergillus* and *Candida albicans* may also cause otitis externa.

Clinical features and therapy

Acute localized otitis externa may be due to a pustule (*S. aureus*) or erysipelas (group A streptococci) involving the canal. There may be regional lymphadenopathy. Systemic antibiotics are usually curative; surgical drainage is rarely necessary.

Acute diffuse otitis externa

A large portion of the canal skin becomes edematous, red, itchy, and painful. Gram-negative bacteria (e.g., *P. aeruginosa*) are important causative organisms. Cases occur in humid weather and may be associated with swimming.

Irrigation with saline and alcohol and acetic acid mixes may help. Neomycin/hydrocortisone ear drops or oral antibiotics with topical hydrocortisone reduce inflammation and speed resolution.

Chronic otitis externa

This is due to discharge through a perforated tympanic membrane secondary to chronic suppurative otitis media, which results in irritation of the external canal. Rare causes are TB, leprosy, and sarcoid.

Invasive otitis externa

This severe, necrotizing infection is usually caused by *P. aeruginosa*. It is seen in the elderly, diabetics, and immunocompromised patients and is characterized by infection spreading from the skin of the external auditory canal to the tissue, vessels, and bone beneath.

Symptoms include pain and tenderness of the tissue around the ear, and pus discharging from the canal. Disease may be life threatening in those cases where the sigmoid sinus, skull base, and meninges become involved. Cranial nerves 7, 9, 10, and 12 may be affected (sometimes permanently).

Diagnosis can be confirmed and the extent of tissue damage ascertained on CT or MRI. Necrotic tissue may need removing and topical steroids and antipseudomonal antibiotics combined with systemic therapy for 4–6 weeks. Underlying disease should be identified and treated.

Otitis media

Otitis media is an acute inflammatory condition characterized by fluid in the middle ear. It is a common cause of fever, pain, and hearing impairment in children and may cause sequelae in adults.

Epidemiology

The most frequent diagnosis made by general practitioners is in those <15 years old. By the age of 3 years, two-thirds of children have had at least one episode. It complicates one-third of respiratory infections and occurs at higher rates in children attending daycare centers.

Most children with recurrent or severe disease have no obvious predisposition. There is increased risk in those with anatomical abnormalities (e.g., cleft uvula) and immune deficiency (e.g., HIV infection).

It is more common in males and tends to be more severe in Native Americans and Australian aborigines.

Pathogenesis

Dysfunction of the Eustachian tube, e.g., due to mucosal congestion, leads to accumulation of middle ear secretions, which provide a hospitable environment for bacteria.

S. pneumoniae is the most frequent bacterial cause of otitis media. *H. influenzae* is the second most common cause, of which only 10% are caused by type B. Other bacterial causes include group A streptococci and *Moraxella catarrhalis*.

Causes of chronic suppurative otitis media are *P. aeruginosa*, *S. aureus*, *Corynebacterium* spp., and *Klebsiella pneumoniae*. Uncommon causes include *Chlamydia trachomatis* (in infants <6 months of age), diphtheria, and TB.

Respiratory viruses (e.g., rhinovirus, RSV, influenza) cause up to 25% of clinical cases and may coinfect with bacteria.

Clinical features

Acute otitis media

There is fluid in the middle ear with features of acute illness such as ear pain, discharge, hearing loss, fever, and lethargy. Vertigo, nystagmus, and tinnitus may occur. Tympanic erythema is an early feature but is not specific to middle ear infection. Otitis media with effusion ("glue ear") is seen in 10% of children (90% of those with cleft palates).

The presence of fluid is associated with hearing impairment, and children with a history of recurrent episodes of acute otitis media show delay in speech and language abilities.

Chronic suppurative otitis media

In this condition, inflammation of the middle ear lasts ≥6 weeks and is associated with discharge. Some authorities consider a single infection that resolves leaving a persistent effusion to be "chronic otitis media."

Diagnosis

- *Detecting fluid:* use techniques that assess the mobility of the tympanic membrane (e.g., pneumatic otoscopy, tympanometry) or the difference in acoustic reflectivity between a fluid-filled or air-filled middle ear.
- *Culture* is not usually attempted. Causative organisms are well defined and routinely covered in antibiotic therapy. Take blood cultures and local samples if patients are severely unwell or have infection elsewhere.

Even after therapy and the resolution of acute features, fluid persists for some weeks (10% of children still have fluid at 3 months after infection). Tympanocentesis may be warranted in those with immune impairment, those unresponsive to antibiotic therapy, or the critically ill.

Management

Acute otitis media

Uncomplicated cases with no systemic features usually resolve without antibiotic therapy (~25% are viral). Consider antibiotics after 72 hours if there is no improvement or if symptoms worsen. Agents must achieve good middle ear penetration, e.g., oral amoxicillin (erythromycin if allergic). Amoxicillin-clavulanate or ceftriaxone should be considered if there is no improvement after 24–48 hours.

Ensure gram-negative coverage in newborn infants or the immunosuppressed or for suppurative chronic otitis media. If the tympanic membrane has perforated, culture and sensitivity testing of discharge may guide antibiotic choice.

Recurrent episodes of acute infection

Antibiotic prophylaxis (e.g., oral amoxicillin) may benefit those experiencing well-documented recurrent episodes. Consider it in those patients experiencing two episodes in the first 6 months of life or three episodes in 6 months for older children. It reduces the number of febrile episodes attributable to otitis media. There is a risk of side effects and selection of resistant organisms. Patients should be reviewed monthly and assessed for the presence of an asymptomatic effusion

Xylitol is a polyol sugar alcohol that inhibits bacterial colonization and, used by children in chewing gum form (5 times a day!), has been shown to reduce the number of episodes of acute otitis media

The Advisory Committee on Immunization Practices (ACIP) recommends pneumococcal conjugate vaccine (PCV13) for all children aged 2–59 months. The ACIP also recommends PCV13 for children aged 60–71 months with underlying medical conditions that increase their risk for pneumococcal disease or complications. Hib vaccination prevents only 10% of cases caused by *H. influenzae* (90% are non-type B).

Persistent effusion

Systemic antibiotics are not usually indicated. Refer patient to ENT if glue ear persists for >1–2 months. Interventions include the following:

- *Myringotomy*, once commonplace, is now used only in cases of intractable pain, for drainage of a persistent effusion unresponsive to medical therapy, or to speed the resolution of mastoid infection
- *Adenoidectomy* may improve Eustachian tube function in selected children and reduce the time spent with effusion.
- *Tympanostomy tubes* are placed in the tympanic membrane to allow ventilation and drainage in cases of persistent effusions unresponsive to medical therapy over 3 months.

Chronic suppurative otitis media

Thorough cleaning with microsuction may resolve long-standing infection. Acute exacerbations of chronic infection will require systemic therapy with broad cover (e.g., amoxicillin and metronidazole) and may need to be given parenterally.

Dental infections

Pathogenesis

Fermentation of dietary carbohydrates by bacteria (e.g., *S. mutans* and lactobacilli) leads to acid production and dental caries.

Dental caries erodes protective enamel, allowing bacteria access to the dentin and pulp. In the pulp, infection may track through the root, reaching the medullary cavity of the maxilla or mandible.

Advanced infection perforates the bony cortex, draining into tissues of the oral cavity or deep fascial planes. Neutropenic patients are at particular risk of sepsis and airway compromise.

Clinical features

Local infections

There is local pain, edema, and sensitivity to percussion and temperature. Severe local infections may be associated with abscess formation.

Mandibular infection

This involves pain and local swelling (e.g., infection of the mandibular incisors causing submental space infection may produce midline swelling beneath the chin; sublingual space infection may cause swelling of the floor of the mouth and tongue elevation). Retropharyngeal infection may follow molar infection (p. 533). Horner's syndrome or cranial nerve palsies may follow involvement of deep areas of the neck.

Buccal space infection

Buccal space infection due to infection of posterior teeth may cause facial edema. Masticator space infection causes trismus, is typically indicated by cheek edema, and is due to infection of posterior teeth, usually premolar or molar.

Ludwig's angina

This is a severe cellulitus of the floor of the mouth; 75% of odontogenic cases follow infection of the second or third mandibular molars. Features include elevation and swelling of the tongue, drooling, airway obstruction, and sensation of choking or suffocating (from which it gets its name). It is polymicrobial in nature and can cause widespread infection.

Vincent's angina

This is an acute necrotizing ulcerative gingivitis that presents with oral pain, bleeding gums, fetid breath, fever, anorexia, and lymphadenopathy. It is caused by invasive fusiform bacteria and spirochetes. On examination patients have ulcerated interdental papillae, with necrosis and pseudomembrane formation over the tonsils and gums.

Differential includes candidiasis, HSV stomatitis, and diphtheria. Material swabbed from the affected area should be cultured.

Treatment is with penicillin V and metronidazole or amoxicillin-clavulanate.

Risk factors include poor dental hygiene, smoking, and severe intercurrent illness. A rare complication in the immunocompromised is progression to noma, a gangrenous stomatitis.

Management

Airway protection is paramount.

Dental X-ray, facial series, or soft tissue X-ray of the neck may help localize the region involved. A CT scan is necessary in more advanced infections.

Localized infections may respond to oral antibiotics. Patients who appear unwell should be given IV antibiotics initially. More extensive infection and abscesses may require surgical intervention.

Lateral pharyngeal abscess

Infection of the lateral pharyngeal space may complicate pharyngitis, tonsillitis, mastoiditis, and dental abscesses.
- Caused by mixed organisms
- Anterior infection may present with fever, pain, trimus, swelling below the mandible, dysphagia, and displacement of the tonsil

toward the midline. Posterior infection may present with sepsis and little pain
- Complications include systemic sepsis, respiratory obstruction (laryngeal edema), thrombosis of the internal jugular, and erosion of the internal carotid.
- Management is with airway protection, parenteral antibiotic, and surgical drainage.

Acute bronchitis

This is a syndrome of tracheal and bronchial inflammation associated with respiratory infection. Diagnoses peak in the winter months and are made most frequently in children less than 5 year of age.

Etiology
Viral causes are most common: rhinoviruses, coronaviruses, adenovirus, and influenza (acute bronchitis cases are common during flu outbreaks). Other viruses (e.g., measles) are uncommon but produce severe disease.

Less common bacterial causes include *Mycoplasma pneumoniae*, *Chlamydophila pneumoniae*, and *Bordetella pertussis*.

Pathogenesis
The exact nature of pathogenesis varies among viruses. Some (e.g., influenza) invade the lower respiratory tract. Others (e.g., rhinovirus) do not, and symptoms may be secondary to inflammatory mediators. Either way, the outcome is an inflamed edematous tracheobronchial tree with increased secretions. The extent of epithelial damage varies with the etiological agent.

Attack severity may be increased by exposure to irritants such as cigarette smoke and may lead to long-term airway damage. Patients with acute bronchitis are more likely to have a history of atopic disease, which may be associated with airway hyperreactivity.

Some cases progress to develop adult-onset asthma.

Clinical features
Severe, prolonged cough distinguishes acute bronchitis from other respiratory syndromes such as the common cold. It lasts over 4 weeks in over 40% of patients. Cough may be productive early on but is typically dry.

Cough and respiration may be associated with retrosternal pain in those cases with severe tracheal inflammation. Dyspnea and more severe respiratory symptoms are seen only in those with underlying chest disease. Fever is seen in some cases, most frequently with agents such as influenza or *M. pneumoniae*.

Diagnosis
Bronchitis is a diagnosis of exclusion, and a complete history and examination should be performed, seeking any more serious cause of cough.

Vaccination and exposure histories may point to a specific etiological agent, e.g., influenza or pertussis infection (a common cause of bronchitis in adults whose childhood vaccine immunity is waning).

Cultures of respiratory secretions may be useful in looking for specific viruses or agents such as *M. pneumonia* or *B. pertussis*, but routine bacteriological culture is unhelpful in defining a cause of bronchitis.

Those in whom cough persists beyond a reasonable duration of illness should be investigated for other causes (e.g., foreign body, tuberculosis, malignancy).

Treatment

Healthy patients do not usually require any therapy other than management of cough.

Those with severe bronchitis (particularly those with underlying heart or lung disease) may develop respiratory impairment and require oxygen or ventilatory assistance.

Cough suppression has traditionally been attempted with codeine-based agents such as dextromethorphan. However randomized controlled trials (RCTs) (albeit small) have found no significant difference in cough severity between such agents and placebo in children or adults with acute bronchitis. The FDA recommends that children under age 2 not receive decongestants or cough suppressants and that children under the age of 6 should not receive medications containing hydrocodone.

The FDA review conducted in 2007 found 54 reports of deaths in children associated with decongestant medicines made with pseudoephedrine, phenylephrine, or ephedrine. It also found 69 reports of deaths associated with antihistamine medicines containing diphenhydramine, brompheniramine, or chlorpheniramine.

NSAIDs, sedating antihistamines such as diphenhydramine (the cough suppressant component of many commercial "cough mixtures"), and short courses of inhaled steroids are widely used but, their efficacy remains unproven.[1]

Antibiotics should be used only in those cases in which a bacterial cause is suspected. There is no evidence that extended-spectrum agents are more effective than amoxicillin or doxycycline. Specific therapies for viral and bacterial causes are covered in the appropriate sections.

Smoking should be actively discouraged.

Reference

1. Schroeder K, Fahey T (2003). Over the counter medications for acute cough in children and adults in ambulatory settings (Cochrane review). *The Cochrane Library*, Issue 1. Oxford: Update Software.

Chronic bronchitis

Chronic bronchitis is defined as a cough productive of sputum on most days during at least 3 months of two successive years that cannot be attributed to other specific diseases (e.g., TB, bronchiectasis). When airflow obstruction exists, the patient has chronic obstructive pulmonary disease (COPD), which may coexist with emphysema.

Epidemiology

Chronic bronchitis is common, affecting 10–25% of the adult population. Men are affected more than women and it is more common in those >40 years of age.

Associations include cigarette smoking (although only 15% of smokers develop chronic bronchitis), pollution, and exposure to allergens.

Pathogenesis

Even modest smoking is associated with increased alveolar macrophages, inflammation of the respiratory bronchioles, epithelial hyperplasia, and fibrosis of the bronchiolar and alveolar walls.

The inflammation and edema seen in patients with chronic bronchitis results from the interaction between exogenous irritants and the pathological response, including: an increase in bronchial mucus-secreting cells, granulocytic infiltration in response to chemokines produced by epithelial cells, increased airway secretions, and the production of neuropeptides promoting bronchospasm.

Acute exacerbations of disease may be related to bacterial infections. Pathogenic bacteria can be cultured from the bronchi of most chronic bronchitics (as well as those with other lung pathologies such as TB), and the development of purulent sputum is not associated with the appearance of specific organisms but does correlate with an increase in number.

H. influenza and *S. pneumoniae* are found in half of chronic bronchitics. Organisms such as *M. pneumoniae, Staphylococcus aureus,* and gram-negative organisms are identified infrequently. One-third of acute exacerbations are thought to be due to viral infections.

Clinical features

There is frequent productive cough, which is most severe in the morning, when patients may produce large amounts of sputum that may be mucoid and white or obviously purulent in appearance.

Patients may be incapacitated only when they develop acute infections; however, most patients have some degree of airflow limitation. COPD exists as a spectrum of clinical disease, with emphysema predominant at one end (breathless, less sputum, fewer infections, barrel-chest with hyperexpanded clear lungs) and bronchitis predominant at the other (productive coughing, frequent infections, wheeze, widespread crepitations, and right heart failure in severe cases).

Diagnosis

Acute exacerbations of chronic bronchitis can be difficult to identify. Most patients do not develop fever or leukocytosis. Diagnosis is made on symptoms such as an increase in sputum production or a change in color with increasing cough and breathlessness.

CXR is useful only in the exclusion of other illnesses.

Treatment

General measures

- Exclude other causes of recurrent chest infections and have a high index of suspicion for lung malignancy.

- Smoking cessation, weight control, avoidance of environmental irritants, and assessment for allergic disease
- Record of baseline spirometry, arterial blood gas (ABG) and oxygen saturations
- Pneumococcal and influenza vaccinations
- Pulmonary rehabilitation program and postural drainage when appropriate

Maintenance therapy to improve airflow obstruction symptoms

For example, regular inhaled steroids, B_2-agonists, and anticholinergic agents can be used. Give oral steroids as required.

Prophylactic antibiotics may be useful in selected patients with very frequent exacerbations (four or more per year). Most specialists believe they do not have a role in routine treatment because of concerns over the development of resistance.

RCTs prior to 1970 demonstrated that chronic bronchitis patients using prophylactic antibiotics had a small but significant reduction in exacerbations compared to placebo, and antibiotics significantly reduced the number of days of disability per person per month treated. There are no contemporary studies.

Intensive therapy for acute exacerbations

- Intensification of normal therapy (e.g., course of oral steroids)
- *Antibiotic therapy:* infection can cause respiratory decompensation (a common cause of death in these patients), and despite difficulties in assessing their efficacy, antibiotic therapy does improve clinical outcome. They are usually given orally for 7–10 days. Specific agents are best determined locally and with reference to previous microbial sensitivities.

Bronchiolitis

Bronchiolitis is an acute infection of the lower respiratory tract characterized by the acute onset of wheeze and associated with cough, nasal discharge, breathlessness, and respiratory distress.

Etiology

RSV (see Respiratory synctial virus, p. 21) accounts for up to 75% of cases. Other viruses, e.g., parainfluenza types 1–3, adenoviruses, rhinoviruses, influenza, and *Mycoplasma pneumoniae* have been implicated.

Epidemiology

In temperate regions, cases peak in winter and early spring (RSV) with small peaks in autumn (parainfluenza). Most cases occur in children aged between 2 and 10 months.

Estimated incidence varies widely; 80% of children have evidence of previous RSV infection by their second birthday. A UK study estimated the total mean annual incidence of hospital admissions of children aged <1 year attributable to RSV at 28.3 per 1000.

Factors associated with high rates of hospitalization with bronchiolitis are young age, young maternal age, living in crowded or polluted areas, a large number of siblings, airway hyperreactivity, and RSV identified as the cause.

Pathogenesis

Virus infects the upper respiratory mucosa and spreads to the lower airways. Bronchial and bronchiolar inflammation and necrosis follow with edema and peribronchiolar mononuclear cell infiltration. In severe cases, interstitial pneumonitis may develop.

Inflammation and edema reduce airway caliber. Necrotic material may block small airways. Distally trapped air is later absorbed, resulting in multiple areas of atelectasis and a low ventilation/perfusion ratio. Children become breathless and tachypnoeic, developing respiratory distress and respiratory failure in severe cases.

Infants who develop wheeze with respiratory virus infection in early life are more likely to have some form of recurrent lower respiratory tract disease. Whether this is related to a propensity to atopy or to pre-existing lung dysfunction or has a viral etiology is not clear.

Clinical features

Mild fever and signs of URTI occur. This progresses after 2–3 days to lower respiratory tract features, with cough, a raised respiratory rate, anorexia, lethargy, and wheeze. Fever may resolve.

Severe cases develop tachypnea, tachycardia, and signs of increased breathing work (nasal flaring, chest wall retraction, grunting). Cyanosis is rare, even in the presence of hypoxia. Apnea is relatively common in young infants hospitalized with RSV infection.

Auscultatory findings are variable: wheeze, crepitations, and decreased breath sounds in severe cases. Other findings are dehydration, otitis media, and diarrhea. Symptoms begin to settle after 2–3 days, with recovery taking 2 weeks or more.

Diagnosis

General features: the white cell count may be elevated in severe cases. CXR findings include hyperinflation, hyperlucent parenchyma, and multiple areas of atelectasis; pneumonia may be present. Findings do not correlate with clinical severity.

Diagnosis is usually clinical in the setting of a seasonal outbreak. Other causes of wheeze and dyspnea must be considered (e.g., a first episode of asthma, gastric reflux and aspiration, congestive cardiac failure, or airway obstruction by a foreign body).

The specific agent may be identified from respiratory secretions (preferably a nasopharyngeal aspirate) by tissue culture or PCR. Positive predictive value diminishes outside the setting of an epidemic. Serology is rarely helpful.

Treatment

General measures include providing oxygen to maintain the saturation above 92% and ventilation if indicated. Bronchodilators are often given but are of limited benefit. Corticosteroids are often used and have been reported to bring about a modest improvement in symptoms but with no effect on the duration of hospitalization.

Ribavirin may be given to hospitalized infants at risk of severe disease by aerosol for 8–12 hours a day for 2–5 days. Such children include those with underlying cardiac or respiratory disease or the premature. Although ribavirin has been shown to speed the improvement in oxygenation, its use does not result in shorter hospital stays.

Prevention

Palivizumab is a humanized monoclonal antibody directed against the F glycoprotein of RSV. It is indicated for the prevention of respiratory syncytial virus infection in infants at high risk of severe disease. It may also be given to at-risk exposed pediatric inpatients.

The American Academy of Pediatrics has issued guidelines for palivizumab administration. Children at risk are those who are younger than 2 months of age with chronic lung disease or prematurity receiving medical care within the 6 months prior to RSV season; infants born before 32 weeks of gestation; infants born at 32 to <35 weeks of gestation, particularly when one of the following risk factors is present: the infant attends child care or one or more children under age 5 live in the same household; infants with congenital abnormalities of the airway or neuromuscular disease; and infants or children younger than 24 months of age with hemodynamically significant congenital heart disease.

Prophylaxis for premature infants should extend until the infant reaches 90 days or a maximum of 3 doses. For infants with congenital heart disease, congenital lung disease, or birth before 32 weeks gestation, only 5 total doses are recommended.

Palivizumab is given IM monthly during the RSV season, the first dose being given prior to the start of the season.

Complications

Infants with underlying cardiac or pulmonary disease or immunodeficiency are at greatest risk of severe disease with respiratory failure and prolonged hypoxia.

Although up to 75% of infants requiring hospital admission have recurrent episodes of bronchospasm within the first 2 years after recovery, the number continuing to experience such episodes drops year by year. The majority with long-term problems tend to either have a predisposition to atopy or have reduced lung function at birth.

Community-acquired pneumonia

Epidemiology

Incidence is 71 per 100 people per year; 20–40% of cases require hospital admission. Mortality varies with the patient group (overall, 5–10%; 50% in those requiring ICU admission).

Peak age is 50–70 years and onset is mid-winter and early spring; 58–89% have underlying disease (e.g., COPD, diabetes, cardiovascular disease, immunosuppression).

Some organisms are acquired by person-to-person spread or are existing commensals (S. pneumoniae, H. influenzae). Others are acquired from the environment (L. pneumophilia) or animals (C. psittaci).

About 80% of community-acquired pneumonia (CAP) cases are managed in primary care. Viruses, S. pneumoniae, and M. pneumoniae are the most common causes.

Risk factors include extremes of age, smoking, COPD, diabetes, cardiovascular disease, severe intercurrent illness, recent anesthesia or intubation, and immunosuppression (see Table 4.2).

Table 4.2 Epidemiological conditions and/or risk factors related to specific pathogens in community-acquired pneumonia

Condition	Commonly encountered pathogen(s)
Alcoholism	Streptococcus pneumoniae, oral anaerobes, Klebsiella pneumoniae, Acinetobacter species, Mycobacterium tuberculosis
COPD and/or smoking	Haemophilus influenzae, Pseudomonas aeruginosa, Legionella spp, S. pneumoniae, Moraxella cararrhalis, Chlamydophila pneumoniae
Aspiration	Gram-negative enteric pathogens, oral anaerobes
Lung abscess	CA-MRSA, oral anaerobes, endemic fungal pneumonia, M. tuberculosis, atypical mycobacteria
Exposure to bat/bird droppings	Histoplasma capsulatum
Exposure to birds	Chlamydophila psittaci (if poultry: avian influenza)
Exposure to rabbits	Francisella tularensis
Exposure to farm animals or parturient cats	Coxiella burnetti (Q fever)
HIV infection (early)	S. pneumoniae, H. influenzae, M. tuberculosis
HIV infection (late)	Pathogens listed for early infection plus Pneumocystis jirovecii, Cryptococcus, Histoplasma, Aspergillus, atypical mycobacteria (especially Mycobacterium kansasii), P. aeruginosa, H. influenzae
Hotel or cruise ship stay in previous 2 weeks	Legionella species

Table 4.2 (*Contd.*)

Condition	Commonly encountered pathogen(s)
Travel to or residence in southwestern United States	*Coccidioides* species, *Hantavirus*
Travel to or residence in Southeast and East Asia	*Burkholderia pseudomallei*, avian influenza, SARS
Influenza active in community	Influenza, *S. pneumoniae*, *Staphylococcus aureus*, *H. influenzae*
Cough >2 weeks with whoop or posttussive vomiting	*Bordetella pertussis*
Structural lung disease (e.g., bronchiectasis)	*Pseudomonas aeruginosa*, *Burkholderia cepacia*, *S. aureus*
Injection drug use	*S. aureus*, anaerobes, *M. tuberculosis*, *S. pneumoniae*
Endobronchial obstruction	Anaerobes, *S. pneumoniae*, *H. influenzae*, *S. aureus*
In context of bioterrorism	*Bacillus anthracis* (anthrax), *Yersinia pestis* (plague), *Francisella tularensis* (tularemia)

CA-MRSA, community-acquired methicillin-resistant *Staphylococcus aureus*; COPD, chronic obstructive pulmonary disease; SARS, severe acute respiratory syndrome.

Reprinted with permission from the Infectious Diseases Society of America/American Thoracic Society Consensus Guidelines on the Management of Community-Acquired Pneumonia in Adults. CID 2007; 44(Suppl 2):S27–S72. Copyright The University of Chicago Press.

Etiology

Organisms vary by country, study, age, and patient group (e.g., *Moraxella* and *H. influenzae* are more common in COPD). Pneumonia in childhood is usually viral.

Common bacterial isolates vary with age:
- 0–1 month: *E. coli*, group B *Streptococcus*, *Listeria monocytogenes*
- 1–6 months: *Chlamydia trachomatis*, *S. aureus*, RSV
- 6 months to 5 years – RSV, parainfluenza viruses
- 5–15 years: *Mycoplasma pneumoniae*, influenza
- 16–30 years: *M. pneumoniae*, *S. pneumoniae*
- Older adults: *Streptococcus pneumoniae*, *Haemophilus influenzae*

Some infections, e.g., *M. pneumoniae*, are associated with epidemics. *S. pneumoniae* infection is associated with viral illness, e.g., influenza.

Mixed infections are more common in the elderly; *S. aureus* and gram-negatives are seen more frequently among those in residential care.

Severe disease occurs with *S. pneumoniae*, MRSA, *L. pneumophilia*, and gram-negative organisms. Mortality is 20–53%.

Rare causes of pneumonia include anthrax, plague, and melioidosis.

Pneumocystis jiroveci (p. 439) is an important cause in HIV-infected patients, who are also at increased risk of infection with mycobacteria, *C. neoformans*, and viruses (e.g., CMV).

Clinical features

History

Most patients present with sudden-onset chills, fever, cough, mucopurulent sputum, pleuritic chest pain, fatigue, anorexia, sweats, and nausea; 20% do not have cough. Ask about predisposing conditions, travel, and exposure to animals.

Symptoms and signs

These include fever, tachypnea, tachycardia, postural blood pressure drop (may indicate dehydration), and consolidation (absent in ~70%). Signs of respiratory distress occur in severe cases. All findings are less pronounced in the elderly, in whom presentation may be insidious (confusion, abdominal pain).

Other findings include herpes labialis (40% of pneumococcal pneumonia patients) and bullous myringitis (*Mycoplasma Pneumoniae*).

Investigations

Blood tests

Full blood count shows neutrophilia, or neutropenia if very unwell. Biochemical abnormalities include raised urea, hyponatremia (especially in the elderly due to syndrome of inappropriate antidiuretic hormone secretion [SIADH]), abnormal LFTs, (especially *legionella*), and raised CRP.

CXR changes are nonspecific:
- Lobar consolidation, cavitation, and effusions suggest a bacterial cause
- A CXR worse than examination findings suggests mycoplasmal or viral pneumonia.
- Diffuse bilateral involvement may suggest pneumocystis pneumonia (PCP), *Legionella* infection, or primary viral pneumonia.
- Pneumatoceles may be seen in pneumonia caused by *S. aureus*, *K. pneumoniae*, *H. influenzae*, and *S. pneumoniae*.

CT is useful in recurrent pneumonias or those unresponsive to therapy (e.g., to identify a tumor). In immunocompromised patients, some pathogens (e.g., *Aspergillus*) have typical CT appearances that aid in diagnosis.

Microbiological investigations

Microbiological tests are not routinely recommended for patients managed in the community. Consider them in those who do not respond to empirical antibiotic therapy or in whom unusual pathogens are suspected.
- *Blood culture:* positive in only 1–16% of hospitalized patients with CAP (≤25% of cases of pneumococcal pneumonia)
- *Sputum examination* has low sensitivity; ~50% of sputum cultures are negative even in proven bacterial cases. Sputum examination is, however, useful in the identification of organisms such as *Legionella* spp., *Pseudomonas* spp., *Burkholderia* spp., *M. tuberculosis*, and *P. carinii*.

- *Serology:* severely ill patients with symptoms for 5–7 days should have serum tested for antibodies to atypical pathogens (*Legionella, Mycoplasma, Chlamydia* spp.). Take a second specimen 7–10 days later.
- *Antigen testing:* urinary *Legionella* antigen testing should be performed on all patients with severe disease and at least 5 days of symptoms. Some authorities also recommend pneumococcal antigen testing.
- *Bronchoalveolar lavage (BAL):* a bronchoscope is used to instill sterile fluid into a segment of lung and the fluid examined microscopically and cultured. A threshold of 10^4 colony-forming units (CFU)/mL is used to define significant isolates. It is particularly useful in diagnosis of *M. tuberculosis, Pneumocystis jiroveci,* CMV, and ventilator-associated pneumonia (VAP).
- *Pleural fluid sampling:* where positive, pleural fluid cultures are specific for the organism causing the underlying pneumonia. Fluid analysis helps differentiate other causes of lung disease (e.g., TB, tumor).
- *Other tests:* immunofluorescence or PCR for respiratory viruses; immunofluorescence for *Chlamydia* spp.; cold agglutinins for *M. pneumoniae* (<25% positive), lung biopsy (e.g., immunosuppressed patients with no diagnosis)

Severity assessment

The CURB-65 score (**C**onfusion, **U**rea, **R**espiratory rate, **B**lood pressure, age **65** or over) enables rapid assessment of severity and guides initial management (Fig. 4.1).

Additional adverse features include hypoxia regardless of oxygen therapy (arterial oxygen saturation [SaO_2] <92% or partial pressure of arterial oxygen [PaO_2] <8 kPa), bilateral or multilobe involvement on CXR, positive blood cultures, and WCC <4 x 10^9/L or >20 x 10^9/L.

Severity should be reassessed regularly during the course of the illness. Other scoring systems include the PORT Severity Index (PSI). Use of scoring systems to determine the site of care should be supplemented by physician assessment of factors such as ability to safely and reliably take oral medication and availability of outpatient resources (ATS/IDSA Guidelines on Community Acquired Pneumonia; www.idsociety.org).

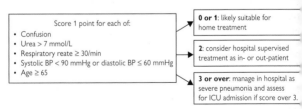

Fig. 4.1 The CURB-65 severity-assessment tool. DBP, diastolic blood pressure; SBP, systolic blood pressure.

Management

Antimicrobial guidelines from the American Thoracic Society/Infectious Diseases Society of America 2007 Guidelines are shown below. See also Table 4.2.

Table 4.3 Recommended empirical antibiotics for community-acquired pneumonia

Outpatient treatment

1. Previously healthy and no use of antimicrobials within the previous 3 months
   - A macrolide (strong recommendation; level I evidence)
   - Doxycyline (weak recommendation; level III evidence)
2. Presence of comorbidities such as chronic heart, lung, liver, or renal disease; diabetes mellitus; alcoholism; malignancies; asplenia; immunosuppressing conditions or use of immunosuppressing drugs; or use of antimicrobials within the previous 3 months (in which case an alternative from a different class should be selected)
   - A respiratory fluoroquinolone (moxifloxacin, gemifloxacin, or levofloxacin [750 mg]) (strong recommendation; level I evidence)
   - A β-lactam **plus** a macrolide (strong recommendation; level I evidence)
3. In regions with a high rate (>25%) of infection with high-level (MIC ≥16 mg/mL) macrolide-resistant *Streptococcus pneumoniae*, consider use of alternative agents listed above in (2) for patients without comorbidities (moderate recommendation; level III evidence)

Inpatients, non-ICU treatment

- A respiratory fluoroquinolone (strong recommendation; level I evidence)
- A β-lactam **plus** a macrolide (strong recommendation; level I evidence)

Inpatients, ICU treatment

- A β-lactam (cefotaxime, ceftriaxone, or ampicillin-sulbactam) **plus** either azithromycin (level II evidence) **or** a respiratory fluoroquinolone (level I evidence) (strong recommendation) (for penicillin-allergic patients, a respiratory fluoroquinolone and aztreonam are recommended)

Special concerns

If *Pseudomonas* is a consideration:
- An antipneumococcal, antipseudomonal β-lactam (piperacillintazobactam, cefepime, imipenem, or meropenem) plus either ciprofloxacin or levofloxacin (750 mg)

or
- The above β-lactam plus an aminoglycoside and azithromycin

or
- The above β-lactam plus an aminoglycoside and an antipneumococcal fluoroquinolone (for penicillin-allergic patients, substitute aztreonam for above β-lactam) (moderate recommendation; level III evidence)

If CA-MRSA is a consideration:
- Add vancomycin or linezolid (moderate recommendation; level III evidence)

CA-MRSA, community-acquired methicillin-resistant *Staphylococcus aureus*; ICU, intensive care unit.

Reprinted with permission from the Infectious Diseases Society of America/American Thoracic Society Consensus Guidelines on the Management of Community-Acquired Pneumonia in Adults. CID 2007: 44(Suppl 2): S27–S72. Copyright The University of Chicago Press.

- IV antibiotics should be switched to oral therapy as soon as there is evidence of clinical improvement (preferably within 48 hours). However, IV treatment may be continued in patients with severe infections caused by Legionella, S. aureus, or aerobic gram-negatives.
- 3 to 5 days' therapy is usually sufficient in uncomplicated cases. Treatment duration may be prolonged to 7–21 days in severe disease.
- CXR should be repeated at 6 weeks if symptoms persist or in those at increased risk of lung cancer (e.g., smokers).
- Failure to respond: adequately treated pneumonia will resolve clinically over 7–10 days. Older patients and those with underlying disease may take longer. CXR findings should normalize within 4 weeks but may take longer in the elderly, those with multilobe involvement, and those with pre-existing pulmonary disease. Consider infection with resistant organisms, underlying malignancy, empyema, or lung abscess. Additionally consider IV catheter infection or antibiotic-associated diarrhea in those with prolonged fever.

Complications
- Parapneumonic effusion
- Empyema (p. 563)
- Adult respiratory distress syndrome (ARDS)
- Sepsis syndrome
- Metastatic infection (meningitis, arthritis, endocarditis)
- Rare neurological sequelae may follow M. pneumoniae infection, e.g., meningoencephalitis, cranial nerve palsies, and Guillain–Barré syndrome (GBS).

Prevention
There is a pneumococcal polysaccharide vaccine available, made from the 23 capsular serotypes that cause over 90% of invasive infections.

References

British Thoracic Society (BTS) guidelines for community-acquired pneumonia 2004 update. Available from www.brit-thoracic.org.uk

Infectious Diseases Society of America (IDSA)/ American Thoracic Society (ATS) Consensus Guidelines on Management of Community Acquired Pneumonia in Adults (2007). Available from www.idsociety.org

Atypical pneumonias
These account for 7–28% of CAP. The term was originally used to describe cases that failed to respond to penicillin or sulfa drugs and in which no organism was identified. More recently it has meant those cases that start with an apparently mild respiratory tract illness (which may last up to 10 days) followed by pneumonia with dyspnea and cough with or without sputum.

Clinical signs tend to be milder than the CXR would suggest. It usually involves the lower lobes and may be unilateral or bilateral. The clinical course is usually benign, although certain organisms may cause extrapulmonary symptoms (e.g., mycoplasmal infection and neurological sequelae)

or severe disease (e.g., *Legionella*). CXR tends to improve faster than typical pneumonia.

It is good practice to avoid the term *atypical pneumonia*, although it is still useful to refer to *atypical organisms*, as they have certain features in common: they tend not to be respiratory tract colonizers, they affect healthy individuals of all age groups, they occur in epidemics, and they do not respond to penicillin.

Mycoplasma pneumoniae (p. 301)

This causes autumn epidemics every 4–8 years (more frequently within closed populations such as prisons). Infection is most common in children > 4 years and young adults.

Certain respiratory viruses cause a similar clinical picture (e.g., influenza, parainfluenza, adenovirus, RSV).

It resolves without complications in most cases, although the illness may last a few weeks, with a protracted cough.

It is difficult to culture; diagnosis is usually retrospective by serology.

Serum cold agglutination is a nonspecific test (positive in 50–70% of patients after 7–10 days of infection).

CXR appearance is of basal atelectasis or involvement of a single lower lobe, sometimes a nodular infiltration resembling that associated with other diseases with granulomatous pathology, such as TB, mycoses, and sarcoidosis.

Treatment is with erythromycin or azithromycin.

Rare complications include pericarditis, arthritis, Stevens–Johnson syndrome, hemolytic anemia, thrombocytopenia, CNS infections, GBS, peripheral neuropathy, other neurological manifestations, and ocular complications.

Legionella pneumophila (p. 268)

This accounts for 1–20% of CAP cases. It is more common in summer.

The organism colonizes water piping systems, and outbreaks are associated with acquisition from contaminated water sources, including cooling systems, showers, decorative fountains, humidifiers, respiratory therapy equipment, and whirlpool spas.

Risk factors include smoking, diabetes, malignancy, AIDS, end-stage renal disease (ESRD), and alcohol abuse.

Clinical features are a 1–2-day prodrome (mild headache and myalgias) followed by high fever, chills, and rigors, cough (nonproductive becoming productive as the disease progresses), dyspnea, pleuritic chest pain, hemoptysis, nausea, vomiting, diarrhea, abdominal pain, altered mental status, arthralgias, and myalgias. Consider it in those with a high fever, multilobar involvement, a need for ICU care, and rapidly evolving gastrointestinal (GI), neurological, and radiographic abnormalities.

Laboratory abnormalities include DIC, SIADH, abnormal LFTs, and renal impairment.

Treatment is with azithromycin or respiratory fluoroquinolone.

It has a 25% mortality rate (may be related to comorbidities).

Chlamydophila pneumoniae **(p. 306)**

This accounts for 3–10% of CAP cases in adults. It causes mild pneumonia or bronchitis in adolescents and young adults.

Incidence is highest in the elderly, who may experience more severe disease and repeated infections.

Mortality rate is ~9%.

Chlamydophila psittaci **(p. 305)**

This is usually associated with exposure to birds; pet shop employees and poultry industry workers are at risk.

The clinical spectrum ranges from an asymptomatic infection to fulminant toxicity.

Consider infection in those patients with pneumonia, splenomegaly, and a history of bird exposure (especially sick birds). Patients may develop rash, hepatitis, hemolytic anemia, DIC, meningoencephalitis, or reactive arthritis.

Treatment is with tetracycline.

The mortality rate is <1%.

Coxiella burnetii **(p. 298)**

This intracellular pathogen is found worldwide, with the exception of New Zealand. It is highly prevalent in parts of Spain and France (the second-most common cause of CAP in some regions).

The reservoir is primarily farm animals (e.g., cattle, goats, sheep). It is excreted in urine, milk, and feces and attains high concentration in birth products.

Rare human-to-human transmission occurs from exposure to the placenta of an infected woman and from blood transfusions.

Acute Q fever may cause a febrile illness, a pneumonia, or hepatitis. Most cases of acute Q fever resolve spontaneously within 2 weeks, although 14–21 days of treatment with doxycycline reduces symptom duration.

Aspiration pneumonia

Elderly patients, those with neurological impairment (e.g., acute phase of stroke), and others with altered consciousness (e.g., alcoholics) and abnormal swallow or gag reflexes are at risk of aspiration.

Acid aspiration results in the release of proinflammatory cytokines, which recruit neutrophils into the lung. These are thought to be the key mediators of acute lung injury, with bacterial pneumonia developing several days later, perhaps facilitated by bronchial obstruction by inhaled debris (e.g., peanut).

Abscess and empyema are not uncommon. Anaerobes on their own or mixed with aerobes are the most common bacteriological findings (e.g., *Bacteroides*, *Fusobacterium*).

Bronchoscopy may be indicated to provide material for culture and exclude foreign bodies.

Hospital-acquired pneumonia

Hospital-acquired pneumonia (HAP) is the leading cause of infection-related deaths in the hospital. HAP is defined as pneumonia developing more than 48 hours after admission. Hospital-acquired-type organisms should also be considered when choosing empiric therapy for individuals having frequent contact with the health care system (hemodialysis, chronic home infusion therapy, nursing home residents).

Sixty percent of cases are caused by aerobic gram-negatives, the majority being enterobacteria and *Pseudomonas* spp. Other causes include *S. aureus* and *S. penumoniae* and anaerobes.

Nosocomial outbreaks of viral pneumonia are not uncommon.

Risk factors include the following:

- *Patient related*: age >70 years, severe underlying disease, malnutrition, coma, metabolic acidosis, and possibly sinusitis
- *Infection control related*: poor health care worker hand hygiene, contaminated respiratory equipment
- *Intervention related*: sedatives, corticosteroids and cytotoxic drugs, prolonged antibiotic use, ventilation (risk of acquiring pneumonia 20 times that of unventilated patients)

Ventilator-associated pneumonia

Ventilator-associated pneumonia (VAP) complicates the course of 8–28% of patients receiving mechanical ventilation.[1]

Causes

The predominant organisms responsible for infection are *P. aeruginosa*, *S. aureus*, enterobacteria, *Haemophilus* spp., and *Acinetobacter* spp., but etiological agents vary according to ICU, duration of inpatient stay, and prior antibiotic use. Polymicrobial infections are common.

Pathogenesis

Intubation compromises the natural barrier between the orphraynx and the trachea and also facilitates entry of bacteria into the lung by polling and leakage of contaminated secretions around the endotracheal tube cuff.

Risk factors

These include hypoalbuminemia, age ≥60 years, ARDS, COPD, coma, burns, trauma, organ failure, gastric aspiration, gastric colonization and pH, upper respiratory tract colonization, sinusitis, H_2 receptor antagonists, paralytic agents, prior antibiotics, continuous sedation, mechanical ventilation >2 days, reintubation, tracheostomy, nasogastric tube, and supine position.

Clinical features

The diagnosis of VAP is based on three features: systemic signs of infection, new or worsening pulmonary infiltrates, and bacteriological evidence of parencyhmal infection. Patients present with purulent secretions, CXR changes, neutrophilia, fever, and increased ventilatory requirements.

The differential includes pulmonary embolism (PE), ARDS, and aspiration (chemical pneumonitis).

Diagnosis

Diagnosis can be difficult. Quantitative cultures of endotracheal aspirates may be misleading, as they may only reflect upper respiratory tract colonizers. Bronchoscopic sampling provides lower respiratory tract samples for microbiological analysis. This may be directed (i.e., in area of maximal pulmonary infiltrate) or nondirected.

Quantitative BAL cultures indicate the likelihood of infection, with >10^4 organisms/mL being diagnostic of infection. Some authorities recommend surveillance BALs in patients on ICU.

Treatment[2]

This should be targeted against the likely organism and antimicrobial susceptibility pattern. In early-onset VAP (≤4 days after hospital admission), the organisms are community acquired and unlikely to be multi-drug resistant. Treatment should be with ceftriaxone or fluoroquninolone or amoxicillin-clavulanate or ertapenem.

In late-onset VAP (>4 days after hospital admission), organisms are likely to be hospital flora and multi-drug resistant. Treatment is with an antipseudomonal cephalosporin or antipseudomonal penicillin (piperacillin) or carbapenem plus a fluoroquinolone or an aminoglycoside. Vancomycin should be added if there is a possibility of MRSA, which is a common cause of nosocomial pneumonia in many hospitals.

Prognosis

Mortality ranges from 24% to 76%. An update to the American Thoracic Society Guidelines for the Management of Hospital Acquired Pneumonia was released in fall 2010.

References

1. Chastre J, Fagon JY (2002). Ventilator associated pneumonia. *Am J Respir Crit Care Med* 165:867–903.

2. American Thoracic Society guidelines for hospital acquired, ventilator associated and health care associated pneumonia. *Am J Respir Crit Care Med* 2005;171:388–416.

Pulmonary infiltrates with eosinophilia

The differential diagnosis is broad and includes the following:
• Tropical eosinophilia
• Parasitic infections e.g., *Ascaris* or *Strongyloides*
• Tuberculosis
• Brucellosis
• Psittacosis
• Coccidioidomycosis
• Histoplasmosis

- Bronchopulmonary *Aspergillus*
- Drug allergy
- Sarcoidosis,
- Churg–Strauss syndrome
- Eosinophilic leukemia
- Hypersensitivity pneumonitis.

Empyema

Empyema is microbial infection of the pleural space. Prognosis can be poor in those cases where diagnosis is missed or therapy inadequate.

Etiology

Empyem is usually secondary to pneumonia. Cases may occur with no evidence of pneumonia (primary empyema). Other precipitants include surgery, trauma, esophageal perforation, and chest drains.

Common organisms in cases secondary to pneumonia are *S. aureus*, *S. pneumoniae*, and *S. pyogenes*. Incidence of *H. influenzae* has declined since the introduction of the Hib vaccine.

Cases associated with aspiration or arising from gastrointestinal sites are more likely to be due to anaerobic organisms. Those associated with subdiaphragmatic disease are often polymicrobial. Aerobic gram-negative organisms are common in cases complicating trauma or surgery and those associated with serous effusions.

Immunocompromised patients have higher rates of gram-negative and fungal empyema generally in the context of disseminated disease.

Clinical features

- Chest pain, breathlessness, weight loss, night sweats, fever.
  Examination reveals only the signs of the effusion in most cases.
- Consider in patients with persistent fever who are already receiving antibiotics for pneumonia.
- Consider esophageal rupture in those who develop a pleural effusion soon after significant retching or vomiting.

Diagnosis

See the BTS guidelines for the management of pleural infection.[1]

- *Radiology:* CXR shows pleural effusion. Ultrasound enables diagnostic aspiration and identification of loculated effusions. Contrast CT distinguishes empyema from most lung abscesses and is used to monitor treatment.
- *Diagnostic sampling* should be performed in all patients with a pleural effusion in the context of pneumonia or sepsis. Samples should be kept tightly sealed on ice to prevent changes in pH and glucose. Presence of pus cells or high numbers of microorganisms on Gram stain confirms diagnosis. Cultures may be negative in patients receiving antibiotics.
- *Biochemical tests:* empyema is confirmed by measurement of pH (<7.2), glucose (<2.2 mmol/L), and lactate dehydrogenase (LDH)

Table 4.4 Pleural fluid characteristics in empyema

Stage	Pleural fluid findings	Comments
Simple parapneumonic effusion	Clear fluid; pH > 7.2; LDH <1000 IU/L, glucose >2.2 mmol/L; no organisms on culture or Gram stain	Will usually resolve with antibiotics alone. Perform chest tube drainage for symptom relief if required
Complicated parapneumonic effusion	Clear or cloudy fluid; pH <7.2, LDH >1000 IU/L, glucose >2.2 mmol/L; may be Gram stain- or culture-positive	Requires chest tube drainage
Empyema	Purulent fluid; may be Gram stain- or culture-positive	Requires chest tube drainage

(>1000 IU/L). Low pH values (pH 6–6.7) should raise the suspicion of esophageal rupture or chronic empyema. See Table 4.4.

- *Culture-negative cases:* consider blood culture, urine antigen testing for legionella or histoplasmosis; pleural biopsy in suspected TB (95% positive on histology compared to 23% by pleural fluid culture and microscopy); serology for *E. histolytica* (positive in 98% of patients with pleural amebiasis); microscopy and culture of empyema pus for acid-fast bacilli (AFB) in those at risk of nocardiosis; examination of stool and sputum for eggs in cases with pleural or blood eosinophilia suggestive of paragonimiasis.

Management

Empyema requires prompt treatment to prevent complications and the need for surgical drainage. Involve a respiratory specialist.

- *Drainage:* indications for chest tube insertion are (1) purulent pleural fluid; (2) pleural fluid pH <7. 2; (3) positive pleural fluid Gram stain or culture; (4) loculated pleural collections; (5) large nonpurulent pleural effusions; and (6) poor response to antimicrobial therapy alone.
- *Antibiotics:* the regimen should be guided by culture results. Culture-negative cases should receive antibiotics covering community-acquired and anaerobic organisms (e.g., ceftriaxone and metronidazole). Broader-spectrum cover should be initiated in cases of hospital-acquired empyema. Consider adding a macrolide in cases of suspected *Legionella* infections. Once the fever has settled, convert to oral antibiotics and continue treatment for at least 3 weeks.
- Intrapleural thrombolytic therapy (e.g., urokinase 100,000 IU od for 3 days) has been recommended, although it was not associated with improved radiological appearance and demonstrated no improvement in mortality rate, rate of surgical intervention, or length of hospital stay.[2]
- Consider bronchoscopy if there is a high index of suspicion of bronchial obstruction.

- In patients with persistent sepsis and/or residual pleural effusion, review the diagnosis and perform a CT chest to confirm chest tube position and effusion anatomy and look for obstructing lesions.
- Patients should be considered for surgery if they have ongoing sepsis with persistent pleural collection by day 7 despite chest tube drainage and antibiotics. Modalities include video-assisted thoracoscopic surgery (VATS), open thoracic drainage, or thoracotamy and decortication.

References

1. British Thoracic Society (2003). Guidelines for the management of pleural infection. *Thorax* 58(Suppl II):ii18–ii28.

2. Maskell NA, Danei CWH, Numa AJ, et al. (2005). UK controlled trial of intrapleural strep for pleural infection. *N Engl J Med* 1352:865–874.

Lung abscess

This is a suppurative lung infection that destroys lung parenchyma, producing a pus-filled cavity with an air–fluid level.

Etiology

The risk of pneumonia progressing to lung abscess in the absence of effective therapy relates to the size of the inoculum and state of host defense mechanisms. Anaerobic organisms are the most common causes.

Some cases follow primary pneumonia (e.g., *S. aureus*, *Klebsiella pneumoniae*, *Pseudomonas aeruginosa*). Most follow aspiration in the context of states of altered consciousness (e.g., alcoholism, stroke) or dysphagia (e.g., neurological disease).

Other associations include intestinal obstruction, periodontal disease or gingivitis, septic embolization, bronchiectasis, immunosuppression, and pharyngeal instrumentation (e.g., endotracheal intubation). Up to 5% of pulmonary emboli may become secondarily infected.

Pathogenesis

Bacteria are usually endogenously acquired from the flora of the upper respiratory tract. Some may be acquired nosocomially.

Lung regions that are dependent when lying flat are commonly affected: the posterior segment of the right upper lobe and apical segments of the lower lobes. Bases may be affected in cases of subdiaphragmatic extension (e.g., amebic liver abscess).

Multiple abscesses follow septic embolization (e.g., *S. aureus* right heart endocarditis) or emiabacteremia (enteric gram-negatives and anaerobes).

Microbiology

- *Community-acquired aspiration:* mixed anaerobic infections: gram-negatives (*Prevotella oralis*, *Bacteroides fragilis*, *Fusobacterium nucleatum*) and gram-positives (*Peptostreptococcus* and *Clostridium perfringens*). α-Hemolytic streptococci are the most common aerobes.
- *Hospital-acquired infection:* *S. aureus*, *Klebsiella*, *Pseudomonas*, and *Proteus* in combination with anaerobes

- *Necrotizing infection*: S. aureus, S. pyogenes, K. pneumonia, P. aeruginosa, E. coli, Legionella pneumonphilia, and certain mycobacteria and fungal infections in combination with anaerobes. Uncommon causes of cavitating pneumonia include: Nocardia, Burkholderia, and melioidosis.

Clinical features

Cases diagnosed late may present with several weeks or months of cough, low-grade fever, weight loss, anemia, and clubbing. Sputum is copious and may be foul smelling. Findings are those of a severe pneumonia with or without effusion.

In cases of secondary lung abscess, the primary lesion may also be apparent (endocarditis, subphrenic infection, etc.) as well as multiple lung lesions (e.g., S. aureus in intravenous drug users) with pain and hemoptysis.

Necrotizing pneumonia is seen in severe cases of anaerobic infection and may affect a single segment or extend to involve one or both lungs with associated empyema. Disease rapidly spreads, destroying large volumes of parenchyma. Patients appear ill with a pronounced leukocytosis. Pulmonary actinomycosis may present similarly.

Amebic lung abscess shows features of the coexistent liver abscess and presents with cough productive of brown-red (anchovy sauce) sputum.

Complications include empyema (one-third of cases), brain abscess, and localized bronchiectasis. Tuberculosis should be considered in the differential diagnosis.

Diagnosis

- *Radiology:* CXR may reveal a cavity with an air–fluid level. CT scanning facilitates the detection of smaller lesions.
- *Microbiology:* sputum culture is helpful only in the diagnosis of amebic infection. Culture of empyema fluid or percutaneous transtracheal aspiration (CT guided) is useful where possible. Quantitative culture of bronchoscopic sampling can provide good results. It is essential that samples be placed in anaerobic conditions for transport to the laboratory. Blood cultures may be positive but not reveal the entire infecting flora.

Treatment

Empirical therapy is needed while awaiting culture in community-acquired cases, e.g., ceftriaxone and metronidazole, and in nosocomially acquired infection (cover for S. aureus and P. aeruginosa), e.g., piperacillin/tazobactam plus vancomycin.

Consideration of community-acquired MRSA (CA-MRSA) should be maintained, as this pathogen is associated with necrotizing pneumonia, particularly following viral URTI.

Antibiotics should be given for 2–4 months. Patients should be monitored carefully for relapse.

Bronchoscopy and postural physiotherapy may facilitate drainage.

Surgical resection is rarely required outside the context of malignancy.

Prognosis

Overall mortality is <15% for anaerobic lung abscesses and ~25% for anaerobic necrotizing pneumonia.

Mortality is higher in acute pneumonias caused by organisms such as *S. aureus*.

Cystic fibrosis

Cystic fibrosis (CF) is a recessive genetic disorder with complex pathogenesis and a variable clinical syndrome. One-third of patients are adults.

Pathogenesis

The *CF* gene (chromosome 7) codes for the cystic fibrosis transmembrane regulator (CFTR), a plasma membrane cAMP-regulated chloride channel. Defective CFTR chloride channel function has been identified in epithelial cells of the airways, sweat ducts, and small intestine in CF patients, resulting in viscous secretions.

Microbiology

The colonizing organisms and antimicrobial resistance patterns change over time:

- *S. aureus* colonizes in childhood.
- *P. aeruginosa* colonizes in childhood or early adolescence; >80% are infected by adulthood. Early nonmucoid isolates can be eradicated. Later isolates produce large amounts of mucoid polysaccharide (alginate), are difficult to eradicate, and are associated with greater mortality than nonmucoid strains. Chronic infection is associated with rapid decline in lung function and increased mortality.
- *Burkholderia cepacia* complex is an important and highly transmissible group of pathogens, intrinsically resistant to aminoglycosides and polymixins. It may be difficult to identify, requiring specific isolation media ± referral to reference laboratory. Colonized patients should be separated from the noncolonized. Infection with *B. cenocepacia* can lead to a rapid deterioration in pulmonary function, emiabacteremia, and even death among adolescents and young adults (cepacia syndrome).
- Other organisms include *H. influenzae*, *Aspergillus* spp., and non-tuberculous mycobacteria (clinical significance is unknown).

Clinical features

Features reflect obstruction of organs by viscous secretions and the presence of chronic bacterial lung infection.

- *General features:* chronic cough, wheeze, recurrent pneumonia, sinusitis, clubbing, hemoptysis, pneumothorax, signs of respiratory impairment. Hypoxia and CO_2 retention are uncommon. The CXR may show airway thickening, retained secretions, and bronchiectasis.
- *Acute respiratory infections:* patients often produce a large amount of purulent sputum even when well. Episodes of deterioration are associated with increased volume and purulence of sputum, dyspnea,

wheeze, chest ache, anorexia, and malaise. High fever or sepsis is unusual despite the large number of organisms in the secretions (10^8 organisms/mL of sputum). CXR may be unchanged from the patient's normal film. Forced expiratory volume in 1 second (FEV_1) falls, returning to preinfection levels with successful antibiotic therapy.

- *Other:* diabetes mellitus, pancreatic insufficiency, and urogential and gastrointestinal features

Management

The aims are to slow lung damage by removing viscous airway secretions, control bacterial infection, and monitor the appearance of highly transmissible or antibiotic-resistant organisms.

Antibiotics need to be given to CF patients for longer and at frequent, higher doses than those for non-CF patients. Outpatient IV antibiotic therapy may be given via a long line. Those requiring very frequent antibiotics may require insertion of a tunneled catheter.

General measures

These include postural drainage, deep breathing, coughing, exercise, aerosolized DNase I (reduces mucus viscosity, clears airway secretions), inhaled steroids, and bronchodilators (helpful in some patients). Pneumococcal and annual influenza vaccinations are recommended.

Lung transplantation should be considered if life expectancy is less than 2 years and quality of life is severely impaired despite medical therapy.

Antimicrobial prophylaxis

This is controversial. A Cochrane review[1] found that antibiotic prophylaxis against *S. aureus* infection reduced isolation of *S. aureus* from sputum but had no impact on lung function.

Whereas the U.S. guidelines do not recommend it, the UK Cystic Fibrosis Trust recommends oral flucloxacillin from diagnosis until age 2 years, and some UK clinics promote lifelong prophylaxis.[2]

Eradication of Pseudomonas colonization

The first isolation of a nonmucoid *Pseudomonas* strain should be treated with the aim of eradication (e.g., 6 weeks of PO ciprofloxacin 750 mg bid with nebulized colistin 1 mega unit bid).

Long-term management of Pseudomonas colonization

Patients with established colonization may benefit from long-term nebulized antibiotics (e.g., colistin or tobramycin) to reduce the bacterial burden. Studies have shown improved lung function and reduced episodes of respiratory illness in such patients.

Some centers advocate elective courses of IV antipseudomonal therapy every 3 months to reduce the frequency of exacerbations and consequent lung damage. There is no evidence to support this.

Treatment of acute exacerbations

The patient's most recent sputum culture result should be used to guide therapy. Broad-spectrum oral agents are beneficial despite the presence of resistant *P. aeruginosa*. High doses and prolonged therapy (3–4 weeks) are recommended.

Aggressive IV therapy is indicated in those patients who do not respond to oral treatment. Such therapy is usually directed at *P. aeruginosa*, e.g., ceftazidime and an aminoglycoside. Once-daily aminoglycoside dosing is as effective as three times a day and is associated with reduced toxicity in children.

Haemophilus influenzae and *S. aureus* should be treated if isolated, even if the patient is asymptomatic.

Burkholderia cepacia is very resistant and should be treated with a combination of two or three agents such as ceftazidime and an aminoglycoside. Nebulized vancomycin can be used to treat MRSA colonization of sputum, but IV therapy is required for exacerbations. Parenteral therapy may be given on an outpatient basis and should continue for 10–14 days or longer.

Aspergillus is frequently cultured from sputum. Treatment (steroidsor, antifungals) is indicated only for allergic bronchopulmonary aspergillosis, if present.

Reference

1. Smyth A, Walteo S (2003). Phophylatic anti-staphylococcal antibies for cystic fibrosis. *Cochrane Database of Systematic Reviews* Issue 3. Art. No. CDøø1912.

2. UK Cystic Fibrosis Trust (2002) Antibiotic treatment for cystic fibrosis, second edition. September 2002. http://www.cytrust.org.uk/aboutof/publication/consensusdor

Infective endocarditis

Infective endocarditis (IE) is characterized by infection of the endocardial surface of the heart. It may be classified as acute, subacute, or chronic, depending on the time course of the infection.

It is now more commonly classified according to the type of valve (native or prosthetic) and the etiological agent (e.g., staphylococcal, streptococcal, enterococcal, fungal, culture negative).

Epidemiology

The incidence of IE is estimated to be 0.16–5.4 cases per 1000 hospital admissions. Most patients are aged 30–60 years, men more than women. It is uncommon in children in the absence of a predisposing condition.

Risk factors include congenital heart disease, rheumatic heart disease, degenerative heart disease, prosthetic valves, intravenous catheters, intravenous drug use, and mitral valve prolapse.

Pathogenesis

The development of IE requires the simultaneous occurrence of a number of events: alteration of the valvular surface, deposition of platelets and fibrin, colonization by bacteria, bacterial multiplication, and development of a vegetation.

Etiology

- 80% of cases of native-valve endocarditis are due to streptococci (viridans group, *S. bovis*) or staphylococci.
- *S. aureus* is the most common isolate in IV drug users and tricuspid-valve IE.

- *S. epidermidis* is the most common isolate in early (<2 months) prosthetic-valve endocarditis (PVE).
- Enterococcal endocarditis is usually associated with malignancy or manipulation of the genitourinary (GU) or GI tracts.
- Other organisms, e.g., *Corynebacteria*, *Listeria*, *Bacillus*, *Salmonella*, *E. coli*, *Enterobacter*, *Citrobacter*, *Pseudomonas* spp., are uncommon.
- HACEK organisms or fungi are associated with large vegetations.
- Culture-negative endocarditis (~5%) may be caused by *Coxiella burnetii*, *Chlamydia* spp., *Legionella* spp., *Mycoplasma pneumoniae*, *Bartonella* spp., or *Brucella* spp.
- Polymicrobial infections occur in 1–2% of patients.

Clinical features

The incubation period may vary from days to weeks. Symptoms are protean and include fever, chills, weakness, dyspnea, sweats, anorexia, weight loss, malaise, cough, skin lesions, stroke, nausea, vomiting, headache, myalgia, arthralgia, edema, chest pain, abdominal pain, delirium, coma, hemoptysis, and back pain.

Physical findings include fever, cardiac murmur, Roth spots, clubbing, splinter hemorrhages, Osler's nodes, Janeway lesions, petechiae, peripheral emboli, splenomegaly, and septic complications (pneumonia, meningitis, mycotic aneurysms; see Endovascular infections, p. 574).

Laboratory diagnosis

Blood cultures are positive in ~2/3 of cases. Three blood culture sets should be obtained in the first 24 hours and incubated for 3 weeks.

Blood tests may show elevated ESR (90–100%), anemia (70–90%), leukocytosis (20–30%), leukopenia (5–15%), and thrombocytopenia (5–15%). Hypergammaglobulinemia (20–30%) may result in false-positive results for rheumatoid factor and Venereal Disease Research Laboratory (VDRL) (syphilis) testing. Renal impairment and hypocomplementemia occur in 5–15%.

Urinalysis is frequently abnormal with proteinuria (50–60%), microscopic hematuria (30–60%), gross hematuria, pyuria, bacteriuria, red cells casts, and white cell casts.

Serology is useful for diagnosis of culture-negative endocarditis.

Transthoracic echocardiography (TTE) allows visualization of vegetations in 60–75% of cases, compared with >95% with transesophageal echocardiography (TEE).

Electrocardiography – lengthening of the PR interval in aortic valve endocarditis indicates aortic root involvement.

Duke criteria

This schema stratifies patients with suspected IE into three categories:
- *Definite:* identified by histopathologically or clinical criteria. Clinical diagnosis requires the presence of two major criteria, one major and two minor criteria, or five minor criteria:
  - *Major criteria:* ≥2 positive blood cultures (or single positive culture for *C. burnetii*), echocardiographic evidence for endocardial involvement

- *Minor criteria:* predisposing condition (heart condition, IV drug user), temperature >38°C, vascular phenomena, immunological phenomena, microbiological evidence (not satisfying major criteria)
- *possible:* one major and one minor criterion, or three minor criteria
- *rejected:* firm alternative diagnosis, rapid resolution with no or short course antibiotics, no pathological evidence of IE

Management

Antimicrobial therapy is targeted at the causative organism.
- UK endocarditis guidelines[1]
- U.S. endocarditis guidelines[2]

Surgery is indicated in patients with life-threatening congestive cardiac failure or cardiogenic shock due to surgically treatable valvular disease, if the patient has a reasonable prospect of recovery. Surgery is recommended for annular or aortic abscesses, heart block, recurrent emboli on therapy, antibiotic-resistant infections, and fungal endocarditis.

Prevention

There are few data to support antimicrobial prophylaxis for the prevention of IE. For detailed recommendations, see the American Heart Association guideline for prevention of endocarditis.[3]

References

1. Elliott TS, Foweraker J, Gould FK, et al: Working Party of the British Society for Antimicrobial Chemotherapy (2004). Guidelines for the antibiotic treatment of endocarditis in adults: report of the Working Party of the British Society for *Antimicrobial Chemotherapy. J Antimicrob Chemother* 54:971–81.

2. Bonow RO, Carabello BA, Chatterjee K, et al. (2006). ACC/AHA 2006 guidelines for the management of patients with valvular heart disease: a report of the American College of Cardiology/American Heart Association Task Force on Practice Guidelines (writing Committee to Revise the 1998 guidelines for the management of patients with valvular heart disease) developed in collaboration with the Society of Cardiovascular Anesthesiologists endorsed by the Society for Cardiovascular Angiography and Interventions and the Society of Thoracic Surgeons. *Circulation* 114: e84

3. Wilson W, Taubert KA, Gemitz M, et al. (2007). Prevention of infective endocantitis: guidelines from the American Heart Association. *Circulation* 116:1736–1794.

Intravascular catheter—related infections

Definitions

- *Catheter colonization:* significant growth of organism in quantitative or semiquantitative culture from catheter tip, subcutaneous segment, or catheter hub
- *Phlebitis:* induration, erythema, pain, or tenderness around exit site
- *Exit site infection:* exudate at exit site yielding microorganism or phlebitis <2 cm from exit site + signs of infection (fever, pus) ± bloodstream infection
- *Tunnel infection:* phlebitis ≥2 cm from exit site, along subcutaneous tract of catheter ± bloodstream infection

- *Pocket infection:* infected fluid in subcutaneous pocket of implanted intravascular device, often associated with local erythema, induration, tenderness, rupture and drainage, and necrosis of skin, ± bloodstream infection
- *Bloodstream infection:* bacteremia or fungemia in a patient who has an intravascular device and ≥1 positive blood culture obtained from a peripheral vein and no obvious source (apart from the device)

Epidemiology

In the United States, >200,000 nosocomial bloodstream infections occur per year; most of these are related to intravascular devices. Risk factors for intravenous catheter (IVC)-related infections include type of catheter, site of catheter, duration of placement, and hospital demographics.

Etiology

- Staphylococci, e.g., coagulase-negative staphylococci, *S. aureus*
- Aerobic gram-negative bacilli, e.g., *E. coli*, *Klebsiella* spp., *Pseudomonas* spp., *Enterobacter* spp., *Serratia* spp., *Acinetobacter* spp.
- Fungi, e.g., *Candida albicans*, *Candida* spp., *Malassezia furfur*

Clinical features

The clinical features are unreliable. The most sensitive clinical features, e.g., fever and chills, lack specificity, whereas inflammation and purulence at the catheter site are specific but not sensitive.

Diagnosis

Rapid diagnostic techniques, e.g., Gram stain or acridine orange stain, may be used for diagnosis of exit site infections but have poor sensitivity.

Cultures of IVC samples—semiquantitative (roll plate method) or quantitative (flush, vortex or sonication methods)—have greater specificity than that of qualitative methods.

For paired blood cultures drawn through the IVC and percutaneously, all patients with suspected IVC-related infections should have two sets of blood cultures drawn, at least one peripherally. A positive culture from a line requires clinical interpretation, whereas a negative culture virtually excludes catheter-related bloodstream infection.

In quantitative cultures of central venous catheter (CVC) and peripheral blood samples, a 5- to 10-fold difference in colony count between the central and peripheral culture or an absolute colony count of 100 CFU/mL from a central culture supports the diagnosis of catheter-related bloodstream infection.

Measurement of differential time to positivity for CVC and peripheral cultures takes advantage of continuous blood culture monitoring, e.g., by radiometric methods, to compare differential times to positivity between central and peripheral cultures. It correlates well with quantitative methods and is suitable for use in routine labs.

Management

See the Infectious Diseases Society of America (IDSA) guidelines for management of IVC-related infections.[1]

Peripheral venous catheters

Remove the IVC, swab the exit site if pus is present, and take two sets of blood cultures before starting antimicrobial therapy.

Non-tunneled CVCs

If there are local or systemic signs or positive blood cultures, the CVC should be removed, antimicrobial therapy started, and the CVC replaced at a new site:

- Complicated infections (septic thrombosis, endocarditis, osteomyelitis): remove the CVC and treat with systemic antimicrobials for 4–6 weeks.
- Uncomplicated coagulase-negative staphylococcal infection: remove the CVC and treat with 5–7 days of systemic antibiotics.
- Uncomplicated *S. aureus* bacteremia: remove the CVC and treat with 14 days' systemic antibiotics (if negative TEE) or 4–6 weeks antibiotics (if positive TEE).
- Uncomplicated gram-negative bacteremia: remove the CVC and treat with 10–14 days of systemic antibiotics.
- Uncomplicated candidemia: remove the CVC and treat with antifungals for 14 days after last positive blood culture

Tunnelled CVCs and implanted devices (IDs)

Investigations should be performed to establish the CVC or ID as the source of infection:

- Tunnel infection or port abscess: remove the CVC/ID and treat with systemic antibiotics for 10–14 days.
- Complicated infections (septic thrombosis, endocarditis, osteomyelitis): remove the CVC/ID and treat with systemic antibiotics for 4–6 weeks.
- Uncomplicated coagulase-negative staphylococcal infection: retain the CVC/ID and treat with 7 days of systemic antibiotics plus antibiotic lock therapy for 10–14 days. Remove the CVC/ID if there is persistent bacteremia or clinical deterioration.
- Uncomplicated *S. aureus* bacteremia: remove the CVC/ID and treat with 14 days of systemic antibiotics (if negative TEE) or 4–6 weeks of antibiotics (if positive TEE). For salvage therapy, see IDSA guidelines.[1]
- Uncomplicated gram-negative bacteremia: remove the CVC/ID and treat with 10–14 days of systemic antibiotics.

Prevention

See IDSA guidelines for the prevention of intravascular catheter–related infections.[2]

References

1. Mermel LA, Farr BM, Sherertz RJ et al. (2001). Guidelines for management of intravascular catheter-related infections. *Clin Infect Dis* 32:1249–1272.

2. O'Grady NP, Alexander M, Dellinger EP, et al. (2002). Guidelines for the prevention of intravascular catheter-related infections. *Clin Infect Dis* 35:1281–1307.

Endovascular infections

Persistent bacteremia (i.e., multiple blood cultures taken on different occasions that are positive for the same isolate) suggests endovascular infection. These infections include endocarditis, IVC-related infections, mycotic aneurysms, pacemaker infections, and vascular graft infections.

Mycotic aneurysm

Definition

A mycotic aneurysm may be any extra- or intracardiac aneurysm of infectious origin, except syphilitic aortitis.

Etiology

In the pre-antibiotic era, mycotic aneurysms were usually associated with infective endocarditis and caused by streptococci and staphylococci. Today, mycotic aneurysms are usually due to hematogenous seeding of atherosclerotic vessels or trauma. Pathogens include *S. aureus*, *Salmonella* spp., aerobic gram-negative bacilli, *L. monocytogenes*, *B. fragilis*, group A and C streptococci, *C. septicum*, enterococci, and pneumococci.

Clinical features

Symptoms and signs of infective endocarditis (p. 569) may be present. Intracranial mycotic aneurysms are usually silent but may present with headache, homonymous hemianopia, or focal neurological symptoms and signs. Symptomatic intracranial hemorrhages carry a high mortality.

Visceral mycotic aneurysms are uncommon. The most common location is the superior mesenteric artery, but other sites include the hepatic artery, celiac artery, external iliac artery, and femoral, peripheral, and carotid arteries. Aortic aneurysms are usually associated with infected atherosclerotic lesions and present with fever, back or abdominal pain ± draining cutaneous sinus.

Diagnosis

Blood cultures may identify the causative organism. Echocardiography is useful to visualize aortic valve mycotic aneurysms. CT brain scan may show intracerebral hemorrhages, although cerebral angiography is the investigation of choice for intracranial mycotic aneurysms. MR angiography is less invasive but less sensitive.

Abdominal X-ray may show calcified abdominal aorta. CT and MRI abdomen are less sensitive than angiography for intra-abdominal aneurysms.

Management

Intracranial mycotic aneurysms should be treated with antimicrobial therapy, monitored by angiography, and excised if they enlarge or bleed.

Infected atherosclerotic aneurysms should be operated on before rupture occurs and systemic antibiotics continued for 6–8 weeks postoperatively. Peripheral vessel mycotic aneurysms are managed by surgical resection and reconstruction and antibiotic therapy.

Pacemaker infections

Pacemaker infections affect 1–7% of procedures. Superficial infections involve the generator pocket and/or subcutaneous electrode. Deep infections involve the transvenous intravascular electrode ± generator.

Etiology

Coagulase-negative staphylococci and S. aureus are the most common isolates. Other organisms include *Enterobacteriaceae* spp., *P. aeruginosa*, *C. albicans*, streptococci, enterococci, *Corynebacteria* spp., *Listeria* spp., and *Aspergillus* spp.

Clinical features

Infections confined to the generator pocket usually present with local swelling, erythema, tenderness ± discharge through the incision site or fistula ± systemic symptoms. Infection of the epicardial electrodes may be associated with pericarditis (p. 578), mediastinitis (p. 579), bacteremia, and systemic symptoms.

Infection of the intravascular portion presents with clinical features of endocarditis (p. 569).

Management

Superficial infection confined to the subcutaneous elements may be treated by a one-stage exchange under antimicrobial cover.

For pacemaker endocarditis, the generator and electrodes should be removed transcutaneously, if possible, but surgical extraction may be required. A temporary pacing system is inserted and at least 2 weeks' systemic antimicrobial therapy is given before insertion of a permanent system. A full course of endocarditis therapy should be given; this may need to be extended if there is evidence of metastatic infection.

Vascular graft infections

Epidemiology and pathogenesis

The incidence of vascular graft infection is 1–5%. Three mechanisms are thought to be responsible for infection: intraoperative contamination (most common), extension from adjacent infected tissue, and hematogenous seeding.

Etiology

S. aureus is the most common cause. However, a wide range of organisms may cause infection, e.g., *Enterobacteriaceae* spp., coagulase-negative staphylococci, enterococci, streptococci, *P. aeruginosa, Bacteroides* spp., and corynebacteria.

Clinical features

These depend on the site of the graft infection:
- Inguinal graft infections present with an inguinal mass ± pain, erythema, fever, and sinus formation.
- Abdominal graft infections present with fever, abdominal pain or mass, retroperitoneal bleeding, lower extremity emboli, and GI bleeding due to erosion into the GI tract.

Diagnosis
Superficial graft infections may be readily diagnosed clinically. Deep grafts may require radiological imaging (e.g., CT or MRI abdomen) to confirm the infection. Blood cultures are often negative, unless infection involves the graft lumen.

Management
Surgical resection of the infected graft and revascularization (preferably through an extra-anatomic, uninfected route) is the treatment of choice.

Systemic antimicrobial therapy is given for 4–6 weeks postoperatively If the arterial stump is infected at the time of surgery, culture-specific antimicrobial therapy is given for 6 months postoperatively.

Salvage therapy with long-term suppressive antibiotic therapy is sometimes given for vascular graft infections that are not surgically resectable.

Myocarditis

Myocarditis is an inflammation of the myocardium. Most cases are viral Up to 4% of unselected postmortems reveal unsuspected myocarditis especially in young people dying abruptly. There is histological evidence of myocarditis in up to 20% of cases of idiopathic dilated cardiomyopathy.

Etiology
Myocardial injury may be a consequence of direct cell damage by an infectious agent, by a circulating toxin, or by immune reactions following infection. The cause is not identified in most cases.

Viruses are the most common agents in the developed world, e.g., measles, influenza, polio, mumps, adenovirus, and the group B Coxsackie viruses.

Bacterial infection may cause myocarditis through immunological mechanisms (e.g., Lyme disease, acute rheumatic fever) or through direct myocardial infection with associated inflammation (e.g., brucellosis, meningococcal, streptococcal and staphylococcal sepsis, *Legionella* spp., *M. pneumoniae*, and *C. psittici* infection). Toxin-mediated damage is seen in infection by *C. diptheriae* (blocks cellular protein synthesis) and *C. perfringens*.

Parasitic causes include trypanosomal disease; e.g., *T. cruzi* is a common cause in South America.

Disseminated infection in the immunocompromised may lead to myocarditis (e.g., *Toxoplasma*, *Aspergillus*, and *Cryptococcus* spp.). Cardiac dysfunction may be clinically apparent in up to 20% of AIDS patients, with echocardiographic abnormalities in up to 65% of AIDS patients.

Pathogenesis
The pathological process varies according to the mechanism of the injury and whether it is acute or chronic. All lead to an inflammatory infiltrate and damage to adjacent myocardial cells. In addition, some agents damage vascular endothelial cells. Routine histology rarely gives a definitive etiological diagnosis.

When normal cardiac function is regained, histological abnormalities may lag behind clinical improvement. Cases that leave permanent damage are marked by interstitial fibrosis and a loss of muscle fibers.

Clinical presentation

Myocarditis may be asymptomatic or result in severe heart failure or sudden death. Myocarditis should be considered in a young person developing cardiac abnormalities in the context of a recognized systemic illness or in an otherwise well individual developing unexpected heart failure or arrhythmias (e.g., supraventricular tachycardia [SVT] or extrasystoles).

Fever, malaise, upper respiratory tract symptoms, tachycardia, dyspnea, and chest pain may precede Coxsackie virus myocarditis.

On examination there may be cardiomegaly, murmurs, and signs of cardiac failure. Pericarditis may coexist.

Diagnosis

Diagnosis can be difficult in those cases occurring in the context of fulminant systemic infection.

Electrocardiogram (ECG) changes are nonspecific (e.g., sequential ST elevation and T-wave inversion).

Around one-third of patients with biopsy-proven myocarditis have raised troponin levels.

Echocardiography may demonstrate systolic dysfunction and can be used to track the progression of disease. MRI scanning is a sensitive means of detecting myocardial inflammation.

Endomyocardial biopsy is considered the gold standard for diagnosis but can miss cases in which disease is focally distributed, and timing is critical. Most experts believe it is not warranted in most cases.

Demonstrating a viral cause requires isolation of the virus or viral material from myocardium. Generally, diagnosis is inferred by serology (e.g., Lyme disease) or detection of the organism in other specimens (e.g., stool or blood).

Treatment

Therapy should be directed at the causative agent, where possible.

General measures include bed rest (exercise is associated with increased death in mouse models) and management of heart failure and arrhythmias. Most patients recover completely. Severe cases may require cardiac-assist devices.

Steroids are of no benefit and are probably deleterious overall. Immunoglobulin administration may help certain subgroups (e.g., CMV myocarditis). Antivirals may be of benefit in the future.

Differential diagnosis

This includes pericarditis, idiopathic congestive cardiomyopathy, acute rheumatic fever, and noninfectious myocarditis (collagen vascular disease, thyrotoxicosis, drug or radiation induced).

Pericarditis

Pericarditis is an inflammation of the pericardium that may be acute or chronic

Etiology

Idiopathic cases account for up to 86% of cases and are probably viral.

- *Viruses:* enteroviruses (particularly Coxsackie viruses) are the most common cause. Others include echoviruses, adenovirus, mumps, influenza, EBV, varicella, CMV, HSV, and hepatitis B virus.
- *Bacteria:* before antibiotics became widely available, bacterial pericarditis (e.g., *S. aureus* and *S. pneumoniae*) was a recognized complication of pneumonia. Bacterial pericarditis is now uncommon and tends to occur following gram-negative infection in older people with predisposing conditions, e.g., esophageal perforation, head and neck infections (usually anaerobes), and in cases of meningococcal septicemia. Other bacterial causes include *M. pneumoniae*, *Legionella pneumophilia*, and *Haemophilus influenzae*. Tuberculous pericarditis is a major cause of heart failure in Sub-Saharan Africa; chronic disease is associated with a constrictive pericarditis.
- *Fungi* include *H. capsulatum*, *C. immits*, *Aspergillus* spp., *C. neoformans*, and *Candida* spp.
- *Parasites* include *T. gondii*, *E. histolytica*, and *T. canis*.

Pathogenesis

Viruses reach the pericardium hematogenously, and infection results in inflammation of both the visceral and parietal pericardium, with or without a pericardial effusion. Most patients recover; some may experience episodes of relapse, a phenomenon that is probably related to immune mechanisms rather than to persistent viral infection. It is rare that viral pericarditis leads to constriction.

Bacterial infection may occur as a result of direct inoculation (trauma or surgery), contiguous spread (e.g., endocarditis or untreated pneumonia), or bacteremia. Fluid is usually grossly purulent, and subsequent organization with adhesions may lead to constriction.

TB pericarditis may arise from hematogenous spread (during primary infection), lymphatic spread (from the regional lymph nodes), or contiguous spread (from infected lung or pleura). Initial fibrin deposition, granuloma formation, and polymorphonuclear cell infiltration is followed by the development of a serous or serosanguinous effusion in lymphocytes and plasma cells.

Later, the pericardium is thickened by fibrin deposition and granulomas. In late disease, the pericardial space is taken up with adhesions and fibrous tissue, leading to constriction.

Clinical presentation

Idiopathic or viral pericarditis presents with retrosternal chest pain, radiating to the shoulder and neck and aggravated by breathing or lying flat. Fever may be present along with flu-like features.

Bacterial pericarditis is usually seen in the context of severe systemic infection in an acutely ill patient. Chest pain and pericardial rubs may be reported in less than one-third of patients. Bacterial pericarditis may be recognized late, after the onset of hemodynamic complications.

TB pericarditis has an insidious onset with chest pain, weight loss, night sweats, cough, and breathlessness. The classic clinical finding is a pericardial rub. Where the effusion is significant, there may be jugular venous distension, pulsus paradoxus.

Diagnosis

Diagnosis is often made clinically and depends on the history.

The ECG is abnormal in 90% of cases (due to diffuse subepicardial inflammation), with 50% showing the classic findings of early ST-elevation in multiple leads, resolving over a few days and replaced with T-wave flattening or inversion.

Echocardiography is useful in diagnosing and assessing effusions and the extent of any compromise.

Virus isolation from throat swabs or stool, or acute and convalescent viral serology, may lead to a diagnosis but rarely affect management.

Diagnostic sampling may be indicated if the effusion persists for >3 weeks, when TB, fungal infection, malignancy, or connective tissue disorders should be considered.

Pericardiotomy with biopsy is preferable to pericardiocentesis, as it has a higher diagnostic yield and fewer complications.

Treatment

- *Viral/idiopathic:* bed rest, analgesia, and monitoring for hemodynamic complications. Steroids should be avoided in the acute phase due to the frequent concomitant myocarditis in which steroids are contraindicated. They may, however, have a role in preventing recurrent pericarditis once a patient has recovered. Colchicine may also be useful.
- *Purulent bacterial:* surgical drainage and appropriate antibiotic therapy are essential. Early pericardiocentesis may be life saving, but fluid often reaccumulates. Overall mortality, however, remains at around 30%, particularly in those cases associated with endocarditis or following surgery.
- *TB:* antituberculous therapy should be initiated. Constrictive pericarditis may develop in up to half of patients despite this. Steroids (prednisolone 60 mg for 4 weeks, then reducing over 7 weeks) in addition to antituberculous therapy reduce the need for repeat drainage, as well as resulting in a modest reduction in those developing constriction. Those developing hemodynamic compromise secondary to effusion reaccumulation or progressive pericardial thickening benefit from early surgery (pericardectomy).

Mediastinitis

Acute mediastinitis is an uncommon but potentially devastating infection involving the mediastinal structures.

Epidemiology and pathogenesis

Primary infection is rare. Almost all cases are secondary to
- Esophageal perforation, e.g., iatrogenic, trauma, spontaneous
- Head and neck infections, e.g., odontogenic, Ludwig's angina, phayngitis, tonsillitis, epiglottitis, parotitis
- Spread from other infections, e.g., pneumonia, empyema, subphrenic abscess, pancreatitis, skin or soft tissue infections of chest wall, osteomyelitis of sternum, clavicle, ribs or vertebrae, hematogenous seeding
- Cardiothoracic surgery,now the most common cause.

Etiology

The spectrum of organisms causing infection varies strikingly according to the underlying cause.

Esophageal perforation or head and neck infections are usually polymicrobial and caused by oral streptococci (e.g., viridans streptococci peptococci, peptostreptococci) and anaerobic gram-negative bacilli (e.g. *Bacteroides* spp., *Fusobacterium* spp., *Prevotella* spp., *Porphyromonas* spp.).

Cardiothoracic surgery–related infections are primarily due to gram-positive cocci (e.g., *S. aureus*, *S. epidermidis*, enterococci, streptococci), with lesser contributions from gram-negative bacilli (e.g., *E. coli*, *Enterobacter* spp., *Klebsiella* spp., *Proteus* spp. *Pseudomonas* spp.).

Clinical features

The clinical manifestations also depend on the underlying cause:
- Head and neck infections usually present with fever, pain, and swelling of the affected site.
- Esophageal perforation may be obvious or clinically inapparent.
- Symptoms include chest pain (site depends on location of infection), respiratory distress, and dysphagia.
- Physical signs include fever, tachcycardia, crepitus, and edema of the head and neck. Hamman's sign (a crunching sound heard over the precordium synchronous with the cardiac rhythm) is due to emphysema of the mediastinum.
- Post-cardiothoracic mediastinitis usually presents within 2 weeks of surgery, with fever, wound erythema and discharge, and chest pain (often pleuritic). Sternal instability, wound dehiscence, and chest wall emphysema may occur.

Diagnosis

Blood tests show leukocytosis and raised inflammatory markers. Blood cultures may yield the causative organism(s).

Chest X-ray may show mediastinal widening, air–fluid levels, and subcutaneous or mediastinal emphysema.

CT thorax is particularly useful in postoperative mediastinitis to distinguish superficial wound infections from deep retrosternal infections.

Management

Prompt surgical intervention is required with drainage, debridement, and repair (in cases due to esophageal perforation). Postoperative mediastinitis may be managed by the open technique (wound debrided and left open to heal by secondary intention) or the closed technique (debridement, primary closure, and irrigation through drains).

Appropriate parenteral antibiotic therapy should be initiated as soon as the diagnosis is made. Empiric therapy should cover the most likely organisms (e.g., penicillin and metronidazole or clindamycin for head and neck or esophageal infections, and vancomycin and meropenem for postoperative mediastinitis).

Complications

- Pericardial effusion and cardiac tamponade
- Pleural effusions and empyema
- Peritonitis
- Sternal osteomyelitis (postoperative mediastinitis)

Esophagitis

Inflammation of the esophagus is generally noninfectious (e.g., gastroesophageal reflux) but may also be caused by a variety of infectious agents, usually in the context of impaired immunity (HIV, transplant recipients, or those receiving cancer chemotherapy).

Etiology

Candida

C. albicans is the most common cause of esophagitis. Other *Candida* species are less commonly isolated. Colonization is seen in 20% of the population (particularly those receiving antacid therapy). Infection follows when breakdown of local and systemic defenses permit invasion to the deeper epithelial layers.

Endoscopy reveals yellow-white plaques adhering to a hyperemic esophagus (usually the distal third). Removal of these reveals an inflamed friable surface. Perforation occurs rarely.

Predisposing factors include acute or advanced HIV infection, diabetes mellitus, hematological malignancy, broad-spectrum antibiotic therapy, corticosteroid therapy, conditions that impair esophageal motility (systemic sclerosis, achalasia), and reflux esophagitis.

Cytomegalovirus

CMV is seen usually in AIDS (the cause in ~30% of such patients reporting esophageal symptoms) or severely immunosuppressed patients. Endoscopy may demonstrate large (10 cm^2), shallow, "punched-out" ulcers.

Diagnosis is best made by histopathological examination of biopsies obtained from the ulcer edge and base, which show enlarged endothelial cells with large intranuclear inclusions. Isolation of CMV in culture is not reliable because of contamination from blood or saliva.

Coinfection with HSV or *Candida* is common.

Herpes simplex virus

HSV is usually seen in those with significant immunosuppression; it is rare in healthy adults. HSV-1 is more common than HSV-2, which is rarely implicated. HSV-1 accounts for up to 16% of HIV patients with esophageal symptoms.

Presentation may be with odynophagia, chest pain, fever, nausea, and vomiting; <25% may develop clinically significant GI bleeding. Oral and labial or cutaneous HSV infection may also be apparent (<38% of cases).

Endoscopy reveals multiple small superficial ulcers in the distal third of the esophagus. Large confluent ulcers and denuded epithelium may be seen as infection progresses.

Viral culture of brushing or biopsy is most sensitive for diagnosis.

Idiopathic ulceration

Extensive ulceration may occur in those with acute or advanced HIV or in mild form in otherwise healthy individuals. These cases may be attributed to unrecognized infectious agents. A course of prednisolone (40 mg a day for 14 days then tapered to stop) improves symptoms in most cases of HIV-related aphthous ulceration.

Clinical features

Patients present with difficulty in, or pain on, swallowing. Liquids may be better tolerated than solids. Pain may be worse with acidic substances.

Severe ulcerative esophagitis can cause such severe pain that oral intake is limited, causing weight loss and dehydration. GI bleeding can occur. Esophagitis can exist in the absence of symptoms (<41%).

Fever may be seen in those with CMV or mycobacterial infection. Vomiting is more common with CMV than with other causes. The presence of oral lesions may be indicative of the cause of esophagitis (e.g., oral thrush or herpetic ulceration).

Diagnosis and treatment

Accurate diagnosis of esophageal candidiasis requires endoscopic brushing (with a sheathed cytology brush) and biopsy. The gross appearance can mislead: white lesions may be seen with HSV, CMV, and candidal infection. Histopathological examination and viral culture or PCR may identify viral causes. Fungal culture is useful only in the management of refractory cases, e.g., to identify the species and sensitivities.

Management

Diagnostic endoscopy may not always be feasible (bleeding, severe pain, critical illness), particularly in those patients developing esophagitis secondary to cancer chemotherapy. Empirical treatment for *Candida* and HSV infection may be appropriate (e.g., intravenous fluconazole or echinocandin and acyclovir), particularly if symptoms are very severe or oral thrush and HSV stomatitis are apparent.

Patients receiving immunosuppressant therapy may need drug level monitoring if treated with antifungals such as fluconazole.
- *Candida:* fluconazole PO or IV for 14–21 days
- *HSV:* acyclovir IV for 7–14 days or PO for 14–21 days
- *CMV:* ganciclovir IV for 14–21 days

Esophagitis in AIDS patients

Esophageal symptoms are seen in 40–50% of patients with AIDS at some point in their illness and affect nutritional status and morbidity.

Candida esophagitis is most common and can be treated empirically with fluconazole in mild cases if oral thrush is observed in a symptomatic patient (70% of such cases will have esophageal involvement); 5% of patients with proven Candida esophagitis do not respond to fluconazole therapy because of resistance. This is more common in those with previous exposures to fluconazole. Some may respond to itraconazole (see Triazoles, p. 75) or amphotericin B (see Polyenes, p. 73) or echinocandins (see Echinocandins, p. 77).

Viruses cause one-third of cases (often in association with candidiasis). Three-quarters will have a partial or complete response to induction therapy with antiviral drugs, but relapses are common without maintenance treatment; 70% of HSV esophagitis cases respond to acyclovir, but relapse is seen in 15% within 4 months.

Other rare causes of esophagitis in HIV are EBV, *Mycobacterium avium* complex, *Cryptococcus neoformans*, *Cryptosporidium,* and *Actinomyces*.

Peptic ulcer disease

Heliobacter pylori is a motile, curved, gram-negative rod that lives within the mucous layer overlying the gastric (and occasionally duodenal or esophageal) mucosa. It is present in most people with peptic ulcer disease, increasing the risk of several inflammatory and neoplastic processes.

All clinical isolates of *H. pylori* produce urease. It has been isolated from people in all parts of the world. Humans appear to be the major reservoir, with transmission likely to be via feco-oral and possibly oral-oral routes. Rates of colonization are equal between men and women.

Carriage is near universal by age 20 years in developing countries. Prevalence is over 50% by age 50 years in the UK; 1–3% of those who remain free of the organism by adulthood acquire the bacteria each year.

Clinical features

- *Acute acquisition* may cause an acute upper GI illness with nausea and abdominal discomfort with vomiting, burping, and fever lasting 3–14 days. However, infection is clinically silent in most individuals. There have been some documented cases of acute self-limited infection.
- *Persistent colonization: H. pylori* persists for decades in most people. Acute symptoms do not recur in most, although the incidence of non-ulcer dyspepsia is slightly higher in colonized individuals.
- *Duodenal ulceration:* 90% of those with such ulceration carry *H. pylori,* and it is usually associated with cases occurring in the absence of aspirin or NSAID use. The organism is found only in areas of metaplastic gastric-type epithelium, and its presence is associated with an over 50 times greater risk of duodenal ulceration.
- *Gastric ulceration:* 50–80% of patients with benign gastric ulceration are colonized. This is less than duodenal ulceration, as a greater proportion of gastric ulcers are due to NSAID or aspirin use.

- *Gastric carcinoma:* the presence of *H. pylori* has been identified as a risk factor for gastric carcinoma. It induces a chronic gastritis, which is thought to lead to atrophic and metaplastic changes over decades. However, *H. pylori* is neither necessary nor sufficient for oncogenesis.
- *Gastric lymphoma:* colonization is strongly associated with mucosa-associated lymphoid tumors (MALT; lymphomas arising from B lymphocytes). There is evidence to suggest that eradication may lead to improvement in tumor histology.
- *Esophageal disease:* as the incidence of *H. pylori* colonization falls, it appears that incidence of gastroesophageal reflux disease (GERD), Barrett's esophagus, and esophageal adenocarcinoma is on the rise. Certain *H. pylori* strains may have an inverse association with Barrett's esophagus. Eradication of *H. pylori* in those with duodenal ulceration doubles the rate of GERD development, and patients with GERD are less likely to be colonized with *H. pylori* than controls.

Pathogenesis

Several features help the organism survive in the hostile gastric environment: its microaerophilic characteristics (enabling its survival within the mucus layer), its motility, and its urease activity (allowing it to generate ammonium ions to buffer the acidity).

It colonizes gastric mucosa (stomach or ectopic cells in the duodenum and esophagus) and induces a cellular infiltrate (lymphocytes, monocytes, plasma cells, neutrophils). It does not appear to invade tissue, and damage is due to either contact with the organism or its extracellular products (ammonia and proteins).

The presence of *H. pylori* induces the production of proinflammatory cytokines, and colonized persons have higher gastrin levels than those in individuals who are not colonized.

Diagnosis

Endoscopy with biopsy

This is expensive and invasive but allows the examination of pathology (e.g., if a neoplasm is considered in the differential). Specimens may be cultured on selective media (e.g., Skirrow's media) in microaerobic conditions for up to 5 days at 37°C. This allows determination of antibiotic sensitivities. Histology is generally more sensitive than culture. The organism may be visualized in biopsy specimens with Gram or silver stains or by immunofluorescence.

Antibody tests

IgG is positive in nearly all colonized patients and may be more sensitive than biopsy. The organism may be present in focal regions of the stomach. Antibody levels decline 3–6 months after successful eradication.

Urease breath test

Patients fast and are then given a meal containing ^{13}C- or ^{14}C-urea. Over the next hour, their breath is examined for $^{13}CO_2/^{14}CO_2$. Results may be falsely negative after therapy that suppresses but fails to eradicate the organism, and it should not be performed within 4 weeks of treatment with an antibacterial agent, or within 2 weeks of treatment with anti-secretory drug.

Commercial test kits are available: collected breath samples are sent to an appropriate laboratory for analysis.

Treatment

Antibiotic therapy aimed at eradicating *H. pylori* is associated with significantly lower recurrence rates than those with acid suppression alone in the treatment of duodenal and gastric ulcers associated with the organism. Eradication is associated with tumor regression in patients with gastric MALTomas.

Treatment is with a combination of antimicrobials; single agents are rarely effective. They are given in combination with an acid suppressant. Proton pump inhibitors are directly inhibitory to *H. pylori* and appear to be potent urease inhibitors. Example regimes are 7 days of either omeprazole 20 mg bid, amoxicillin 1 g bid, clarithromycin 500 mg bid, or ranitidine bismuth citrate 400 mg bid, clarithromycin 500 mg bid, and metronidazole 400 mg bid. (see *BNF* 1.3 for detailed regimes and cost).

Acquired resistance may develop after therapy with certain agents (e.g., quinolone, imidazoles, macrolides).

True eradication has not been achieved if the biopsy or breath test is negative at 1 month, or serology at 6 months.

Infectious diarrhea

Definitions

- *Gastroenteritis* is inflammation of the stomach and intestinal epithelium.
- *Diarrhea* is the passage of ≥3 loose or liquid stools within 24 hours.
- *Food poisoning* is vomiting and/or diarrhea caused by eating food contaminated with microorganisms or toxins (bacterial or otherwise, e.g., poisonous mushrooms).
- *Dysentery* is bloody diarrhea with mucus, tenesmus, pain, and fever usually caused by bacterial, parasitic, or protozoan infection.

Etiology

Some individuals are at higher risk (e.g., previous gastric surgery, immunodeficiency), and recent antibiotic use predisposes to antibiotic–associated diarrhea. Bacterial infections are more common in the tropics. In the U.S., causes of gastroenteritis include the following:

- *General patients:* viruses (50–70% cases e.g., rotavirus, norovirus), *Campylobacter, Shigella, Salmonella, C. perfringens, S. aureus, B. cereus, E. coli, C. difficile,* parasites (10–15% e.g., *Giardia, Cryptosporidium*)
- *Immunosuppressed patients:* general causes plus increased *E. coli, Cryptosporidium,* mycobacteria, *Microsporidia,* CMV and HSV (especially HIV patients with CD4 count <200/mm³)
- *Returning travelers:* enterotoxigenic *E. coli* (30–70%), *Shigella* spp. (5–20%), *Salmonella* spp. (5%), *Campylobacter* (5–20%), *V. parahaemolyticus* (shellfish), viral (10–20%), protozoal (5–10%)

Clinical features

History

- *Nature of the diarrhea:* blood, mucus or pus? Is it painful? Watery diarrhea with blood or mucus implies large bowel pathology; fatty or smelly diarrhea suggests small bowel involvement.
- *Timing (acute or chronic):* an abrupt onset suggests bacterial and viral infections. Chronic diarrhea is more characteristic of parasites and may also occur with noninfectious causes, e.g., inflammatory bowel disease or malignancy.
- *Food history:* specific restaurant, reheated food, unusual diets, fish
- Are other people affected? Is it an outbreak, and if so, what was the source?
- Recent antibiotic use (in community or hospital)
- *Foreign travel:* country, city or rural, with reference to timing of possible exposures, e.g., food from a street vendor
- Risk factors for immunosuppression

Examination

- Is the patient, febrile, systemically unwell, and in shock? Consider infection as well as surgical causes, e.g., diverticulitis.
- Wasting implies a longer-standing problem, e.g., small bowel malabsorption, immunosuppression, or malignancy.
- *Rectal examination:* blood, mucus, fecal occult blood, impacted feces causing overflow diarrhea, rectal carcinoma

When gastrointestinal symptoms are followed by neurological signs, think of *C. botulinum* (nausea, dry mouth, cranial nerve palsies, and descending weakness with respiratory and autonomic dysfunction) or *C. jejuni* infection-associated GBS (occurs 1–3 weeks after GI symptoms).

Differential diagnosis

Noninfectious causes of food poisoning include mushrooms and metal poisoning. Noninfectious causes of diarrhea include perforation, appendicitis, diverticulosis, inflammatory bowel disease (IBD), colonic malignancy, ischemic colitis, malabsorption, irritable bowel syndrome, constipation with overflow, thyrotoxicosis, drugs, and autonomic neuropathy.

Investigations

- *Blood tests:* anemia or macrocytosis may be due to malabsorption. Renal failure may occur with dehydration or hemolytic uremic syndrome (HUS). Blood film shows red cell fragmentation in HUS.
- Sigmoidoscopy may show inflamed colonic mucosa ± pseudomembranes (*C. difficile* colitis). Biopsies may be taken to exclude IBD.
- Abdominal X-ray or CT abdomen may be necessary to exclude surgical causes.

Stool samples should be sent to the laboratory for the following:

- *Microscopy:* blood and pus cells indicate infectious diarrhea (e.g., *Salmonella*, *Shigella*, or *Campylobacter* spp.) or IBD. Ova, cysts, and parasites may be diagnostic in patients with a history of foreign travel.

Modified Ziehl–Neelsen (ZN) stain for *Cryptosporidium* (preschool children and the immunocompromised)
• *Culture* detects specific pathogens such as *Salmonella* spp., *Shigella* spp., *Campylobacter jejuni*, *E. coli* O157, *Yersinia* spp., and *Vibrio* spp. Special media are required.
  • *Toxin detection:* either the toxin itself within stool (e.g., *C. difficile*), or the toxin gene in isolated organisms (e.g., *E. coli* O157)

Management

Oral rehydration is sufficient in mild cases. Oral rehydration salts are commercially available. Patients with moderate or severe dehydration require IV replacement or fluid and electrolytes.

Antibiotics are not generally indicated in immunocompetent patients. The exceptions are early *C. jejuni* enteritis, *Y. enterocolitica* infections (children and immunocompromised patients), *S. dysenteriae*, severe *S. enteritidis* and *S. typhimurium* infections (e.g., bacteremia), *Giardia lamblia*, and *Entamoeba histolytica*.

Antispasmodic agents are useful for mild diarrhea without blood. Do not use these if there is a suggestion of dysentery.

Public health aspects

All cases of suspected food poisoning or dysentery should be notified to the local health department. Reportable causes include cholera, *Cryptosporidium*, *Giardia*, *Salmonella*, *Shigella*, and *E. coli* O157.

In outbreaks, save culture plates, isolates, and relevant food and water (−70°C).

References

Thielman NM, Guerrant RL (2004). Clinical practice. Acute infectious diarrhea. *N Engl J Med* 350:38.

Working Group of the Former PHLS Advisory Committee on Gastrointestinal Infections. Preventing person-to-person spread following gastrointestinal infections: guidelines for public health physicians and environmental health officers. *Commun Dis Public Health* 2004;7:362–384.

Enteric fever

The clinical and pathological features of typhoid fever were first described in the 19th century by Louis (1829) and then by Jenner (1850). The term *enteric fever* was proposed by Wilson in 1869.

The species that cause enteric fever are *Salmonella enterica* serovar *typhi* (typhoid fever)[1] and *Salmonella enterica* serovar *paratyphi* A, B, or C (paratyphoid fever).[2]

Epidemiology

Enteric fever is a global health problem, affecting an estimated 12 to 33 million people per year. The disease is endemic in many developing countries, e.g., Indian subcontinent, Asia, Africa, and Central and South America.

The organisms are usually spread by ingestion of fecally contaminated food or water. Direct person-to-person spread is rare, and laboratory transmission has been reported.

Outbreaks in developing countries may result in high morbidity and mortality, especially when caused by multi-drug-resistant strains. In developed countries, infection is usually associated with international travel, although food-borne outbreaks do occur.

Pathogenesis

Data from volunteer studies and outbreak investigations suggest that inoculum size and decreased gastric acidity are important determinants of disease severity. The ability of the organisms to survive within macrophages is essential to disease pathogenesis and spread. Organisms multiply in Peyer's patches then enter the bloodstream and re-invade the small bowel, causing bleeding and peritonitis.

The Vi antigen of *S. typhi* prevents antibody-mediated opsonization, increases resistance to peroxide, and confers resistance to complement-mediated lysis.

Clinical features

The incubation period ranges from 5 to 21 days, depending on the inoculum size and host immune status.

Abdominal symptoms (e.g., diarrhea, constipation, or abdominal pain) may initially develop then resolve. This is followed by nonspecific symptoms (e.g., chills, diaphoresis, headache, anorexia, cough, weakness, sore throat, muscle pains, dizziness, delirium, or psychosis) prior to the onset of fever.

On examination, patients are acutely ill with fever, relative bradycardia (<50%), rose spots, abdominal tenderness, and hepatosplenomegaly. Cervical lymphadenopathy, respiratory crepitations, cholecystitis, pancreatitis, seizures, or coma may also occur.

Complications occur in the third or fourth week of illness and include intestinal perforation or hemorrhage, endocarditis, pericarditis, hepatic or splenic abscesses, and oorchitis.

Mortality rates are <1% in developed countries but may be as high as 10–30% in developing countries, as a result of delayed treatment or multi-drug-resistant strains.

Long-term carriage (presence of salmonellae in stool or urine for >1 year) occurs in 1–4% of patients with *S. typhi*. It is associated with biliary abnormalities, concurrent infection with *Schistosoma haematobium*, and an increased risk of developing cholangiocarcinoma.

Diagnosis

Definitive diagnosis requires isolation of the organism from cultures of blood (50–70% sensitivity) or bone marrow (>90% sensitivity). Other diagnostic samples include stool, urine, rose spots, peripheral blood mononuclear cells (PBMCs) or gastric or intestinal secretions. A combination of specimens increases the likelihood of diagnosis.

A number of serological tests exist (e.g., Widal test), but none are sensitive, specific, or rapid enough for clinical use.

DNA probes for *S. typhi* have been developed, but these are not as sensitive as culture nor commercially available.

Management

The management of enteric fever depends on the clinical severity and drug susceptibility of the isolate.

Uncomplicated typhoid (community to outpatient)

- *Fully susceptible:* fluoroquinolone 15 mg/kg/day for 5–7 days
- *Multi-drug resistant:* fluoroquinolone (ciprofloxacin) 15 mg/kg/day for 5–7 days
- *Nalidixic acid resistant:* azithromycin 8–10 mg/kg/day for 10 days

Severe typhoid (hospitalized)

- *Fully susceptible:* fluoroquinolone 15 mg/kg/day for 10–14 days
- *Multi-drug resistant:* fluoroquinolone (ciprofloxacin) 15 mg/kg/day for 10–14 days
- *Nalidixic acid resistant:* ceftriaxone 60 mg/kg/day or cefotaxime 80 mg/kg/day for 10–14 days

Prevention

Immunization may be used to prevent enteric fever in travelers to endemic areas, in laboratory personnel who work with *S. typhi*, and in household contacts. The available vaccines include: heat-killed or inactivated whole-cell vaccines, the Vi capsular polysaccharide vaccine (Typhim Vi), and the live attenuated oral vaccine Ty21a.

Food handlers may return to work after symptoms have resolved. Two negative stool samples are recommended for food handlers who prepare foods that are consumed raw.

While Typhoid Mary Mallon worked as a cook in New York in the early 1900s, she infected almost 50 people with typhoid. Three of them died from the disease. In the end, she was forcibly quarantined and, ultimately, died. Some commentators say the problem was exacerbated by the prejudice against working-class Irish immigrants at that time.

Typhoid Mary is probably the most famous disease-carrier of all time. Her name is often used as a generic term for a disease-carrier who is a danger to the public because they refuse to take appropriate precautions.

References

1. Parry CM, Hien TT, Dongan G, et al. (2002). Typhoid fever. *N Eng J Med* 347(322):1770–1782.

2. Bhan MK, Bahl R, Bhatnagar S (2005). Typhoid and paratyphoid fever. *Lancet* 366:749–762.

Cholera

Cholera is an epidemic diarrheal disease caused by *Vibrio cholerae*. *V. cholerae* is a curved gram-negative rod that belongs to the family *Vibrionaeceae*.

The bacterium has a single polar flagellum that causes erratic movement, visible on microscopy. It has a flagellar H antigen and a somatic O antigen; the latter enables differentiation of the two types that cause cholera (O1 and O139).

V. cholerae O1 can be classified into three serotypes (Inaba, Ogawa, and Hikojima) based on the presence of somatic antigens and two biotypes (classic and El Tor) based on phenotypic characteristics.

Epidemiology

Cholera has the ability to both cause epidemics with pandemic potential and remain endemic in affected areas.

Epidemic cholera affects nonimmune individuals of all ages, occurs after a single introduction, spreads by the feco-oral route, and has high secondary spread.

Endemic cholera affects children aged 2–15 years, has an aquatic or asymptomatic human reservoir, and is spread by water or food or feco-orally. Immunity increases with age, and secondary spread is variable.

Seven pandemics occurred between 1817 and 1961. The first six were caused by *V. cholerae* O1 classic biotype, originated from the Indian subcontinent, and spread to Europe and the Americas. The seventh pandemic originated in Indonesia in 1961 and was caused by *V. cholerae* O1 El Tor biotype. This pandemic was the most extensive and is still ongoing in some countries.

Finally, in 1992, a new epidemic caused by *V. cholerae* O139 occurred in India and Bangladesh.

Pathogenesis

V. cholerae causes disease by secreting an enterotoxin that induces secretion of fluid and electrolytes by the small intestine. The toxin consists of five B subunits (which bind to a ganglioside receptor on the mucosal surface) and two A subunits.

Activation of the A1 subunit by adenylate cyclase results in an increase in cyclic AMP, which blocks absorption of sodium and chloride by the microvilli and promotes secretion of chloride and water by crypt cells. The infectious dose varies with route of transmission: 10^2–10^6 organisms. Reduced gastric acidity is associated with an increased severity of disease.

Clinical features

Cholera is characterized by the sudden onset of profuse watery diarrhea ("rice water" stool) and vomiting, accompanied by varying degrees of dehydration. Fever is uncommon (<5% of patients) but the pulse may be rapid and weak and the blood pressure unrecordable.

Patients may be anxious, restless, or obtunded, with sunken eyes, dry mucous membranes, and loss of skin elasticity.

Hypoglycemia, seizures, coma, and fever are more common in children. Hypoglycemia in children carries a higher risk of death.

Severe disease is more common in pregnancy and associated with fetal loss in up to 50%

Laboratory diagnosis

- *Microscopy and culture:* dark-field microscopy shows large numbers of vibrios moving chaotically; their movement may be blocked by specific antisera. The organism is cultured on selective media (thiosulfate citrate bile salts sucrose agar, or tellurite taurocholate gelatin agar) and its identity confirmed using specific antisera.
- *Laboratory abnormalities* include raised urea and creatinine, normal or low serum sodium and potassium levels, a metabolic acidosis with high anion gap, raised white cell count, packed cell volume, and

serum-specific gravity total protein. Hyperglycemia is more common than hypoglycemia.

Management[1,2,3]

The goal of therapy is to restore fluid losses rapidly and safely.

Evaluate the patient for degree of dehydration: mild (<5% fluid loss), moderate (5–10% fluid loss), or severe (>10% fluid loss). Rehydrate the patient in two phases: intensive phase (2–4 hours) and maintenance phase (until diarrhea resolves).

Use intravenous fluids only for severely dehydrated patients in rehydration phase (50–100 mL/kg/h), moderately dehydrated patients who cannot tolerate oral fluids, and high stool volumes (>10 mL/kg/h) in maintenance phase. Use oral hydration salts (OHS) for patients in maintenance phase (800–1000 mL/h) matching input with output.

Discharge patients when all of the following criteria are fulfilled: oral intake ≥1000 mL/h; urine volume ≥400 mL/h; stool volume ≤400 mL/h.

Antimicrobial agents play a secondary role in treatment and have been shown to reduce duration and volume of diarrhea. Oral tetracycline (500 mg qid [four times a day] PO for 3 days) or doxycycline (300 mg stat PO) are the agents of choice in adults with sensitive strains. Alternative agents include trimethoprim/sulfamethoxazole (TMP-SMX; 960 mg bid PO for 3 days), ciprofloxacin (20 mg/kg stat), or azithromycin (20 mg/kg stat).

Prevention

Provision of uncontaminated water and good sanitation prevents cholera transmission. Active surveillance for *Vibrio* organisms in the environment and at-risk populations can aid in predicting the onset of an epidemic.

Parenteral cholera vaccines have proved disappointing. Oral cholera vaccines (e.g., oral inactivated whole cell plus B subunit [WCBS] or live attenuated oral vaccines) look more promising.

References

1. Seas C, Du Pont HL, Valdez LM, et al. (1996). Practical guidelines for the treatment of cholera. *Drugs* 51:966–973.

2. Morris JG (2003). Cholera and other types of vibriosis: a story of human pandemics and oysters on the half shell. *Clin Infect Dis* 37:272–280.

3. Sack DA, Sack RB, Nair GB, Siddique AK (2004). Cholera. *Lancet* 363:223–233.

Antibiotic-associated colitis

Diarrhea is the most common complication of antibiotic therapy, occurring in up to 15% of those receiving β-lactams and 25% of those receiving clindamycin. Predisposing factors include increased age, underlying illness, recent surgery, and recent use of bowel motility–altering medications (e.g., GI stimulants, enemas).

Etiology

Clostridium difficile is a frequent cause (20–30% of antibiotic-associated diarrhea (*C. difficile*-associated diarrhea [CDAD], 50–75% of antibiotic-associated colitis) and is associated with higher death rates and an increase in hospital cost and length of stay.

Other causes include *Candida*, enterotoxigenic *Clostridium perfringens*, and salmonellosis. The etiology of diarrhea and colitis not caused by *C. difficile* is not well understood.

Epidemiology

Incidence varies with antibiotic and epidemiological setting. Toxigenic *C. difficile* is the most common cause of hospital-acquired diarrhea. Rates vary with prescribing patterns, endemic strains, and the clinical setting; 3% of healthy adults carry *C. difficile*. Asymptomatic carriage rates rise to 20% among hospitalized adults receiving antibiotic therapy. Such patients rarely harbor significant quantities of toxin in their stool.

The most frequently implicated inciting agents are clindamycin and the cephalosporins (particularly third generation), penicillins, fluoroqunolones, and proton pump inhibitors. Certain antineoplastic agents have also been associated with *C. difficile* diarrhea, including doxorubicin, cyclophosphamide, and methotrexate.

Most disease-causing organisms are likely acquired from the environment. *C. difficile* may be cultured from surfaces, the hands of hospital personnel, soil, swimming pools, beaches, and tap water. Many outbreaks feature a predominant strain or related group of strains.

Clinical features

Infection with toxigenic *C. difficile* may be asymptomatic (particularly neonates), mildly symptomatic, or cause fulminant and occasionally fatal colitis. Symptoms commonly start 5–10 days after antibiotic therapy (<10 weeks after therapy has finished). Features include fever, abdominal pain, nausea, dehydration, and leukocytosis.

Severe cases involve perforation and toxic megacolon (acute dilatation of the colon to a diameter >6 cm with systemic toxicity with no mechanical obstruction, with mortality >64%) in the absence of diarrhea.

Extraintestinal complications (e.g., splenic abscess, osteomyelitis, Reiter's syndrome) are rare.

Differential diagnosis include other infectious causes of diarrhea, adverse drug reaction, ischemic colitis, and inflammatory bowel disease.

Pathogenesis

The complex ecosystem of the normal gut flora confers resistance to *C. difficile*. Antibiotics or antineoplastic agents disrupt this and render the colon more susceptible to *C. difficile* colonization.

The organism is acquired feco-orally; spores survive the acidic environment of the stomach. They convert to the vegetative form in the small intestine and begin to produce two toxins, A and B. These cause intestinal fluid secretion, mucosal injury, and inflammation. The resulting neutrophilic infiltrate with mucin, fibrin, and nuclear debris produces raised white/yellow plaques, thus the name *pseudomembranous colitis*.

The severity of disease seen in the UK has increased dramatically with the introduction of a strain originally identified in the U.S. (ribotype 027).

Diagnosis

Toxin detectionfrom stool samples is the most widely used means of diagnosis. ELISA-based tests for toxins A or B are rapid and specific but not as sensitive as the slower, more cumbersome cytotoxicity tests (in which filtered stool is incubated with a mammalian tissue culture cell line and assessed for its cytotoxic effect).

Rare isolates produce toxin B alone, thus testing for A only will miss some. Combined with strict clinical criteria and positive culture, ELISA sensitivity ranges from 63% to 94%, with specificity from 75% to 100%.

Cultureis sensitive and essential in the assessment of an outbreak, but most hospital microbiology labs cannot distinguish between toxigenic and nontoxigenic strains. PCR-based assays for toxins A and B are available but not yet in widespread use.

Endoscopyis usually reserved for specific situations: when a rapid diagnosis is required, if a patient has ileus and cannot produce stool, or when the differential diagnosis includes disease that could be confirmed endoscopically.

Management

- *General measures:* isolate the patient, implement infection control measures, discontinue the precipitating drug, replace fluid and electrolyte losses, and avoid antimotility agents.
- *Specific treatment:* oral metronidazole (500 mg PO qid for 10 days), or oral vancomycin (125 mg qid for 10 days). Patients unable to take oral antibiotics should receive antibiotics via a nasogastric (NG) tube or intravenously. Other antibiotics with activity against *C. difficile* infection include teicoplanin, fusidic acid, tigecycline, and nitazoxanide. Ribotype 027 may be less sensitive to metronidazole.
- *Recurrent disease:* CDAD recurs in 8–50% of cases. Re-treat with the original drug, e.g., metronidazole. If this fails, try the alternative, e.g., vancomcyin. In cases of multiple recurrence or refractory disease, consider the use of probiotics, immunoglobulins, or corticosteroids.
- Surgery is rarely necessary but is life saving in cases of toxic megacolon or perforation. Mortality in such cases is around 35%.
- Do not treat asymptomatic carriers. Vancomycin suppresses the organism but may cause prolonged carriage; metronidazole is ineffective.

Prevention

Limit the use of inciting agents, e.g., antibiotics and proton pump inhibitors. Infection control measures such as handwashing, universal precautions, and phenolic disinfectants for environmental cleaning are of proven benefit in reducing *C. difficile* transmission in health care settings.

Acute cholecystitis

This is inflammation of the gall bladder, usually secondary to cystic duct obstruction. Acute cholecystitis usually occurs on the background of chronic cholecystitis; most gall bladders removed at cholecystectomy exhibit fibrosis and other histological changes indicative of chronic inflammation.

Pathogenesis

Ninety percent of patients have gallstones impacted in the cystic duct. The consequent increase in intraductal pressure impairs blood supply and lymphatic drainage. Tissue necrosis and bacterial proliferation follow within the gall bladder.

Complications occur in 10–15% of cases: gall bladder empyema, emphysematous cholecystitis (elderly diabetic men), gall bladder perforation and peritonitis, pericholecystic abscess, intraperitoneal abscess, cholangitis, liver abscess, pancreatitis, and bacteremia.

The differential diagnosis includes myocardial infarction, ulcer perforation, intestinal obstruction, and right lower lobe pneumonia.

Clinical features

Early obstruction may cause only mild epigastric pain and nausea. Transient cases may settle in 1–2 hours. Persistent obstruction sees the symptoms localize to the right upper quadrant and increase in severity with signs of peritoneal irritation (shoulder tip pain). The gall bladder may be palpable in 30–40% of cases. Fever may occur.

Most patients settle within 4 days, with 25% requiring surgery or developing complications.

Severe fever with jaundice or hypotension should raise the suspicion of suppurative cholangitis (and obstruction of common bile duct [CBD]).

Diagnosis

- *Blood tests:* WCC is usually raised. 50% of patients have mild elevations of bilirubin, 40% have raised aspartate transaminase (AST), and 25% raised alkaline phosphatase (ALP).
- *Microbiology:* bacteria may be isolated from bile even in asymptomatic cases of cholecystitis. Rates of bile infection rise with the duration of symptoms and age of the patient and in jaundiced patients (particularly with CBD obstruction). The organisms isolated are those of the intestinal flora: enteric gram-negative bacilli (*E. coli*, *Klebsiella*, *Enterobacter*, *Proteus* spp.), enterococci, and anaerobes (*Bacteroides*, *Clostridia*, *Fusobacterium* spp.). Anaerobic organisms may be found in polymicrobial infection and are often isolated following biliary tract procedures.
- *Radiology:* CXR is of limited use. Gas in the gall bladder wall or lumen is diagnostic of emphysematous cholecystitis. Ultrasound is the diagnostic study of choice, showing a sensitivity of around 90% (presence of stones, thickened gall bladder wall, dilated gall bladder lumen, pericholecystic collection). Other useful modalities include nuclear medicine hepatobiliary scanning, CT, and MRI.

Treatment

Antibiotics

Elderly or severely ill patients with signs of infection or complications should be treated empirically, e.g., an aminoglycoside (gentamicin) with ampicillin and metronidazole. Therapy should be altered when culture results are available.

Antibiotics do not affect the outcome or incidence of infectious complications (e.g., empyema) in uncomplicated cases, perhaps because of poor penetration into gall bladder bile due to obstruction. Perioperative antibiotics reduce postoperative infectious complications such as wound infection and are recommended in the elderly, those with jaundice, CBD obstruction, or fever (cases associated with significant bactobilia).

Surgery
- *Acute uncomplicated cholecystitis:* some surgeons advocate delayed surgery after acute infection has settled. However, there is no difference in morbidity between early and delayed surgery and presentations can be deceptively benign, leading to urgent surgery under less favorable conditions
- Gangrenous/emphysematous cholecystitis, perforation, and percholecystic abscess all require urgent surgery.

Acute cholangitis

Obstruction of the common bile duct (by gallstones, tumor, parasite etc) leads to inflammation and infection of the biliary tree. Patients usually have a history of gall bladder disease.
- *Etiology:* similar to that seen in acute cholecystitis
- *Clinical features:* onset is acute with high fever, sweating, jaundice (Charcot's triad is seen in 85% of cases), and diffuse right upper quadrant pain. Gram-negative sepsis with shock is common
- *Diagnosis* is similar to that of cholecystitis. WCC, bilirubin, and ALP are high. However, patients with cholangitis have a high rate (50%) of bacteremia: *E. coli*, then anaerobes are the most frequently isolated organisms. Those patients with biliary stents are more likely to grow *Pseudomonas* spp.
- *Treatment:* antibiotic therapy, e.g., amoxicillin-clavulanate and gentamicin, should be commenced immediately as there is a high incidence of septic shock. Therapy is aimed at managing the bacteremia. Prompt decompression of the CBD by endoscopic retrograde cholangiopancreatography (ERCP) or surgery is essential. Intraoperative cholangiography should be performed.

Primary peritonitis

This is inflammation of the peritoneum due to infection not directly related to other intra-abdominal abnormalities. It occurs in all age groups.

Etiology
- *Children:* associated with postnecrotic cirrhosis, nephrotic syndrome, and urinary tract infection but can occur in those with no predisposing condition. Its incidence has fallen in children with the use of antibiotics.

- *Adults:* at-risk groups include those with ascites associated with alcoholic cirrhosis, chronic active hepatitis, congestive cardiac failure (CCF), metastatic malignancy, SLE, or HIV. It is a cause of decompensation in those with previously stable chronic liver disease.

Pathogenesis

Infection is acquired via the lymph nodes or blood (particularly in those with portosystemic shunting in association with cirrhosis which may increase the rates and duration of bacteremia), by bacterial transmural migration from the gut lumen, or via the Fallopian tubes in women (e.g., gonococcal or chlamydial perihepatitis).

Enteric organisms account for nearly 70% of infections in cirrhotic patients (*E. coli*, *Klebsiella pneumoniae*, enterococci, and other streptococci). *S. aureus* and anaerobes are less commonly isolated. Bacteremia may occur in up to 75% of those with aerobic organisms.

Unusual causes of peritonitis include *M. tuberculosis* and *Coccidioides immitis;* such organisms are usually found in disseminated infection. *S. pneumoniae* is the most common cause in HIV patients.

Clinical features

This is an acute febrile illness with fever, diffuse abdominal pain, nausea and vomiting, diarrhea, and rebound tenderness on examination. It resembles acute appendicitis. The onset may be insidious and patients can present with signs of infection or sepsis and no localizing features.

Cirrhotic patients may have other features of chronic liver disease.

Tuberculous peritonitis is gradual in onset with fever, weight loss, night sweats, and abdominal distension.

Gonococcal or chlamydial perihepatitis is usually seen in women. It presents with pain, guarding, and tenderness in the right upper quadrant.

Diagnosis

Abdominal paracentesis is indicated in all cirrhotic patients with ascites. Peritoneal fluid should be sent for cell count, Gram stain, culture, and protein concentration. Culture yield is improved by the direct inoculation of 10 mL fluid into blood culture bottles at the bedside. A positive Gram stain is diagnostic but is negative in 60% of cirrhotics with infection.

Ascitic fluid neutrophil count of over 500/microliter is the best single predictor of peritonitis (86% sensitive, 98% specific); generally a threshold of 250/microliter is used (93% sensitive, 94% specific). Improved diagnostic accuracy is achieved by combining cell counts and the ascitic fluid pH (neutrophil count >500/microliter and an ascitic fluid pH <7.35 gives 100% sensitivity and 96% specificity).

Blood cultures may be positive in about one-third of patients. The diagnosis of primary peritonitis can be made only after other potential primary sources of infection have been excluded.

Contrast-enhanced CT can help identify intra-abdominal sources of infection.

Some surgeons will exclude appendicitis in children only at operation. Tuberculous peritonitis may be confirmed at operation or histology and culture of peritoneal biopsies.

Treatment

Treat those patients with positive cultures or Gram stain regardless of the cell count (nearly 40% of those with positive cultures and normal cell counts go on to develop peritonitis) and all culture-negative patients with raised cell counts.

Initial treatment is empirical while culture results are awaited: ampicillin in combination with an aminoglycoside, or a third-generation cephalosporin (avoids the risks of nephrotoxicity). Patients with primary peritonitis respond within 48 hours to appropriate antibiotic therapy. Antibiotics are usually given for 10–14 days.

Follow-up peritoneal fluid cell counts are useful but not essential.

In those who do not respond, another primary source of infection should be considered (e.g., perforation, intra-abdominal abscess).

Prevention

Antimicrobial prophylaxis (e.g., ciprofloxacin) decreases the frequency of primary peritonitis in certain high-risk groups (patients with ascites admitted with GI bleeds, those awaiting liver transplantation, those with ascitic protein levels <1 g/dL), but does not confer a survival advantage.

Secondary peritonitis

Secondary peritonitis occurs as a result of a breach in the mucosal barrier, leading to spillage of organisms from the GI or GU tracts into the peritoneal cavity. This normally occurs in the context of intra-abdominal infections (e.g., appendicitis, diverticulitis) or surgery (abdominal, gynecological, or obstetric).

Etiology

Most cases are due to infection by the commensal flora of the mucous membranes within the abdominal cavity. Peritonitis also complicates an exogenously acquired visceral infection (e.g., *S. aureus, M. tuberculosis*).

Infection is usually polymicrobial. The most common isolates are *E. coli, B. fragilis*, enterococci, other *Bacteroides* spp., *Fusobacterium, C. perfringens, Peptococcus,* and *Peptostreptococcus.*

Antibiotic-resistant organisms are more likely to be found among those patients who acquire peritonitis while receiving antibiotics in the hospital (e.g., *Candida,* enterococci, *Enterobacter, Serratia, Acinetobacter* spp.). Vaginal flora, e.g., group B streptococci, may be present after vaginal surgery or labor.

Pathogenesis

Many anaerobic infections are synergisitic, e.g., facultative anaerobes providing a sufficiently reduced environment for the establishment of obligate anaerobic organisms.

Leaking bile or acid may cause a chemical peritonitis that leads to inflammation, necrosis, and further intra-abdominal damage, facilitating the establishment of bacterial infection.

Local inflammatory response of peritoneum leads to fluid production and granulocyte entry to the peritoneal cavity. The exudate contains fibrinogen, which forms plaques around inflamed surfaces aimed at localizing infection and may later lead to adhesions. Some instances of infection may be contained and resolve. Others may lead to local abscess formation. If localization fails completely, diffuse peritonitis may result.

Clinical features

- *Symptoms:* initial features are those of the primary disease process (e.g., appendicitis). Moderate abdominal pain, aggravated by movement, becomes more severe and diffuse as infection spreads throughout the abdomen. Pain may reduce in intensity and become more focal if localization strategies are effective. Other symptoms include vomiting, fever, distension, anorexia, unable to pass flatus, and thirst.
- *Signs:* patient lying still, alert, and restless at first, later becoming listless. Fever is usually present. Hypothermia may be noted in early chemical peritonitis and is a severe sign late in the course of patients presenting with sepsis. Tachycardia, hypotension, tachypnea, and abdominal tenderness (maximal over primarily affected organ) with rebound and guarding can occur; bowel sounds present initially later disappear. Some of these features may be masked in patients receiving glucocorticoids or whose abscess has been localized away from the anterior abdominal wall (e.g., subphrenic).

Diagnosis

- *Lab tests:* peripheral WCC 17,000–25,000 cells/mL with a left shift (in some situations, massive peritoneal inflammation may lead to low peripheral WCC with an extreme shift to immature forms), hemoconcentration, elevated amylase, acidosis in late disease, features of underlying condition (diabetic ketoacidosis [DKA], hematuria, pyuria, pancreatitis).
- *Radiology:* contrast CT is the preferred initial study. Plain XR: signs of inflammation, free air, distended loops of adynamic bowel, signs of the underlying condition (obstruction, volvulus, intussusception, gall bladder calcification). Ultrasound may be limited by the presence of air-filled loops of bowel.
- Blood cultures
- Peritoneal lavage or aspiration may be appropriate in some situations.
- *Differential diagnosis:* pneumonia, sickle cell anemia, herpes zoster, DKA, porphyria, familial Mediterranean fever, SLE, uremia

Treatment

General measures include fluid resuscitation, circulatory and respiratory support, and appropriate surgical interventions.

Antimicrobial therapy

Broad spectrum antimicrobial therapy should be started right after taking blood cultures. Combinations of two or three antibiotics provide good activity against aerobes and anaerobes, e.g., IV cephalosporin, metronidazole ± gentamicin, or IV amoxicillin-clavulanate ± gentamicin.

Detailed culture and sensitivity results may take several days, as cultures are often mixed and some organisms are slow growing. Antibiotics may not need to be active against every organism isolated. The elimination of the majority may allow host defenses to eliminate the remainder.

Antifungal therapy (e.g., fluconazole or echinocandin) should be used if *Candida* spp. are isolated; 5 to 7 days of treatment should be sufficient after adequate surgical intervention depending on the severity of infection and clinical response. Conversion to oral therapy may be indicated in those patients with a good response.

Prognosis

Survival depends on age, comorbid conditions, duration of peritoneal contamination, the primary process, and microorganisms involved.

Mortality ranges from 3.5% in those with early infection from penetrating trauma to 60% in those with established infection and secondary organ failure. Death is thought to follow uncontrolled cytokine release.

Prevention

Pre- and perioperative antibiotics reduce infections in clean, contaminated surgery (e.g., appendectomy for appendicitis without rupture, penetrating wounds of the abdomen, vaginal hysterectomy in premenopausal women). Postoperative infection rates fall from 20–30% to 4–8% with prophylactic antibiotic use in such infections.

Continuous ambulatory peritoneal dialysis peritonitis

Peritonitis was a common complication of peritoneal dialysis until Tenckhoff introduced his improved catheter in 1968. Rates fell further as techniques and bag adapters improved. However, it still occurs at around one episode per patient year, with up to 70% of patients experiencing an episode of infection in their first year of dialysis.

Recurrent infection is one of the most common reasons for discontinuing continuous ambulatory peritoneal dialysis (CAPD) (20–30% of patients). Prognosis is good; mortality is less than 1%.

Pathogenesis

Infection is commonly acquired by contamination of the catheter by skin organisms. Enteric organisms may be cultured from the skin of some CAPD patients. Organisms can also enter via the catheter exit site and through contamination of the dialysate delivery system, as well as transmurally in the manner seen in some cases of primary peritonitis.

Host defenses are impaired in CAPD patients by the low pH, high osmolality, and low IgG and C3 levels of dialysate (the addition of IgG to the fluid has been shown to have a prophylactic effect). Gram-positive organisms account for over 60% of isolates (CoNS, *S. aureus,* streptococcal species, and diphtheroids).

Other organisms include Gram negatives (*E. coli, Klebsiella, Enterobacter,* and *Pseudomonas*). Anaerobic organisms and yeasts are uncommon isolates. *Pseudomonas aeruginosa* peritonitis is associated with high treatment failure rates, and organisms such as *S. aureus, Streptococcus,* and fungi are associated with more severe disease.

Clinical features
Features include abdominal pain, tenderness (up to 80% of patients), nausea and vomiting, fever (10%), and diarrhea.

Diagnosis
Fluid should be taken from the catheter under sterile technique. It is usually cloudy in appearance. A WCC above 100/microliter is indicative of infection (neutrophils dominate). Peritoneal eosinophilia may be seen after tube placement (represents an allergic reaction to the tubing) and in some cases of fungal infection.

Gram stain is positive in less than half the cases. Blood cultures are rarely positive. Fluid should be inoculated into blood culture bottles. Yield can be improved by culturing the sediment of 50 mL of centrifuged fluid.

Treatment
- *Bacterial:* intraperitoneal antibiotics are preferred; there is no advantage to IV therapy. This allows for ambulatory treatment. Therapy should be started empirically then guided by the Gram stain and culture results. Treatment should continue for 10–21 days, or for 1 week after catheter removal. Most patients improve within 2 to 4 days. Those who do not should be re-evaluated and unusual (e.g., fungi) or resistant organisms considered, as well as alternative diagnoses.
- *Fungal:* most cases can be treated with amphotericin B, which can be given intraperitoneally but may cause abdominal pain. Most patients with fungal infections will require catheter removal and IV therapy. Flucytosine may be used, but levels must be carefully monitored. Some *Fusarium* species are resistant to amphotericin.
- *Catheter removal:* up to 20% of patients require catheter removal due to persistent skin or tunnel infection, intractable infections (fungal, mycobacterial, or *P. aeruginosa* infection), recurrent infections with the same organism, or catheter failure.

Prevention
Good technique helps reduce infection rates, e.g., exit site care, connection methods, patient training. Antibiotic prophylaxis may be of some benefit in those patients undergoing extensive dental procedures or lower GI endoscopy.

Further details are available in the guidelines produced by the International Society for Peritoneal Dialysis.[1]

Reference
1. ISPD Guidelines. www.ispd.org/lang-en/treatmentguidelines/guidelines (accessed August 12, 2008).

Diverticulitis

Pathogenesis

Diverticulae are small mucosal herniations that protrude through the intestinal layers and smooth muscle along openings created by the nutrient vessels in the wall of the colon. They are associated with a low-fiber diet, constipation, and obesity. Diverticulosis affects >10% of those over 45 years of age and 80% of those over 85 years.

Inflammation occurs in 20% of patients with diverticulae. It is more common in the elderly and those with extensive disease. Inflammation may remain confined to the bowel wall or be complicated by the formation of fistulae or perforation.

Presentation

Uncomplicated sigmoid diverticulitis can resemble appendicitis, but with left-side findings: fever, tenderness and guarding in the lower left quadrant of the abdomen, a mass, and raised WCC. Urinary symptoms may reflect inflammation close to the bladder, and fistulae may form (pneumaturia, fecaluria). Severe disease may present with peritonitis.

Diagnosis

Diagnosis is often made clinically acutely; patients should be managed medically with investigations following symptom resolution. CT has replaced barium enema for the diagnosis of diverticulosis and is also useful in guiding the drainage of any abscesses. Sigmoidoscopy may help exclude other pathology.

Differential diagnosis includes malignancy, IBD, pelvic inflammatory disease, and mesenteric ischemia.

Management

- *First attacks of acute uncomplicated diverticulitis* are managed medically if tolerated: oral antibiotics (e.g., amoxicillin-clavulanate) and liquid diet. Otherwise, patients require admission and IV antibiotics.
- *Complicated disease:* intravenous antibiotics (as for secondary peritonitis), nasogastric tube, and surgery may be indicated. Small abscesses may resolve with IV antibiotics alone or be amenable to guided percutaneous drainage. Abscesses containing gross fecal material require surgical intervention. Fistulae may need repairing.
- *Perforated diverticulitis:* a two-stage procedure is commonly performed with resection of the diseased bowel and proximal colostomy to decompress the bowel and divert the fecal stream, followed by reanastomosis a few months later. A single-stage procedure may be appropriate in certain patients. Intravenous antibiotics should be started preoperatively.
- Consider surgery for those patients failing to respond to conservative therapy within 72 hours or with persistent obstruction or if malignancy is suspected.

Intra-abdominal abscess

Intra-abdominal abscesses may complicate peritonitis of any cause. Primary abscesses develop following primary peritonitis. Secondary abscesses may follow appendicitis, diverticulitis, biliary tract lesions, pancreatitis, IBD, perforated peptic ulcers, trauma, and surgery.

Pathogenesis

Infections are usually polymicrobial, with anaerobes isolated in up to 70% of cases. Other organisms include enterococci, *Enterobacteriaceae*, *P. aeruginosa*, and *S. aureus*. Abscess location is related to that of the primary disease and the direction of peritoneal drainage (e.g., most appendicitis-related abscesses occur in the right lower quadrant or pelvis).

Clinical features

These include high or fluctuating fever, rigors, abdominal pain, and tenderness over the affected area. Specific features will vary with the location—e.g., subphrenic abscesses may cause costal tenderness and chest signs on examination.

Presentation can be acute or chronic (particularly subphrenic abscesses where the patient has been receiving antibiotics) and may follow primary abdominal disease (e.g., pancreatitis) or abdominal surgery with a prolonged recuperation.

Diagnosis

Ultrasound, CT, or MRI scans are the most effective means of identifying abscesses. A pleural effusion on chest X-ray may indicate a subphrenic abscess. The diagnosis is confirmed by radiologically guided diagnostic aspiration. Samples should be sent to the lab for microscopy, culture, and sensitivity (MC&S) testing.

Treatment

Drainage is key: percutaneous drainage (radiologically guided) is suitable for unilocular collections that are readily accessible, are not vascular, and are likely to drain easily by simple dependent drainage. Repeat scanning should be used to confirm resolution following adequate drainage. Surgical drainage is usually required for multiple or loculated abscesses or in those with very viscous pus.

Antibiotic agents should be directed against the most likely organisms, e.g., *Enterobacteriaceae* and anaerobes. Therapy should be started immediately after blood cultures have been taken. The antimicrobial regimen should be tailored to culture results. Repeat samples may be required in patients with prolonged antimicrobial therapy.

Retroperitoneal abscess

Abscesses may form in the retroperitoneal space following direct extension of infection from a retroperitoneal structure (e.g., pyelonephritis, spinal osteomyelitis), intra-abdominal sepsis, traumatic hemorrhage, or bacteremia.

Common organisms include *S. aureus* and coliforms. Anaerobes and polymicrobial infections are less common. *M. tuberculosis* may be seen in endemic areas. Patients present with fever, abdominal, flank, and lumbar pain, and a palpable mass. If the psoas sheath is involved, there may be pain on hip flexion.

Diagnosis is made by CT or MRI scan. Blood cultures and aspirated pus should be sent to the lab for culture.

Management is by surgical drainage and empirical broad-spectrum IV antibiotic therapy while awaiting results of cultures. Treatment should be tailored to culture results.

Pancreatic abscess

Up to 9% of patients with acute pancreatitis develop a pancreatic abscess. Abscesses may also develop following penetration by a peptic ulcer or secondary infection of a pancreatic pseudocyst. Up to 50% of abscesses are polymicrobial. Hematogenous seeding of bacteria may explain those abscesses caused by single organisms.

- *Clinical features:* patients present with failure to improve or abrupt deterioration following initial recovery from acute pancreatitis. Most patients experience abdominal pain radiating to the back, with fever and vomiting. Rarer manifestations include jaundice, distension, peritonitis, and abdominal mass. Serum amylase may be elevated.
- *Diagnosis:* ultrasound and CT demonstrate the abscess in most cases, but distinguishing abscess from pseudocyst may require guided diagnostic needle aspiration.
- *Treatment:* surgical drainage or debridement is essential (53–86% survival). Percutaneous drainage may be helpful in some patients requiring stabilization prior to surgery but is rarely sufficient. Initial antibiotic therapy needs to be broad and can later be adjusted according to sensitivity testing.
- *Complications:* retroperitoneal extension of infection; fistula formation between the abscess and stomach, duodenum or colon; erosion of major blood vessels causing intra-abdominal hemorrhage

Splenic abscess

This is uncommon and may be due to bacteremic seeding of infection (e.g., bacterial endocarditis, IV drug user), splenic infarction (e.g., blunt trauma, sickle cell disease), or direct extension of intra-abdominal infection. Abscesses are usually multiple.

- *Etiology:* causes include *S. aureus*, streptococci, *Enterobactericeae*, anaerobes, and *Candida* spp. Around a quarter are polymicrobial.
- *Clinical features:* left upper quadrant pain with shoulder tip discomfort and fever. Multiple small abscesses may not cause spleen enlargement.
- *Diagnosis:* chest X-ray may demonstrate an elevated hemidiaphragm, basal pulmonary infiltrates, or pleural effusion. Ultrasound, CT, or MRI scanning confirms the diagnosis.
- *Treatment:* initial antibiotic therapy must be broad spectrum (e.g., cephalosporin and metronidazole) and modified following culture results. Multiple or large single abscesses may necessitate splenectomy. Incision and drainage may be preferred in cases where the spleen is held by extensive adhesions.

Hepatic abscess

Etiology

Bacterial liver abscesses are relatively uncommon. They are associated with liver transplantation, chronic granulomatous disease, and sickle cell anemia. Infection may be acquired by the biliary tract (may cause multiple abscesses), the portal vein (e.g., in appendicitis or IBD), from an adjacent structure (e.g., gall bladder), hematogenous seeding of infection from elsewhere in the body, and trauma to the liver.

Bacterial abscesses are usually polymicrobial e.g., enterobacteriaceae and anaerobes. *S. aureus* is found in <20% of cases, many of these young children. Other organisms identified in the context of liver abscess include *Y. enterocolitica* and *Candida* spp. (patients are often immunosuppressed).

Amebic liver abscess is caused by *Entamoeba histolytica*. It complicates <10% of cases of amebic colitis. It occurs in males more than females. Abscesses are usually solitary and more common in the right lobe.

Presentation

Bacterial abscesses present with fever over days or weeks. Ascending cholangitis causing multiple abscesses presents with characteristic spiking temperatures. Abscesses in the upper right lobe may cause cough and pleuritic and shoulder pain; <70% of patients have hepatomegaly. Jaundice is unusual out of the context of ascending cholangitis or in cases of extensive hepatic involvement (e.g., multiple abscesses).

Amebic liver abscess is particularly suggested by a history of diarrhea with point tenderness over the right chest wall.

Diagnosis

- *Radiology:* plain CXR may reveal elevation of the right diaphragm, with a right pleural effusion or gas in the abscess cavity. Ultrasound or CT are most useful and may be used to guide diagnostic aspiration.
- *Blood tests:* WCC, CRP, and ALP may be raised.
- *Blood cultures* are positive in 50% of patients with bacterial abscesses.
- *Amebic serology* is useful outside endemic areas and is positive in 90% of those with amebic abscess. Aspirated material should be cultured aerobically and anaerobically and examined for *E. histolytica* on direct microscopy. Brown, sterile fluid without a foul odor suggests an amebic abscess, although secondary infection with bacteria is common.

Treatment

Bacterial abscesses

Broad-spectrum IV antibiotic therapy should be started as soon as the diagnosis is suspected. Although there are reports of successful resolution in the absence of drainage, most experts recommend percutaneous drainage. Material should be cultured to guide specific therapy. Antibiotics should be continued for at least 1 month and often as long as 4 months in the case of multiple abscesses.

Most fevers resolve within 2 weeks; some may take up to 4 weeks. The rate of resolution may be assessed with serial scans.

Surgical drainage should be considered in those cases that fail to respond, in loculated or viscous abscesses, and in those resulting from biliary obstruction. Cure rates may be >90% in cases where the diagnosis is made early and the abscess is not associated with serious underlying disease.

Amebic abscesses

Metronidazole is active against both the intestinal and hepatic stages of the organism. Aspiration is probably not necessary unless the lesion is very large, threatens to rupture, or fails to respond to medical therapy. Large lesions may require repeated aspiration.

The mortality rate of uncomplicated amebic abscesses is under 1%. Higher mortalities are associated with those abscesses that rupture into the peritoneum (18%), pericardium (30%), or pleura/bronchi (6%).

Acute hepatitis

This is a self-limiting inflammation of the liver, which may be caused by a broad range of infectious or noninfectious agents.

Etiology

- *Hepatitis viruses:* e.g., hepatitis A (HAV, p. 358), hepatitis B (HBV, p. 359), hepatitis C (HCV, p. 362), hepatitis D (HDV, p. 362), hepatitis E (HEV, p. 365). Novel candidate viruses include hepatitis GB virus C (HGBV-C), hepatitis G (HGV), and transfusion transmissible virus (TTV).
- *Other viruses:* Epstein–Barr virus (p. 347), cytomegalovirus (p. 351), herpes simplex virus (p. 341), varicella zoster virus, measles (p. 330), rubella (p. 335), adenovirus (p. 379), Coxsackie B, enterovirus, and yellow fever virus (p. 399)
- *Nonviral infectious diseases:* spirochetes (p. 284), *Coxiella* (p. 298), *Legionella, Ponicella, Franciscella, Yersinia,* syphilis, (p. 642), leptospirosis (p. 292), Q fever (p. 298), sepsis (p. 523), legionellosis (p. 268), tuberculosis (p. 307), brucellosis (p. 261), tularemia (p. 266), plague (p. 263)
- Drug-induced hepatitismay be caused by a variety of drugs. Common culprits include aspirin, paracetamol, isoniazid, rifampicin, pyrazinamide, phenytoin, and halothane.
- Alcoholic hepatitis may mimic acute viral hepatitis.
- Anoxic liver injury may be caused by hypotension, cardiac failure, or cardiopulmonary arrest.
- Other liver diseases include Wilson's disease and Budd–Chiari syndrome.

Clinical features

There are no clinical features that distinguish the various causes.

Acute viral hepatitis can be divided into four clinical stages: incubation period, preicteric phase, icteric phase, and convalescence.

Clinical features may range from asymptomatic disease to anorexia, malaise, abdominal pain, and jaundice to fulminant hepatic failure.

Hepatitis B and C may cause immune complex–mediated diseases, e.g., serum sickness, polyarteritis nodosa (HBV), glomerulonephritis, and mixed cryoglobulinemia.

Fulminant viral hepatitis, characterized by liver failure and hepatic encephalopathy, occurs within 8 weeks after onset of symptoms.

Diagnosis

- *Routine blood tests:* AST and alanine aminotransferase (ALT) are usually dramatically elevated and bilirubin may be variably elevated. A prolonged prothrombin time (PT) is rare and suggests severe hepatic necrosis.
- *Serology:* anti-HAV IgM, HBsAg and anti-HBc IgM, anti-HCV should be performed initially. If these are negative, other diagnoses should be considered (see above).
- *Liver ultrasound* is usually normal in acute viral hepatitis. Abnormalities, e.g., hepatic lesions, cirrhosis, portal hypertension, or ascites, suggest alternative diagnoses (see above).
- *Liver biopsy* may be performed to establish the diagnosis in acute hepatitis with negative serology.

Management
Supportive care
Most patients with acute viral hepatitis do not require hospitalization unless they are at risk of dehydration, have clinical evidence of liver failure, or have a rising bilirubin or PT. Bed rest and alcohol avoidance are recommended while patients are symptomatic. Most medications should be avoided, but symptomatic therapy for nausea or pain may be required. Vitamin K may be given if the PT is prolonged.

Treatment
There is no specific treatment for acute viral hepatitis. Corticosteroids have been recommended for cholestatic hepatitis and fulminant hepatic failure, although clinical trials have failed to show benefit.

Interferon-A has also been used in fulminant HBV but the evidence is poor. There is some evidence that treatment of acute HCV infection with interferon-B may prevent chronic infection.

Monitoring
Inpatients should be monitored regularly for signs of liver failure and with blood tests (bilirubin, AST, ALT, and PT). Hepatitis serology should be rechecked after 6 months to determine chronicity.

Liver biopsy and transplantation
Liver biopsy may be performed for various reasons, e.g., diagnostic uncertainty, if more than one cause is a possibility, or if specific treatment is being considered.

Liver transplantation is the only available treatment for fulminant hepatic failure, and patients should be promptly referred for consideration of transplantation.

Chronic hepatitis

Chronic hepatitis is a descriptive term used to denote ongoing inflammation (>6 months) of the liver.

Causes
- Chronic viral hepatitis: hepatitis B virus (p. 359), hepatitis C virus, hepatitis D virus, hepatitis E virus (p. 365)
- Autoimmune hepatitis
- Hereditary hemochromatosis
- Wilson's disease
- A_1-antitrypsin deficiency
- Fatty liver and non-alcoholic steatohepatitis (NASH)
- Alcoholic liver disease
- Drug-induced liver disease
- Hepatic granulomas: infectious, drug induced, neoplastic, idiopathic

Clinical features
There are no specific clinical features, and most patients remain asymptomatic until they develop end-stage liver disease. Nonspecific features (e.g., fatigue and right upper quadrant discomfort) are common. Symptoms such as jaundice, weight loss, abdominal distension, or confusion suggest decompensation.

Examination may show signs of chronic liver disease (e.g., palmar erythema, Dupytren's contractures, jaundice, spider nevi, hepatosplenomegaly, caput medusa, ascites).

Clinical features of hepatic encephalopathy include confusion, drowsiness, asterixis, ophthalmoplegia, and ataxia.

Diagnosis
- *Routine blood tests:* AST and ALT are usually dramatically elevated and bilirubin may be variably elevated. A prolonged PT suggests hepatic failure. A low albumin occurs in cirrhosis.
- *Serology:* HBsAg and anti-HCV should be performed for patients with suspected chronic viral hepatitis. If these are negative, other diagnoses should be considered (see above).
- Liver ultrasound may show hepatomegaly or cirrhosis, portal hypertension, or ascites. Hepatic lesions may be due to hepatocellular carcinoma.
- Liver biopsy may be performed to establish the diagnosis in chronic hepatitis with negative serology or to determine the degree of fibrosis in patients with suspected cirrhosis. In patients with deranged clotting this may be performed by the transjugular route.

Management
Chronic HBV infection is usually treated with antiviral agents (see Antivirals for chronic viral hepatitis, p. 85), e.g., interferon-α lamivudine, adefovir dipivoxil, and entecavir. Tenofovir (TDF) also has anti-HBV activity and should be used to treat HIV/HBV coinfected patients.

Liver transplantation may be performed for patients with end-stage liver disease. However, the risk of reinfection is 20% even with prophylaxis (lamivudine and polyclonal anti-hepatitis B immunoglobulin [HBIG]).

Chronic HCV infection is also treated with antiviral therapy, e.g., pegylated interferon-α and ribavirin (see Antivirals for chronic viral hepatitis, p. 85). End-stage liver disease secondary to chronic HCV is the leading indication for hepatic transplantation. HCV recurrence occurs in >90% by 1 year after transplantation.

The best strategy to prevent or treat reinfection has not yet been established. At present, combination therapy with interferon-α and ribavirin may be given in the following situations: before transplantation to prevent complications, e.g., hepatoma; prophylactically just before transplantation to prevent recurrence; pre-emptively just after transplantation; and when HCV recurs after transplantation.

Other gastrointestinal infections

Mesenteric adenitis

Inflammation of the mesenteric lymph nodes may be acute or chronic depending on the infecting agent. Organisms are thought to pass through intestinal lymphatics to the lymph nodes where they produce inflammation and sometimes suppuration. This is most common in children <15 years of age.

- *Causes* include *Yersinia* species, *Staphylococcus* spp., *E. coli*, *Streptococcus* spp., *M. tuberculosis*, *Giardia lamblia*, nontyphoidal salmonellae and viruses (e.g., Coxsackie and adenovirus).
- *Clinical features:* fever, abdominal pain, and tenderness. It may be difficult to distinguish clinically from appendicitis.
- *Diagnosis:* CT scan may demonstrate enlarged mesenteric lymph nodes. The key feature in diagnosis is to recognize appendicitis and other problems requiring surgical intervention; <20% of appendectomies may reveal evidence of nonspecific mesenteric adenitis. Blood cultures may be positive in those bacterial cases that progress to sepsis. Serological tests may demonstrate evidence of *Y. enterocolitica* infection.
- *Treatment:* patients with mild symptoms need only supportive care. Ill patients with more obvious evidence of infection require antibiotic treatment.
- *Complications:* abscess formation, sepsis, peritonitis

Typhlitis

This is inflammation of the cecum. It may occur in patients with HIV or severe neutropenia. It is thought that bacteria from the lumen invade ulcerations in the bowel wall during periods of neutropenia, proliferate, and produce exotoxins causing damage to the gut wall.

- *Clinical features* resemble those of acute appendicitis, with fever, pain, and rebound tenderness in the right iliac fossa. Rapid progression to an acute abdomen may occur.

- *Treatment:* broad-spectrum IV antibiotic therapy (aerobic and anaerobic cover) with surgical resection of necrotic bowel is recommended, as the mortality rate of severe cases of neutropenic enterocolitis is >50%.

Tropical sprue and enteropathy

This is a syndrome of acute or chronic diarrhea, weight loss, and malabsorption of at least two nutrients, which is believed to follow an intestinal microbial infection that causes enterocyte injury and bacterial overgrowth. Villous destruction and demonstrable nutrient malabsorption occur in varying degrees. It has been described in tropical climates throughout the world but primarily Southeast Asia and the Caribbean.

- *Clinical features:* symptoms develop over months after several years' residence in an affected area. It presents with weight loss, fatigue, and features of the loss of specific nutrients, most commonly folate, vitamin B_{12}, and iron.
- *Diagnosis:* there are no specific tests. Laboratory studies reveal the features of the specific nutritional deficiencies (e.g., megaloblastic emiaanaemia). Stool studies may demonstrate fat malabsorption, and small bowel biopsy may show villous atrophy. The diagnosis is one of exclusion.
- *Treatment:* management is with nutritional support and antibiotic therapy (e.g., tetracycline or metronidazole for 6–12 months).

Whipple's disease

This is a rare, chronic, and systemic infectious disorder caused by a gram-positive bacterium, *Tropheryma whippelii*. Clinical manifestations probably follow a disordered host response to the organism's infiltration of various body tissues. The organism is taken up into tissue macrophages that may be seen with periodic acid–Schiff (PAS) staining.

It predominantly affects middle-aged Caucasian men. Patients with HIV infection do not develop the disease, and one small study found *T. whippelii* DNA in 35% of healthy volunteers.

- *Clinical features:* presents with arthritis, fever, diarrhea, abdominal pain, and weight loss (90%). Malabsorption follows disruption of the villous architecture. Cardiovascular (endocarditis), respiratory, and central nervous system (supranuclear ophthalmoplegia, cerebellar ataxia, disinhibition, meningoencephalitis) involvement may occur.
- *Diagnosis:* biopsy of affected organs (small bowel, synovium, brain, endocardium) to demonstrate the typical histopathology (not pathognomic and may be seen with *Mycobacterium avium intracellulare* [MAI], cryptococcosis, or other parasitic infections usually observed in patients who are immunosuppressed with HIV disease) and DNA testing for *T whippelii*. The disease is almost universally fatal within 12 months if untreated.
- *Treatment:* prolonged course of antibiotics, e.g., 2 weeks of IV ceftriaxone followed by 1 year of TMP-SMX. PCR may be the best way to demonstrate remission; therapy should be continued if patients remain positive, perhaps with an alternative regime. Malnourished patients will need nutritional support and vitamin supplementation.

Urinary tract infections: introduction

Definitions

The term *urinary tract infection* (UTI) covers the whole spectrum of infection, from asymptomatic bacteriuria to severe pyelonephritis.

Uncomplicated UTI is considered to be infection of a structurally and functionally normal urinary tract, e.g., acute cystitis in women.

Complicated UTI is infection of a urinary tract that is abnormal, either structurally (obstruction, stents, medullary scars), functionally (vesicoureteral reflux, incomplete bladder emptying), or neurologically.

All UTIs in men, pregnant women, and children are considered complicated. Any patient with a complicated UTI should be referred to a specialist for assessment and follow-up.

Epidemiology

Asymptomatic bacteriuria occurs in all age groups and does not necessarily result in clinical infection.

- *Infants:* incidence of UTI is 1–2%, more common in males.
- *Children:* asymptomatic bacteriuria and UTI are more common in girls. UTI is rare in boys and suggests a structural abnormality.
- *Women:* asymptomatic bacteriuria occurs in 1–3% of nonpregnant women and 2–9.5% of pregnant women; 10–20% of women experience symptomatic UTI during their life. Risk factors include frequent sexual intercourse, diaphragm use, spermicide use, lack of urination after intercourse, and history of recurrent infections; 20–30% of pregnant women with untreated asymptomatic bacteriuria go on to develop acute pyelonephritis.
- *Men:* asymptomatic bacteriuria <0.1%. Circumcision is associated with a decreased risk of UTI.
- *Elderly:* 10% of men and 20% of women aged >65 years have bacteriuria. Risk factors include prostatic disease, poor bladder emptying, perineal soiling, and urinary tract instrumentation.
- *Hospitalized patients:* high rates of bacteriuria; 10% of catheterized patients develop UTI. Other risk factors include female diabetics, pregnant black women with sickle cell trait, those with interstitial renal disease, renal transplant recipients.
- *Renal transplant patients:* asymptomatic bacteriuria is associated with a high incidence of pyelonephritis and the risk of graft loss.

Etiology

From 70 to 95% of acute community infections are due to *E. coli*. Recurrent UTIs or nosocomial infections are associated with *Proteus, Pseudomonas, Klebsiella, Enterobacter,* enterococci, and staphylococci.

Polymicrobial infections are common in those with structural abnormalities, as are antibiotic-resistant organisms (secondary to antibiotic exposure and instrumentation).

Fungi (particularly *Candida*) occur in patients with indwelling catheters receiving antimicrobial therapy.

Coagulase-negative staphylococci (CoNS) are a common cause among young sexually active women.

S. aureus infection is usually hematogenous and associated with renal or perinephric abscesses.

Adenoviruses (especially type 11) are implicated in acute hemorrhagic cystitis in children and allogenic bone marrow transplant recipients.

Pathogenesis

Host factors

The urinary tract is normally sterile and fairly resistant to bacterial colonization (except the urethra). Host antibacterial mechanisms include urinary flow and pH, bactericidal cytokines, inhibitors of bacterial adherence, local immune responses, and the inhibitory effect of prostatic fluid secretions. Individuals who are particularly susceptible to UTIs may have defects in these mechanisms.

Abnormalities of the urinary tract may also undermine the effectiveness of the host response.

Organism factors

Infection may be caused by many bacterial species, each of which has its own virulence factors, e.g., *E. coli* has P fimbriae that facilitate adherence to the uroepithelium. Bacteria enter the urethra tract by (a) ascending the urethra or (b) hematogenously. The urethra is normally colonized with bacteria, which may be forced into the bladder by sexual intercourse or catheterization.

Women have shorter urethras and thus higher rates of UTI. Hematogenous spread is less common but occurs in the context of staphylococcal bacteremia or endocarditis or candidemia.

Diagnosis

Specimen collection

Urine may be collected by midstream clean catch (to reduce the number of urethral organisms collected), by catherization, or by suprapubic aspiration of the bladder.

Urine dipstick analysis

Pyuria (10–50 white cells/mm^3 urine) is nonspecific and does not necessarily indicate infection, but most patients with UTI have pyuria. The leukocyte esterase test is sensitive (75–96%) and specific (94–98%) for detecting >10 white cells/mm^3 urine.

Hematuria may be seen in certain infections, but calculi, tumor, vasculitis, glomerulonephritis, and renal TB should be considered. Proteinuria is common in UTI and should be <2 g/24 hours.

The dipstick nitrite test detects the products of bacterial nitrate reduction. It may be falsely negative in the presence of diuretic use, low dietary nitrate, or organisms that do not produce nitrate reductase (e.g., *Enterococcus*, *Pseudomonas*, and *Staphylococcus*). The combined sensitivity and specificity of dipstick leukocyte and nitrite testing is 79.2% and 81%, respectively.

Urine culture

Patients with UTI usually have ≥10^5 organisms/mL urine in properly collected specimens. Patients without infection will have counts of <10^4

organisms/mL urine. However symptomatic infections can result in counts of 10^4–10^5 organisms/mL urine. These criteria apply to gram-negative organisms. Infection caused by gram-positive organisms, fastidious bacteria, and fungi rarely measures over 10^4 bacteria/mL.

Blood cultures should be taken if systemic infection is a possibility.

Urological assessment
Exclude anatomical abnormalities, stones, and tumors in patients with recurrent UTIs; complicated UTIs; or UTIs in men, pregnant women, infants, and children.

Cystitis

Cystitis is a superficial mucosal infection confined to the lower urinary tract and characterized by dysuria, frequency, and urgency. These symptoms may also be related to urethritis or inflammation without infection.

Nonbacterial causes of cystits include infectious agents (viral, mycobacterial, chlamydial, and fungal species) and noninfectious precipitants (radiation, chemical, autoimmune, hypersensitivity, and interstitial cystitis). Consider these nonbacterial causes in cases of cystitis that are culture negative and fail to respond to antibiotic therapy.

Clinical features
These include dysuria, urgency, hesitancy, polyuria, incomplete voiding, urinary incontinence, hematuria, and suprapubic or low back pain.

Elderly patients may present with confusion and no localizing features.

Constitutional symptoms such as fever are mild or absent.

Management[1]
General measures include hydration, management of diabetes, investigation, and management of obstruction or structural abnormalities.

Antibiotic therapy
All symptomatic infections should be treated and empirical regimes based on local resistance data. The resolution of bacteriuria is related to the concentration of the antimicrobial agent achieved in the urine; dosage modifications are necessary in patients with renal insufficiency for agents excreted primarily by the kidney.

- *Uncomplicated lower urinary tract infections in women:* 3-day treatment courses are as effective as 7-day schedules and have as few side effects as less effective 1-day regimens, e.g., nitrofurantoin 60 mg qid
- *Lower urinary tract infection in other groups:* short courses have not been evaluated in men and are not suitable for children or women with a history of previous UTI caused by antibiotic-resistant organisms. These groups should receive 7–10 days' treatment.
- *Complicated infection:* 7–14 days' treatment

Recurrent infection
This may follow relapse (bacteriuria with the same organism that was present when treatment was started) or reinfection (bacteriuria with a

different organism from that before treatment). Reinfection with the same organism may occur if it has persisted in nearby areas, e.g., vagina.

Relapse

Consider renal involvement (necessitating a longer course of therapy, 2–6 weeks), a structural abnormality (e.g., calculi, obstruction; consider urological investigation), or chronic prostatitis (p. 622).

Patients with repeated relapses in whom surgical correction is not indicated or is not feasible may be appropriate for long-term antibiotic therapy. Such patients should have regular urine cultures (looking for antibiotic resistance), assessment of renal function, and renal imaging.

There is no consensus on how long prophylaxis should last. Rates of infection return to pretreatment levels once therapy is stopped. Cranberry juice *does* reduce the frequency of episodes compared to placebo.

Reinfection

Certain patients experience repeated reinfections (with successful clearance following appropriate therapy between each episode). Those cases related to sexual intercourse may benefit from postcoital voiding. One RCT demonstrated reduced recurrence rates on taking a single dose of antibiotic (TMP-SMX) up to 2 hours after intercourse.[2]

When no associated precipitating event can be identified, long-term chemoprophylaxis may be appropriate, particularly in children who may be at risk of renal damage.

Prognosis

Children

Those without obstruction (e.g., urethral valves) or vesicoureteric reflux (VUR) have a good prognosis. Obstruction can lead to severe destruction of the renal parenchyma. VUR is seen in 30–50% of children with bacteriuria and can lead to renal scarring. Infants and preschool children are at the greatest risk.

Severe reflux may lead to repeated infection and renal impairment. Reflux alone, particularly intrarenal reflux, may be capable of causing renal scarring even in the absence of infection. Infection exacerbates reflux, which reduces with the elimination of bacteriuria.

Adults

Once a woman has had a UTI, she is more likely to go on have further episodes. There may be a role for prophylactic antibiotic therapy in women with recurrent uncomplicated UTIs.

Urethral syndrome

This is seen in women with acute onset of urinary symptoms (dysuria, etc.) but with <10^5 bacteria/mL. Studies have shown that most of these patients have genuine infection with a low number of organisms confined to the lower urinary tract. Others may represent patients with sterile pyuria and urethritis secondary to infection with *Chlamydia trachomatis* or *N. gonorrhoeae*.

However, some patients with the syndrome have no pyuria and persistently sterile cultures. The cause of their symptoms is not clear, but vaginitis and genital herpes should be excluded.

References

1. Guidelines for antimicrobial treatment of uncomplicated acute bacterial cystitis and acute pyelonephritis in women. *Clin Infect Dis* 1999;29:745–758.

2. http://www.clinicalevidence.com (accessed August 12, 2008).

Acute pyelonephritis

Acute pyelonephritis is infection and inflammation of the renal parenchyma, characterized by flank pain and fever with or without dysuria, frequency, and urgency. It is potentially organ threatening, and each episode of infection may scar the kidney, impairing renal function.

Complications are renal failure, abscess formation (nephric, perinephric), sepsis, or shock and multi-organ failure.

Clinical features

Symptoms develop over hours to (rarely) days and vary greatly in severity. Symptoms of lower UTI may be present: dysuria, frequency, hesitancy, lower abdominal pain, urgency, hematuria (hemorrhagic cystitis), and suprapubic pain.

Symptoms of pyelonephritis include flank pain, back pain, fever, rigors, chills, weakness, and anorexia. Signs are fever, tachycardia, hypotensive if shock, suprapubic tenderness, and flank tenderness.

Diagnosis

Pyelonephritis is usually easily diagnosed in women but may be less obvious in men, the elderly, and hospitalized patients, in whom infection may develop insidiously. See general points on diagnosis of UTI (p. 110).

- *Urinalysis:* macroscopic hematuria is unusual in pyelonephritis and is seen more commonly in lower UTI (hemorrhagic cystitis). Consider calculi, cancer, glomerulonephritis, tuberculosis, trauma, and vasculitis.
- *Urine culture:* all patients with presumed pyelonephritis should be tested because of the possibility of antibiotic resistance.
- *Blood cultures* are indicated for hospitalized patients. Up to 20% are positive.

Imaging

Imaging is rarely indicated in the diagnosis of those presenting with typical signs. It is useful in those with atypical features and in those who deteriorate or do not respond to therapy (e.g., fever and positive blood cultures >48 hours after therapy initiated, complicated UTIs) for the purposes of identifying organ- or life-threatening complications.

Contrast-enhanced spiral CT is the study of choice (more sensitive than ultrasound). Dimercaptosuccinic acid (DMSA) scanning is used in children to lessen radiation exposure.

Other patients in whom early imaging may be useful are those at increased risk of complications: patients with AIDS, the immunosuppressed, and those with poorly controlled diabetes, sepsis, or shock.

Management[1]

General management includes rehydration, antipyretics, and analgesics.

Antibiotic therapy

Start antibiotics empirically as guided by local resistance patterns, while awaiting culture and sensitivity testing. Most community-acquired cases are due to *E. coli* or other enterobacteriaceae. Appropriate therapy would include IV amoxicillin-clavulanate or ceftriaxone ± a single dose of gentamicin. Treatment duration is usually 14 days; 7 days' ciprofloxacin is sufficient in healthy young women with uncomplicated disease.

Consider the addition of vancomycin in those at risk of MRSA infection (e.g., recent instrumentation, previous MRSA isolation in urine). Hospitalized patients or those from residential institutions may require enterococcal coverage.

Surgery

Surgery may be required in some patients with predisposing conditions who fail to respond to therapy and in those developing certain complications, e.g., renal cortical abscess, corticomedullary abscess, emphysematous pyelonephritis.

Patients with complicated infection

Obtain follow-up urine cultures, consider for follow-up urinary tract imaging, and refer for specialist management. Such cases would include the first episode in a child, those presenting with renal impairment, pregnant patients, those with unusual organisms, and immunocompromised patients.

Prevention

- *Cases with an obvious precipitant:* practice changes (e.g., different means of contraception, administration of prophylactic antibiotics, early identification and treatment of lower UTIs) may prevent UTIs. If they do not, consider an underlying structural abnormality.
- *Long-term catheter-related infections:* ensure a closed system, consider intermittent or suprapubic catheterization.
- *Renal transplant recipients:* antibiotic prophylaxis may be given to some groups of patients in the first 6–12 months after transplantation.

Prognosis

Acute renal failure (ARF) is rare in children, healthy adults, and pregnant women outside the context of hypovolemia, obstruction, or sepsis. ARF may follow papillary necrosis (sloughing necrotic renal papillae cause ureteric obstruction), which may be seen in those with diabetes mellitus, sickle cell disease, or urinary tract obstruction.

Renal scarring

- *Children:* seen in 6–15% of children after a febrile UTI. This is often associated with a degree of VUR (thought to be congenital), and patients with scarring are at risk of hypertension and renal impairment in later life. This risk increases with delayed treatment in those experiencing recurrent infection.
- *Adults:* a single episode of acute pyelonephritis in an adult woman leads to renal scarring in 46%, as demonstrated by Tc99m-labeled DMSA scanning 10 years later. Acute pyelonephritis in pregnancy may lead

to acute renal impairment, ARF, ARDS, low-birth-weight children, preterm delivery, and sepsis. Renal scarring is four times more likely after pyelonephritis in pregnant women than in nonpregnant women. Renal impairment is seen particularly in infections causing severe papillary necrosis.

• Pyelonephritis becomes potentially fatal when secondary conditions develop, such as emphysematous pyelonephritis (20–80% mortality rate), perinephric abscess (20–50% mortality rate), or sepsis. Severe sepsis mortality is higher in those with chronic renal disease or acute renal impairment and in the elderly.

• Acute renal transplant pyelonephritis occurring in the first 3 months after transplant has a significant association with graft loss (>40%) by 96 months as compared to all renal transplant cases with or without the occurrence of pyelonephritis at any time after the transplant up to 96 months (25–30%).

Reference

1. Warren JW, Abrutyn E, Hebel JR, et al. (1999) Guidelines for Antimicrobial Treatment of uncomplicated acute bacterial cystitis and acute pyelonephritis in women. *Clin Infect Dis* 29:745–758.

Chronic pyelonephritis

The chronic condition is not as well defined as acute pyelonephritis but is generally considered to refer to the pathological changes of diffuse interstitial inflammation that can be caused by several conditions, including obstruction, calculi, analgesic nephropathy, hypokalemic nephropathy, and renal TB, and following acute pyelonephritis in childhood in the context of VUR.

Chronic pyelonephritis secondary to VUR

VUR is congenital incompetence of the ureterovesical valve due to an abnormally short intramural segment of the ureter. The condition is present in 30–40% of young children with symptomatic UTIs and in almost all children with renal scars.

VUR may also be acquired by patients with a flaccid bladder due to spinal cord injury. This may lead to impaired renal function (reflux nephropathy). Sometimes this diagnosis is established on the basis of radiological evidence obtained during an evaluation for recurrent UTI in young children. Infection without reflux is less likely to produce injury.

• *Symptoms:* patients with chronic pyelonephritis present with fever, lethargy, nausea and vomiting, flank pain, and dysuria, and children may fail to thrive. Hypertension may be noted.

• *Investigations:* proteinuria (negative prognostic feature), urine cultures (negative cultures do not exclude the diagnosis), demonstration of renal stones and dilatation (intravenous urogram, renal ultrasound), reflux (voiding cystourethrogram, cystoscopy), and renal scarring (radioisotopic scanning with technetium DMSA).

• *Management:* infection should be treated and underlying structural abnormalities corrected (e.g., ureteric reimplantation).

- *Complications:* proteinuria, focal glomerulosclerosis, renal impairment secondary to scarring (rate of progress of scars can be slowed by speedy institution of appropriate antibiotic therapy), pyonephrosis (if obstructed), nephrosis (may occur in cases of obstruction), hypertension (increases rate of decline in renal function), xanthogranulomatous pyelonephritis

Emphysematous pyelonephritis

This is a severe, necrotizing, acute multifocal bacterial nephritis with extension of the infection through the renal capsule. Gas is found in the renal substance and perinephric space.

- 85–100% cases are seen in patients with diabetes.
- Most cases are due to enterobacteriaceae.
- Patients present with fever, chills, pain, flank mass (50%), crepitation (over thigh or flank), and urinary symptoms.
- Diagnosis is best confirmed by CT.
- Treatment is with antibiotics, drainage, and nephrectomy.
- Mortality is 60% in those with gas within the kidney alone and managed with antibiotics and drainage, 80% in those with gas extending to the perinephric space and managed by antibiotic therapy alone, and 20% in those managed by nephrectomy.

Xanthogranulomatous pyelonephritis

This rare, serious, debilitating illness is characterized by a chronic inflammatory mass originating in the renal parenchyma. Gross appearance is a mass of yellow tissue composed of lipid-laden macrophages and inflammatory cells (perhaps with an abscess cavity), regional necrosis, and hemorrhage.

- *Causes* are often associated with infection by *Proteus*, *E. coli*, or *Pseudomonas* spp. in the context of chronic obstruction (stones are seen in 75% of patients, e.g., staghorn calculus).
- Patients are often immunocompromised or diabetic, and it is four times more common in women than in men.
- *Clinical features:* patients appear chronically ill, with dull, persistent flank pain, fever, weight loss, fistulae (pyelocutaneous and ureterocutaneous fistulae have been described). It can present acutely with fever and flank pain. Renal function is reduced in almost all cases.
- *Diagnosis:* CT scan helps in the diagnosis. The mass resembles a neoplastic lesion in its radiographic appearance and has a tendency to involve adjacent structures, including the psoas muscle and perirenal space. Renal pelvis is dilated. Many are confirmed only at operation. Bacteria are not typically cultured from urine, but if culture is positive the most common organisms are *Proteus mirabilis*, *E. coli*, and *Pseudomonas* spp.
- *Treatment:* appropriate antibiotic therapy may be important in initial stabilization but definitive therapy is always surgical, usually nephrectomy. Other factors complicating response to therapy include obstructing calculus and renal papillary necrosis.

Renal abscess

Perinephric abscess

This follows chronic or recurrent pyelonephritis, rupture, or extension of suppuration within the kidney, or dissemination or direct extension from another site. The abscess is located between the renal capsule and surrounding fascia and may extend to involve the GI tract, groin, lung (pleuritic pain, raised hemidiaphragm, pleural effusion), and psoas (there may be signs of psoas irritation, e.g., scoliosis, pain on hip flexion).

- *Clinical features:* presentation is insidious with fever, chills, unilateral flank pain (70%), dysuria (40%), nausea, vomiting, weight loss (25%), flank tenderness, abdominal tenderness (60%), referred pain (i.e., hip, thigh, or knee), flank or abdominal mass (<50%), pyuria (70%), sterile urine (40%), and bacteremia (40%).
- *Diagnosis* is often not apparent; one-third of patients are diagnosed at autopsy. CT helps confirm the diagnosis. Ultrasound may be falsely negative. MRI defines extension.
- *Treatment:* drainage is always required. Specific agents providing pseudomonal or enterococcal coverage may be indicated. Other organisms that have been reported include tuberculosis and fungi. Nephrectomy may be necessary.
- Mortality is <50%, and lower if recognized early and managed appropriately (e.g., surgery and aminoglycoside with antistaphylococcal agent).

Renal corticomedullary abscess

This is usually associated with urinary tract abnormalities and commonly caused by the *Enterobacteriaceae*. Disease is part of a spectrum that ranges from acute focal bacterial nephritis affecting a single lobe to severe emphysematous pyelonephritis. Males and females are equally affected in most cases.

- *Clinical features:* fever, chills, flank pain, nausea, vomiting (usually absent in cortical abscesses), flank mass, hepatomegaly. Urinary symptoms may be absent (but are seen more frequently than with cortical abscesses), and urinalysis is normal in 30%.
- *Diagnosis* is best confirmed with CT. Microbiology: midstream urine (MSU), blood cultures, culture of pus obtained by CT- or ultrasound-guided aspiration or drainage.
- *Treatment* is with antibiotic therapy (e.g., ciprofloxacin and gentamicin) and drainage or surgical intervention. Structural abnormalities should be corrected, e.g., obstruction relieved.

Renal cortical abscess

This is uncommon and usually due to the hematogenous spread of *S. aureus*, most commonly from a skin infection. Risk factors include IV drug use, diabetes mellitus, and hemodialysis. Microabscesses forming in the cortex coalesce to form a circumscribed abscess over days to months. This abscess is more common in men than in women.

- *Clinical features:* onset is often insidious. Symptoms include fever, chills, back pain, abdominal pain, flank mass, and, rarely, urinary symptoms (if the abscess communicates with and involves the collecting system).
- *Diagnosis* is best confirmed by CT, and this or ultrasound may be used to guide aspiration or drainage.
- *Microbiology:* MSU (culture is usually normal), blood cultures (often negative), culture of aspirated pus
- *Treatment:* IV antibiotics (e.g., high-dose flucloxacillin for 4 weeks) and drainage (for all but the smallest abscesses), which may be successfully achieved percutaneously. Nephrectomy is rarely required.

Catheter-associated UTI

Urinary tract infection (UTI) is the most common nosocomial infection, accounting for 40% of hospital-acquired infections, 80% of which occur in association with the use of catheters and related devices.

Pathogenesis of UTI

Catheterization thwarts a number of defense mechanisms that reduce the incidence of UTI in healthy individuals.

Organisms may be introduced from the perineum or urethra at the time of insertion, contaminate the collecting device (greatly reduced following the introduction of closed drainage systems in the 1950s), or enter via the space between the catheter and the urethral mucosa.

Once in the urinary tract, organisms are not eliminated as efficiently as is usual and can reach large numbers within a couple of days. Some are capable of producing biofilms that facilitate their growth. An inflammatory response may result in cystitis and pyuria. Organisms may ascend and cause upper urinary tract infection.

Risk factors for catheter-associated bacteriuria are duration of catheterization, absence of a drip chamber, microbial colonization of collection system, diabetes mellitus, quality of catheter care, and being female.

Short-term catheterization

Up to 25% of patients have a catheter placed at some point during a hospital stay, most for less than 4 days; 10–30% of catheterized patients develop bacteriuria. Common organisms include *E. coli* (24%), *Candida* spp. (26%), *Pseudomonas aeruginosa*, *Klebsiella pneumoniae*, *Proteus mirabilis*, enterococci, and CoNS.

Most bacteriuric episodes in this group are caused by a single organism. Organisms isolated from the catheter may not be found in the urine (due to sequestration of the bacteria within catheter-related biofilm). Most episodes of bacteriuria are asymptomatic, but 5% of such patients develop fever. Bacteremia is uncommon but occurs at higher rates in bacteriuric patients undergoing instrumentation (e.g., prostatectomy).

Long-term catheterization

The two most frequent indications are urinary incontinence (women) and outflow obstruction (men). Patients may be catheterized for months to years. All develop bacteriuria at some point, and certain species have adhesins enabling them to persist in the catheterized urinary tract. Polymicrobial bacteriuria is seen in 95% of long-term catheterized patients.

Mildly symptomatic UTIs occur fairly regularly, most lasting only a day and resolving without treatment. Bacteremia occurs in 4–10% of institutionalized patients undergoing catheter removal or replacement, often following the development of acute pyelonephritis.

Other complications include symptomatic UTI, catheter obstruction (by bacteria, crystals, particularly with *Proteus* infection, protein, glycocalyx), urinary stones, chronic renal inflammation, periurinary infection, bladder metaplasia, and malignancy (in very long-term patients).

Some of the complications of long-term catheterization once seen in spinal-injury patients are now seen much less frequently, as these individuals manage themselves with intermittent catheterization.

Prevention

Patients should be catheterized for clear indications only. Incontinence in particular may be more appropriately managed by other means.

When urethral catheterization cannot be avoided, caregivers should be meticulous in maintaining a closed collection system and the catheter should be used for as short a period as possible.

Alternatives to indwelling urethral catheterization are conveens (lower incidence of bacteriuria but have infection risks and other complications of their own), intermittent catheterization, and suprapubic catheterization (cleaner skin region is associated with lower rate of infection).

A single dose of gentamicin at insertion may reduce infection.

Treatment

Asymptomatic bacteriuria

There is no evidence that treating catheterized patients with bacteriuria in the absence of symptoms significantly reduces the number of people who go on to develop symptoms. Long-term catheterized patients treated with antibiotics for bacteriuria regardless of symptoms showed no difference in the number of febrile episodes.

Certain situations do warrant treatment: identification of organisms with a high incidence of bacteremia (e.g., *Serratia marcescens*), control of organisms associated with an outbreak of UTI in an institution and with bacteriuria in those patients at high risk of serious complications (e.g., pregnant women, immunosuppressed patients), or patients undergoing urological surgery.

Symptomatic catheter-associated UTI

Cultures of blood and urine should be taken, and most patients should be treated with empirical parenteral antibiotics based on locally known organisms and previous infections the patient might have experienced. These can be modified once culture results are available and be given orally once afebrile.

Bacteria may persist in catheter biofilm, and it is sensible to replace or remove the catheter prior to treatment. Antiseptic or antibiotic irrigation is of no benefit. Treatment duration is usually 7–10 days. Rule out obstruction and renal stones.

Candiduria

This is seen in many catheterized patients and is particularly related to hospitalization and previous antibiotic exposure. It is usually asymptomatic. Catheter removal resolves it in 40%; changing the catheter resolves it in 20%. Patients who must remain catheterized and continue to have candiduria may benefit from a course of fluconazole if they have a non-*krusei* candidal cystitis. Systemic therapy with IV amphotericin B or fluconazole and possibly surgery may be indicated.

Complications include fever, renal or perirenal abscess, fungus balls in the bladder and renal pelvis, and dissemination.

Prostatitis

Up to 50% of men will experience symptoms of prostatitis at some time in their lives. The key clinical issue is to distinguish patients with bacteriuria and bacterial prostatitis from the larger number of patients without bacteriuria.

Acute bacterial prostatitis

- *Clinical features:* symptoms are those of a lower UTI (dysuria, frequency) and possibly obstruction (due to prostatic edema) and fever. On examination there is lower abdominal, suprapubic discomfort, and an extremely tender, firm prostate on per rectum (PR) exam.
- *Investigations:* urinalysis shows pyuria and cultures are positive; blood cultures may be positive either spontaneously or following vigorous PR.
- *Management:* response to antimicrobial therapy is usually rapid; agents should provide good coverage of pseudomonads, enterococci, and the enterobacteriaceae. Urinary retention is best managed by suprapubic catheterization to avoid obstructing drainage of prostatic secretions.
- *Complications:* prostatic abscess, prostatic infarction, chronic prostatitis

Chronic bacterial prostatitis

This is an important cause of bacterial persistence in the lower urinary tract. Gram-negative organisms are the most important causes.

Patients often experience repeated infections with the same organism and are asymptomatic between episodes with a normal prostate on examination.

Long treatment courses fail in one-third of patients, cure one-third, and bring about resolution while on treatment but with subsequent relapse in one-third. These poor results may be a consequence of poor drug penetration into the prostatic parenchyma or perhaps of infected calculi serving as persistent foci for infection. Those not cured may remain asymptomatic on long-term, low-dose suppressive antibiotic therapy despite the persistence of prostatic bacteria.

Chronic prostatitis/chronic pelvic pain syndrome

The largest subset of patients with symptoms of prostatitis has this syndrome. There is no history of bacteriuria or evidence of infection.

Symptoms include difficulty voiding, erectile dysfunction, and a dull, aching pain that may be pelvic, perineal, suprapubic, scrotal, or inguinal and is exacerbated by ejaculation. Examination is unremarkable.

Some patients may have leukocytes in semen or prostatic secretions (expressed by digital massage), whereas others have no evidence of inflammation. Although the reason for this is not known, patients with leukocytes are more likely to have bacteria in their prostatic parenchyma. It may be that those without leukocytes are experiencing a noninfectious disease.

Asymptomatic inflammatory prostatitis

This is prostate inflammation with no symptoms. These patients may be identified through assessment of the cause of a raised prostate-specific antigen (PSA) level, with prostate biopsy showing a simple inflammatory process.

Granulomatous prostatitis

This is a histological reaction that may follow acute bacterial prostatitis, tuberculous prostatitis (and that following bacillus Calmette–Guérin therapy for transitional cell carcinoma of the bladder), or systemic mycoses. It may cause an indurated, firm, or nodular prostate, clinically indistinguishable from that caused by malignancy.

Prostatic abscess

This is a rare complication of acute bacterial prostatitis. Patients most commonly affected are those with urinary tract obstruction or foreign bodies, those with diabetes, the immunocompromised, and those not adequately treated for their acute episode.

Most cases are caused by the common uropathogens acquired by the ascending route and, rarely, organisms such as *S. aureus*.

Symptoms resemble those of acute bacterial prostatitis: fever, dysuria and signs of urinary sepsis. A fluctuant area of the prostate may be apparent on PR exam.

Definitive diagnosis can be made by ultrasound, CT, or MRI of the pelvis.

Treatment is with drainage and appropriate antibiotics.

Epididymitis

Epididymitis is an inflammatory reaction of the epididymis to infection or trauma. There are two distinct patterns of infective epididymitis: sexually transmitted and nonspecific (nonsexually transmitted) bacterial epididymitis. Underlying genitourinary tract abnormalities are common only in the latter group.

General features

- *Symptoms:* painful swelling of the scrotum, which may be acute (over 1–2 days) or more gradual in onset; dysuria with or without urethral discharge. Fever may be present, particularly in hospitalized patients who develop the condition following urinary tract manipulation.
- *Examination:* tender swelling and erythema of the scrotum, usually unilateral. Early in the disease course, swelling may be localized to one portion of the epididymis. Consequent involvement of the associated testis is common, producing epididymo-orchitis. Secretion of inflammatory fluid can lead to the development of a hydrocele.

Nonspecific bacterial epididymitis

The most common pathogens in men >35 years are coliforms and *Pseudomonas* spp. Other infectious agents are *M. tuberculosis* (tuberculous epididymitis is the most common form of male genital TB) and systemic mycoses (e.g., blastomycetes).

Patients often have underlying urinary tract pathology or a history of recent genitourinary tract manipulation (cases may occur weeks or months after the intervention), particularly if bacteriuric at the time. Bacterial prostatitis or long-term urethral catheters are other important predisposing factors.

Complications include testicular infarction, scrotal abscess, pyocele, scrotal sinus, infertility, and chronic epididymitis.

Management is with empirical antibiotics aimed at covering gram-negative rods and gram-positive cocci while awaiting urinary cultures. Bed rest, scrotal elevation, and analgesics are recommended. Some complications may require surgical intervention.

Sexually transmitted epididymitis

This is the most common form of epididymitis in young men. Major pathogens are *C. trachomatis* and *N. gonorrheae*

Many patients do not complain of discharge. *Chlamydia* spp. may be carried for prolonged periods (≥1 month) before developing symptoms

Diagnosis requires a high index of suspicion and appropriate cultures. Patient should be evaluated for the presence of other sexually transmitted infections, and sexual partners should be followed up. Underlying genitourinary abnormalities are uncommon in this group

Treatment is with specific therapy covering both chlamydial and gonococcal infections. If symptoms do not subside within 3 days of therapy, or tenderness or swelling persists on completion, the diagnosis should be reviewed. Consider abscess, infarction, malignancy, and tuberculous or fungal epididymitis

Complications include abscess, testicular infarction, infertility, and chronic epididymitis.

Orchitis

Orchitis is less common than epididymitis or prostatitis. Blood-borne dissemination is the major route of infection.

Viral orchitis

Viruses are by far the most common cause, e.g., mumps, Coxsackie B virus. Mumps rarely causes orchitis in prepubescent males but is seen in 20% of postpubertal patients.

Testicular pain and swelling follows 4–6 days after parotitis and may be seen even in the absence of parotitis; 70% of cases are unilateral. Contralateral involvement may occur a few days after the first testicle. Symptoms range from mild discomfort to severe pain with nausea, vomiting, prostration, fever, and constitutional symptoms.

Mild cases resolve within 4–5 days, severe ones may take 3–4 weeks; 50% of patients experience some degree of testicular atrophy. Contrary to previous belief, mumps orchitis rarely results in infertility.

Bacterial orchitis

Isolated bacterial orchitis is extremely rare. It usually follows from contiguous spread from an infected epididymis. Most cases of pyogenic orchitis are caused by *E. coli*, *K. pneumoniae*, *P. aeruginosa*, staphylococci, and streptococci.

Patients are acutely ill with a high fever, marked discomfort, testicular swelling, and nausea and vomiting. Pain radiates to the inguinal canal. There is usually an acute hydrocele, and the testis is swollen and tender. Overlying skin may be erythematous and edematous.

Treatment is as for bacterial epididymitis. Complications (e.g., infarction, abscess) may require surgery.

Sexually transmitted infections: introduction

Sexually transmitted infections (STIs) have been on the rise in recent years, fuelled by a decline in the practice of safer sex. The most severely affected groups are teenage females and MSM.

Risk factors

The risk factors that influence an individual's chance of acquiring a particular STI are broadly the same for all STIs. This means that patients with one STI should be assessed for the presence of others, including syphilis and HIV.

Risk factors include the number of sexual partners an individual has, failure to use barrier contraception, frequency of partner change, lower socioeconomic status, age <25 years, residence in an inner city, symptomatic partner, sexual orientation (syphilis, gonorrhea, HIV, and hepatitis B are more prevalent among men who have sex with men), and sexual practices (orogenital and anogenital contact).

Contact tracing

Health departments in the United States participate in contact tracing and partner notification programs, however the rate of utilization of such programs varies by disease (ranging from 89% for syphilis to 17%

for gonorrhea).[1] Recommendations for contact tracing and partner notification can be found in a 2008 report.[2]

Patient assessment

- *History:* last intercourse, contraceptive method, nature of sexual contacts and number, frequency of partner change, sexual orientation, sexual practices, previous history of STI, previous treatments received, menstrual history, drug use, foreign travel
- *Examination:* skin (rashes, lesions), lymphadenopathy, hair loss, jaundice, mucosal lesions, conjunctivitis, urethritis, arthritis, detailed examination of the genitalia, including a speculum examination of women and the subpreputal space and male urethra in men. A rectal examination and proctoscopy may be indicated.
- *Tests:* samples of genital secretions should be taken; in practice this will usually done by an experienced individual in the genitourinary medicine clinic. In men, take urethral swab (*Chlamydia*) and smear for Gram stain and culture (*N. gonorrhoea*); in women, take high vaginal swab in Stuart's media for microscopy and culture (*Candida, G. vaginalis,* anaerobes, *Trichomonas*) and endocervical swab (*C. trachomatis*). Other tests include swab ulcers for HSV culture, dark microscopy for syphilis, and blood serology for syphilis, hepatitis, and HIV.

Differential diagnoses

The differential diagnosis includes the following*:
- *Men with urethritis:* N. gonorrheae, nongonococcal urethritis (chlamydia, trichomoniasis, UTI)
- *Balanitis:* if associated with ulcers or blisters consider causes of genital ulceration. If associated with erythema or excoriation consider chlamydia, causes of urethritis, trichomoniasis, *Candida,* bacterial infection. For non-STI causes consider dermatological causes such as dermatitis, lichen simplex, and lichen planus.
- *Vulval irritation and pain:* if associated with ulcers and blisters consider causes of genital ulceration. Otherwise, consider candidiasis (especially if pregnant, diabetic, have discharge, or on recent antibiotics), trichomoniasis, and bacterial vaginosis. Non-STI causes include dermatological conditions, especially atopic vulvitis, and consider vulval intraepithelial neoplasia.
- *Abnormal vaginal discharge:* if watery white/gray with fishy smell, consider bacterial vaginosis; if white curdy discharge with vulval rash, consider candidiasis; if malodorous green/yellow discharge, consider trichomoniasis. Other causes are gonorrhea, chlamydia, and cervical herpes simplex. Non-STI causes are retained foreign body (e.g., tampon)
- *Anogenital ulceration:* herpes (preceded by vesicles), syphilis, tropical. Non-STI causes are neoplasia, drug reactions, Behcet's disease, and trauma.
- *Genital lumps:* genital warts, molluscum contagiosum, condylomata lata. Non-STI causes are folliculitis, lichen planus, keratoacanthoma, and carcinoma.

* This list is reproduced from Pattman R, Snow M, Hardy P, Sarkar KN, Elawad B, et al. *Oxford Handbook of Genitourinary Medicine, HIV and AIDS.* Oxford: Oxford University Press, 2005, with permission from Oxford University Press.

Infestations that may be transmitted sexually include pubic lice and scabies.

References

1. Golden MR, et al. (2003). Partner notification for HIV and STD in the United States: low coverage for gonorrhea, chlamydial infection and HIV. *Sex Transm Dis* 30(6):490–496.

2. Recommendations for partner services programs for HIV infection, syphilis, gonorrhea and chlamydial infection. *MMWR Recomm Rep* 2008;57(RR-9):1–83.

Bacterial vaginosis

Bacterial vaginosis (BV) causes vaginal discharge in ≤50% of symptomatic women (the other causes are vulvovaginal candidiasis and trichomoniasis) and is termed *vaginosis* rather than *vaginitis* because of the absence of inflammation. Rather than being due to a single organism, BV is caused by complex changes in the balance of the microbiological flora.

Epidemiology

Worldwide prevalence ranges from 11% to 48% in women of child-bearing age.

Risk factors for acquisition are having new or multiple sexual partners, vaginal douching, and smoking. It can occur in women who have never had vaginal intercourse.

Pathology

There is a reduction in the normally dominant lactobacilli and an increase in other organisms, especially anaerobes such as *G. vaginalis* and *Bacteroides* spp. The mechanism by which this change occurs is not certain.

Lactobacilli produce hydrogen peroxide, which lowers the pH; the loss of these organisms permits an increase in pH and overgrowth of vaginal anaerobes. These produce proteolytic enzymes that degrade vaginal peptides into offensive-smelling products and promote discharge and exfoliation of the epithelial layers.

Clinical features

- <75% of cases are asymptomatic.
- Thin, white, fishy smelling discharge, most noticeable after intercourse
- May be associated with cervicitis, which may or may not occur in the presence of simultaneous chlamydial or gonococcal infection
- Vaginal pain or vulval irritation is uncommon.
- *Complications:* pregnant women with BV have a higher rate of pre-term delivery. BV is associated with endometritis, postpartum fever, and infections following gynecological surgery. It is a risk factor for HIV acquisition and transmission, and acquisition of HSV-2, chlamydia, and gonorrhea.

Diagnosis

The Amsel criteria have a sensitivity of 90% and specificity of 77% if three of the four criteria are present. Trichomonal infection may cause the first three findings:

- Homogeneous, watery white-gray discharge coating the vaginal walls
- Vaginal pH >4.5
- Positive amine test: add 10% KOH to sample of discharge: it is positive if it produces a fishy odor.
- Presence of "clue cells" (epithelial cells studded with adherent coccobacilli) on a saline wet mount is the single best predictor of BV. At least 20% of epithelial cells should be clue cells in women with BV. Gram staining is most sensitive but impractical in standard clinical practice.

No bacteria are specific for BV, and bacterial culture is not useful. Diagnostic card tests for pH indicate the presence of amines.

Differential diagnosis

This includes trichomoniasis and atrophic vaginitis (dyspareunia and inflammation are present in these cases).

Management

Infection resolves spontaneously in one-third of cases. Treatment may reduce the risk of acquiring other STIs. The following should be treated:

- All women presenting with symptoms. Oral treatment is safe in pregnancy and not associated with adverse fetal effects.
- Asymptomatic women proceeding to abortion or hysterectomy. Treatment reduces the risk of postoperative infection.
- Asymptomatic pregnant women with previous preterm delivery may also benefit from treatment. BV is associated with a higher rate of pre-term birth (perhaps due to chorioamnionitis) but studies have not demonstrated that treating it brings about a significant reduction. However, treatment of BV in those women with a history of preterm delivery is associated with reduced rates of preterm pre-labor rupture of membranes and low-birth-weight babies. Consider screening those women with a history of preterm labor for BV.

Regimes

- Metronidazole: 500 mg bid PO for 7 days (single 2 g dose has lower efficacy and is no longer recommended), or 5 g od PV (per vagina) 0.75% metronidazole gel for 5 days. Early cure rates are >90%; 80% at 4 weeks.
- Clindamycin: 300 mg bid PO for 7 days, or 100 mg ovules od PV for 3 days. The use of clindamycin may be associated with acquisition of clindamycin-resistant anaerobes. No resistance to metronidazole has been demonstrated.

Thirty percent of patients experience recurrence within 3 months. A prolonged (e.g., 14 days) or alternative treatment course should be used in such patients. Those who experience multiple relapses may benefit from a long-term maintenance regime of twice-weekly PV metronidazole gel. Clindamycin should not be used for this purpose.

Treating sexual partners does not appear to reduce recurrence.

Vulvovaginal candidiasis

Vulvovaginal candidiasis accounts for one-third of cases of vaginitis.

Epidemiology

Candida species may be found in the lower genital tract of up to 50% of asymptomatic women.

It is common, with <75% of premenopausal women reporting at least one episode. It is less common in postmenopausal women.

Candidal infection is uncommon in prepubertal women but does occur in children who have had recent antibiotic therapy, wear diapers, or are immunosuppressed.

There is an increase in incidence when women begin regular sexual activity.

Pathology

Candida albicans is the cause of around 90% of cases, but the incidence of other *Candida* species, such as *C. glabrata*, may be increasing as a result of increasing use of over-the-counter drugs.

Sporadic episodes usually occur with no identifiable predisposing factor. Risk factors include diabetes mellitus, immunosuppression, recent antibiotic use, oral contraceptive use, and estrogen therapy.

Clinical features

Features include pruritus, dysuria, dyspareunia, and soreness. There may be discharge, which might be white and clumpy or thin and watery, but it is often absent with only vulvar and vaginal erythema on examination

Recurrent infection is defined as ≥4 episodes a year and is seen in 5–8% of women. Predisposing factors such as diabetes are seen in a minority of patients, and susceptibility seems to be largely determined genetically. Behavioral factors seem to play a part: a two-fold increase in risk has been associated with the consumption of cranberry juice and use of sanitary towels and sexual lubricants.

Diagnosis

Self-diagnosis is unreliable; one study demonstrated that only 34% of those women self-diagnosing candidal infection actually had it.

A wet mount of the discharge with 10% KOH may enable recognition of yeast and hyphae, but microscopy is negative in around 50%. Vaginal pH is around 4–4.5 (unlike trichomonal infection or bacterial vaginosis).

Perform culture in patients with persistent discharge or recurrent symptoms unresponsive to azole treatment; they may have non-*albicans Candida* infection. Routine culture is unhelpful.

As well as other infective causes, consider allergic reactions and contact dermatitis in the differential.

Management

Treatment is indicated for symptoms. Asymptomatic carriage does not require therapy.

Ninety percent of cases represent uncomplicated infection (healthy nonpregnant women with mild to moderate symptoms, infrequent episodes, and infection with *C. albicans*). Oral and topical treatments are similarly effective, with topical therapy relieving symptoms more rapidly but oral therapy being preferred by women, e.g., PO fluconazole.

Ten percent of cases are complicated (infection with non-*albicans* species, severe symptoms, four or more episodes per year, and those cases occurring in pregnant women, uncontrolled diabetics, or the immunosuppressed).

Immunosuppressed patients and those with severe symptoms are unlikely to respond to short treatment courses; 7–14 days of topical therapy or two doses of oral fluconazole (150 mg) 72 hours apart is indicated.

Half of women infected with *C. glabrata* fail treatment with azoles. Moderate success may be seen with intravaginal boric acid, and >90% cure may be seen with topical flucytosine cream.

In pregnant women, treat only for symptoms using a topical imidazole for 7–14 days (e.g., clotrimazole). Oral azoles are contraindicated in pregnancy. Vaginal candidiasis is not associated with adverse outcomes in pregnancy.

With recurrent infection (four or more episodes per year), aim to eliminate risk factors (e.g., better glucose control, lower estrogen-containing contraceptives, behavioral changes where appropriate). After the initial treatment course, long-term suppressive therapy (e.g., fluconazole 150 mg PO weekly for 6 months) is effective at preventing relapses. However, more than half of patients are likely to experience further infections in the months following cessation of suppressive therapy. These patients should be treated acutely once again, and then be given a year of suppressive treatment after culture confirmation of relapse. Development of azole resistance has not yet been associated with long-term therapy in this setting.

Most experts do not recommend treatment of asymptomatic sexual partners.

Genital warts

Anogenital warts are one of the most common sexually transmitted viral infections. They are caused by human papilloma virus (HPV), a highly infectious, double-stranded DNA virus of which there are over 100 serotypes (see p. 383); 90% of cases are related to serotypes 6 and 11 (the least likely to exhibit malignant potential). Serotypes 16 and 18 have a strong association with malignancy.

Epidemiology

Exposure is usually sexual, and incubation is from a few weeks to several months. The risk of disease increases with the number of sexual partners. Women tend to be affected more than men in most settings.

Anal disease can occur in women as a result of extension of perineal infection or receptive anal intercourse. Men usually experience lesions on the shaft of the penis or the preputial cavity. Anal lesions are more common among men who have sex with men but also occur among heterosexual men.

The prevalence of anogenital warts is higher among those who are HIV positive or have other sexually transmitted disease. The risk increases with lower CD4 counts and decreases with antiretroviral treatment.

Most infections are cleared within 2 years, but persistent infections can occur and are associated with the development of squamous cell carcinoma.

Clinical features

Those with a small number of lesions may experience no symptoms.

A larger number of lesions may be associated with pruritus, bleeding, dysuria, PV discharge, pain, and tenderness.

Rarely, warts may form larger exophytic masses that can interfere mechanically with intercourse, defecation, and even child birth.

Anal disease may cause strictures.

Diagnosis

Diagnosis is usually made visually. Lesions are pink and can take the form of flattened papules or more classic verrucous papilliform warts. Application of 5% acetic acid causes lesions to turn white. This is not specific for anogenital warts, however.

Anoscopy and colposcopy allow the extent of disease to be assessed.

Biopsy should be performed when the diagnosis is in doubt, in immunocompromised patients (higher risk of malignancy), and in cases that do not respond to therapy.

The differential includes condyloma lata (flat, velvety lesions of secondary syphilis), anogenital squamous cell carcinoma (may coexist with genital warts), vulvar intraepithelial neoplasia, skin tags, and molluscum contagiosum.

Management

Spontaneous regression is seen in up to 30% of immunocompetent cases by 3 months. The choice of therapy where indicated is governed by the number and extent of the lesions. All modalities have high rates of recurrence.

Women should have a pap smear. Small external lesions can be managed by application of a topical treatment either in the clinic or by the patient, when appropriate.

Large, multiple, or internal lesions should be referred to a surgeon or gynecologist and pathological studies undertaken where indicated.

Chemical agents

Podophyllin contains an antimitotic agent that stops the cell cycle in metaphase, causing cell death; 25% solution is administered 1–2 times per week, usually at a clinic, and achieves clearance rates of 20–50% at 3 months. It should be applied to small areas of skin, allowed to dry, and washed off 6 hours later. It should not be used on the cervix or vaginal epithelium (burns). It is contraindicated in pregnancy (teratogenic).

Podophyllotoxin is a related agent that can be self-administered to external warts with similar rates of success.

Trichloroacetic acid acts by protein coagulation and has similar rates of success and similar side effects to those of podophyllin. It can be used on internal lesions and during pregnancy. Neighboring skin can be protected from its caustic effects by the application of petroleum jelly prior to use.

5-fluorouracil/adrenaline gel injected intralesionally can achieve an initial cure rate of up to 60%, but half of patients relapse by 3 months.

Immunomodulation

Imiquimod is applied topically as a cream to external lesions only and acts by cytokine induction. It achieves high rates of clearance (over 80%) and low rates of recurrence (under 20%).

Interferon-A given systemically achieves rates of clearance similar to those with thermocoagulation but has higher rates of recurrence.

Surgery

Ablation or excision should be performed when medical therapies have failed or are not indicated (e.g., due to size). Cryotherapy with liquid nitrogen or a cryoprobe is safe in pregnancy and achieves clearance rates of over 90% at 3 months. Repeated applications are required.

Laser therapy is expensive, requires anesthesia, and places the operator at risk of developing warts. It achieves cure rates of almost 100% at 1 year.

Surgical excision has clearance rates of 36% at 3 months. As well as the standard risks associated with anesthesia and surgery, patients may develop strictures. Excised lesions should be examined pathologically for signs of malignancy.

Newer therapies

These include topical cidofovir, topical BCG, and infra-red coagulation.

Tropical genital ulceration

Genital ulceration is much more common in patients presenting with STI in the developing world and an important factor in the spread of HIV.

The common causes of genital ulcers in the developed world (HSV and syphilis) remain common in developing regions (e.g., HSV remains the top cause in Jamaica and South Africa) but may be pushed out of top place by certain other infections (e.g., chancroid in Rwanda).

Diagnosing lesions clinically can be difficult; syphilis classically causes a single painless ulcer, but so may HSV and lymphogranuloma venereum (LGV). Where facilities allow, investigations should include: serological testing for syphilis, a diagnostic evaluation for herpes, and, where appropriate, Gram-stain and culture on selective media (for *H. ducreyi*).

Chancroid

This is caused by *Haemophilus ducreyi*,a fastidious gram-negative rod. It produces a potent cytolethal distending toxin that is likely to contribute to both the formation of ulcers and their slow healing.

Incubation after infection is around 1 week, following which painful erythematous papules develop on the external genitalia (prepuce, corona, or glans in men; the labia, vagina, and perianal areas in women), develop into pustules, and then erode into sloughy, non-indurated hemorrhagic ulcers. Lesions are usually multiple, often developing on adjacent skin surfaces (thigh, scrotum), and suppurative inguinal lymphadenopathy is common (sometimes forming fluctuant buboes).

Coinfection with HIV may result in atypical presentations with multiple lesions, extragenital involvement, and delayed response to treatment.

Diagnosis is by clinical appearance and culture and Gram stain (organisms clump in parallel strands, appearing like a school of fish) of material from the ulcer or aspirated lymph nodes. Enriched culture media are required. PCR-based tests are in development.

Treatment is with erythromycin 500 mg qid for 1 week or azithromycin 1 g PO stat or ceftriaxone 250 mg IM stat. Fluctuant buboes should be aspirated (risk of fistulae).

Lymphogranuloma venereum (LGV)

This genital ulcer disease is caused by the L1, L2, and L3 serovars of *C. trachomatis*. It is endemic in areas of East and West Africa, India, Southeast Asia, and the Caribbean. Since 2003, a series of outbreaks of LGV have been reported in men who have sex with men (MSM).

Asymptomatic infection in women is common and may serve as a reservoir. Incubation is 3–12 days.

Primary infection is characterized by a transient, painless genital ulcer. Direct local extension leads to a secondary lesion 2–6 weeks later. There is an inflammatory reaction in the inguinal lymph nodes with fever, headache, weight loss, ± pneumonia, meningoencephalitis, and arthritis.

Lymphadenopathy may be so severe as to bulge each side of the inguinal ligament ("groove sign"). An inflammatory mass may form in the rectum, leading to pain, constipation, tenesmus, and rectal discharge.

LGV proctitis may be confused with inflammatory bowel disease. Late disease may lead to fibrosis and strictures in the anogenital tract, genital elephantiasis, anal fistulae, frozen pelvis, and infertility.

Diagnosis is based on clinical features. Culture of pus from lesions and nodes is possible but rarely practical in regions where the disease occurs. chlamydial serology is useful but not specific for serovars. PCR-based tests are available.

Treatment is with doxycycline or erythromycin for 3 weeks.

Granuloma inguinale (*Klebsiella granulomatis*)

Endemic in western New Guinea, the Caribbean, southern India, South Africa, Southeast Asia, Australia, and Brazil, granuloma inguinale (or donovaniosis) is a primarily sexually transmitted infection causing indolent, painless, nonpurulent ulceration. Infection may also be acquired fecally and by passage through an infected birth canal.

After an incubation of 1–3 months, the "beefy red" ulcers appear on the prepuce or labia and enlarge over months to 5 cm diameter or more. Autoinoculation may see ulcers forming on adjacent skin. Local extension and fibrosis occur, and late lesions may cause elephantiasis-like swelling of the external genitalia. Regional lymphadenopathy is rare, but metastatic spread to the bones, joints, and liver has been reported.

Diagnosis is clinical and by microscopy of Giemsa-stained material from ulcers, which may demonstrate bipolar intracellular bacteria ("Donovan bodies," a characteristic safety-pin appearance). Culture is extremely difficult and rarely performed.

Treatment is with TMP-SMX or doxycycline for 3 weeks. Alternatives include azithromycin 1 g weekly or erythromycin (again for 3 weeks). An aminoglycoside may be added if there is no initial response (which may be seen in HIV-positive patients).

Genital herpes

Genital herpes simplex infections are a major public health problem across the world. Like all herpes viruses, herpes simplex establishes a latent state following primary infection and may reactivate, causing episodic local disease.

Epidemiology

HSV-2 is the most common cause of genital herpes, but an increasing number of cases are due to HSV-1 infection.

Asymptomatic HSV-2 infection is more likely in those previously infected with HSV-1 and vice versa.

The incidence of genital herpes has been increasing in the U.S. and the presence of HSV-related ulcers is associated with an increased risk of HIV transmission.

Clinical features

Incubation is usually 3–7 days. Primary infection is characterized by local burning followed by a painful genital vesicular eruption. These vesicles then rupture, forming ulcers. Other symptoms include fever, dysuria, tender inguinal lymphadenopathy, headache, and herpetic proctitis. New lesions appear for around a week.

Resolution occurs over 1–3 weeks. Up to 60% of primary cases are asymptomatic, thus the first clinical attack may actually represent the first reactivation.

Recurrent attacks tend to be less severe with a shorter duration of symptoms and infrequent systemic features. Up to half of patients with reactivation experience prodromal symptoms (local tingling, shooting pains). Most patients developing primary infection will experience a recurrence within the first year. Prolonged first episodes are associated with earlier and more frequent relapses. Recurrence rates are much higher with HSV-2 infection and in immunosuppressed patients.

Rare extragenital features of primary infection include meningitis, urinary retention due to autonomic dysfunction, and distant skin lesions.

Subclinical viral shedding can occur in the absence of lesions. This is of importance, as it leads to unrecognized transmission to neonates and sexual partners. It is more common with HSV-2.

Diagnosis

Type-specific antibodies to HSV develop in the first few weeks of infection and are maintained indefinitely. Commercial tests are available, but a positive test does not allow one to distinguish present from previous infection.

Viral culture from lesions allows definitive diagnosis; it is more likely to be positive if the fluid is taken from vesicles that have not yet ruptured. Viral-antigen detection tests are available and allow rapid, type-specific diagnosis.

PCR-based viral detection is rapid and specific and allows recognition of asymptomatic viral shedding.

Management

Antiviral treatment includes acyclovir, valacyclovir, and famciclovir, which reduce the severity of episodes but do not alter the course of the disease. Treatment should be commenced as soon as possible, ideally within 24 hours, for maximum benefit. Systemic antivirals are less useful in recurrent attacks which are in any case shorter and milder. Topical acyclovir is of little benefit; IV acyclovir is indicated in neonatal infection or severe disease. Drug treatment reduces but does not eliminate viral shedding.

Patients with frequent recurrences (more than four per year) may benefit from prophylactic acyclovir. HIV-positive patients developing severe genital herpes should be given prophylactic therapy if their CD4 count is under 100 cells/mm^3.

If catheterization is required (e.g., autonomic disturbance or pain), the suprapubic route may be better to reduce pain, aid recognition of return of normal micturition, and reduce the risk of ascending infection.

Pelvic inflammatory disease

Pelvic inflammatory disease (PID) is an acute infection of the female upper genital tract that may involve the uterus, Fallopian tubes, ovaries, and even adjacent pelvic structures. It occurs when organisms, either transmitted sexually or constituting part of the normal vaginal flora, breach the barrier of the endocervical canal and gain access to the upper genital organs. Such a breach may be precipitated by infection with organisms such as *N. gonorrheae* or *C. trachomatis*.

Epidemiology

Most cases present within 1 week of menses, which is thought to enhance the ascension of vaginal organisms.

Those at greatest risk of PID are those with multiple sexual partners. It is rarely seen in celibate women and those in longstanding monogamous relationships.

Other risk factors include age (highest incidence in those aged 15–25 years), presence of symptomatic STI in the partner, previous PID, and possibly vaginal douching.

Microbiology

PID is a polymicrobial infection. Species identified include streptococci, *E. coli*, *Klebsiella* spp, *Proteus mirabilis*, *Haemophilus*, *Bacteroides*, *Peptococcus*, and *Peptostreptococcus* spp. Around 15% of those acquiring endocervical gonorrhea go on to develop PID, and it accounts for one-third of PID presentations worldwide (less in Europe).

C. trachomatis serovars D–K account for another one-third of cases overall (much more in Western Europe), and as with gonococcus, around 15% of endocervical *Chlamydia* infections produce PID. Studies have demonstrating that screening for chlamydial infection reduces the rate of PID (see p. 634).

Clinical features

Infection of the upper genital structures may precipitate any or all of endometritis, salpingitis, oophoritis, peritonitis, and perihepatitis.

Symptoms include lower abdominal pain that may start during or shortly after menses, vaginal discharge, and abnormal uterine bleeding. Rebound tenderness is common in the lower quadrants, and fever is seen in half of patients. Those with perihepatitis may also develop upper-abdominal pain. The uterus and adnexae will be tender on pelvic examination.

PID can be a subclinical disease and cause of infertility; one-third of women with no history of PID were found to have *C. trachomatis* in the upper genital tract with no clinical findings except infertility.

Diagnosis

No test for PID achieves high sensitivity or specificity. It is appropriate to initiate empirical antibiotic therapy when clinical suspicion in strong.

Consider the diagnosis in patients with abdominal pain *and* one of the following: cervical or uterine/adnexal tenderness, fever >38°C, raised WCC, abnormal cervical or vaginal discharge, or raised inflammatory markers. Have a low threshold for treating such individuals empirically.

Investigations include the following:

- *Microscopy of vaginal discharge*: if this demonstrates gram-negative intracellular diplococci, the probability of PID is high.
- *Laparoscopy*: although specificity approaches 100%, laparoscopy has been found to be only around 50% sensitive in the diagnosis of PID. It should be considered in patients who do not respond to empirical therapy within 72 hours (less if acutely ill) and those in whom there is a high suspicion of an alternative diagnosis (e.g., appendicitis).
- *Endometrial biopsy*: the demonstration of plasma cell endometritis is a common finding in cases of clinical PID, but it is also found in asymptomatic women with no other evidence of PID.
- *Other tests*: transvaginal ultrasound has a low specificity and sensitivity for PID but is useful in identification of pelvic abscesses; positive DNA testing for gonococcus and chlamydia increases clinical probability.

Confirmed cases are those with pelvic pain or tenderness *and* one of the following: endometritis/salpingitis on biopsy, *N. gonorrheae* or *C. trachomatis* in the genital tract, salpingitis seen on laparoscopy or laparotomy, isolation of pathogenic bacteria from the upper genital tract, or inflammatory pelvic peritoneal fluid with no other cause.

All patients should have a pregnancy test and urinalysis.

Differential diagnosis includes appendicitis, cholecystitis, IBD, UTI, dysmenorrhea, ectopic pregnancy, and ovarian cyst, torsion, or tumor.

Treatment

Most people can be treated as outpatients. Consider admitting pregnant women, those failing to respond to oral medications, those with severe clinical features (high fever, vomiting, severe pain), and those with abscesses or likely to require surgical intervention.

Selected antibiotics should cover *N. gonorrhea*, *C. trachomatis*, group A and B streptococci, anaerobes, and the common gram-negative enterics. Avoid fluoroquinolones (they have increasing *N. gonorrhea* resistance). Suitable regimes include the following:

- *Inpatient therapy:* cefoxitin 2 g IV qid *and* doxycycline 100 mg PO or IV bid; or clindamycin 900 mg IV tid *and* gentamicin 5–7 mg/kg IV od. Patients should be moved to an oral regime within 24–48 hours and complete 14 days of therapy (as below but omitting the IM stat dose).
- *Outpatient therapy:* single dose ceftriaxone 250 mg IM stat then doxycycline 100 mg PO bid 14 days *and* metronidazole 500 mg tid PO 14 days
- *Penicillin-allergic patients* in whom it is considered too risky to use ceftriaxone should be admitted and given the clindamycin regime described above, for 48 hours. If improving, they can then complete treatment on metronidazole 500 mg tid PO *and* clindamycin 450 mg PO qid *or* doxycycline 100 mg PO bid for 14 days.

As with all STIs, contacts should be traced and patients should be counseled and screened for HIV and hepatitis when indicated.

Toxic shock syndrome

This syndrome of fever, skin rash, and shock is due to toxins produced by certain strains of infecting *S. aureus*. Classically, it is associated with menstruation and the use of highly absorbent tampons. Around half of cases are now nonmenstrual (e.g., surgical and wound infections, osteomyelitis, septic arthritis, burns).

Pathogenesis

S. aureus establishes infection and produces toxins. The first of these to be identified, toxic shock syndrome toxin-1 (TSST-1), was first isolated in the 1970s when a series of cases of toxic shock syndrome (TSS) occurred in association with the use of highly absorbent tampons. It remains commonly associated with menstrual-related cases.

Nonmenstrual cases are more likely to be associated with other toxins, e.g., staphylococcal enterotoxin B. These exotoxins are superantigens, capable of activating a large number of T cells simultaneously, resulting in massive cytokine production that leads to fever, muscle proteolysis, and shock.

Epidemiology

Menstrual cases of TSS fell rapidly following the withdrawal of certain types of highly absorbent tampons in the 1970s, but they still occur. Women who develop the syndrome are more likely to have used tampons of high absorbancy and kept individual tampons in place for longer periods.

Nonmenstrual TSS accounts for half of reported cases. Patients tend to be slightly older, and studies imply an equal incidence in men and women if vaginal and postpartum cases are excluded.

Clinical features

Symptoms, which develop rapidly, 1–2 days post-menstruation or post-surgery, include fever, hypotension (may be unresponsive to fluid therapy), skin lesions (erythroderma resembling sunburn, conjunctival bleeds, petechiae, mucosal ulceration and vesicles), myalgia (due to cytokine-mediated muscle damage), headache, sore throat, vomiting, diarrhea, and abdominal pain.

Certain skin manifestations may occur late in disease, with itchy maculopapular rash appearing 1–2 weeks later, desquamation up to 3 weeks later, and even nail loss 1–2 months later.

Multiple organ systems may be involved: renal failure (of both pre-renal and renal etiology), gastrointestinal symptoms (diarrhea), encephalopathy (due to cerebral edema), cardiac depression, liver function impairment, and anemia or thrombocytopenia.

Recurrent disease can occur if an episode is not adequately treated with antistaphylococcal antibiotics. A subacute form of TSS may occur in patients with HIV, with symptoms occurring over weeks.

Diagnosis

Isolating *S. aureus* is not a prerequisite for the diagnosis of TSS. It is rarely isolated in blood cultures (<5%) but frequently grown from swabs of wounds or mucosal sites; the toxin produced may be identified by specialist laboratories. The CDC has produced clinical criteria for the diagnosis of TSS. These were designed for epidemiological surveillance and should not be used to exclude the diagnosis in a patient in whom TSS is considered likely.

A confirmed case is a patient with fever of 39°C or more, hypotension, diffuse erythroderma, involvement of three organ systems, and desquamation (if the patient survives). A probable case lacks one of these symptoms.

Differential diagnosis includes streptococcal TSS (which is important to recognize, as urgent surgical debridement may be required), meningococcal disease, leptospirosis, dengue, and typhoid fever.

Management

- *Supportive:* hypotension can be difficult to manage and may not respond to fluid therapy alone, necessitating the use of vasopressors such as dopamine.
- *Surgical:* foreign bodies should be removed in the case of menstrual TSS, and wound debridement may be required in postsurgical cases.
- *Antibiotics:* while it is not clear whether antibiotics are required in the acute management of TSS, they are important in preventing recurrent disease. Clindamycin *may* be more effective than antibiotics acting solely on the bacterial cell wall, as it suppresses protein synthesis (and therefore potentially toxin production). MRSA should be covered in any regime. Recommended empirical treatment is clindamycin 600 mg IV tid and vancomycin 30 mg/kg/day in two divided doses IV. Treatment should be for 10–14 days.
- *Intravenous immunoglobulin:* there are no trials to demonstrate the effectiveness of immunoglobulin in the management of staphylococcal TSS. Case reports suggest it may be of benefit in severe cases that fail to respond to fluids and vasopressors.
- *Corticosteroids:* there is no evidence to suggest that the use of steroids affects outcome.

Prognosis

Death usually occurs within a few of days of presentation but can occur up to 2 weeks later. Causes of death include cardiac arrhythmias, respiratory failure, and bleeding. Mortality in menstrual cases is around 1.8%; nonmenstrual cases, 6%.

Gonorrhea

This purulent infection of mucous membranes (e.g., urethra, rectum, cervix, conjunctiva, pharynx) is caused by sexually transmitted *Neisseria gonorrhoeae*.

Epidemiology

Infection is common across the world. In the developing world, perinatal transmission and neonatal eye infections remain a significant problem.

Following a 74% decline in the rate of reported gonorrhea from 1975 to 1997, rates of gonorrhea have plateaued in the United States from 1998 to 2008 (approximately 111 cases per 100,000 population).[1]

The recent increase in incidence (probably related to an increase in unsafe sexual practices) and growing prevalence of antimicrobial resistance have made it a major public health concern.

Resistance to first-line antibiotic treatment is related to an increased risk of treatment failure (with consequent disease complications) and onward transmission within a community. In 2005, 21% of isolates were resistant to ciprofloxacin overall (42.4% among gay men and 11.3% among heterosexual men), and 17.9% of isolates were resistant to penicillin. Therefore, first-line therapy should be ceftriaxone or cefixime.

Clinical features

Incubation is 2–5 days. Lower genital tract infection may be asymptomatic or cause urethritis with purulent discharge and dysuria in men, and endocervicitis with PV discharge, itch, and dysuria in women. Although infection of the female urethra, the pharynx, and rectum (seen in MSM) can cause discharge and tenesmus, they are usually asymptomatic.

Retrograde spread may occur, causing salpingitis and endometritis, PID, and tubo-ovarian abscesses in up to 20% of women with cervicitis. In rare cases, frank peritonitis or perihepatitis (Fitz-Hugh–Curtis syndrome) are seen. Men with gonococcal urethritis can develop epididymitis or epididymo-orchitis.

Disseminated gonococcal infection may follow around 1% of genital infection; 75% of such cases occur in women who are at increased risk if mucosal infection occurs during menstruation or pregnancy. Features include rash, fever, arthralgias, migratory polyarthritis, septic arthritis, endocarditis, and meningitis.

Neonates acquiring infection intrapartum present with ophthalmia neonatorum, and disseminated infection. Conjunctivitis can also occur in adults after direct inoculation of organisms and may lead to blindness.

Diagnosis

- *Gram stain:* highly sensitive from swabs of urethral discharge (the presence of gram-negative diplococci within leukocytes is 95% sensitive for gonococcal infection). Sensitivity and specificity are less good for endocervical or pharyngeal specimens.
- *Culture* is the gold standard. All infected areas should be swabbed and cultured both to confirm diagnosis and to provide sensitivity data.
- *Disseminated infection:* joint effusions, blood, and CSF should be sent for culture and Gram stain when appropriate. Negative cultures do not rule out disseminated infection.

Management

First-line therapy is with a cephalosporin: ceftriaxone 250 mg IM single dose, or cefixime 400 mg PO single dose for uncomplicated infection.

Coinfection with other STIs is common, and patients and their sexual partners should be screened. Some physicians treat patients empirically for associated chlamydial infection; chlamydial urethritis can present as apparent treatment failure after confirmed gonorrhea.

A pregnancy test should be performed on all women with suspected gonococcal infection.

References

1. CDC Sexually Transmitted Diseases Surveillance 2008. www.cdc.gov/std/stats08/toc.html

Chlamydia

Epidemiology
Chlamydia is the most common sexually transmitted infection in the United States, with rates highest in those under 25. A significant number of cases are asymptomatic, and 10–40% of untreated infected women develop pelvic inflammatory disease, making it an important reproductive health issue. The responsible organisms are *Chlamydia trachomatis* serovars D–K (p. 304).

Clinical features
The incubation period is 1–3 weeks. Around 50% of infected males and 80% of infected females are asymptomatic. Such infection may persist for many years if untreated.

Symptoms include mucopurulent cervicitis in females and urethritis with dysuria and discharge in males. Ascending genital tract infection may lead to pelvic inflammatory disease in women and is the most common cause of epididymitis in men under 35 years. Proctitis and pharyngitis occur in men and women.

Other presentations are LGV (the cause of 10% of genital ulcers in tropical countries; see p. 632), neonatal conjunctivitis (p. 304), and neonatal pneumonia, which may occur in children born to infected mothers.

Complications include PID (p. 634), Reiter's disease (urethritis, conjunctivitis, reactive arthritis), perihepatitis, and conjunctivitis.

Coinfection of chlamydia and gonorrhea is common (40% of women and 20% of men with chlamydia also have gonorrhea).

Diagnosis
Culture is not performed routinely. Enzyme immunoassay is available and cheap but is only 40–60% sensitive.

DNA testing is widely available and highly sensitive and specific. It may be performed on cervical swabs, urine, and vulvovaginal swabs (it is best on urine in men and endocervical swab in women) and is the first-line investigation for all specimens.

Management
Antibiotics include azithromycin 1 g single dose (the drug of choice for reasons of compliance) or doxycycline 100 mg bid for 7 days. Alternative regimens are erythromycin 500 mg bid for 10–14 days or ofloxacin 200 mg bid or 400 mg od for 7 days. First-time cure rates are over 95%.

Patients should be thoroughly worked up for other STIs and contacts traced.

Recurrent infection is usually due to reinfection by untreated partners. Female partners of men with urethritis should be treated regardless of whether there is evidence of infection, given the high risk of asymptomatic disease.

Trichmoniasis

This infection is caused by the flagellated protozoan, *Trichomomas vaginalis* (p. 482), which may be asymptomatic (particularly in men) or lead to vaginal discharge, dysuria, and lower abdominal pain in women, or to urethritis in men.

Epidemiology

Transmission is by sexual contact and its incidence in highest in women with multiple sexual partners and those with other STIs, including HIV. Vertical transmission may take place during delivery.

Nonsexual transmission (e.g., by contact with contaminated linen in institutions) occurs but is very rare.

Clinical features

Incubation is 5–28 days. Infection is asymptomatic in most men and 50% of women.

Symptoms tend to develop during menstruation or pregnancy (higher vaginal pH provides a favorable environment for parasite replication) and include yellow vaginal discharge (may be itchy and smelly), dyspareunia, dysuria, and lower abdominal pain.

On examination, the vulva may be erythematous with obvious discharge, vaginal inflammation, and punctuate hemorrhages on the cervix ("strawberry cervix"). Symptomatic men experience a urethritis indistinguishable from other causes of nongonococcal urethritis.

Complications include vaginitis emphysematosa (gas-filled blebs in the vaginal wall), vaginal cuff cellulitis after hysterectomy, premature labor, and low-birth-weight infants.

Diagnosis

Phase-contrast or dark-ground microscopy of wet preparation of genital specimens will demonstrate the motile flagellated protozoans in 48–80% of infected women and 50–90% of infected men.

Culture is the most sensitive technique; modified Diamond's media produce the best results.

Other methods such as ELISA, DNA probe, PCR, and fluorescent antibody staining are more sensitive than wet prep microscopy but less sensitive than culture.

Management

Give metronidazole 2 g stat dose. The main disadvantage of single-dose treatment is the risk of reinfection should the partner not be treated simultaneously. Metronidazole is relatively contraindicated in the first trimester of pregnancy. Treatment should be deferred until the start of the second trimester if symptoms are severe. Partners and asymptomatic individuals should be treated.

Syphilis

Syphilis is caused by *Treponema pallidum* subspecies *pallidum* (see *Treponema* species, p. 286).

Epidemiology

It is generally transmitted by sexual contact; it can also be transmitted vertically and via blood transfusions. Highest rates are seen in adults.

HIV infection is associated with treatment failures and more frequent, earlier neurological disease.

Clinical features

Primary syphilis

After an incubation period of 14 days to 3 months, a painless, erythematous papule develops. This ulcerates, forming a painless punched-out chancre on the genitalia (rarely on the mouth, hands, anus). It is associated with regional lymphadenopathy.

Multiple chancres can occur, particularly in HIV-infected patients. They are highly infectious and heal spontaneously after 1–2 months.

Secondary syphilis

Organisms disseminate from the chancre, causing symptoms 1–6 months later:

- *Rash:* localized or diffuse mucocutaneous rash may be macular, papular, pustular, or mixed. It involves the trunk, limbs, palms, and soles. Mucosal ulcers may occur. Condylomata lata occur in warm, moist areas (e.g., skin folds) and are highly infectious.
- *Early neurosyphilis* (more common in HIV) may be asymptomatic (CSF findings: pleocytosis, raised protein, decreased glucose, reactive CSF VDRL test), present with syphilitic meningitis (chronic basal meningitis with headache and cranial nerve palsies; fever is usually absent), or cause meningovascular syphilis (headache, fits, limb paralysis). It may also present with stroke, cervical myelopathy, and hemiplegia.
- *Other features* include fever, sore throat, "snail-track" ulcers in the mouth, lymphadenopathy, malaise, hepatitis, periostitis, iritis, arthritis, and glomerulonephritis.

Latent infection

Spontaneous resolution of secondary syphilis occurs at 3–12 weeks. During the latent period, infectivity is low, but up to one-quarter of patients experience recrudescence of disease.

Tertiary syphilis

This is rare and follows a latent period of up to 20 years. It is characterized by chronic inflammation.

- *Gummatous syphilis:* granulomatous lesions usually affecting skin, mucous membranes, and bone or organs causing local destruction (e.g., saddle nose). Gummata may be indurated, nodular, or ulcerated and can be painful
- *Cardiovascular syphilis* – endarteritis of the aorta leads aortic regurgitation (may present with angina and left ventricular failure

(LVF)) and aneurysm formation (ascending aorta). Other large arteries may be affected. VDRL can be negative

- *Late neurosyphilis* – two forms: (1) general paresis of the insane (presents with gradual confusion, hallucinations, delusions, fits, cognitive impairment, tremor of lips and tongue, brisk reflexes, extensor plantars, Argyll–Robertson pupils), and (2) tabes dorsalis (atrophy of the dorsal columns of the spinal cord with autonomic neuropathy and cranial nerve lesions). Presents with ataxia, sensory loss, sphincter disturbance, shooting pains, sensory loss, arreflexia.

Diagnosis

- *Microscopy:* detection of organisms on dark-field microscopy, or immunofluorescence of samples taken from chancre exudates
- *PCR-based tests* can be used to confirm the diagnosis or to test samples taken from oral lesions, which may be contaminated by commensal spirochaetes, e.g., *T. macrodentium* and *T. microdentium.*
- *Serology*[1] tests fall into two groups: nontreponemal (e.g., VDRL) and treponemal (e.g., treponema pallidum hemagglutination assay [TPHA]). They may be negative in HIV (see p. 287).
- *CSF findings* in asymptomatic neurosyphilis include pleocytosis, low glucose, raised protein, and a positive VDRL test (may be negative in HIV). Symptomatic patients have more severe CSF changes and the CSF VDRL is almost always positive. CSF changes occur in general paresis (elevated lymphocytes, raised protein, and positive CSF VDRL), but are variable in tabes (may be normal; 25% of CSF VDRL tests are nonreactive).
- *Primary syphilis:* dark-field or immunofluorescent microscopy of samples taken from chancre exudates. PCR-based tests are for oral lesions or to confirm microscopy findings. VDRL may be positive in around 75%, TPHA in around 90%.
- *Secondary syphilis:* VDRL is present at high titer in almost 100%, TPHA is positive in 100%. CSF-VDRL is usually positive in early neurosyphilis.
- *Latent infection:* VDRL falls with time and following treatment, so a negative test does not rule out infection. TPHA remains positive.
- *Tertiary syphilis:* in gummatous syphilis, both VDRL and TPHA are positive. In contrast, in syphilitic aortitis and late neurosyphilis, VDRL may be only weakly positive or even negative. TPHA is positive.

Management

All patients should be tested for HIV infection.

- *Early syphilis:* benzathine penicillin G 2.4 million IU IM stat as two injections into separate sites, or doxycycline 100 mg bid for 14 days or erythromycin 500 mg qid for 14 days. Penicillin treatment may be complicated by the Jarisch–Herxheimer reaction.
- *Late syphilis:* benzathine penicillin G 2.4 million IU IM as two injections into separate sites weekly for 3 weeks, or doxycycline 100 mg bid PO for 28 days
- *Neurosyphilis:* benzylpenicillin G 3–4 million IU IV every 4 hours for 14 days, or procaine penicillin G 2.4 million IU IM daily with probenecid 500 mg PO qid for 14 days, or ceftriaxone 2 g IV od for 14 days, or doxycycline 200 mg PO bid for 28 days.

Treatment success is assessed by symptoms and repeat VDRL. Repeat lumbar puncture in patients with neurosyphilis at 3–6 months and every 3 months thereafter until CSF is normal and CSF VDRL is nonreactive. Failure to achieve resolution by 2 years should prompt re-treatment.

Reference

1. Egglestone SI, Turner AJ (2003). Serological diagnosis of syphilis. PHLS Syphilis Serology Working Group *Common Dis Public Health* 3:158–162.

Acute meningitis

Definition

Acute meningitis is defined as a syndrome characterized by the onset of meningeal symptoms (headache, neck stiffness, vomiting, photophobia) and cerebral dysfunction (confusion, coma) over hours to days. It is identified by an abnormal number of white blood cells in the CSF. Table 4.5 summarizes the causes.

Table 4.5 Causes of acute meningitis

Category	Causes
Bacteria	Group B streptococcus, E. coli, L. monocytogenes, K. pneumoniae, H. influenzae, S. pneumoniae, N. meningitidis, E. coli, Klebsiella spp., Salmonella spp., Serratia marcescens, Pseudomonas aeruginosa, Enterobacter spp., S. aureus, S. epidermidis, P. acnes
Viruses	Enteroviruses, mumps virus, measles virus, herpes viruses, influenza and parainfluenza viruses, HIV, arboviruses, lymphocytic choriomeningitis virus
Rickettsia	R. rickettsii, R. conorii, R. prowazekii, R. typhi, R. tsutsugamushi, Erlichia spp.
Protozoa	Naegleria fowleri, Acanthamoeba spp., Angiostrongylus cantonensis
Helminths	Strongyloides stercoralis
Other infectious diseases	Infective endocarditis, parameninigeal foci of infection, viral postinfectious syndromes, post-vaccination
Medications	Antimicrobials, nonsteroidals, azathioprine, OKT-3, cytosine arabinoside, carbamazepine, immune globulin, ranitidine
Systemic diseases	Systemic lupus erythematosus
Procedure related	Post-neurosurgery, spinal anesthesia, intrathecal injections
Miscellaneous	Seizures, migraine, Mollaret's meningitis

Bacterial meningitis

The cause of acute bacterial meningitis depends on the age, immune status, and whether there has been recent head trauma or neurosurgery (see Table 4.6). The initiation of infection usually begins with nasopharyngeal colonization by a new organism, followed by systemic invasion. Important bacterial virulence factors include fimbriae, bacterial capsule, and production of IgA proteases. Host factors that predispose to meningitis include splenectomy and complement deficiencies.

Clinical features

Classical features include fever, headache, meningism (neck stiffness, photophobia, positive Kernig's and Brudzinski's signs), and cerebral dysfunction (confusion and/or reduced conscious level).

Seizures occur in 30% of patients. Cranial nerve palsies (especially III, IV, VI, and VI) and focal signs are seen in 10–20% of cases. Hemiparesis may be due to a subdural effusion.

Papilledema is rare (<1%). Skin rash (initially macular then petechial) occurs in patients with meningococcal septicemia but can occur in pneumococcal, *H. influenzae*, or *S. suis* septicemia.

Rhinorrhea or otorrhea suggests basal skull fracture.

Table 4.6 Causes of bacterial meningitis

Age/condition	Common organisms
0 to 4 weeks	Group B streptococcus, *E. coli*, *L. monocytogenes*, *K. pneumoniae*, *Enterococcus* spp., *Salmonella* spp.
4 to 12 weeks	Group B streptococcus, *E. coli*, *L. monocytogenes*, *K. pneumoniae*, *H. influenzae*, *S. pneumoniae*, *N. meningitidis*
3 months to 18 years	*H. influenzae*, *N. meningitidis*, *S. pneumoniae*
18 to 50 years	*N. meningitidis*, *S. pneumoniae*, *S. suis*
>50 years	*S. pneumoniae*, *N. meningitidis*, *L. monocytogenes*, aerobic gram-negative bacilli, *S. suis*
Immunocompromised	*S. pneumoniae*, *N. meningitidis*, *L. monocytogenes*, aerobic gram-negative bacilli (e.g., *E. coli*, *Klebsiella* spp., *Salmonella* spp., *Serratia marcescens*, *Pseudomonas aeruginosa*)
Basal skull fracture	*S. pneumoniae*, *H. influenzae*, group A streptococci
Head trauma, post-neurosurgery	*S. aureus*, *S. epidermidis*, aerobic gram-negative bacilli
CSF shunt	*S. aureus*, *S. epidermidis*, *P. acnes*, aerobic gram-negative bacilli

Patients with *L. monocytogenes* have an increased risk of seizures and focal signs; some patients present with ataxia, cranial nerve palsies, and nystagmus caused by rhomboencephalitis.

Neonates may present with nonspecific symptoms—e.g., temperature instability, listlessness, poor feeding, irritability, vomiting, diarrhea, jaundice, and respiratory distress. Seizures occur in 40%, and a bulging fontanelle is a late sign.

Elderly patients may present insidiously with confusion, lethargy, obtundation, no fever, and variable signs of meningeal inflammation.

Diagnosis

The diagnosis is confirmed by examination and culture of the CSF. In bacterial meningitis the following are typically seen:

- Opening pressure >18 mm CSF
- CSF white cell count 1000–5000 cells/mm³ (range 100–10,000)
- CSF neutrophils ≥80%
- CSF protein 0.1–0.5 g/dL
- CSF glucose ≤40 mg/dL or ≤2.2 mmol/L
- CSF lactate ≥35 mg/dL or ≥1.9 mmol/L
- Gram stain positive in 60–90%
- Culture positive in 70–85%
- Bacterial antigen detection positive in 50–100%
- Bacterial PCR positive in 90%.

Management

For acute management, see flowchart on the back cover.

Empirical antimicrobial therapy should be commenced immediately, pending investigations (Table 4.7).

If the CSF Gram stain or culture is positive, treatment should be tailored to the infecting organism (Table 4.8).

Adjunctive corticosteroids have been recommended for treatment of acute bacterial meningitis.[1] The recommended regimen was

Table 4.7 Empirical antibiotic therapy for bacterial meningitis

Age/condition	Empiric therapy
Age 0–4 weeks	Ampicillin + cefotaxime or aminoglycoside
Age 4–12 weeks	Ampicillin + cefotaxone or ceftriaxone
Age 3 months–18 years	Cefotaxime or ceftriaxone
Age 18–50 years	Cefotaxime or ceftriaxone
Age >50 years	Ampicillin + cefotaxime or ceftriaxone
Immunocompromised	Ampicillin + ceftazidime ± vancomycin
Basal skull fracture	Cefotaxime or ceftriaxone
Head trauma/neurosurgery	Vancomycin + ceftazidime
CSF shunt	Vancomycin + ceftazidime

Table 4.8 Specific antibiotic therapy for bacterial meningitis

Organism	Antimicrobial therapy
H. influenzae type b	Ceftriaxone or cefotaxime for 7 days
N. meningitidis	Penicillin G or ampicillin or ceftriaxone for 7 days
S. pneumoniae	Ceftriaxone ± vancomycin for 10–14 days
L. monocytogenes	Ampicillin or penicillin G for 21 days
Group B streptococcus	Ampicillin or penicillin G for 14–21 days
E. coli	Ceftriaxone or cefotaxime for 21 days

dexamethasone 10 mg qid for 4 days, administered before or with the first dose of antibiotic. However, more recent data from the developing world do not support this recommendation.[2,3]

Reduction of raised intracranial pressure (ICP) may be achieved by various methods: elevating the head of the bed to 30 degrees to maximize venous drainage, hyperventilation to cause cerebral vasoconstriction, and use of hyperosmolar agents, e.g., mannitol.

Neurosurgery may be required in certain circumstances: persistent CSF leak after basal skull fracture, congenital defects leading to recurrent meningitis, or subdural empyema.

Prevention

Vaccination

H. influenzae type B is part of the routine childhood immunization schedule in the United States. The quadrivalent meningitis vaccine (ACYW135 or MCV4) is recommended for children 11–18 years of age (usually given at the 11- to 12-year-old visit) and for college freshmen living in dormatories, microbiologists routinely exposed to meningococcal bacteria, military recruits, travelers to Sub-Saharan Africa, anyone with terminal complement deficiency, and others who may have been exposed during an outbreak (www.cdc.gov).

S. pneumoniae vaccination is recommended in certain high-risk groups, e.g., those >65 years of age; those with chronic cardiovascular, pulmonary, renal, or liver disease, diabetes mellitus, alcoholism, CSF leak, asplenia, HIV, or hematological and other malignancies; bone marrow transplant patients; and those undergoing immunosuppressive therapy.

Chemoprophylaxis

Chemoprophylaxis should be given within 24 hours to household contacts, kissing contacts, and medical personnel involved in resuscitation of the index case. Rifampicin is the agent of choice for H. influenzae type B meningitis.

For N. meningitis, the agents used are rifampicin (600 mg bid for 2 days), ciprofloxacin (500 mg stat), or ceftriaxone (250 mg IM). Rifampicin interacts with the oral contraceptive pill and may reduce its efficacy.

Penicillin is not recommended to prevent secondary cases of S. pneumoniae meningitis but is recommended for children with sickle cell disease, although the optimum duration is unknown.

Intravenous ampicillin, penicillin, clindamycin, or erythromycin is recommended for pregnant women colonized with group B streptococci or with obstetric risk factors for invasive disease.

Meningitis C vaccination should be given for unvaccinated close contacts of meningitis C cases.

Reference

1. de Gans J, van de Beck D (2002). Dexamethasone in adults with bacterial meningitis. *N Engl J Med* 347:1549–1556.

2. Mai NTH, Chau TTH, Thuastas G, et al. (2007). Dexamethadone in Vietnamese adolescents and adults with bacterial meningitis. *N Engl J Med* 357:2431–2440.

3. Scarborough M, Gordan SB, Whitty CJ, et al. (2007). Corticosteroids for bacterial meningitis in adults in Sub-Saharan Africa. *N Engl J Med* 357:2441–2450.

Viral meningitis

Viruses are the major cause of the aseptic meningitis syndrome. This is usually characterized by lymphocytic pleocytosis in the CSF and sterile bacterial cultures.

Causes

Enteroviruses are the leading cause of viral meningitis, e.g., echoviruses, Coxsackie viruses, enteroviruses 70 and 71.

Arboviruses that cause meningitis include St. Louis encephalitis virus, California, Eastern equine, Western equine, Venezuelan equine, and Colorado tick fever.

Mumps virus is a common cause in unimmunized populations. CNS disease may occur in the absence of parotitis and is usually a benign self-limited disease.

Herpes viruses include herpes simplex viruses (HSV-1 and HSV-2), varicella zoster virus (VZV), cytomegalovirus (CMV), Epstein–Barr virus (EBV), and human herpes viruses. Although all of these can cause meningitis, herpes simplex viruses are the most common cause and are often associated with primary genital HSV-2 infection.

HIV may cause meningitis as part of primary infection.

Lymphocytic choriomeningitis virus (LCMV) is a rare cause of aseptic meningitis. It usually occurs in laboratory personnel, pet owners, or persons living in unsanitary conditions.

Pathogenesis

After colonization of mucosal surfaces, the virus invades and replicates prior to hematogenous dissemination. CNS invasion may occur through several mechanisms: via the cerebral microvascular endothelial cells, via the choroid plexus epithelium, or by spread along the olfactory nerve.

Once CNS invasion occurs, inflammatory cells accumulate, leading to the release of inflammatory cytokines, e.g., IL-6, IFN-G, IL-1B, and synthesis of immunoglobulins, e.g., oligoclonal IgG.

Clinical features

Enterovirus

In neonates, fever is accompanied by vomiting, anorexia, rash, and upper respiratory tract symptoms. Meningeal signs (nuchal rigidity, bulging anterior fontanelle) may be present or absent, and focal signs are uncommon. A severe form may occur in the early neonatal period with hepatic necrosis, myocarditis, necrotizing enterocolitis, and encephalitis.

In older children and adults, symptoms are milder with fever, headache, neck stiffness, and photophobia. There may be nonspecific symptoms, e.g., anorexia, vomiting, rash, diarrhea, cough, phayngitis, and myalgia. Other clues are community enteroviral epidemics, maculopapular or pustular rashes, conjunctivitis, pleurodynia, pericarditis, and herpangina.

Mumps virus

CNS symptoms usually occur 5 days after the onset of parotitis. Other findings include salivary gland enlargement (50%), neck stiffness, lethargy, and abdominal pain.

Herpesviruses

HSV-2 meningitis presents with classical symptoms. Complications include urinary retention, dysesthesia, paresthesia, neuralgia, motor weakness, paraparesis, difficulties in concentration, and impaired hearing; these usually resolve within 3–6 months.

EBV meningitis is associated with pharyngitis, lymphadenopathy, and splenomegaly.

VZV meningitis is associated with a characteristic, diffuse vesicular rash.

HIV

HIV-infected patients may present with a typical aseptic meningitis syndrome associated with acute primary HIV infection.

LCMV

LCMV is usually a biphasic illness that starts with nonspecific viral symptoms, followed by improvement; 15% of patients develop severe headache, photophobia, lightheadedness, myalgia, and pharyngitis. Occasionally, arthritis, oorchitis, myopericarditis, and alopecia may occur.

Diagnosis

CSF examination

CSF pleocytosis (100–1000 cells/mm^3) usually occurs. This may show a neutrophil predominance initially but becomes lymphocytic over 6–48 hours. CSF protein level may be normal or mildly elevated. CSF glucose level is normal or mildly reduced.

Viral culture

Enteroviral meningitis may be identified by tissue culture, although sensitivity is only 65–75%. Prolonged or asymptomatic viral shedding may occur. LCMV is diagnosed by means of viral culture of blood or CSF (early infection) or urine (later infection). HSV-2 has been cultured from CSF and buffy coat of some patients. HIV has been isolated from the CSF of some patients with neurological disease. Arboviruses may be cultured from blood and CSF.

Serology
Rapid diagnosis of enteroviral infections is possible by detection of enteroviral IgM antibodies; the specificity of some tests is unsatisfactory. A four-fold rise in mumps antibody titers confirms the diagnosis of mumps meningitis. A salivary antibody test has been developed that looks promising. LCMV and arboviral infections are usually diagnosed serologically.

Molecular methods
cDNA nucleic acid probes for enteroviruses have been developed but have poor specificity (≤33%). PCR-based assays for enteroviruses are more promising with higher sensitivity and specificity than that of tissue culture. PCR-based assays are the diagnostic test of choice for herpes virus infections, e.g., HSV-2, CMV, and VZV. HIV-RNA has been isolated from the CSF of some patients with meningitis.

Management
Treatment of viral meningitis is mainly supportive, with, e.g., analgesics, antipyretics.

Pleconaril has been used for enteroviral meningitis. Intravenous acyclovir is used for meningitis associated with HSV infection.

No specific antiviral therapy exists for arboviruses, mumps virus, or LCMV. Antiretroviral therapy may be indicated for HIV infection.

Chronic meningitis

Chronic meningitis is a syndrome characterized by the subacute onset of meningoencephalitic symptoms (fever, headache, nausea, vomiting, neck stiffness, lethargy, and confusion) and CSF abnormalities that persist for at least 4 weeks There are a large number of infectious and noninfectious causes (Table 4.9).

Clinical features

History
An exposure history may suggest certain infections, e.g., tuberculosis, brucellosis, cysticerocosis, coccidiodomycosis, histoplasmosis, Lyme disease, syphilis, or HIV infection. In noninfectious cases, there may be a history of pre-existing systemic disease.

Examination
Diagnostic physical findings are rare. Skin lesions may be found in cryptococcosis, sarcoidosis, *Acanthamoeba* infection, coccidioidomycosis, blastomycosis, and secondary syphilis. Subcutaneous nodules may be found in cysticercosis and metastatic carcinoma. Lymphadenopathy and hepatomegaly suggest systemic disease.

Table 4.9 Causes of chronic meningitis

	Syndrome	Causes
Infectious	Meningitis	*Acanthamoeba* spp., *Angiostrongylus cantonensis*, brucellosis, candidiasis, coccidioidomycosis, cryptococcosis, histoplasmosis, Lyme disease, sporotrichosis, syphilis, tuberculosis
	Focal lesions	Actinomycosis, blastomycosis, cysticercosis, aspergillosis, nocardiosis, schistosomiasis, toxoplasmosis
	Encephalitis	African trypanosomiasis, cytomegalovirus, enterovirus (hypogammaglobulinemia), measles (subacute sclerosing panencephalitis [SSPE]), rabies
Noninfectious	Meningitis	Behçet's disease, benign lymphocytic meningitis, granulomatous angiitis, malignancy, sarcoidosis

Eye examination may show choroidal tubercles, sarcoid granulomas, papilledema, iritis, or uveitis.

Neurological examination is nondiscriminatory: focal signs indicate a cerebral mass lesion; hydrocephalus and cranial nerve palsies indicate basal meningitis; peripheral neuropathy suggests sarcoidosis or Lyme disease.

Laboratory diagnosis

Blood tests

In addition to routine blood tests (CBC, ESR, CRP, creatinine, liver function tests), the following may be indicated: Mantoux test, blood culture for fungi and mycobacteria, serology for HIV and syphilis, serum cryptococcal antigen, ANA, and ANCA. Depending on the patient's exposure history, the following tests may be indicated: serology for *Brucella*, *Borrelia burgdorferi*, *Histoplasma*, and *Coccidiodes*.

Radiology

A chest X-ray and CT or MRI brain scan should be performed in all cases. Meningeal enhancement and hydrocephalus are common findings.

CSF examination

This should be performed in all cases (unless contraindicated by scan findings). The CSF should be analyzed for cell count and differential, protein, glucose, and lactate (Table 4.10).

Diagnostic tests include Gram stain and culture, Ziehl–Neelsen stain for mycobacteria, India ink and cryptococcal antigen, and syphilis serology. Depending on the patient's exposure history, the following tests may be indicated: CSF antibodies to *Histoplasma*, *Coccidiodes*, *Blastomycosis*, *Taenia solium*, *Brucella*, and measles virus.

Table 4.10 CSF findings in chronic meningitis

CSF characteristic	Causes
Lymphocytic pleocytosis	Viral causes, TB meningitis
Neutrophilic pleocytosis	Actinomycosis, nocardiosis, HIV-associated CMV, early *M. tuberculosis* infection, aspergillosis, candidiasis
Eosinophilic pleocytosis	*Angiostrongylus*, *Coccidioides*, cysticercosis, schistosomiasis, lymphoma, chemical
Pleocytosis <50 cells/μl	Behçet's disease, benign lymphocytic meningitis, carcinoma, HIV-associated cryptococcosis, sarcoidosis, vasculitis
Low CSF glucose	Actinomycosis, nocardiosis, carcinoma, cysticercosis, fungi, tuberculosis, syphilis, toxoplasmosis, chronic enterovirus, HIV-associated CMV, sarcoidosis, subarachnoid hemorrhage

In cases where the diagnosis remains obscure, the following tests may be helpful: repeat Mantoux test or TB IFN-γ release assay; immunoglobulins, serum ACE; CSF antibody for *Sporothrix schenkii*, enteroviral culture, and PCR. Biopsy of the brain or other tissues may also be indicated.

Management
Specific therapy is tailored according to the cause of chronic meningitis (for further details, see Table 4.9).

Therapeutic trials may be indicated when a specific cause is not found despite comprehensive evaluation. Response to treatment may be slow, making interpretation difficult. Attempts to establish a diagnosis should be continued during the therapeutic trial.

In areas where tuberculosis is endemic, tuberculous meningitis (see next section) is the most common cause of chronic meningitis, and empirical therapy is often initiated if the clinical presentation and CSF indices are compatible. Positive cultures or a clinical response to treatment are indications for continuing therapy. In areas where TB is not endemic, chronic meningitis is usually not infectious.

Tuberculous meningitis

Tuberculous meningitis is caused by *M. tuberculosis* (see *Mycobacterium tuberculosis*, p. 307).

Clinical features
Features are nonspecific with gradual onset of meningeal symptoms, cranial nerve palsies (III, IV and VI), hemiplegia or paraplegia, and urinary retention. CXR is abnormal in 50% of cases and may show pulmonary or miliary tuberculosis. CT or MRI brain scan may show hydocephalus, basal meningeal enhancement, infarcts, or tuberculomas.

Laboratory diagnosis

CSF findings include a lymphocytic pleocytosis (100–500 cells/mm³), increased CSF protein, and decreased CSF glucose levels. Neutrophils may predominate in early disease and in HIV-infected patients.

Diagnosis is confirmed by detection of *M. tuberculosis* by CSF Ziehl–Neelsen smear or culture. Smear positivity rates are generally low (10–22%) but may be increased to >50% if the spun deposit of a large volume of CSF (5–10 mL) is examined meticulously.

PCR detection of mycobacterial DNA has a sensitivity of 27–85% and a specificity of 95–100%. CSF cultures are positive in 38–88% of cases.

Management

The optimum drug choice and duration of treatment have not been established in clinical trials. The UK and U.S. TB treatment guidelines both recommend a four-drug initiation phase (rifampicin, isonazid, pyrazinamide, and ethambutol) for 2 months, followed by a two-drug continuation phase (rifampicin and isoniazid) for 10 months.

As isoniazid and pyrazinamide are the only two drugs that have good CSF penetration, some experts recommend continuing pyrazinamide during the continuation phase. Studies from India and South Africa suggest that 6 months of therapy may be adequate. Adjunctive dexamethasone has been shown to reduce mortality by 30%.

Cryptococcal meningitis

This is caused by *Cryptococcus neoformans* (see Cryptococcus neoformans, p. 426). *C. neoformans* var. *neoformans* has a worldwide distribution and tends to cause disease in immunocompromised patients. *C. neoformans* var. *gatii* occurs in tropical and subtropical climates and in areas near Vancouver Island and tends to affect non-immunocompromised patients.

Clinical features

There is subacute presentation with fever, meningoencephalitis, visual loss, and focal signs (<30%).

Laboratory diagnosis

CSF findings include raised CSF pressure, lymphocytic pleocytosis (40–400 cells/mm³), low CSF glucose (55%), and positive India ink stain (≤50%). CSF findings may be normal in HIV patients.

Serum and CSF crypococcal antigen tests can increase the diagnostic rate to ≥90%. CSF cultures are positive in 75% of patients. Cultures of blood, urine, and sputum may increase the diagnostic rate.

Management

Immunocompetent patients are treated with amphotericin (0.4 mg/kg/day) and flucytosine (150 mg/kg/day) for 6 weeks. Alternatives include amphotericin alone (0.5–0.7 mg/kg/day) or fluconazole (200–800 mg/day).

Treatment of HIV-associated cryptococcal meningitis is with amphotericin ± flucytosine for 2 weeks followed by fluconazole or itraconazole

400 mg/day for 8 weeks. Higher doses of fluconazole (800–2000 mg/day) have been tried, with or without flucytosine.

Lifelong maintenance therapy with fluconazole 200 mg is indicated in all patients until immune reconstitution is achieved (CD4 cell cont >100 cells/μl and undetectable VL sustained for >3 months; minimum of 12 months antifungal therapy) with highly active antiretroviral therapy.

Raised ICP may benefit from serial lumbar punctures, diuretics (e.g., acetazolamide), or venticuloperitoneal shunts, although comparative evidence is lacking.

Reference

Clinical Practice Guidelines for Management of Cryptococcal Disease: 2010 Updated by the Infectious Diseases Society of America. http://www.idsociety.org

Coccidioidal meningitis

Coccidiodes immitis (see *Coccidioides immitis*, p. 457) is endemic in the arid and semi-arid regions of the western hemisphere, e.g., southwest United States, Mexico, and Central and South America.

Clinical features

CNS involvement may be part of generalized coccidiodomycosis or may be the only site of extrapulmonary disease. Meningitis usually occurs within 6 months of pulmonary infection, but can occur up to 12 years after primary infection.

Headache is the most prominent symptom, but the clinical syndrome is indistinguishable from other causes of chronic meningitis.

Laboratory diagnosis

CSF findings resemble those of cryptococcal meningitis, but eosinophilia may be seen. CSF cultures are positive in 30% and spherules are sometimes seen on CSF smear. CSF antibodies are positive in 55–95% of patients; ELISA to spherule is more sensitive than complement fixation tests (CFTs). A serum CFT titer of 1:16 is supportive of the diagnosis.

Skin tests with spherulin are positive in 33–55% of patients.

Management

Fluconazole (400 mg/day) is associated with a 70% response rate. Higher fluconazole doses may be used in patients who do not respond initially. Ketoconazole is an alternative. Intrathecal amphotericin B is used in patients who do not respond to oral azole therapy.

Hydrocephalus may require a ventriculoperitoneal shunt.

Histoplasma meningitis

This is caused by *Histoplasma capsulatum* (see *Histoplasma capsulatum*, p. 448).

Clinical features are nonspecific with fever and gradual onset of meningitic symptoms over weeks or months. Oral mucosal lesions occur in 16% of patients and are more common than skin lesions.

Laboratory diagnosis

CSF cultures are positive in 27–65% of cases. Blood cultures should also be done. Serum and CSF antibody detection is the most sensitive test, but problems occur with cross-reactivity to other fungi. Histoplasma polysaccharide antigen may be detected in blood, urine, or CSF in 61%.

Management

Treatment is with amphotericin (0.7–1.0 mg/kg/day). Lumbar punctures should be performed weekly for 6 weeks, then every 2 weeks, to assess response. Initial response rates are good, but relapse rates are high, resulting in an overall cure rate of 50%.

Neuroborreliosis

This is caused by *Borrelia burgdorferi* and transmitted to humans by the asymptomatic bite of the deer tick *Ixodes scapularis*.

- *Clinical features:* early infection presents with flu-like symptoms and a characteristic rash (erythema chronicum migrans). Neuroborreliosis is characterized by fever, headache, cranial nerve palsies, and peripheral neuropathy ~4 weeks after primary infection.
- *Laboratory diagnosis:* CSF examination shows a lymphocytic pleocytosis. Diagnosis is confirmed by positive serology in the context of an appropriate exposure history. Serology is insensitive in early disease, and false-positive and -negative results are a considerable problem. The most specific test is detection of *B. burgdorferi* antibodies in the CSF and comparison of CSF and serum antibody levels by an immunocapture assay. PCR detection of *B. burgdorferi* has poor sensitivity (25–38%) but high specificity.
- *Management:* IV ceftriaxone 2 g/day for 2–4 weeks. Alternatives include cefotaxime 2 g q8 hours or penicillin G 3 g IV q6 hours.

Neurocysticercosis

Caused by *Taenia solium* (p. 505), this is the most common parasitic disease of the CNS. Infection is endemic in Mexico, Central and South America, the Caribbean, Sub-Saharan Africa, India, and China.

- *Pathogenesis:* infection is acquired by the ingestion of *T. solium* eggs. Larvae hatch in the small intestine, invade the bloodstream, and disseminate to the muscle, eye, and brain, where they encyst. Symptoms occur when the larvae die, causing an inflammatory response.
- *Clinical features:* seizures, focal neurological deficits, chronic basilar meningitis, and hydrocephalus. CT or MRI scans show multiple cystic and calcified lesions in the brain parenchyma. Skeletal muscle calcification may also be seen (<10%).

- *Laboratory diagnosis:* CSF examination shows a lymphocytic or eosinophilic pleocytosis, low CSF glucose (25%), and elevated CSF protein. Positive serology is supportive of the diagnosis, but there is considerable cross-reactivity with other helminth infections. Immunoblotting techniques, using the purified glycoprotein fraction of cyst fluid, appear sensitive and specific. Sensitivity of antibody testing appears higher in patients with multiple cysts.
- *Management* remains controversial, as the benefit of anthelmintic therapy has not been firmly established. If the decision is made to treat, albendazole (15 mg/kg/day for 7–30 days) or praziquantel (50 mg/kg/day for 1–21 days) may be given. More recent studies have recommended a single day regimen of praziquantel. Seizures should be controlled with anticonvulsants and symptomatic hydrocephalus relived by shunting. Corticosteroids may be given to reduce CNS inflammation but can reduce praziquantel levels.

Encephalitis

Encephalitis is an inflammation of the brain that is usually caused by viral infections or noninfectious agents (Table 4.11). It is often accompanied by meningeal inflammation and is therefore referred to as *encephalomyelitis*.

Table 4.11 Viral causes of encephalitis

Family	Viruses
Togaviridae	Eastern equine, Western equine, Venezuelan equine viruses
Flaviviridae	St Louis, Murray Valley, West Nile, Japanese B encephalitis, dengue
Bunyaviridae	La Crosse, Rift Valley, Toscana
Paramyxoviridae	Mumps, measles, Hendra, Nipah
Arenaviridae	Lymphocytic choriomeningitis, Machupo, Lassa, Benin
Picornaviridae	Polio, Coxsackie, echovirus, hepatitis A
Reoviridae	Colorado tick fever
Rhabdoviridae	Lyssavirus, rabies
Filoviridae	Ebola, Marburg
Retroviridae	HIV
Herpesviridae	HSV-1, HSV-2, VZV, HBV, CMV, HHV-6, HHV-7, EBV
Adenoviridae	Adenovirus

Pathogenesis

Infectious agents cause clinical symptoms and signs in the CNS, either by direct invasion or indirectly, without invading the parenchyma. Viruses enter the CNS in one of two ways: via the bloodstream (most viruses) or via the peripheral nerves (e.g., HSV, VZV, polio, rabies). Once the infectious agent enters the brain, only certain cells will become infected. This results in variable clinical manifestations, e.g., seizures, demyelination, impaired consciousness, coma, and respiratory failure.

In fatal viral encephalitis, an inflammatory reaction is usually prominent in the meninges and in a perivascular distribution in the brain. Neural cells may show degenerative changes and apparent phagocytosis of neural cells by macrophages. Intranuclear inclusion bodies are seen in herpesvirus and adenovirus infections.

When acute demyelinating disease complicates viral infections outside the brain, damage is thought to be related to induction of an immune response against CNS myelin rather than invasion on the brain.

Clinical features

Patients usually present with signs and symptoms of meningeal irritation: headache, neck stiffness, and a CSF pleocytosis.

Viral encephalitis is characterized by alterations in consciousness, progressing from mild lethargy to confusion, to stupor and coma.

Focal neurological signs frequently develop and seizures are common.

Motor weakness, attenuation of reflexes, and extensor plantar responses may be seen.

Some viruses may cause CNS symptoms as part of a postinfectious encephalomyelitis, e.g., mumps, measles, rubella, influenza.

Certain diseases are associated with characteristic symptoms or signs:

- HSV encephalitis: personality change, hallucinations, aphasia
- VZV encephalitis: acute contralateral hemiparesis after herpes zoster ophlamicus (due to frontal infarct)
- Japanese B encephalitis: Parkinsonian syndrome
- Rabies: local paresthesia at the site of the bite; history of bat bite
- Polio: flaccid paralysis
- Rocky Mountain spotted fever: rash on palms and soles
- Enteroviral infections: viral exanthems
- Tick-borne encephalitis: history of tick bite

Diagnosis

CSF examination is essential. CSF pleocytosis is variable (10–2000 cells/mm^3) and lymphocytes usually predominate. However, in early disease, there may be no cells in the CSF or neutrophils.

Red cells may be found in HSV encephalitis.

CSF protein is usually increased. CSF glucose is usually normal or slightly low.

Detection of viral nucleic acids in the CSF by PCR is useful for the diagnosis of a number of infections, e.g., herpesviruses and enteroviruses. PCR may be negative in early disease so should be repeated after 48–72 hours.

Acute and convalescent serology may help to confirm the diagnosis. An electroencephalogram (EEG) is often abnormal.

Treatment

Treatment is mainly supportive Specific treatment is only available for some of the causes of viral encephalitis:

- Acyclovir for HSV encephalitis
- Ganciclovir and foscarnet for CMV disease
- Antiretroviral therapy for HIV disease

Prevention

Some diseases may be prevented by vaccination, e.g., mumps, measles, polio, and Japanese B encephalitis.

Cerebral abscess

A focal intracerebral infection begins as a local area of cerebritis and develops into a collection of pus surrounded by a well-vascularized capsule. The introduction of surgical drainage and antimicrobial therapy has transformed this condition from an almost uniformly fatal disease to a treatable condition.

Epidemiology

Brain abscesses are an uncommon but severe disease. They tend to occur more frequently in males, with a median age of presentation of 30–40 years.

In the original site of infection is the paranasal sinuses, most of the patients are 10–30 years old. If the initial site of infection is the ear, then patients are generally <20 or >40 years of age; 75% of cerebral abscesses occur in adults. Case fatality rates range from 0% to 24%.

Etiology

Cerebral abscesses may be caused by a broad spectrum of pathogens. Some pathogens are associated with certain predisposing conditions (Table 4.12).

Pathogenesis

Bacteria reach the brain through several different mechanisms:

- Contiguous spread, e.g., from the ear or sinuses
- Hematogenous spread, e.g., bloodstream infections, pulmonary sepsis
- Direct inoculation, e.g., trauma or surgery.

The brain may be more susceptible to infection than other tissues such as the skin. It may also have different susceptibilities to infection by different organisms. The role of bacterial virulence factors in brain abscess formation has not been adequately studied.

Clinical features

Cerebral abscesses may present with a gradual decline or a rapid deterioration. The presenting symptoms and signs include the following:

Table 4.12 Factors predisposing to cerebral abscess

Predisposing condition	Microorganisms
Otitis media/mastoiditis	Streptococci, *Bacteroides* spp., *Prevotella* spp., *Enterobacteriaceae*
Sinusitis	Streptococci, *Bacteroides* spp., *Enterobacteriaceae*, *S. aureus*, *Haemophilus* spp.
Dental sepsis	*Fusobacterium*, *Prevotella*, *Bacteroides* spp., streptococci
Trauma or neurosurgery	*S. aureus*, streptococci, *Enterobacteriaceae*, *Clostridium* spp.
Pulmonary/pleural sepsis	*Fusobacterium*, *Actinomyces*, *Bacteroides*, *Prevotella* spp., streptococci, *Nocardia* spp.
Endocarditis	*S. aureus*, streptococci
Congenital heart disease	Streptococci, *Haemophilus* spp.
Neutropenia	Aerobic gram-negative bacilli, *Aspergillus* spp., *Mucorales*, *Candida* spp.
Transplantation	*Candida* spp., *Aspergillus* spp., mucorales, *Enterobacteriaceae*
HIV	*T. gondii*, *Nocardia* spp., *Mycobacterium* spp., *L. monocytogenes*, *C. neoformans*

- Headache
- Altered mental status
- Focal neurological deficits
- Fever
- Seizures
- Nausea and vomiting
- Neck stiffness
- Papilledema

The location of the abscess defines the clinical symptoms:
- *Frontal:* headache, drowsiness, inattention, altered mental state, hemiparesis, speech disorder
- *Temporal:* ipsilateral headache, aphasia, visual field defect
- *Cerebellar:* ataxia, nausea, vomiting dysmetria.

Certain pathogens may have specific characteristics:
- *Nocardia spp.:* chronic pulmonary condition and skin nodules
- *Rhinocerebral mucormycosis:* eye and sinus pain, nasal stuffiness

Diagnosis

An urgent CT scan of the brain enables rapid diagnosis. Cerebral abscesses appear as ring-enhancing lesions surrounded by edema. MRI is more sensitive than CT, enabling the early detection of cerebritis.

If single or multiple ring-enhancing lesions are seen, the patient should be referred to neurosurgery for a diagnostic aspirate.

Treatment[1]

A diagnostic aspirate should be obtained and the patient started on broad-spectrum empiric therapy (e.g., ceftriaxone and metronidazole).

Once culture results are available, treatment can be rationalized according to antimicrobial sensitivities. Antimicrobial therapy is given for 2–4 weeks intravenously followed by 2–6 months orally.

Adjunctive corticosteroids should be given to patients with significant edema and mass effect.

Reference

1. de Louvois J, Brown EM, Bayston RN, et al. (2000). The rational use of antibiotics in the treatment of brain abscess. *Br J Neurosurg* 14(6):525–530.

Subdural empyema

Subdural empyema is a collection of pus in the space between the dura and the arachnoid.

Epidemiology

Subdural empyema accounts for 15–20% of localized intracranial infections.

Risk factors include sinusitis, otitis media, mastoiditis, skull trauma, neurosurgery, infection of pre-existing subdural hematoma, cranial traction devices, nasal surgery, ethmoidectomy, or polypectomy. Metastatic infection accounts for ~5%. It is a complication of meningitis in infants.

Spinal subdural empyema is rare and occurs secondary to metastatic infection.

Etiology

Causative organisms include streptococci, staphylococci, aerobic gram-negative bacilli, and anaerobes. Polymicrobial infections are common. Postoperative or traumatic empyemas are usually caused by staphylococci or aerobic gram-negative bacilli.

Unusual causes include Salmonella spp., Propionobacterium acnes, M. tuberculosis, and Candida spp.

Clinical features

An acute onset of fever occurs, along with headache (may be localized to infected sinus or ear), vomiting, altered mental state (disorientation, drowsiness, coma), and focal neurological signs (hemiparesis, cranial nerve palsies, dysphasia, homonymous hemianopia, cerebellar signs); ~80% of patients have meningeal symptoms or signs. Seizures occur in ≤50% of cases. There may be rapid neurological deterioration with signs of raised intracranial pressure and cerebral herniation.

Complications include septic venous thrombosis, cerebritis, and cerebral abscess. In infants with subdural empyema, persistent fever, decline in neurological status, and seizures are seen. Spinal epidural abscess presents with radicular pain and signs of spinal cord compression.

Diagnosis

Consider the diagnosis in any patient with meningism and focal neurological signs. Lumbar puncture is contraindicated because of the risk of cerebral herniation.

CT or MRI brain shows a crescentic or elliptical area of hypodensity below the cranial vault adjacent to the falx cerebri. After administration of contrast, a fine line of enhancement is seen between the subdural collection and the cerebral cortex. MRI is more sensitive than CT and is considered the investigation of choice.

Management

Subdural empyema is an emergency requiring immediate surgical and medical management. Samples should be sent for urgent microscopy and culture. Start IV antibiotics immediately after aspiration, based on the likely infecting organisms, e.g., ceftriaxone and metronidazole. Vancomycin should be added for suspected staphylococcal infection. Tailor treatment to culture results once available.

Outcome is related to conscious level at presentation (>90% for patients who are awake and <50% in patients who are unresponsive to pain); 10–44% of survivors experience permanent neurological sequelae.

Epidural abscess

Epidural abscess is a localized collection of pus between the dura mater and the overlying skull or vertebral column. It may be complicated by subdural empyema.

Epidemiology

The epidemiology of cranial epidural abscess is similar to that of subdural empyema. Spinal epidural abscess usually occurs following hematogenous spread from another site of infection (e.g., bacteremia) or by extension of vertebral osteomyelitis.

Risk factors include bacteremia, diabetes mellitus, skin infections, spinal trauma or surgery, decubitus ulcers, lumbar puncture, and epidural anesthesia or analgesia.

Etiology

The causes of cranial epidural abscess are similar to those of subdural empyema. *S. aureus* is the most common cause of spinal epidural abscess. Others include aerobic and anaerobic streptococci, aerobic gram-negative bacilli (especially *E. coli* and *P. aeruginosa*); 5–10% are polymicrobial. Unusual causes include *Nocardia* spp., *M. tuberculosis*, and fungi.

Clinical features

The presentation of cranial epidural abscess may be insidious, masked by the primary focus of infection, e.g., sinusitis, otitis media. Headache is common and focal neurological signs and seizures eventually develop, followed by signs of raised intracranial pressure.

Gradenigo's syndrome, characterized by unilateral facial pain and V and VI cranial nerve palsies, may occur if abscess is close to the petrous bone.

Spinal epidural abscess may present acutely (hours to days with hematogenous seeding) or chronically (weeks to months with vertebral osteomyelitis). Pain is the most common symptom (70–90%), followed by fever (60–70%). There are four clinical stages: (1) back pain and tenderness; (2) nerve root pain; (3) spinal cord symptoms, e.g., motor or sensory deficits, sphincter dysfunction; and (4) paralysis.

Diagnosis

Gadolinium-enhanced MRI is the diagnostic investigation of choice; abscesses appear as low-density lesions with linear enhancement.

Management

Epidural abscess is an emergency and requires immediate surgical and medical management. Management of cranial epidural abscess is similar to that of subdural empyema: surgical drainage and antibiotics (3–6 weeks after drainage). Management of spinal epidural abscess is urgent surgical decompression (laminectomy) and antibiotics. Empirical therapy should cover staphylococci (e.g., vancomcyin) and aerobic gram-negative bacilli (e.g., ceftazidime or meropenem).

The outcome of spinal epidural abscess depends on the level of neurological deficit before decompression. Complete recovery is possible if neurological signs have been present for <24 hours.

CSF shunt infections

Infection is a frequent complication of neurosurgical procedures used to treat hydrocephalus, occurring in approximately 10% of cases. The types of device that may become infected are as follows:
- Ventriculoatrial (VA), ventriculoperitoneal (VP), or ventriculopleural shunt
- Ommaya drains
- External ventricular drains (EVDs)
- Lumbar-peritoneal or lumbar-pleural shunt

Shunt infections may be classified as follows:
- Internal (associated with CSF abnormalities)
- External (associated with soft tissue abnormalities)

Etiology
- *S. epidermidis* is the most common isolate.
- *S. aureus,* including MRSA
- Streptococci, enterococci
- Corynebacteria, e.g., *Propionobacterium acnes*
- Gram-negative organisms
- Mycobacteria
- Fungi

Pathogenesis

The mechanisms of infection are as follows:

- Contamination (at implantation of device)
- Externalization (erosion of shunt through skin)
- Retrograde (perforation of VP shunt through bowel)
- Hematogenous (rare)

Clinical features

These depend on age of the patient, site of infection, and whether there is raised intracranial pressure.

Symptoms include fever, headache, vomiting, neck stiffness, impaired conscious level, endocarditis (VA shunts), and abdominal pain (VP or lumbar-peritoneal shunts).

External shunt infections are associated with erythema, abscess, or shunt erosion.

Laboratory diagnosis

- *Blood tests:* full blood count, differential WCC, urea and electrolytes (U&Es), glucose, and liver function tests, ESR, CRP. A normal WCC, ESR, and CRP do not exclude shunt infection.
- *Blood cultures:* 90% positive with VA shunt infections
- *CT/MRI* brain to look for raised intracranial pressure
- *Urine dipstick for hematuria and proteinuria:* VA shunts may be associated with shunt nephritis.
- CSF examination should be performed by a neurosurgical team. CSF samples should be taken for urgent MC&S, protein, and glucose. All abnormal results should be confirmed by a second sample within 24 hours, unless clinical condition mandates immediate treatment.
- Obtain a chest X-ray if there is a VA or ventriculopleural shunt.
- Consider abdominal ultrasound or CT if there are abdominal symptoms or signs and VP or lumbar-peritoneal shunt.
- Consider an echocardiogram if there is a VA shunt.

Management[1,2]

CSF shunt infections should be managed by neurosurgeons with infectious disease and microbiology experts' input.

External shunt infectionsshould be managed bydrainage of pus, removal of infected device and bone flap if present, soft tissue closure if possible, insertion of temporary device at a new site, and interval antibiotics for 7–14 days, followed by replacement with a new permanent device.

Internal shunt infectionsshould be managed with shunt removal, external ventricular drainage placement or ventricular taps, and interval antibiotics for 7–14 days, followed by insertion of a new device when CSF sterility is achieved.

Empiric antibiotic therapy should entail vancomycin intravenously (1 g bid IV, monitor levels) and intrathecally (10 mg od intrathecal). Intravenous meropenem (2 g q8 hours) should be added if there are abdominal symptoms or if gram-negative organisms are seen in the CSF. Consider gentamicin intravenously (5 mg/kg qid IV) and intrathecally (1–5 mg od, monitor levels) if there is evidence of endocarditis.

Specific antibiotic therapy should be tailored according to culture results and clinical response.

In some cases, e.g., coagulase-negative staphylococcal infections where shunt removal is not possible, salvage therapy may be tried with vancomycin and rifampicin (there are insufficient data to support this strategy).

Prognosis

Prognosis of internal shunt infections varies with management strategy:
- Intravenous + intrathecal antibiotic therapy with two-stage exchange: 90% cure
- Intravenous antibiotic therapy with one-stage exchange: 70% cure
- Intravenous + intrathecal antibiotic therapy: 40% cure
- Intravenous antibiotic therapy alone: 20% cure
- Salvage therapy (for coagulase-negative staphylococcal infection only) without shunt exchange (but with an Ommaya reservoir) using intrathecal vancomycin and oral rifampicin: 40–99% cure.

References

1. Treatment of infections associated with shunting for hydrocephalus. Working party on the use of antibiotics in Neurosurgery of the British Society of Antimicrobial Chemotherapy. *Br J Hosp Med* 1995; 53:368–373.

2. Management of neurosurgical patients with postoperative bacterial or aseptic meningitis or external ventricular drain-associated ventriculitis. Infection in Neurosurgery Working Party of the British Society of Antimicrobial Chemotherapy. *Br J Neurosurg* 2000; 14(1):7–12.

Periorbital infections

Blepharitis

Blepharitis is inflammation of the lid margins. Bacterial infection is usually secondary to minor trauma and often occurs in association with seborrheic dermatitis, acne rosacea, and pubic lice infestations.

Anterior blepharitis

This affects the lid where eyelashes attach and is usually caused by bacteria colonizing the base of the eyelashes (e.g., *S. aureus*). Infection of the pilosebaceous glands of Zeiss and Moll may result in an abscess (a stye). Anaerobic infection may follow certain injuries, e.g., bites. Symptoms are erythema, pruritus, and crusting of lid margins.

Chronic infections are caused by infection with *S. aureus,* CoNS, and, more rarely, *Pseudomonas* spp., *Proteus mirabilis*, or *Capnocytophaga ochracea*. Clinical features include hyperemia, crusted exudates around the base of the lashes, and lash loss. Exclude the presence of lice and their eggs. Cell-mediated immunological mechanisms have been implicated in the pathogenesis of chronic blepharitis.

Posterior blepharitis

This affects the inner portion of the eyelid where it contacts the eye and is due to Meibomian gland dysfunction and infection. It may present acutely as an internal stye or hordeolum (pain and swelling are usually apparent on the conjunctival surface of the lid) or chronically as a painless cyst (chalazion).

Symptoms include eye watering, foreign body, or burning sensation. An internal stye may rarely progress to cause preseptal cellulitus.

Treatment

Eyelid hygiene may be sufficient in most cases. Blepharitis thought to be infectious in nature should be treated with a topical antibiotic; frequency and duration of treatment are determined by severity (chloramphenicol, bid for up to 2 weeks).

A chalazion may require incision and drainage. Cases following trauma may require oral therapy with anaerobic cover, e.g., animal bites.

Predisposing conditions should be treated, e.g., lice (malathion), acne rosacea (oral tetracycline), seborrheic dermatitis (topical antifungal and steroid combinations).

Other causes of lid inflammation are cosmetic contact allergy, molluscum contagiosum, louse infestation (e.g., *Phthirus pubis*), dermatoblepharitis secondary to HSV infection, or spread of adjacent impetigo.

Infections of the lacrimal apparatus

The lacrimal gland is found at the lateral upper lid margin. It produces around 10 mL of tears a day, the act of blinking serving to smear the tear film from the lateral to the medial edge of the eye surface.

Drainage is via the puncta at the inner canthus into the canaliculi, and from here to the lacrimal sac, the nasolacrimal duct, and out into the nose.

Canaliculitis

Low-grade inflammation of the canaliculi is usually chronic and due to infection by *Propionibacterium* spp. or *Actinomyces*. Gritty casts form that obstruct the lacrimal duct, leading to eye-watering, chronic conjunctivitis and nasal lid swelling. Treatment is with antibiotic irrigation with canaliculotomy and curettage, where necessary.

Dacryocystitis

Inflammation of the lacrimal sac is usually in the setting of obstruction of the sac or duct (congenital, secondary to infection, tumor, or trauma). It is common in infants, resolving spontaneously by 12 months of age.

Organisms include *S. penumoniae*, *S. aureus*, and *P. aeruginosa*. Recurrent cases may be seen with sarcoidosis or *Chlamydia trachomatis*. The only symptom may be eye-watering. Acute cases follow obstruction of both the proximal and distal ends of the drainage system, e.g., sarcoidosis, trauma.

The main symptom is pain in the region of the tear sac. It may be possible to express purulent material through the lacrimal puncta. Cases may require dacryocystorhinostomy. Orbital cellulitis is a serious complication of acute dacrocystitis.

For treatment in newborns, lacrimal sac massage may be sufficient to resolve the blockage and most cases will resolve with time. If not, probing may resolve the problem. Adults can be treated with systemic antibiotics.

Dacryoadenitis

This is inflammation of the lacrimal gland. Symptoms include localized tenderness and swelling of the outer upper eyelid, with conjunctivitis and periorbital edema.

Pyogenic bacteria are the usual causes. Viral infections may be seen in children, e.g., mumps. Ocular motility defects may occur. Chronic infections may be caused by TB, syphilis, leprosy, or fungi.

Treatment is with systemic antibiotics. Drainage is needed if a collection develops.

Mikulicz syndrome

This is dacryoadenitis associated with inflammation and swelling of the salivary glands (of any etiology).

Orbital infections

The orbital septum is a fibrous sheet lying beneath orbicularis oculi. It extends from the periosteum of the orbit and fuses to the levator aponeurosis in the upper lids and orbital retractor in the lower lids. It acts as a physical barrier to infection.

Orbital cellulitis (infection within the septum) is an ophthalmic emergency and must be differentiated from the less devastating preseptal cellulitus (see Table 4.13). Early involvement of an ophthalmologist is essential.

Children with preseptal infection are at high risk of progressing to orbital cellulitis because of the undeveloped nature of the orbital septum. Preseptal infection should be managed as orbital cellulitis.

Preseptal cellulitis

In this condition, an infection of the superficial skin develops around the eyes anterior to the orbital septum. It may follow infection of adjacent structures (e.g., dacryocystitis) or trauma.

- *Etiology: S. aureus,* group A streptococci, *H. influenzae* (if unvaccinated)
- *Clinical features:* hyperemia of eyelid skin, soft tissue distention, low-grade fever. Proptosis and impairment of ocular motility are not seen,

Table 4.13 Orbital vs. preseptal cellulitis

	Preseptal	Orbital
Proptosis	Absent	Present
Ocular motility	Normal	Painful and restricted
Visual acuity	Normal	Reduced in severe cases
Color vision	Normal	Reduced in severe cases
Relative afferent pupillary defect	Normal	Present in severe cases

Reproduced from Denniston A, Murray P (2005). *Oxford Handbook of Ophthalmology.* Oxford: Oxford University Press, with permission from Oxford University Press.

and their presence suggests orbital cellulitus. Optic nerve function is normal. Complications include CNS infections and progression to orbital cellulitus.

- *Investigations:* Gram stain and culture of any discharge, CT/MRI if any question of orbital involvement
- *Management:* oral antibiotics are sufficient in simple cases (e.g., dicloxacillin 500 mg q6 hours with metronidazole 400 mg q8 hours, both for 7 days). Intravenous antibiotics may be required, particularly if *H. influenzae* is suspected, e.g., a cephalosporin. Ensure anaerobic cover if infection developed following trauma (e.g., bite).

Orbital (postseptal) cellulitus

This is acute infection of orbital contents and is an ophthalmic emergency with the risk of visual loss and posterior extension to the cavernous sinus (leading to possible thrombosis and death). Most cases result from contiguous spread from infected sinuses, e.g., paranasal, ethmoid, frontal. Other causes include trauma, otitis media, and dental infection.

Etiology

The most common causes include *S. aureus, group A streptococci, S. pneumoniae,* anaerobes and gram-negatives (particularly in those cases following chronic sinus infection). Rare causes include TB and fungi (aspergillosis or mucormycosis causes a rare but very aggressive form of orbital cellulitus; see p. 435).

Clinical features

Features include fever, lid edema, rhinorrhea, pain and tenderness over the eye, headache, and limited and painful eye movements. Proptosis (risk of exposure keratopathy) and ophthalmoplegia develop as infection progresses.

Late signs are increased orbital pressure, reduced corneal sensation, and congestion of retinal veins. Cases of very posterior infection (orbital apex syndrome) manifest as visual loss and ophthalmoplegia with very limited external features.

The most serious complication is cavernous sinus thrombosis, which manifests as headache, eye pain, neck stiffness, and swelling over the forehead and eyelids, with papilledema, ophthalmoplegia, and altered level of consciousness.

Other complications are meningitis and cerebral abscess.

Investigations

These include Gram stain and culture of material, if possible (external drainage is rare and aspiration of fluid from the orbit is usually contraindicated except as part of a surgical procedure), blood culture, lumbar puncture if there is meningism, sinus X-rays, and CT or MRI (MRI is preferred for diagnosing cavernous sinus thrombosis).

If surgical intervention (e.g., ethmoidectomy) is performed, the organism may be recovered from material despite empirical antibiotic therapy.

Treatment

Treatment includes urgent antibiotics (e.g., IV ceftriaxone and PO metronidazole), ophthalmology opinion, and ENT review (sinus surgery may be required). Continuing deterioration on therapy suggests the development of an abscess, and a repeat CT should be performed with a view to surgical drainage, if necessary.

The management of fungal orbital cellulitis is a complex mix of surgical debridement and antifungal therapy.

Conjunctivitis

Conjunctivitis is the most common ocular inflammation and may be a primary or local infection or part of a systemic infection (e.g., leptospirosis, measles). Some organisms (e.g., *Chlamydia trachomatis*) cause very specific syndromes, but most cannot be distinguished clinically. Viruses are the most common cause.

Acute conjunctivitis resolves within 4 weeks, chronic conjunctivitis persists for ≥4 weeks. Conjunctivitis is typically self-limiting but can progress to potentially sight-threatening infections.

Etiology

- *Viruses:* the most common cause, e.g., adenovirus, Coxsackie A24, enterovirus 70, herpes simplex virus, varicella zoster virus, smallpox, vaccinia, rubella, rubeola, mumps, influenza, EBV
- *Chlamydia:* C. trachomatis, C. pneumoniae
- *Bacterial:* S. aureus, S. pneumoniae, H. influenzae, Moraxella spp., C, diphtheriae, Neisseria spp., and enteric gram-negative rods
- *Parasitic:* Leishmania spp., Trypanosoma spp., microsporidia, cryptosporidia, fly larvae, loa loa, Phthirus pubis (pubic lice), Demodex (mites)
- *Fungal:* Candida spp., Blastomyces spp., Sporothrix schenkii
- *Allergic or toxic:* cosmetics, soaps, detergents, medications

Clinical features

Irritation and itching are the most common symptoms. Ocular pain is unusual unless there is ulceration, e.g., HSV or corneal involvement. Visual acuity is normal or slightly reduced (unless the cornea is involved).

Skin lesions are seen with HSV, VZV, pox viruses, and immune-mediated diseases, e.g., Stevens–Johnson syndrome.

Conjunctival hyperemia is worse in the periphery than in the limbal region. Saccular aneurysms, petechiae, or subconjunctival or intraconjunctival hemorrhages may be present.

Ocular secretion may be due to increased lacrimal flow or impaired drainage. Conjunctival edema (chemosis) may be marked, resulting in an inability to close the eyelids. Chronic chemosis may lead to conjunctivo-chalasis (laxity of the conjunctiva).

- *Conjunctival papillae:* conjunctival inflammation may result in dilated subepithelial blood vessels that become surrounded by an inflammatory infiltrate to form mounds, called *papillae*. They are more common in bacterial and allergic conjunctivitis.
- *Conjunctival follicles:* small elevated clusters of lymphocytes, similar to papillae but with no central vascular core. They are most commonly associated with viral, chlamydial, or toxic conjunctivitis.

- *Membrane and pseudomembranes:* inflammatory exudate may coalesce, forming a yellow-white membrane overlying the palpebral conjunctiva. Membranes are adherent and cause bleeding when removed; pseudomembranes are not. They are more common in viral and bacterial conjunctivitis.
- *Conjunctival phlyctenules:* a phlyctenule is a whitish, nodular collection located at or near the limbus, often in the center of a hyeremic area. It is a delayed-type hypersensitivity reaction and is associated with *S. aureus* and *M. tuberculosis*. Occasionally it is seen in fungal or parasitic conjunctivitis.
- *Conjunctival granuloma:* a granulomatous nodule of inflammatory cells. It is seen in Parinaud's oculoglandular conjunctivitis, foreign body, tuberculosis, and sarcoidosis, and sometimes in chlamydial or fungal conjunctivitis.
- *Corneal involvement* may be mild (superficial epithelial erosions) or severe (ulceration or perforation). Corneal dendritic ulceration is a feature of HSV conjunctivitis. Symptoms include foreign-body sensation, pain, decreased visual acuity, and photophobia.
- *Lymphadenopathy:* preauricular adenopathy is a nonspecific finding associated with viral, chlamydial, and gonococcal causes of conjunctivitis. Submandibular and submental adenopathy are uncommon but may be present in Parinaud's oculoglandular conjunctivitis.

Diagnosis

Laboratory investigations are not usually performed for most cases of conjunctivitis, especially if a viral etiology is suspected.

All cases of ophthalmia neonatorum (conjunctivitis occurring within the first month of life) should be investigated with smears and cultures for bacteria and viruses. The most common causes are *C. trachomatis* and *N. gonorrheae*. Others causes include *S. aureus*, *S. pneumoniae*, *Pseudomonas* spp., *Shigella flexneri*, *M. catarrhalis*, and HSV.

Swabs and conjunctival scrapings should be taken for Gram stain, culture (on blood, chocolate and Sabouraud agar), and chlamydial and viral diagnostics (e.g., immunofluorescent staining, PCR).

Management

Treatment should be directed at the cause.
- *Viral conjunctivitis* usually resolves spontaneously and is usually treated supportively, e.g., artificial tears and cold compresses.
- *HSV and VZV conjunctivitis:* there is no role for antivirals or corticosteroids, but a prophylactic antibacterial ointment is sometimes given to prevent secondary bacterial infection.
- *Chlamydial conjunctivitis:* trachoma is treated with azithromycin 20 mg/kg stat or doxycycline for 21 days, or erythromycin for 14 days. Adult inclusion conjunctivitis is treated with doxycycline or erythromycin for 3 weeks; sexual partners should be treated simultaneously.
- *Acute bacterial conjunctivitis:* topical antibiotic eyedrops, e.g., chloramphenicol for 7–10 days

- *N. gonorrheae or N. meningitis:* IV ceftriaxone for 1 day (3 days if corneal involvement). Patients with gonococcal conjunctivitis should be screened and treated for other STIs.
- *Chronic bacterial conjunctivitis:* treat with appropriate antibiotic therapy (e.g., against *S. aureus*) and aggressive lid hygiene.
- *Microsporidia:* oral albendazole or topical fumagillin.

Keratitis

Keratitis is an inflammation of the cornea that may be caused by infectious or noninfectious agents. Any corneal inflammation should be considered potentially sight threatening and requires prompt investigation and management. Corneal perforation can occur within 24 hours with certain organisms. Subsequent endophthalmitis may lead to loss of vision or even loss of the eye.

Etiology
Microbial agents do not usually cause keratitis in immunocompetent patients with an intact corneal epithelium. Exceptions include *N. gonorrheae, L. monocytogenes, Shigella* spp., and *Corynebacterium* spp.

Risk factors include trauma, contact lens use, contaminated cleaning fluids, immunological impairment secondary to malnutrition, alcoholism, or diabetes, and recent or pre-existing eye disease (e.g., sicca syndrome, recent topical steroid use).

- *Bacteria:* the most common cause of keratitis. Causes include *Staphylococcus* spp., *Streptococcus* spp., *Corynebacterium* spp., *Bacillus* spp., *Propionobacterium* spp., *Pseudomonas* spp., *Haemophilus* spp., *Moraxella* spp., *N. gonorrheae*, and *Enterobacteriaceae*
- *Myobacteria: M. tuberculosis, M. chelonae, M. gordonae, M. avium intracellulare*
- *Chlamydia trachomatis*
- *Spirochetes: Treponema pallidum, Borrelia burgdorferi*
- *Viruses:* HSV, VZV, vaccinia, adenovirus, enterovirus, molluscum contagiosum, EBV, Coxsackie virus, measles
- *Fungi: Fusarium* (most common), *Aspergillus, Curvularia, Paecilomyces, Phialophora, Blastomyces, Sporothrix, Exophiala, Pseudallescheria, Scedosporium,* and *Alternaria* spp.
- *Parasites: Acanthamoeba, Onchocerca volvulus, Leishmania, Microsporidia,* and *Trypanosoma* spp.

Clinical features
Rapid onset of eye pain is characteristic and may hinder physical examination. Topical anesthesia may facilitate eye examination but can result in further epithelial damage.

Eye pain is accompanied by conjunctival injection, tearing, photophobia, blepharospasm, and decreased visual acuity.

Other features include corneal infiltrate, epithelial defects (visualized by fluorescein stain under cobalt blue light), stromal suppuration, corneal edema, corneal neovascularization, intraocular inflammation (white cells or protein flare in the anterior chamber, hypopyon, synechiae, glaucoma), and loss of corneal tissue (keratolysis).

Diagnosis

Because of the limited amount of tissue available, extreme care must be taken in the collection, transport, and processing of specimens. Discuss this with the microbiology laboratory.

Corneal scrapings (or biopsies) should be taken using sterile technique and transferred to glass slides and appropriate culture media. It may also be helpful to culture material from the conjunctiva, eyelids, and contact lenses, solutions, and storage cases.

For viruses, samples should be collected into viral transport media and inoculated into cell culture the same day. PCR assays enable rapid diagnosis of certain viruses, e.g., HSV and VZV.

Management

Patients may need to be admitted to the hospital for management in order to give immediate therapy and to monitor them, particularly if there is evidence of corneal thinning.

- *Bacterial keratitis:* broad-spectrum topical therapy, e.g., cephalosporin (or vancomycin) and an aminoglycoside (gentamicin or tobramycin) are given for severe keratitis. Topical fluoroquinolones are increasingly being used. The use of topical corticosteroids is controversial. Supportive measures include topical cycloplegics, and temporary soft contact lens for corneal ulceration.
- *Chlamydial keratitis:* systemic antimicrobials, e.g., oral tetracycline, erythromycin or azithromycin. Sexual partners should be treated simultaneously.
- *Interstitial keratitis:* an immune phenomenon associated with syphilis and Lyme disease. Specific therapy may be indicated for the primary disease but has little impact on the cornea. Topical corticosteroids may be helpful.
- *HSV keratitis:* acute infection requires topical (trifluridine 1% eye drops for ≥7 days) or systemic therapy (acyclovir, famciclovir, or valacyclovir for 14–21 days).
- *VZV keratitis:* acute herpes zoster ophthalmicus requires antiviral therapy (acyclovir, famciclovir, or valacyclovir) and pain management (e.g., amitriptyline). Exposure keratopathy requires topical antibiotic ointment (to prevent secondary bacterial infection). For dendritiform keratopathy use 3% vidarabine ointment or 1% trifluridine drops or oral antivirals. For immune keratopathy use topical corticosteroids. General measures include nonsteroidal analgesia and cycloplegics.
- *Ocular vaccinia:* topical 1% trifluridine drops or 3% vidarabine ointment. Intravenous immunoglobulin (IVIG) is not indicated unless required for other reasons, e.g., eczema vaccinatum, progressive vaccinia.
- *Viral keratoconjunctivitis:* no specific treatment required; supportive treatment only, e.g., artificial tears ± cycloplegics. If there are severe symptoms, topical steroids and cycloplegics may be helpful.

- *Fungal keratitis:* topical agents (e.g., amphotericin, flucytosine, fluconazole, and itraconazole) have poor corneal penetration. This may require combined topical and systemic therapy for months.
- *Parasitic keratitis:* optimal treatment for *Acanthamoeba* keratitis is unknown and various agents have been used, e.g., diamidines, biguanides, aminoglycosides, and azoles. Onchocerciasis is treated with ivermectin. Microsporidia may be treated with albendazole.

Uveitis

Uveitis is an inflammation of the uveal tract (iris, ciliary body, choroid) or adjacent ocular structures such as the retina. Inflammation may occur in different anatomical regions of the eye, e.g., anterior (most common), intermediate, posterior, or panuveitis.

Uveitis may be caused by infections, autoimmune conditions, or, rarely, trauma; 50% are idiopathic. Some infectious causes affect specific locations. Aspiration of aqueous or vitreous material may help in identifying the causative organism. Involve an ophthalmologist early in management.

Classification

- *Anterior uveitis:* inflammation affects the iris (iritis), anterior ciliary body (cyclitis), or both (iridocyclitis). It presents with a unilateral red eye, deep ocular pain, a tender eyeball, irregular or constricted pupil, photophobia, and eye-watering. Ocular findings include white blood cells in the aqueous humor, keratitic precipitates, and iris nodules. Most cases are associated with autoimmune conditions (45%) or are idiopathic (40%). Infectious causes include HSV, syphilis, TB, Lyme disease, and leprosy.
- *Intermediate uveitis:* inflammation involves the anterior vitreous and adjacent portion of the retina. Ocular findings include white cells, clumped as "snow balls" in the vitreous, and pars plana white exudates, or "snow bank." Most cases have an unknown etiology (69%) or are due to sarcoidosis or multiple sclerosis. Lyme disease causes <1%.
- *Posterior uveitis:* inflammation involves the choroid (choroiditis), retina (retinitis), or both (choroidoretinitis). Ocular findings include lesions in the choroid, retina, or both. Vitritis sometimes occurs; >40% of cases are due to infection, e.g., *Toxoplasma*, CMV, acute retinal necrosis (HSV), *Toxocara*, syphilis, and *Candida*.
- *Panuveitis:* inflammation involves all parts of the uvea. Ocular findings include white cells in the aqueous and vitreous. Causes are mostly autoimmune, idiopathic (25%), and infections (10%), e.g., syphilis, TB, and *Candida*.

Etiology

- *Tuberculosis:* ocular involvement occurs in ~1% of TB cases and may present without evidence of systemic disease; 50% have a normal CXR. TB can involve any part of the eye, but the most common finding is choroiditis. Other ocular findings include chronic anterior uveitis (usually granulomatous), retinal vasculitis/periphlebitis, scleritis, interstitial keratitis, and optic neuritis.

- *Syphilis:* ocular findings in congenital disease include interstitial keratitis and salt-and-pepper fundi. In secondary syphilis, the most common ocular finding is iritis (>70%). In tertiary syphilis, the main symptom is progressive visual loss. All patients with ocular syphilis should have a lumbar puncture done to exclude concomitant neurosyphilis. HIV-infected patients have higher rates of ocular syphilis and neurosyphilis.
- *Acute retinal necrosis* is a rapidly progressive necrotizing retinitis due to human herpesviruses, e.g., HSV, VZV, and, rarely, CMV. It presents with eye pain, photophobia, and reduced vision. Fundoscopy shows one or more foci of retinal necrosis in the peripheral retina. These extend circumferentially and posteriorly over 3–21 days. Although initially unilateral, bilateral involvement occurs in 70% of untreated patients.
- *CMV retinitis:* prior to highly active antiretroviral therapy, CMV disease occurred in 25–40% of all AIDS patients and its introduction has decreased the incidence of CMV retinitis by 55–83%. Blindness follows the development of retinitis in areas affecting central vision, or retinal detachment, as a result of breaks in the peripheral, necrotic retina. Antiviral therapy (for CMV and HIV) has improved outcome over the last decade; see Antivirals for CMV (p. 81) and HIV treatment (p. 87).
- *Toxoplasma* may be asymptomatic; it is bilateral in 40%. Ocular findings include vitritis, retinitis, retinal vasculitis, anterior uveitis (often with raised intraocular pressure), scleritis, punctate outer retinitis, neuroretinitis, retinal detachment, pigmented retinopathy, endophthalmitis, and systemic features of infection. Complications: glaucoma, cataract
- *Toxocara:* disease is usually unilateral and presentation varies with age. Ocular findings include diffuse chronic endophthalmitis, chronic anterior uveitis, posterior synechiae, granulomas, retinal detachment, cataract, isolated anterior uveitis, intermediate uveitis, optic papillitis, and systemic features of toxocariasis.
- *Microsporidia* affects the immunocompromised and presents with irritation, photophobia, punctate keratopathy, and a follicular conjunctivitis, anterior uveitis.
- *Onchocerchiasis* causes sclerosing keratitis, chorioretinitis, sclerosis of the retinal vessels, optic neuritis, and optic atrophy.
- *Candida:* findings include decreased acuity, floaters, pain, multifocal retinitis (yellow-white fluffy lesions), and vitritis ("cotton-ball" colonies that may be joined, forming a string of pearls). Complications include retinal necrosis and tractional retinal detachment.
- *Aspergillus* usually occurs in immunosuppressed patients with chronic pulmonary disease. Clinical findings are subretinal hypopyon, intraretinal hemorrhages, dense vitritis, and anterior chamber hypopyon.
- *Rare causes* are leptospirosis, Lyme disease, brucellosis, Whipple's disease, leprosy, and *Bartonella henselae.*

Diagnosis

The diagnosis of uveitis is almost always presumptive, as the uvea cannot be biopsied without risking sight. The aqueous and vitreous humors may be sampled, but these samples rarely yield a diagnosis.

Molecular diagnostic techniques may be helpful, e.g., PCR for HSV, VZV, and CMV. Serology is unhelpful apart from in diagnosis of syphilis.

Treatment

The treatment of infectious causes of uveitis is the same as treatment for CNS infection caused by the same pathogen. Systemic corticosteroids may be given in some conditions, e.g., ocular syphilis.

Endophthalmitis

Endophthalmitis is inflammation of the ocular cavity, e.g., aqueous and vit-reous humors. It is usually caused by bacteria or fungi, which may be intro-duced into the eye from an external (exogenous) source (e.g., trauma, surgery, keratitis, bleb related) or enter the eye hematogenously from a distant (endogenous)site of infection, e.g., endocarditis. *Panophthalmitis* refers to inflammation of all ocular tissue.

General features

Symptoms

Symptoms include eye pain, redness, lid swelling, decreased visual acuity, headache, photophobia, and discharge. Fungal endophthalmitis may have a more indolent course with symptoms developing over days to weeks. Consider it in anyone with a history of penetrating injury with a plant substance or soil-contaminated foreign body.

Symptoms of the primary source of infection may be seen in endog-enous cases (e.g., fever, meningism).

Signs

Signs include lid swelling and erythema, inflamed conjunctiva, hypopyon, chemosis, corneal edema, discharge, reduced or absent red reflex, papil-litis, cotton-wool spots, vitritis, fluffy yellow-white retinal or vitreoretinal lesions of growing fungi, fever, and, late in panophthalmitis, proptosis.

Etiology

Bacterial

This is the most common infectious cause. Onset is abrupt and progres-sion is rapid. Most cases are seen after intraocular surgery. Slit-lamp examination is necessary to confirm the diagnosis and detect early signs of infection. There are two types: exogenous and endogenous.

Exogenous

Symptoms develop 24–48 hours after eye trauma, later in patients under-going extracapsular cataract extraction (<5 days postoperative). Ocular surface flora are responsible for most infections, and preoperative con-junctival sterilization may reduce the incidence.

Common postoperative causes include CoNS, coryneforms, and *S. aureus*. Common post-traumatic causes are *S. aureus*, *Bacillus cereus*, group A streptococci, coliforms, anaerobes, and *Pseudomonas* spp. Delayed endophthalmitis after cataract extraction in patients with an intraocular lens may run a chronic course; associated organisms include *P. acnes*, *Corynebacterium* spp., CoNS, and nontuberculous mycobacteria.

Visual outcome after recovery is poor.

Endogenous

This type affects the posterior segment of the eye. Patients are usually very unwell and often immunocompromised. Foci of primary infection include meningitis, endocarditis, pneumonia, abdominal infection, and dental procedures. Causes are *S. aureus*, *S. pneumoniae*,and group A streptococci.

Fungal

Fungal cases are increasing in incidence with the use of immunosuppressive agents and antibiotics. Hematogenous cases are most commonly caused by *Candida* species. Treatment is difficult and the risk of permanent damage is high. Cases have occurred in healthy patients following injections of contaminated anesthetic.

Ocular features may arise many days after *Candida* being recovered from the blood. Patients are often sick (e.g., in the ICU) and may not report early visual symptoms. Have a low threshold for ocular examination of such patients. *Aspergillus* enophthalmitis may occur in seriously immunosuppressed patients and IV drug users.

Other causes are *Cryptococcus neoformans*, *Blastomyces dermatitidis*, *Histoplasma capsulatum*, and *Nocardia* spp.

Viral

HSV, VZV, and CMV cause a spectrum of eye disease ranging from acute retinal necrosis (usually healthy patients) to progressive outer retinal necrosis (severely immunocompromised patients). PCR from vitreal samples may enable identification of the causative virus.

CMV retinitis is seen in patients with AIDS and in those receiving chemotherapy for acute leukemia and malignant lymphomas Measles retinopathy may be seen 6–12 days after skin rash, and chorioretinitis can be a complication of SSPE.

Parasitic

Causes include *Toxoplasma gondii* and *Toxocara canis*.

Diagnosis

Early recognition and prompt microbiological investigations are essential if functional vision is to be salvaged in bacterial endophthalmitis. Samples from the vitreous humor have the greatest yield. It may also be appropriate to obtain material from the anterior chamber and any wound. Surgical specimens should be examined.

Gram, Giemsa, and PAS stains should be performed, and samples cultured for aerobic and anaerobic bacteria, mycobacteria, and fungi. ELISA or PCR testing of samples may also be appropriate. Blood cultures should be taken if the patient is systemically unwell.

Viral retinitis may have a characteristic appearance on fundoscopy, and urgent specialist examination is indicated.

Treatment

Successful outcome depends on having a low threshold of clinical suspicion for diagnosing infectious endophthalmitis. Urgent specialist referral is indicated.

Bacterial

Broad-spectrum intravitreal antibiotics (vancomycin, amikacin, ceftazidime) should be started immediately after urgent diagnostic aspirates. Modify as guided by cultures. Those with visual acuity of light perception or worse benefit from immediate vitrectomy; those with better vision than this do no better with vitrectomy and intravitreal antibiotics than with biopsy and intravitreal antibiotics (unless perhaps they are diabetic).

Outcome is influenced by the time to diagnosis and appropriate treatment and the virulence of the organism: *P. aeruginosa* and *S. aureus* can destroy the eye within 24 hours of presentation. There may be a role for early corticosteroids; much of the damage to the eye is done by the immune response.

Fungal

For *Candida* give systemic antifungals such as fluconazole or an echinocandin (based on susceptibilities) and intravitreal amphotericin B, with vitrectomy in those cases with intravitreal abscess.

For *Aspergillus*, vitrectomy and voriconazole or a lipid formulation of amphotericin B are used. Prognosis is poor. Steroids are contraindicated.

Viral

A combination of systemic and, in some cases, intraocular antiviral agents is indicated. See Cytomegalovirus (p. 351) for details regarding the treatment of CMV retinitis.

Skin and soft tissue infections[1]

Impetigo

Impetigo is caused by *S. aureus* and/or group A streptococci. It commonly affects children in tropical and subtropical regions. It is also prevalent in temperate regions in the summer months.

- *Clinical features:* occurs on the face and extremities. Lesions start as small vesicles that develop into flaccid bullae that rupture, releasing a yellow discharge that forms thick crusts.
- *Treatment:* mupirocin is the best topical agent (although resistance has been described). Patients who have numerous lesions or who do not respond to topical treatment should receive oral antibiotics, e.g., penicillinase-resistant penicillin or a first-generation cephalosporin.

Folliculitis

This is a superficial infection of the hair follicles and apocrine structures.

- *Etiology:* S. aureus (most common), P. aeruginosa (hot-tub folliculitis), Enterobacteriaceae (complication of acne), Candida spp. and Malassezia furfur (in patients taking corticosteroids). Eosinophilic pustular folliculitis occurs in patients with AIDS.
- *Clinical features:* lesions consist of small, erythematous, pruritic papules, often with a central pustule.
- *Treatment:* empiric treatment is with oral flucloxacillin. If the clinical response is slow, consider other pathogens.

Cutaneous abscesses

Collections of pus occur within the dermis and deeper skin structures. They are usually polymicrobial, containing skin or mucous membrane flora. S. aureus is the sole pathogen in ~25% of cases.

- *Clinical features:* painful, tender, fluctuant nodules, usually with an overlying pustule and surrounded by a rim of erythematous swelling
- *Treatment* is with incision and drainage. Antibiotics are rarely necessary unless there is extensive infection or systemic toxicity or the patient is immunocompromised.

Furuncles and carbuncles

A *furuncle* (boil) is a deep inflammatory nodule that usually develops from preceding folliculitis. Furuncles commonly occur in areas of the hairy skin, e.g., face, neck, axillae, and buttocks.

A *carbuncle* is a larger, deeper lesion made of multiple abscesses extending into the subcutaneous fat. They usually occur at the nape of the neck, on the back, or on the thighs. Patients may be systemically unwell.

Outbreaks of furunculosis caused by meticillin-sensitive *S. aureus* (MSSA), and MRSA has been described in groups of individuals with close contact, e.g., families, prisons, and sports teams.

Most furuncles can be treated with application of moist heat, which promotes localization and spontaneous drainage. Large lesions require surgical drainage. Systemic antibiotics are indicated if fever, cellulites, or lesions are located near the nose or lip.

Antimicrobial treatment of community-acquired MRSA infections is indicated and includes oral TMP-SMX or doxycycline for uncomplicated infections and intravenous therapy (vancomycin or daptomycin) for complicated infections.Clindamycin may be used in uncomplicated infections, but the isolate should be tested for inducible erythromycin resistance (D test) prior to selecting this agent for primary therapy.

Control of outbreaks may require washing with chlorhexidine soaps; no sharing of cloths or towels; laundering of clothing, towels, and bedclothes; and eradication of staphylococcal carriage in colonized persons.

Ecthyma

Ecthyma are punched-out ulcers surrounded by raised violaceous margins. They are caused by group A streptococci. Similar lesions (ecthyma gangrenosum) may occur with P. aeruginosa in neutropenic patients.

Empiric treatment is with oral penicillin or clindamycin. Antipseudomonal agents, e.g., piperacillin-tazobactam, should be given for P. aeruginosa infections.

Erysipelas

Erysipelas is an acute spreading skin infection with prominent lymphatic involvement. It usually affects children, infants, and the elderly. Predisposing factors include skins lesions, venous stasis, paraparesis, diabetes mellitus, and alcohol abuse.

- *Causes:* group A streptococci (most common), group C and G streptococci, *S. aureus*, or group B streptococci
- *Clinical features:* painful, erythematous, edematous lesion with an elevated, sharply demarcated border. Usually occurs on the face or legs. Systemic symptoms are common; 5% of cases are bacteremic.
- *Treatment* is with penicillin. If *S. aureus* is suspected, treatment should be with dicloxacillin, cefazolin, TMP-SMX, clindamycin, or erythromycin.

Cellulitis

Cellulitis is an acute, spreading infection of the skin that extends into the subcutaneous tissues.[2] *S. aureus* is the main cause if cellulitis is associated with skin lesions. Other causes are group A, C, G, or B streptococci. Clinical clues to other causes include physical activities, trauma, water contact, and animal, insect, or human bites, and immunosuppression.

Examples include *Enterobacteriaceae, Legionella pneumophila, Aeromonas hydrophila, Vibrio vulnificus, Erysipelothrix rhusiopathiae,* and *Cryptococcus neoformans.*

- *Clinical features:* spreading erythematous, hot, tender lesion, usually accompanied by systemic symptoms
- *Diagnosis* is usually clinical; cultures should only be obtained in patients who do not respond to first-line treatment. If unusual organisms are suspected or in immunocompromised hosts, appropriate culture material should also be obtained. Unfortunately, aspiration of skin is not helpful in 75–80% of cases of cellulitis, and results of blood cultures are rarely positive (<5% of cases).
- *Treatment:* empiric treatment of cellulitis is with dicloxacillin, clindamycin, or erythromycin (unless infections resistant to these agents are common in the community). Vancomycin, linezolid, or daptomycin are indicated for MRSA cellulitis. If a gram-negative organism is suspected, an intravenous cephalosporin, e.g., cefuroxime, may be used. Oral metronidazole should be added for patients with diabetic or vascular ulcers. The affected limb should also be immobilized and elevated and cool sterile saline dressings used to remove any exudate.

References

1. Storers DL, Pislo AL, Chambers HI, et al. (2005). Practice guidelines for the management of skin and soft tissue infections. *Clin Infect Dis* 41:1373–1406.

2. Smartz MN (2004). Cellulitis. *N Engl J Med* 350:904–912.

Bite infections

Animal bites

Etiology

Animal bites are usually caused by domestic pets (e.g., dogs or cats) but may be caused by exotic pets or wild animals. Most infections are polymicrobial. The predominant pathogens are the oral flora of the biting animal, e.g., *Pasteurella multocida, Capnocytophaga canimorsus, Bacteroides* spp., *Fusobacterium* spp., *Prevotella* spp., *Porphyromonas* spp., *Propionobacterium* spp., and peptostreptococci. Secondary bacterial infection with *S. aureus* or group A streptococci may occur.

Clinical features

Patients who present >8 hours after injury usually have established infection that may be nonpurulent, purulent, or abscesses.

Diagnosis is clinical, but samples may be taken to identify the causative organisms. Complications include septic arthritis, osteomyelitis, subcutaneous abscesses, tendonitis, and bacteremia.

Management

Wounds should be irrigated copiously with sterile saline and any debris removed; debridement is rarely necessary. Wounds should be steri-stripped but not sutured (except facial wounds by a plastic surgeon). Empiric antibiotic therapy is with PO amoxicillin/clavulanic acid. Alternatives include PO doxycline or IV piperacillin/tazobactam or carbapenems.

A tetanus booster should be given to those with unknown vaccination status. Rabies vaccination should be considered for animal bites in endemic regions. Prophylactic valacyclovir should be considered for monkey bites (for simian herpes virus).

Human bites

Etiology

Human bites result from aggressive behavior and are often more serious than animal bites. The causative organisms are usually the oral flora of the biter, e.g., oral streptococci, staphylococci, *Haemophilus* spp., *Eikenella corrodens, Fusobacterium* spp., *Prevotella* spp., *Porphyromonas* spp., and, rarely, *Bacteroides* spp. Human bites may also potentially transmit viral infections, e.g., HBV, HCV, and HIV.

Clinical features

Bite wounds may be may be occlusive injuries (where teeth bite the body part) or clenched fist injuries (where one person's fist hits the other person's teeth). Complications of closed-fist injuries include tendon or nerve damage, fractures, septic arthritis, or osteomyelitis.

Management

Principles are the same as for animal bites, e.g., wound irrigation and prophylactic antimicrobial therapy. Hand injuries should be evaluated by a surgeon for complications. Post-exposure prophylaxis of hepatitis B and HIV should be considered if the source is potentially infected.

Surgical site infections

Infections of surgical wounds are common adverse events following surgery.[1,2] The frequency of surgical site infections (SSIs) is related to the category of operation and is highest with contaminated or high-risk surgical procedures. There are three categories of SSI:

- *Superficial incisional SSI* involves subcutaneous tissue and occurs within 30 days of operation.
- *Deep incisional SSI* involves muscle and fascia and occurs with 30 days of surgery (or 1 year if a prosthesis is inserted).
- *Organ/space SSI* involves any part of the anatomy (organs or spaces) other than the incisional site.

Etiology and pathogenesis

The most common organisms are *S. aureus* and MRSA. Others include coagulase-negative staphylococci, aerobic gram-negative bacilli, *Bacillus* spp., and corynebacteria. SSIs that occur after an operation on the GI tract or female genitalia have a high probability of having mixed flora.

The presence of prosthetic material greatly reduces the number of organisms required to initiate infection.

Clinical features

Most SSIs have no clinical manifestations for at least 5 days after the operation, and many may not become apparent for up to 2 weeks later.

Local signs of pain, swelling, erythema, and purulent drainage are usually present. Fever may not be present until a few days later.

In morbidly obese patients or in patients with deep, multilayer wounds, e.g., thoracotomy, the external signs of SSIs may appear late.

Diagnosis

The diagnosis is usually clinical, but samples of fluid or tissue should be sent to the laboratory for Gram stain and culture.

Management

The primary therapy for SSI is to open the incision, debride the infected material, and continue dressing changes until the wound heals by secondary intention.

Although patients commonly receive antibiotics for SSIs, there is little or no evidence to support this practice.

A common practice, endorsed by expert opinion, is to open all infected wounds. If there is minimal evidence of invasive infection (<5 cm of erythema) and if the patient has minimal systemic signs of infection (temperature <38.5°C, pulse rate of <100/min), antibiotics are unnecessary. For patients with a temperature of >38.5°C or a pulse rate of >100 beats/min, a short course of antibiotics (24–48 hours) may be indicated.

References

1. Stevens DL, Bisno AL, Chambers HF, et al. (2005). Practice guidelines for the diagnosis and management of skin and soft tissue infections. *Clin Infect Dis* 41:1373–1406.

2. Health Protection Agency. Surgical Site Infection Surveillance Service (SSISS). http://www.hpa.org.uk/infections/topics_az/surgical_site_infection/default.htm (accessed Aug. 15, 2008).

Gas gangrene

This is a rapidly progressive, life-threatening, skeletal muscle infection caused by *Clostridia* spp. (clostridial myonecrosis).

Etiology and pathogenesis

Gas gangrene usually occurs following muscle injury and contamination of the wound by soil or foreign material containing clostridial spores. *Clostridium perfringens* (see Other clostridia, p. 217) is the predominant cause (80–95%). The pathological effects are mediated by production of A and θ toxins.

Spontaneous or nontraumatic gas gangrene may occur in the absence of an obvious wound. This form is usually caused by *C. septicum* and associated with intestinal abnormalities, e.g., colonic cancer, diverticulitis, bowel infarction, or necrotizing enterocolitis.

Other organisms include *C. novyi*, *C. bifermentans*, *C. histolyticum*, and *C. fallux*. Organisms such as *E. coli*, *Enterobacter* spp., or enterococci may be isolated, reflecting contamination of the wound.

Clinical features

The incubation period is usually 2–3 days but may be shorter. Patients present with acute onset of excruciating pain and signs of shock (fever, tachycardia, hypotension, jaundice, and renal failure).

Local edema and tenderness may be the only early signs, or there may be an open wound, herniation of muscle, a serosanguinous, foul-smelling discharge, crepitus, skin discoloration, and necrosis.

Progression is rapid and death may occur within hours.

Diagnosis

The diagnosis is usually clinical but may be confirmed by Gram stain of the wound or aspirate. Liquid anaerobic cultures may be positive within 6 hours.

Plain radiographs may show gas in the affected tissues.

Management

Emergency surgical exploration and debridement of the affected area may be life saving.

Antimicrobial therapy with intravenous benzylpenicillin and clindamycin is widely recommended (based on animal experimental data). Additional antibiotics (e.g., ciprofloxacin, ceftriaxone, or chloramphenicol) may be given if gram-negative bacilli are seen in the initial Gram smear.

The role of adjunctive hyperbaric oxygen therapy remains controversial; it should never delay surgery.

Necrotizing fasciitis

This is a severe, acute infection involving the superficial and deep fascia.[1]

Etiology and pathogenesis

Type I necrotizing fasciitis involves at least one anaerobic species (e.g., *Bacteroides* or *Peptostreptococcus* spp.) as well as one or more facultative anaerobic species (e.g., non-group A streptococci, E. coli, Enterobacter, Klebsiella, Proteus spp.).

Type II necrotizing fasciitis is caused by group A streptococci alone or in combination with other species (e.g., S. aureus). This form usually occurs after trauma, wounds, or surgery in patients with predisposing conditions (e.g., diabetes mellitus, peripheral vascular disease, hepatic cirrhosis, corticosteroid therapy, IV drug use). There has been a recent increase in cases associated with streptococcal toxic shock syndrome.

Clinical features

Necrotizing fasciitis most commonly affects the lower limbs but may affect any part of the body, e.g., wound sites, abdominal wall, groin, or perianal area. The affected area is usually red, hot, swollen, and exquisitely tender and painful. There is rapid progression with skin discoloration, bulla formation, and cutaneous gangrene. The affected area becomes anesthetic as result of small vessel thrombosis and destruction of superficial nerves. Systemic toxicity is common.

In newborns, necrotizing fasciitis may complicate omphalitis and spread to involve the abdominal wall, flanks, and chest wall.

Fournier's gangrene is a form of necrotizing fasciitis that affects the male genitals and is usually polymicrobial.

Craniofacial necrotizing fasciitis is usually associated with trauma and caused by A streptococci.

Cervical necrotizing fasciitis is usually associated with dental or pharyngeal infections and is polymicrobial.

Diagnosis

Diagnosis is usually clinical but may be confirmed by Gram stain of the exudate. Blood cultures are frequently positive.[2]

CT or MRI scans may demonstrate subcutaneous and fascial edema but should never delay surgical exploration.

Management

Emergency surgical exploration and debridement confirms the diagnosis and is the mainstay of treatment.[2]

Empiric antimicrobial therapy should cover the most likely organisms, e.g., intravenous cefuroxime or amoxicillin-clavulanate, clindamycin, and gentamicin. Adjunctive therapies (e.g., IV immunoglobulin for streptococcal toxic shock syndrome or hyperbaric oxygen) remain unproven.

References

1. Bisno AL, Stevens DL (1996). Streptococcal infections of skin and soft tissues. N Engl J Med 334:240–245.

2. Stevens DL, Bisno AL, Chambers HF, et al. (2005). Practice guidelines for the diagnosis and management of skin and soft tissue infections. Clin Infect Dis 41:1373–1406.

Pyomyositis

Pyomyositis (primary muscle abscess) is an acute bacterial infection of skeletal muscle.

Epidemiology

Most cases occur in the tropics, where it may affect any age group, and accounts for 1–4% of hospital admissions. In temperate climates, pyomyositis usually affects adults or the elderly, 40% of whom have a predisposing condition (e.g., diabetes mellitus, alcoholic liver disease, corticosteroid therapy, hematological malignancies, or HIV infection).

Etiology

S. aureus accounts for 95% of cases in the tropics and 66% of cases in North America. Group A streptococci account for 1–5% of cases. Uncommon causes include groups B, C, and G streptococci, *S. pneumoniae*, and *S. anginosus*. Rare causes include *Enterobacteriaceae*, *Y. enterocolitica*, *N. gonorrhoeae*, *H. influenzae*, *Aeromonas hydrophila*, anaerobes, *Burkholderia mallei*, *Burkholderia pseudomallei*, *Aspergillus fumigatus*, *Candida* spp., *M. tuberculosis*, and *M. avium* complex.

Clinical features

Between 20% and 50% of patients have had recent blunt trauma or vigorous exercise of the affected area. There are three clinical stages:

- *Invasive stage:* subacute onset of fever, local swelling ± erythema, mild pain, and minimal tenderness
- *Suppurative stage* (2–3 weeks later): fever, distinct muscle swelling, and tenderness; pus may be aspirated from muscle
- *Systemic stage:* sepsis syndrome, erythema, exquisite tenderness, and fluctuance. It may progress to metastatic abscesses, shock, and renal failure. Complications include compartment syndrome.

Diagnosis

Early pyomyositis may be difficult to differentiate from a number of other conditions, e.g., thrombophlebitis, muscle hematoma, muscle rupture, fever of unknown origin (FUO), and osteomyelitis. Iliacus pyomyositis may mimic septic arthritis of the hip, and iliopsoas pyomyositis may mimic appendicitis.

CT or MRI scans are useful both to delineate intramuscular abscesses and to aid diagnostic aspiration.

Management

Percutaneous or open drainage of all abscesses is the essential. Fasciotomies and debridement may be required for compartment syndrome.

Empiric antimicrobial therapy should cover *S. aureus* and group A streptococci, e.g., intravenous oxacillin, nafcillin, cefazolin, or vancomycin if MRSA is suspected.

Antibiotic therapy should be modified according to Gram stain or culture results. Ongoing fever despite appropriate therapy should prompt a search for further foci of infection.

Fungal skin infections

Fungi may cause primary infection of the skin or present with cutaneous manifestations of systemic disease.

Candida (p. 417)

- *Localized skin infections:* erosio interdigitalis blastomycetica (between fingers and toes), folliculitis, intertrigo, diaper rash, paronychia, onychomycosis, balanitis
- *Generalized cutaneous candidiasis:* in which lesions spread and become confluent, affecting widespread areas of the trunk, thorax, and extremities (uncommon)

Chronic mucocutaneous candidiasis

This constitutes a group of candidal infections that fail to respond to normally adequate therapy, resulting in complications such as esophageal stenosis, alopecia, and disfigurement of the face, scalp, and hands. These failures seem to be associated with immunological abnormalities. Most cases present in infancy or by the age of 20 years.

There is a wide spectrum of severity. Up to half of patients subsequently develop certain endocrinopathies (e.g., hypoparathyroidism). Most patients have good life expectancies. The most common cause of death is bacterial sepsis rather than disseminated candidiasis.

Chronic mucocutaneous disease is very difficult to treat. Intravenous amphotericin is initially effective, but most patients relapse on its cessation. Months or years of treatment with azoles may be necessary.

Malessezia furfur (p. 425)

This causes pityriasis versicolor (a superficial skin infection characterized by hypopigmented lesions usually confined to trunk and proximal limbs), folliculitis, as well as IV catheter infections. *Malessezia* spp. have been implicated in the pathogenesis of seborrheic dermatitis.

Aspergillus (p. 432)

Cutaneous infection is rare, usually occurring in burn wounds or neutropenic patients at the site of IV catheter insertion. More common is otomycosis, caused by *A. niger* in those with chronic otitis externa. Cleaning and topical therapy with an agent such as amphotericin B 3% or clotrimazole is curative.

Mucormycosis (p. 437)

This is infection by fungi belonging to the order *Mucorales*. Risk factors include immunosuppression, transplantation, diabetes mellitus, and trauma. It presents with chronic ulcer or cellulitis. If unrecognized, the organism penetrates deeper into the skin, with vascular invasion, necrosis, and possible dissemination.

Eumycetoma (p. 440)

This is a chronic, slow-growing, destructive fungal infection of the hands or feet. It is found worldwide in tropical regions but is rare in temperate areas.

Pseudallescheria boydii **(p. 444)**

This may cause eumycetoma, skin, and soft tissue infection, or abscesses.

Scedosporium prolificans **(p. 444)**

This infection is extremely rare. Focal (e.g., osteoarticular) disease occurs in immunocompetent individuals and with disseminated infection (including skin) in the immunocompromised (e.g., those undergoing hematopoietic stem cell transplantation [HSCT]).

Fusarium **species (p. 444)**

This species is rare in immunocompetent people. Skin lesions start as macules and progress to necrotic papules. Systemic infection is seen in patients with acute leukemia with prolonged neutropenia and in those undergoing HSCT.

Sporothrix schenckii **(p. 445)**

The organism is inoculated into skin at sites of minor trauma. It may cause either a fixed plaque, or painless smooth or verrucous erythematous nodular papules with secondary lesions that follow the routes of lymphatic vessels.

Chromomycosis (p. 447)

An itchy small pink papule is followed by crops of either warty, violaceous nodules or firm tumors, which may enlarge, forming groups with ulceration and dark hemopurulent material on the surface. Satellite lesions may occur. Some people develop annular, papular lesions with active edges and healing in the center that can become scarred or form keloid. Fibrosis and edema of the affected limb occur in severe cases.

Dermatophytes (p. 441)

This group of fungi is capable of invading the dead keratin of skin, hair, and nails. Clinical classification is by body area involved: tinea capitis (scalp hair; most common in children), tinea corporis (trunk and limbs), tinea manuum and pedis (palms and soles; most common overall worldwide), tinea cruris (groin), tinea barbae (beard area and neck), tinea faciale (face), tinea unguium (nails; also known as onychomycosis).

Cutaneous manifestations of systemic fungal infection

Systemic fungal infections that present with cutaneous disease include
- Disseminated candidiasis
- Cryptococcosis (p. 735)
- *Penicillium marneffei* (p. 462)
- *Blastomyces dermatitidis* (p. 454)
- *Coccidioides immitis* (p. 457)
- *Paracoccidioides brasiliensis* (p. 460)
- *Fusarium* spp. (p. 444)
- *Scedosporium prolificans* (p. 444)
- Mucormycosis (p. 437).

Viral skin infections

Herpes simplex virus (p. 341)

Cutaneous manifestations of HSV infection include the following:

- *Pharyngitis/gingivostomatitis:* the most common presentation of primary HSV-1, generally seen in children and young adults. General features: fever, malaise, difficulty chewing, cervical lymphadenopathy. Ulcers and exudative lesions are found on the posterior pharynx and sometimes the tongue, buccal mucosa, and gums. Patients with eczema may develop severe orofacial disease (eczema herpeticum) which may disseminate requiring systemic therapy. HSV has been associated with up to 75% of cases of erythema multiforme
- *Recurrent herpes labialis:* the most frequent manifestation of HSV-1 reactivation. May be asymptomatic (viral secretion). Reactivation is usually localized with symptoms that are milder and of shorter duration than primary infection. Mild prodromal tingling is followed by the development of lesions within 48 hours – resolution is quick, usually within 5 days. Immunosuppressed patients may experience severe mucositis with spread to skin surrounding the mouth. AIDS patients can develop persistent HSV ulceration
- *Herpetic whitlow:* HSV infection of the finger which may result from auto-inoculation (existing oral or genital infection), or by direct inoculation from some other environmental exposure – e.g., healthcare workers. Edema, tenderness, and erythema are followed by the development of vesicular lesions. Regional lymphadenopathy may occur. Diagnosis is important if only to prevent unnecessary surgical intervention and onward transmission
- *Herpes gladiatorum:* mucocutaneous infection of surfaces such as chest, ears, face, and hands seen in rugby players and wrestlers.

Varicella zoster virus (p. 343)

Chickenpox

Illness is associated with primary varicella virus infection; 90% of cases occur in children under 13 years of age. Incubation is 10–14 days and may be followed by a 1- to 2-day febrile prodrome before the onset of constitutional symptoms (malaise, itch, anorexia) and rash.

Lesions start as maculopapules (<5 mm across), progressing to vesicles that quickly pustulate and form scabs that fall off 1–2 weeks after infection. They appear in successive crops over 2–4 days starting on the trunk and face and spreading centripetally. They may rarely involve the mucosa of the oropharynx and vagina. Complications are secondary bacterial infection, pneumonitis, and encephalitis.

Disease may be severe in pregnancy and the immunocompromised.

Shingles

Shingles, or herpes zoster, is the localized recurrence of varicella virus. A unilateral vesicular eruption occurs in a dermatomal distribution (most commonly thoracic and lumbar), often preceded by 2–3 days of pain in the affected area. Maculopapular lesions evolve into vesicles, with new crops forming over 3–5 days. Resolution may take 2–4 weeks.

Complications include keratitis (herpes zoster opthalmicus), Ramsay–Hunt syndrome (VIII cranial nerve palsy), encephalitis, and paralysis (anterior horn cell involvement).

Smallpox (p. 389)

Smallpox is caused by variola virus, an orthopoxvirus. There are two strains: variola major (mortality 20–50%) and variola minor (mortality <1%). The last reported case was in Somalia in 1977, and the virus was declared eradicated by the World Health Organization in 1980.

Virus stocks exist in two laboratories. There are concerns about its potential use as a bioterrorism agent (p. 753).

The incubation period is 10–12 days and is followed by a prodromal period of 1–2 days. The centrifugal rash is initially maculopapular and progresses to vesicles, pustules, and scabs over 1–2 weeks. Death may occur with fulminant disease.

Diagnosis may be confirmed by electron microscopy or PCR (to differentiate it from other pox viruses). There is no specific treatment. Management is by isolation of cases to prevent transmission.

Monkeypox (p. 389)

Monkeypox is caused by an orthopox virus. It causes a vesicular illness in monkeys and rodents in West and Central Africa. Infection may sporadically be transmitted to humans. A large outbreak in humans in the United States was traced to the importation and sale of exotic pets. The disease is similar but less severe than smallpox.

Diagnosis is by electron microscopy or PCR (to differentiate it from other pox viruses).

Management is symptomatic, as there is no specific treatment.

Orf (p. 389)

Orf is caused by a parapox virus and primarily affects sheep and cattle. Humans are infected following direct exposure to infected animals. It presents with vesicular rash on sites of contact, e.g., hands and arms. This progresses to pustules that coalesce, scab, and gradually resolve over weeks.

Diagnosis is by virus culture and identification of the virus by electron microscopy. Management is symptomatic; there is no specific treatment.

Molluscum contagiosum (p. 389)

Molluscum contagiosum is caused by a pox virus. It is spread by close human contact and may cause severe, generalized disease in HIV-infected patients. The lesions are small, firm, umbilicated papules that occur on exposed epithelial surfaces or the genitalia. Lesions may resolve spontaneously or persist for months or years.

Diagnosis is confirmed by histology or electron microscopy. Management is with local therapy, e.g., laser, cryotherapy, or incision and curettage. One small uncontrolled study of three patients has shown benefit with cidofovir.

Reference

Toutous-Trellu L, Hirschel B, Piguet V, et al. (2004). Treatment of cutaneous human papilloma virus, poxvirus and herpes simplex virus infections with topical cidofovir in HIV positive patients. *Ann Dermatol Venereol* 131(5):445–449.

Miscellaneous skin infections

Cutaneous anthrax

Cutaneous anthrax is caused by *Bacillus anthracis* (p. 204). It usually affects humans who are in direct contact with infected animals (e.g., cattle and sheep) or animal products.

The lesion begins with a pruritic papule that enlarges to form an ulcer surrounded by vesicles and then develops into an eschar surrounded by edema. There may be regional lymphangitis, lymphadenopathy, and systemic symptoms.

Diagnosis is confirmed by microscopy and culture of vesicle fluid. If the patient has received antibiotics or cultures are negative, a punch biopsy may be taken for immunohistochemistry or PCR.

Antimicrobial therapy does not accelerate healing of the skin lesion but may reduce edema and systemic symptoms. Empiric therapy is with oral ciprofloxacin for 5–9 days; the duration of treatment should be increased to 60 days if inhalational anthrax is a possibility.

Erysipeloid

Erysipeloid is caused by *Erysipelothrix rhusiopathiae* (p. 212). It usually affects people who handle fish, marine mammals, poultry, or swine.

After exposure, a red maculopapular lesion develops, usually on the fingers or hands. Erythema spreads centrifugally with central clearing. A blue ring with a peripheral red halo may appear. Regional lymphangitis or lymphadenopathy occurs in ~1/3 cases. A severe, generalized cutaneous infection may also occur.

Diagnosis is confirmed by culture of a lesion aspirate and/or biopsy specimen; blood cultures are rarely positive.

Untreated erysipeloid resolves during a period of 3–4 weeks, but treatment probably hastens healing and perhaps reduces systemic complications. Treatment is with oral pencillin or amoxicillin for 7–10 days.

Cat scratch disease

Cat scratch disease is mainly caused by *Bartonella henselae* (p. 299). A papule or pustule develops 3–30 days after a scratch or a bite. Regional adenopathy occurs ~3 weeks after inoculation, and ~10% of nodes suppurate. Extranodal disease (e.g., CNS, liver, spleen, bone, and lung) occurs in 2% of cases.

Diagnosis is by serology (poor specificity), PCR, or histology (Warthin–Starry silver stain).

Treatment is with oral azithromycin for 5 days. Clinical response is rarely dramatic, but lymphadenopathy usually resolves by 6 months.

Bacillary angiomatosis

Bacillary angiomatosis may be caused by *Bartonella henselae* or *Bartonella quintana*. It usually occurs in immunosuppressed patients, especially those with AIDS.

Reference

Stevens DL, Bisno AL, Chambers HF, et al. (2005). Practice guidelines for the diagnosis and management of skin and soft tissue infections. *Clin Infect Dis* 41:1373–1406.

Septic arthritis

This is an inflammatory reaction of the joint space caused by an infectious agent.

Etiology

- *Staphylococcus aureus*
- Streptococci, e.g., groups A, B, C, and G streptococci, *S. pneumoniae*
- Coagulase-negative staphylococci
- *E. coli*
- *H. influenzae*
- *N. gonorrhoeae*
- *N. menigitidis*
- *P. aeruginosa*
- *Salmonella* spp.
- Others, e.g., *Pasteurella multocida*, *Capnocytophaga canimorsis*, *Eikenella corrodens*, *Streptobacillus moniliformis*, *Brucella* spp., *Burkholderia pseudomallei*, *Clostridium* spp.
- Polymicrobial infections

Epidemiology

The reported incidence of septic arthritis varies from 2 to 5/100,000 per year in the general population. Risk factors for septic arthritis include rheumatoid arthritis, intra-articular injections, trauma, diabetes mellitus, immunosuppression, intravenous drug use, and human and animal bites.

Pathogenesis

Septic arthritis usually occurs after hematogenous seeding of pathogenic microorganisms but may occur following trauma.

Clinical features

Children and adults with acute septic arthritis usually present with fever (60–80%) and monoarticular involvement (90%).

The knee is the most commonly affected joint, followed by the hip. Clinical features include pain, swelling, and reduced mobility in the joint.

Polyarticular infections occur in 10–20% of patients, especially those with rheumatoid arthritis and viral causes.

Infections with mycobacteria or fungi usually have an insidious onset.

Differential diagnosis
- Inflammatory arthritides
- Postinfectious arthritis
- Chronic bacterial arthritis, e.g., *Borrelia burgdorferi*, *Brucella* spp., *Tropheryma whippelii*, *Nocardia asteroides*
- Viruses, e.g., parvovirus B19, hepatitis B, mumps, rubella, HTLV-1, HIV-1, lymphocytic choriomengitis virus, Chikungunya virus, Ross River virus
- Mycobacteria, e.g., *M. tuberculosis* (most common), *M. kansasii*, *M. marinum*, *M. avium intracellulare*, *M. fortuitum*, *M. haemophilum*, *M. leprae*
- Fungi, e.g., *Sporothrix schenkii*, *Blastomyces dermatitidis*, *Coccidioides immitis*, *Paracoccidiodes braziliensis*, *Candida albicans*, *Pseudallescheria boydii*
- Parasites, e.g., filarial infections, schistosomiasis

Diagnosis

Laboratory investigations

Lab results frequently show a raised white cell count and inflammatory markers. Aspiration of the joint reveals a purulent synovial fluid with high neutrophil count. Gram stain is positive in 50%, and culture is positive in 80–90% of cases. False-positive Gram stains may occur with artifacts from stain, mucin, and cellular debris.

Direct inoculation of the synovial fluid into blood culture bottles may improve recovery of pathogens. Samples should also be sent for microscopy for crystals.

Radiological investigations

Plain radiographs may show periarticular soft tissue swelling, fat pad edema, periarticular osteoporosis, loss of joint space, periosteal reactions, erosions, and loss of subchondral bone. Ultrasound can be used to confirm an effusion and guide aspiration.

CT and MRI are highly sensitive for imaging early septic arthritis. CT is better for imaging bone lesions. MRI may not distinguish septic arthritis from inflammatory arthropathies.

Management

Drainage

Drainage of the joint, either by closed aspiration or arthroscopic washout, should be performed urgently. Open drainage may be required either when repeated drainage has failed to control the infection or for drainage of hip joints. Prosthetic joint infections usually require removal of the prosthesis.

Antimicrobial therapy

This should be guided by the initial Gram stain findings. If the Gram stain is negative, then intravenous ceftriaxone ± vancomycin is a reasonable choice. Definitive therapy should be tailored to the organism isolated and its antimicrobial susceptibility pattern. Treatment is usually for 3–6 weeks.

Adjunctive therapy
Short-course systemic corticosteroid treatment has been shown to be of benefit in children with hematogenous bacterial arthritis.

Septic bursitis

This common condition usually affects the olecranon bursa or the prepatellar bursa. Bacteria are usually introduced following minor trauma but may rarely be inoculated during intrabursal injection of corticosteroids. Infection of the deep bursa is rare but may occur in association with septic arthritis.

S. aureus is the cause in >80% of cases; the remainder are caused by streptococci, various gram-negative bacteria, and fungi.

Diagnosis is made by aspiration of the affected bursa and examination of the synovial fluid for cells, organisms, and crystals.

Treatment is with antibiotics (guided by Gram stain results) and aspiration. Treatment should be tailored to the organism isolated and its antimicrobial susceptibility pattern. The duration of treatment is 14 days.

Reactive arthritis

Also known as Reiter's syndrome, this condition is characterized by arthritis, urethritis, and uveitis, and, often, lesions of the skin and mucous membranes. It complicates 1–2% of cases of non-gonococcal urethritis (NGU) and is the most common inflammatory arthritis in young men.

Etiology
Reiter's syndrome is associated with sexually transmitted infections and gastrointestinal infections:
• *C. trachomatis*
• *N. gonorrhoeae*
• *Salmonella* spp.
• *Shigella* spp.
• *Campylobacter* spp.
• *Yersinia* spp.

It is also reported after antibiotic-associated colitis, cryptosporidiosis, after bladder instillation of BCG, and after respiratory infections with *C. psittaci* and *C. pneumoniae*.

Pathogenesis
The pathogenesis of the condition is not fully understood; it probably represents an abnormal host response to infectious agents.

It is associated with the presence of HLA-B27, which is found in >90% of patients with Reiter's syndrome.

Clinical features
Urethritis is the first symptom and usually occurs 14 days after sexual intercourse. Cystitis has been reported in women. The other features occur after 1–5 weeks.

Arthritis most frequently affects the knees, but other joints may be involved, e.g., ankles, small joints of feet, and sacroiliac joints. Complications include ankylosing spondylitis, calcaneal spurring, and dactylitis.

Ocular findings include conjunctivitis, iritis, keratitis, or uveitis. Skin manifestations include waxy papules, keratoderma blenorrhagica, circinate balanitis.

Initial episode lasts 2–6 months but the disease may recur.

Rare complications include pericarditis, myocarditis, first-degree heart block, and aortic regurgitation.

Diagnosis

There is no diagnostic test. Anemia and raised ESR are common. Synovial fluid shows a raised WCC with a neutrophil predominance and low glucose level. Histology shows nonspecific changes.

Management

Treatment is controversial. Because of the association with STIs, some authorities recommend treatment with antibiotics, but there are limited data to support this. NSAIDS are given for symptomatic relief. Sulfasalazine, methotrexate, or ciclosporin may be used in refractory cases.

Osteomyelitis

Osteomyelitis is an infection of the bone, characterized by progressive bone destruction and formation of sequestra. It may be due to hematogenous seeding, contiguous spread from adjacent infected tissues, or traumatic or surgical inoculation of microorganisms.

Classification

Two classification systems exist.[1]

Cierny–Mader system is functional classification based on the affected portion of bone and physiological status of the host. It is useful in guiding therapy:

- *Anatomical type:* stage 1 = medullary osteomyelitis, stage 2 = superficial osteomyelitis, stage 3 = localized osteomyelitis, stage 4 = diffuse osteomyelitis
- *Physiological type:* A = normal host, B = host with local (BL) or systemic (Bs) compromise, C = treatment worse than disease

Lee and Waldvogel system is essentially an etiological classification based on duration of illness (acute or chronic), mechanism of illness (contiguous or hematogenous), and presence or absence of vascular insufficiency. It is less helpful in terms of treatment.

Pathogenesis

In experimental models, normal bone is highly resistant to infection; osteomyelitis only occurs after inoculation of large inocula, as a result of bone trauma, or in the presence of foreign material. When digested by osteoclasts, *S. aureus* can survive in a dormant state for a long time, making it difficult to treat with antimicrobials and resulting in high relapse rates if short courses of antibiotics are given.

Biofilm formation associated with prosthetic material can also make these infections difficult to treat.

Etiology

S. aureus and coagulase-negative staphylococci are the most common causes of osteomyelitis, accounting for >50% of cases. Less common causes (>25%) include streptococci, enterococci, *Pseudomonas* spp., *Enterobacter* spp., *Proteus* spp., *E. coli*, *Serratia* spp., and anaerobes.

Rare causes (<5%) include *M. tuberculosis*, *M. avium complex*, rapidly growing mycobacteria, dimorphic fungi, *Candida* spp., *Aspergillus* spp., *Mycoplasma* spp., *Tropheryma whipplei*, *Brucella* spp., *Salmonella* spp., and *Actinomyces* spp.

In hematogenous long bone osteomyelitis, the infection is usually monomicrobial, whereas contiguous infection is often polymicrobial.

Clinical features

Osteomyelitis usually presents with subacute to chronic onset of pain around the affected site.

Systemic symptoms and signs are frequently absent, and local erythema and swelling are unusual.

In chronic osteomyelitis, a draining sinus may be present.

Diagnosis

Diagnosis is often suspected clinically and is confirmed by a combination of radiological, microbiological, and histopathological investigations.

- *Blood tests:* the peripheral WCC may be normal or raised; inflammatory markers (ESR and CRP) are often elevated.
- *Radiology:* although insensitive, a plain radiograph is readily available and inexpensive and may show changes after 10–14 days. Bone scans are sensitive but nonspecific. CT or MRI scans are expensive but highly sensitive and specific and have become the investigations of choice. MRI is contraindicated in patients with metal implants; these may also cause artifacts on CT.
- *Biopsy:* radiologically guided or surgical biopsy, preferably taken prior to antibiotic therapy, is essential to identify the causative organism(s). Samples should be sent for microbiology and histology. Sinus tract swabs are of dubious value, as they may represent colonizing flora.

Management

General principles

Owing to the lack of good clinical trial data, most of the recommendations for the management of osteomyelitis come from animal models, retrospective cohort studies, and expert opinion. The goal of therapy is to eradicate infection and restore and preserve function. Osteomyelitis in adults is usually treated with a combination of surgical debridement and antibiotic therapy, preferably started after surgical debridement.

Surgery

The principles of surgical therapy are debridement of infected tissue, removal of metal implants, management of dead space (using a flap), wound closure, and stabilization of infected fractures.

Antimicrobial therapy

Choice of antimicrobial therapy depends on the organism isolated and its drug-susceptibility results. The optimal length of treatment is not known, but most experts advocate 4–6 weeks of IV therapy. The addition of rifampicin to β-lactams has been shown to be effective in animal models of staphylococcal osteomyelitis and is often used in infections, particularly those involving prosthetic material. Once patients are clinically stable, they may be discharged from the hospital and treated with outpatient antimicrobial therapy via a long-term IV catheter, if appropriate.

Adjunctive therapy

Hyperbaric oxygen has been shown to be effective in animal studies, but there are inadequate data to support this approach in humans.

Special situations

- Osteomyelitis after open fracture
- Vertebral osteomyelitis, discitis, epidural abscess
- Osteomyelitis in patients with diabetes or vascular insufficiency
- Acute hematogenous osteomyelitis
- SAPHO (synovitis, acne, plantar pustolsis, hyperosteosis, osteitis)

Reference

1. Mader JT, Shirtliff M, Calhoun JH (1997). Staging and staging application in osteomyelitis. *Clin Infect Dis* 25:1303–1309.

Prosthetic joint infections

Prosthetic joint infections complicate 1–5% of implants, resulting in considerable morbidity. The treatment of prosthetic joint infections is difficult and costly.[1]

Epidemiology

Risk factors for prosthetic joint infection include previous surgery at the same site, rheumatoid arthritis, diabetes mellitus, immunosuppression, poor nutrition, obesity, psoriasis, and being elderly.

Pathogenesis

Infection occurs by one of two mechanisms:

- Local infection (60–80%), e.g., perioperative contamination or local wound infection
- Hematogenous seeding (20–40%), e.g., *S. aureus* bacteremia, dental, genitourinary, or gastrointestinal tract procedures

As foreign bodies, the metallic implant and the cement contribute to infection by reducing the number of organisms required to establish infection and permitting pathogens to establish and survive within biofilms.

Etiology

Prosthetic joint infections are usually monomicrobial but may be mixed. Common causes include coagulase-negative staphylococci (22%), *S. aureus*

(22%), α-hemolytic streptococci (9%), groups A, B, and G streptococci (5%), enterococci (7%), gram-negative bacilli (25%), and anaerobes (10%). Rarer causes include corynebacteria, propionibacteria, *Bacillus* spp., mycobacteria, and fungi.

Clinical features

Cardinal symptoms include joint pain (95%), fever (43%), periarticular swelling (38%), and wound or cutaneous sinus drainage (32%).

Constant joint pain is suggestive of infection, whereas pain that only occurs on motion or weight bearing is more suggestive of prosthetic loosening.

Most patients present with a gradual onset of pain ± discharging sinus. Some patients present acutely with high fever, severe joint pain, swelling, erythema, and systemic toxicity.

The pattern of clinical presentation is determined by the virulence of the infecting pathogen, route of infection, and nature of host tissue.

Diagnosis

- *Blood tests* are nonspecific, and usually show a raised blood WCC, ESR, and CRP.
- *Plain X-rays* may show abnormal lucency (>2 mm) at the bone cement surface, periosteal reaction, cement fractures, changes in position of the prosthetic components, and movement of components on stress views. However, these changes are evident in 50% of cases and may also occur with prosthetic loosening.
- *Radioisotope scans* are generally unhelpful. Technetium diphosphonate scans may show increased uptake in infected joints, but this may also occur in normal joints for up to 6 months after arthroplasty. Sequential technetium gallium bone scans also have poor sensitivity (66%) and specificity (81%).
- *Arthrocentesis* (aspiration of joint fluid) may confirm the diagnosis. Synovial fluid should be aspirated using aseptic technique and sent for cell count, microscopy, and culture. The diagnostic sensitivity of arthrocentesis is 86–92%, and the specificity is 82–97% in larger studies. The Gram stain is only positive in 32%.
- *Operative samples* (arthroscopic or open surgical) are used to make a definitive diagnosis. Several (3 to 6) operative samples of tissue and fluid should be taken, ideally prior to antibiotic therapy, and sent for microbiology and histology. Three positive cultures for the same organism give a 94.8% probability of prosthetic joint infection.[2]

Management

The most successful approach is a two-stage surgical procedure: removal of the prosthesis and cement, then 6 weeks of intravenous antimicrobial therapy, followed by insertion of a new prosthesis. Success rates of 90–97% have been reported. The use of antibiotic-impregnated spacers (prior to reimplantation) and antibiotic-impregnated cement (at reimplantation) is common, although clinical trial data are lacking.

An alternative approach is a one-stage surgical procedure: removal of the infected prosthesis and cement, immediate implantation of a new prosthesis, and antimicrobial therapy. This method is often used in elderly or infirmed patients. Success rates of 80–83% have been reported.

Simple surgical drainage with retention of the prosthesis and antibiotic therapy is only successful in 20–36% of cases. Treatment without prosthesis removal is more likely to be successful in early postoperative (<1 month), in early hematogenous seeding (<1 month symptoms), and with certain pathogens.

Long-term suppressive antibiotic therapy is given in special circumstances: e.g., prosthesis removal is impossible; the prosthesis is not loose; the pathogen is relatively avirulent; the pathogen is highly sensitive to oral antibiotic; the patient is able to tolerate long-term oral antibiotics. If all five criteria are met, a 63% success rate is seen with retained hip arthroplasty and variable success rates with total knee replacements.

Prevention

Prosthetic joint infections may be prevented by perioperative antimicrobial prophylaxis, meticulous surgical technique, filtered laminar airflow systems in operating rooms, early recognition, and prompt treatment of wound infections.

References

1. Lentino JR (2003). Prosthetic joint infections: bane of orthopedists, challenge for infectious diseases specialists. *Clin Infect Dis* 36:1157–1161.

2. Atkins BL, et al. (1998). Prospective evaluation of criteria for microbiologic diagnosis of prosthetic joint infections. *J Clin Microbiol* 36:2932–2939.

Diabetic foot infections

A *diabetic foot infection* may be defined as any inframalleolar infection in a patient with diabetes mellitus. The most common lesion is an infected diabetic ulcer, but the spectrum of infections is broad and may include paronychia, cellulitis, myositis, abscesses, necrotizing fasciitis, septic arthritis, tendonitis, and osteomyelitis.

Epidemiology

Foot infections in diabetic patients are common, debilitating, and difficult to manage. Risk factors include peripheral sensory, motor, and/or autonomic neuropathy, neuro-osteopathic deformity (e.g., Charcot joint), vascular insufficiency, hyperglycemia leading to poor immune function and wound healing, patient disabilities (e.g., poor vision, limited mobility, previous amputations), maladaptive patient behaviors (inadequate foot care or footwear), and health system failure (inadequate education and management of diabetes and footcare).

Etiology

A number of organisms may be associated with various syndromes (see Table 4.14).

Table 4.14 Etiology of diabetic foot infections

Foot infection syndrome	Pathogens
Cellulitis	β-hemolytic streptococci (groups A, B, C, and G), S. aureus
Infected ulcer, antibiotic naive	Often monomicrobial: S. aureus or β-hemolytic streptococci (groups A, B, C, and G)
Infected ulcer, chronic, previous antibiotic therapy	Usually polymicrobial: S. aureus, β-hemolytic streptococci (groups A, B, C, and G), Enterobacteriaceae
Macerated ulcer	Pseudomonas aeruginosa ± other organisms as above
Longstanding, nonhealing wound, prolonged antibiotic therapy	Usually polymicrobial with antibiotic-resistant organisms: aerobic gram-positive cocci (S. aureus), coagulase-negative staphylococci, enterococci), diphtheroids, Enterobacteriaceae, Pseudomonas spp., nonfermentative gram-negative rods, fungi
"Fetid foot": extensive necrosis or gangrene	Mixed aerobic gram-positive cocci (S. aureus, coagulase-negative staphylococci, enterococci), Enterobacteriaceae, nonfermentative gram-negative rods, obligate anaerobes

Pathogenesis

Neuropathy plays the central role, leading to ulceration due to trauma or excessive pressure on a deformed foot that lacks protective sensation. Once the protective layer of skin is breached, underlying tissues are exposed to bacterial colonization. This wound may progress to become actively infected, and, by contiguous extension, the infection can involve deeper tissues.

Clinical features

These can range from mild to severe and life threatening:
- Foot ulcer with no signs of infection
- Foot ulcer with surrounding inflammation or cellulitis <2 cm from edge of wound
- Local complications: cellulitis >2 cm from edge of wound, lymphangitis, spread beneath superficial fascia, deep tissue abscess, gas gangrene, involvement of muscle, tendon, or bone
- Systemic toxicity or metabolic instability: fever, chills, tachycardia, hypotension, confusion, vomiting, leukocytosis, acidosis, hyperglycemia, uremia

Diagnosis

Diagnosis is based on clinical features listed above. It is important to assess perfusion (peripheral pulses) as well as sensation (using a monofilament).

If the peripheral pulses are not palpable, use a Doppler ultrasound to determine ankle/brachial pressure indices (ABPIs).

Imaging, e.g., MRI, may be helpful to determine the extent of infection, e.g., deep collections, osteomyelitis.

Deep tissue specimens (not superficial swabs) should be taken and sent to the laboratory for microscopy and culture prior to starting antimicrobial therapy.

Management

See the IDSA guidelines for management of diabetic foot infections.[1]

- Determine the need for hospitalization.
- Stabilize the patient if systemically unwell and correct any metabolic abnormalities.
- *Antibiotics:* do not give antibiotics for uninfected ulcers. Initial empiric therapy should be based on severity of infection and available microbiological data, e.g., Gram stain. If there are no data, initial therapy should be broad spectrum, e.g., IVpiperacillin-tazobactam, vancomycin.
- *Assess the need for surgery:* patients with severe infections, e.g., necrotizing fasciitis, gas gangrene, extensive tissue loss, critical limb ischemia, should be referred for urgent surgical review.
- *Wound care plan:* the wound should be dressed in a way that allows daily inspection. Special aids may be available to offload pressure on the wound.
- *Adjunctive therapies:* use of granulocyte colony-stimulating factors has not been shown to be beneficial. Hyperbaric oxygen may have a role.

Reference

1. Lipsky BA, Berendt AR, Deery HG, et al. (2004). Diagnosis and management of diabetic foot infections. *Clin Infect Dis* 39:885–910.

Neonatal sepsis

This is defined as sepsis occurring within 4 weeks of birth:

- *Early onset:* within 7 days, associated with microbes acquired from the mother either transplancentally or intrapartum; 85% of early-onset cases present within 24 hours of delivery
- *Late onset:* after 7 days, associated with organisms acquired from the environment (e.g., caregivers or urinary or vascular devices)

Premature infants experience the most rapid onset. Certain viral infections may cause an indistinguishable clinical picture.

Epidemiology

Incidence of culture-proven sepsis is 2/1000 live births in the United States, but up to 7–13% of neonates may be evaluated for sepsis due to the non-specific nature of the early signs. Neonatal sepsis contributes to 15% of all neonatal deaths from meningitis and 4% of all neonatal deaths.

Risk factors

- *Early-onset sepsis:* maternal colonization with group B streptococci, premature rupture of membranes, prolonged rupture of membranes, prematurity, maternal UTI, chorioamnionitis, maternal fever >38°C at delivery, poor maternal nutrition, recurrent abortion, meconium staining, congenital abnormalities
- *Late-onset sepsis:* prematurity, central venous catheterization (duration >10 days), continuous positive pressure nasal cannula, H_2 antagonist/proton pump inhibitor use, GI tract pathology

Etiology

- *Early onset:* group B streptococci, E. coli, H. influenzae, L. monocytogenes
- *Late onset:* coagulase-negative staphylococci, S. aureus, Klebsiella spp., E. coli, Pseudomonas spp., Candida spp., Enterobacter spp., Serratia spp., Acinetobacter spp., group B streptococci, anaerobes

Clinical features

- *Pneumonia:* neonates may aspirate organisms during delivery or have developed intrauterine pneumonia following aspiration of amniotic fluid. Signs are tachypnea, cyanosis, grunting, apnea, costal/sternal retractions, and nasal flaring. CXR may show bilateral consolidation and pleural effusions. *Klebsiella* spp. and *S. aureus* may generate severe lung damage with abscesses and empyema. Early-onset group B streptococcal pneumonia may be fulminant with significant mortality.
- *Cardiac features:* overwhelming sepsis may be associated with pulmonary hypertension, decreased cardiac output, and hypoxia. Late features are overt shock, pallor, poor capillary perfusion, and edema.
- *Metabolic features of sepsis:* hypo/hyperglycemia, acidosis, jaundice
- *Neurological signs:* ventriculitis, meningitis (36% group B streptococci, 31% E. coli, 5–10% Listeria), cerebral vasculitis, cerebral edema, cerebral infarction. Meningitis in early-onset sepsis occurs within 24–48 hours; signs of meningitis are present in only 30% and CSF WCC may be normal. In late-onset disease, 80–90% have neurological features and CSF changes may be markedly abnormal, especially with gram-negative organisms. Neonates with meningitis are likely hypothermic.
- *Hematological abnormalities:* thrombocytopenia, DIC, high or low WCC (50% normal). The immature-to-total neutrophil ratio is a more useful marker of infection.
- *Gastrointestinal:* necrotizing enterocolitis has been associated with the presence of a number of species in immature gut.

Investigations

- *Blood tests:* CBC, urinalysis, liver function tests, CRP
- *Microbiological:* blood, CSF, and urine cultures. Gram stain may provide early identification. Cultures may be negative if the mother received intrapartum antibiotics. If CSF is culture positive, a follow-up lumbar

puncture is often performed at 24–36 hours after initiation of antibiotic therapy to document CSF sterility.
• *Other tests:* infection markers such as IL-6, IL-8, and CD64 have been used in the evaluation of sepsis in neonates.
• *Radiology:* CXR may show lobar changes but usually resembles respiratory distress syndrome, with a diffuse reticulogranular pattern. Cranial ultrasound may show evidence of ventriculitis and chronic changes. CT is used in complex meningitis with obstruction and abscesses.

Management

• *Medical emergency:* IV antimicrobials should be started as soon as cultures are taken. Antibiotic choice should be guided by maternal history and local drug-resistance patterns. A 2004 Cochrane review found no significant difference in outcome between various antibiotic regimes.[1] A glycopeptide is combined with an aminoglycoside. Treatment for 7–10 days may be appropriate even without positive cultures.
• Cardiovascular, respiratory, and nutritional support may be required.
• Infants with bacterial meningitis require antibiotics capable of penetrating the blood–brain barrier to achieve therapeutic concentrations in the CSF and longer courses of treatment (up to 3 weeks). If the CSF is not sterile on a follow-up lumbar puncture 24–36 hours after the initiation of therapy, consider modification of therapy.
• *Surgical interventions:* development of hydrocephalus may require the placement of a ventriculoperitoneal shunt. Abscesses may require surgical drainage.
• Early diagnosis and treatment offer good prognosis, although residual neurological damage affects 15–30% of neonates with septic meningitis.
• *Follow-up:* hearing assessments before discharge and at 3 months if aminoglycosides have been given; follow-up for those at risk of developing neurological sequelae (with a pediatric neurologist)

Prevention

Some authorities recommend that antibiotic prophylaxis should be given to certain groups of women at risk of carriage of group B streptococci.

Reference

1. Mtitimila CL, Cooke RW (2004). Antibiotic regimes for suspected early neonatal sepsis. *Cochrane Database of Systematic Reviews* Issue 4, Article No: CD 004495.

Viral causes of childhood illness

Table 4.15 Viral causes of childhood illness

Virus	Typical age	Features
Herpes simplex virus	Neonate: 90% of infections acquired perinatally, 5% congenitally, and the remainder postnatally (e.g., from an adult with herpes labialis)	Nearly all infected infants manifest disease. Incubation: 3–14 days. May be localized to the eye or CNS. 70% of untreated cases disseminate (hepatomegaly, jaundice, pneumonitis, encephalitis, vesicular rash). Neonates have the highest rates of visceral and/or CNS infection of any patient group.
		70% of infected infants are born to mothers with no apparent disease. 70% of cases are due to HSV-2. 50% of babies delivered via an infected birth canal become infected. Most cases of HSV-1 follow maternal acquisition of genital HSV-1 late in pregnancy, with consequent neonatal contact with infectious secretions during delivery. Untreated, the death rate is 65%. Less than 20% of those with CNS infection develop normally. CNS morbidity is less severe with HSV-1 than HSV-2. Systemic acyclovir is essential and has reduced the death rate of neonatal herpes to < 25%.
	Childhood (highest incidence of HSV-1 infection is seen in children aged 6 months to 3 years)	>80% of primary HSV infections are asymptomatic. Symptoms: fever, anorexia, sore mouth (an ulcerative gingivostomatitis), local lymphadenopathy. Contamination of skin by infectious saliva may lead to secondary lesions on the perioral skin, eye, fingers, and vulva. Those with disseminated infection should be isolated. Topical acyclovir is of no benefit in acute primary infection of children. Systemic treatment can decrease healing time and is important in the immunocompromised.
Varicella zoster virus	90% of cases occur in those under 13 years of age	Primary infection causes chickenpox, a maculopapular rash that forms pustulating vesicles. Complications are bacterial superinfection, cerebellar ataxia, and encephalitis. See pp. 346 and 347 for prevention and management of neonatal disease.
Measles ("first disease")	Uncommon in those populations with vaccination	Acute, highly infectious disease characterized by cough, coryza, fever, and rash. Severe manifestations and complications include pneumonia, encephalitis, bacterial superinfection, and subacute sclerosing panencephalitis.

Table 4.15 (Contd.)

Virus	Typical age	Features
Rubella ("third disease")	Prior to vaccination, incidence was highest in the spring among children aged 5–9 years	Acute, mild, exanthematous viral infection of children and adults resembling mild measles but with the potential to cause fetal infection and birth defects
Parvovirus B19 (slapped-cheek disease, erythema infectiosum, "fifth disease")	Infection common in childhood: 50% are IgG-positive by age 15 years	20% asymptomatic. Prodrome (5–7 days) of myalgia, arthralgia, malaise, rhinorrhea, and fever, then a bright red rash on the cheeks followed 1–2 days later by maculopapular rash on the trunk, legs, arms, and buttocks. This clears after a few days, leaving a characteristic lacey pattern that fades and reappears over the following 3 weeks.
Human herpesvirus 6 (roseola, exanthem subitum, "sixth disease")	Most children acquire infection between 4 months and 3 years of age.	Abrupt onset of fever (± periorbital edema) is followed 3–5 days later by rash (rose-pink papules that are mildly elevated, nonpruritic, and blanche on pressure) on the back and neck and spread to the chest and limbs, sparing the feet and face. It lasts 72 days. Other features are malaise, vomiting, diarrhea, cough, pharyngitis and lymphadenopathy, febrile convulsions (10% of primary infections). Meningitis and encephalitis are less commonly seen.
Mumps	90% of cases occurred in those under 15 years of age prior to introduction of vaccination. Many cases now occur in older children and those in college	Acute, generalized viral infection of children and adolescents, causing swelling and tenderness of the salivary glands and, rarely, epididymo-orchitis
Enteroviral infections	All age groups but more common in younger children	Accounts for most childhood fever–rash syndromes as well as meningitis, myocarditis, sepsis, hand, foot, and mouth disease, and herpangina
Epstein–Barr virus (cause of 90% of infectious mononucleosis)	Approximately 50% of U.S. children are infected by age 5 years, around 80% by age 25 years, although range is affected by socioeconomic status (higher prevalence in low socioeconomic status)	Primary infection in childhood is asymptomatic. Infection in adolescence may present with an acute infectious mononucleosis syndrome.
Other common viral infections of childhood	Adenovirus, molluscum, RSV, metapneumovirus, rhinovirus, rotavirus	

Enteroviral infections

The non-polio enteroviruses (including Coxsackie virus, enterovirus, and echoviruses) cause a large number of different clinical syndromes, accounting for the majority of childhood fever–rash syndromes as well as being important causes of meningitis, myocarditis, and neonatal sepsis.

Of the many clinical syndromes that they cause, only hand, foot, and mouth disease and herpangina have a clinical presentation distinct enough to allow identification.

Epidemiology

Transmission is fecal-oral or via contact with discharging skin lesions. Respiratory and oral-to-oral routes occur in crowded conditions. Viruses can survive at room temperature for several days and tolerate the acidic pH of the gastrointestinal tract.

Found worldwide, infection affects all age groups but highest rates are seen in children (secondary to exposure, hygiene, and immune status). Infection course is benign in older children, more serious in neonates.

Neonatal infections are probably acquired after birth.

Clinical features

Incubation is 3–10 days, and virus may be excreted in stool for weeks. Infection may be asymptomatic (90% of infections) or cause an undifferentiated flu-like illness or a more characteristic syndrome.

Undifferentiated illness

Low-grade fever of sudden onset occurs with or without upper respiratory and gastrointestinal symptoms, e.g., flu-type syndrome of malaise, myalgias, sore throat, headache, conjunctivitis, nausea, vomiting, and diarrhea. Orchitis and epididymitis can occur. Symptoms last 3–7 days.

Herpangina (enteroviral vesicular pharyngitis)

Typically this is seen during the summer in children aged 3–10 years (may occur in young adults). Painful vesicles (usually 3–6) and ulcers of the posterior pharynx and tonsils occur with fever and a sore throat. There are no exudates present. Pain may make the child reluctant to eat. Symptoms last 3–7 days.

The organism is Coxsackie virus group A and sometimes group B.

Hand, foot, and mouth disease (HFM)

HFM is enteroviral vesicular stomatitis with exanthema: fever and vesicular eruption in the anterior pharynx, palms, and soles of toddlers and school-aged children. Oral vesicles are not initially painful but later burst, leaving painful ulcers. Cutaneous vesicles heal by resorption of fluid and do not crust. Patients may develop characteristic rash.

The organism is Coxsackie virus group A, serotype 16 (among others).

HFM caused by enterovirus-71 has been associated with a higher incidence of neurological complications (polio-like syndrome, aseptic meningitis, encephalitis, encephalomyelitis, acute cerebellar ataxia, acute transverse myelitis, Guillain–Barré syndrome, opsomyoclonus syndrome, and benign intracranial hypertension), rare cases of myocarditis, interstitial pneumonitis, and pulmonary edema.

Other features

Viral exanthems (pink, maculopapular, blanching rash, rarely urticarial, vesicular or petechial; it can mimic rubella and roseola but with no significant adenopathy), aseptic meningitis, myocarditis or pericarditis, pleurodynia (lancinating chest-pain attacks with fever and headache, also seen with Coxsackie B infection), and neonatal sepsis can also occur.

Diagnosis and management

Diagnosis of herpangina and HFM is clinical (both are mild self-limiting illnesses that do not warrant laboratory diagnosis) and management is supportive (e.g., soft food for those with painful mouth ulcers, antipyretics, topical analgesics). See individual sections for the diagnosis and management of the more severe clinical presentations.

The virus can be identified from respiratory secretions, cutaneous lesions, and stool. Paired serology will confirm recent infection. PCR tests are available.

Use of good hygiene practices can help prevent continued feco-oral spread (handwashing, etc.).

Bacterial causes of childhood illness

Scarlet fever

Scarlet fever is a syndrome of exudative pharyngitis, fever, and scarlatiniform rash caused by infection with an erythrogenic exotoxin-producing group A β-hemolytic streptococcus. It was once known as "second disease"—the second exanthematous disease of childhood.

Clinical features

Normal inhabitants of the nasopharynx, group A streptococci may cause pharyngitis, skin infections, pneumonia, and bacteremia. Scarlet fever usually occurs in association with pharyngeal infection. It is usually seen in children aged 5–15 years.

Rash appears 1–2 days after onset of sore throat with a diffuse red blush with scattered points of deeper red. First noticed on the chest, it spreads to involve the trunk, neck, and extremities, sparing the palms, soles, and face. The face may, however, be flushed with circumoral pallor. Skin folds in the neck, axillae, groin, elbows, and knees may appear as lines of deeper red. There maybe petechiae and a sandpaper texture to the skin due to sweat gland occlusion.

Examination of the oropharynx may reveal exudative pharyngitis, tonsillitis, and small, red hemorrhagic spots on the palate. The tongue may be coated in early disease but then becomes beefy red ("strawberry tongue"). The skin rash fades over a week and is followed by desquamation that may last several weeks.

Although common and fatal in the 19th and early 20th century, it is rarely considered serious today. Severe scarlet fever may be due to hematogenous spread or systemic toxicity with high fever, which may be complicated by arthritis and jaundice.

Complications include suppurative complications (e.g., abscess), rheumatic fever, poststreptococcal glomerulonephritis, and erythema nodosum.

Diagnosis and management

- Throat swab for culture and anti-streptolysin O titer (ASOT)
- *Treatment:* penicillin V PO or IV benzylpenicillin
- *Differential:* consider measles, infectious mononucleosis, other viral infections with rash, Kawasaki's disease, and staphylococcal infection.

Staphylococcal epidermal necrolysis

Also known as (staphylococcal) scalded skin syndrome (SSSS), this condition is caused by an exotoxin produced by *S. aureus* which leads to exfoliation of the upper layers of the epidermis; 98% of cases occur in children under 6 years of age because of lack of immunity and immature renal clearance capability.

Mortality is low in children (1–5%) but can be higher in adults, who are usually immunocompromised or have renal failure.

Clinical features

An infection commonly occurs at a site such as the oral or nasal cavities, throat, or umbilicus. Epidermolytic toxins are produced locally and act at a remote site, leading to the abrupt onset of generalized skin erythema.

The epidermis beneath the granular cell layer separates because of binding of the toxins to desmoglein 1 in desmosomes. Bullae form, and diffuse, sheet-like desquamation may occur 1–2 days later (Nikolsky sign positive). This leaves a raw and tender exposed surface.

There may be associated conjunctivitis, stomatitis, and urethritis.

Most patients do not appear very ill but significant dehydration can develop. Healing occurs over 1–2 weeks.

Diagnosis and management

S. aureus can usually be cultured from the site of remote infection. The WCC count is usually normal but inflammatory markers may be elevated. A PCR test for the toxin is available. Blood cultures are usually negative in children (but may be positive in adults).

Differential diagnosis includes toxic epidermal necrolysis (part of the disease spectrum that contains bullous erythema multiforme and Stevens–Johnson syndrome and is associated with a deeper epidermal detachment than that of SSSS) erythema multiforme, and burns.

Management

- *Antibiotics:* dicloxacillin, or erythromycin if penicillin allergic
- *Fluids:* patients can leak a lot of proteinaceous fluid through the skin and may require IV supplementation. Wound care is similar to that given for burns, and very severe cases may require specialist burn-unit input. The skin damage can make patients vulnerable to secondary infection.

Pertussis

Pertussis is a highly contagious bacterial infection of the respiratory tract, spread by droplets and characterized by paroxysmal cough (whooping cough). It is caused by *Bordetella pertussis* (p. 259), a gram-negative pleomorphic bacillus of which humans are the sole reservoir, and, less commonly, *B. parapertussis*.

Epidemiology

Infection is worldwide but unusual in countries with widespread vaccination. Neither infection nor vaccination provides complete or lifelong immunity. Protection against typical disease lasts 3–5 years, and immunity is not detectable after 12 years.

The UK introduced a preschool pertussis booster in 2001. Consequently, morbidity has reached the lowest levels yet in both vaccinated groups and infants too young to receive the vaccine.

Most cases occur in infants and children (the majority infected by coughing adults and older children). Adults (10% of cases) experience milder disease. Children <1 year of age are most likely to require hospitalization.

Worldwide, it remains a major cause of death. There are around 50 million cases and 600,000 estimated deaths each year.

Those at risk of severe disease (pneumonia, encephalopathy, death) include premature infants and those patients with underlying cardiac, pulmonary, or neuromuscular or neurological disease.

Clinical features

Incubation is 3–12 days. Patients are infectious from the onset of illness until toward the end of the paroxysmal phase.

Pertussis is a 6-week illness of three stages, each lasting around 2–4 weeks. Older children and adults may not exhibit these distinct stages.

- *Stage 1 (catarrhal phase)* is indistinguishable from the common cold, with congestion, sneezing, mild fever, and rhinorrhea. Patients are at their most infectious during this phase.
- *Stage 2 (paroxysmal phase)* consists of paroxysms of intense coughing that can last several minutes. These may be followed by a loud whoop in older infants and toddlers. Infants <6 months may have apneic episodes but do not whoop. Vomiting is common after coughing. Subconjunctival hemorrhages and facial petechiae may occur. Most deaths occur in infants (coughing leading to choking and apnea).
- *Stage 3 (convalescent phase)* consists of chronic cough, which may last for weeks, triggered by intercurrent viral infections.

Differential diagnosis includes bronchiolitis, mycoplasmal pneumonia, chlamydial pneumonia, and inhaled foreign body.

Complications are pneumonia, secondary bacterial infection, pneumothorax, diaphragmatic rupture, surgical emphysema, and neurological deficits secondary to hypoxia.

Diagnosis

Lab confirmation is usually delayed. Diagnosis should be made clinically.

- *General:* leukocytosis (WBC > 100,000 is associated with an increased risk of death), CXR may be normal or show peribronchial thickening, consolidation (secondary bacterial infection, rarely pertussis pneumonia), pneumothorax, pneumomediastinum, or air in the soft tissues.
- *Microbiological culture* requires special media (e.g., Regan–Lowe or Bordet–Gengou agar). Culture specimens are best obtained by flexible swab or deep nasopharyngeal aspiration during the catarrhal or early paroxysmal phase and should be cultured for 7 days. They are usually negative in those previously immunized or given antibiotics.

Serology is useful to confirm the diagnosis retrospectively. PCR-based tests are available.

Management
- *General:* supportive care is the mainstay. Consider admitting patients at risk of severe disease and complications (see above, plus those younger than 3 months, or 3–6 months with severe paroxysms); 50% of infants require hospitalization. Infection control measures should be taken for those patients in the contagious phase of the disease.
- *Antimicrobial therapy:* erythromycin given early in the catarrhal phase shortens duration of the paroxysmal stage. Once cough is established, antimicrobial agents do not alter the course of the illness but serve to limit the spread of disease. Treatment duration is 14 days. Patients should be isolated. Consider treating close contacts of pertussis cases (including children and staff at daycare centers) who are particularly vulnerable or those who are unvaccinated, partially vaccinated, or under 5 years of age.
- *Other agents:* there is no evidence for any benefit from use of corticosteroids or B$_2$-adrenergic agents. Pertussis-specific immunoglobulin is an experimental therapy that may be effective in decreasing paroxysms of cough.

Prevention
Vaccination is recommended for all babies at 2, 3, and 4 months as part of the DTP (diphtheria, tetanus, polio) vaccine. It may not prevent the illness entirely, but it lessens disease severity and duration.

There is no transfer of protective maternal antibody from mothers with a documented history of infection or vaccination. Nearly all cases of fatal pertussis in developed countries occur in infants too young to be immunized. In the UK and United States, children are given boosters at 3–4 or 11–12 years of age, respectively, with the aim of reducing transmission to prevaccination infants.

Other common causes of bacterial infection in childhood
- Bacterial meningitis, including *N. meningitidis* (p. 222)
- Bacterial causes of pneumonia (p. 190)
- Infectious diarrhea (p. 585)
- Urinary tract infections (p. 610)
- Upper respiratory tract infections (p. 530)
- Superficial bacterial infections of the skin (e.g., erysipelas) (p. 678)

Congenital infections

Congenital infections may be acquired in utero or perinatally. The acronym TORCH has been used to describe a group of infections that generally cause a mild or inapparent infection in the mother yet cause severe disease in the infant:

* **T**oxoplasmosis
* **O**thers (e.g., syphilis, parvovirus, and VZV)
* **R**ubella
* **C**ytomegalovirus
* **H**SV (mother may be asymptomatic)

Long-term consequences include growth retardation, microcephaly, congenital defects with long-term sequelae, and progressive disease in childhood. They may also present with unusual exanthemata, organomegaly, or thrombocytopenia in the neonatal period.

Any infant with features of TORCH illness should undergo thorough serological evaluation for these agents as well as others, e.g., HIV.

Toxoplasmosis

* *Maternal:* may be subclinical or present with an infectious mononucleosis–like illness with lymphadenopathy
* *Fetal:* risk of transmission is lowest in the first trimester (but associated with more severe abnormalities) and highest in the last trimester. Clinical features include chorioretinitis, hydrocephaly, microcephaly, aqueductal stenosis, agenesis of corpus callosum, cerebral calcifications, and nonimmune hydrops. Three-quarters of infants are asymptomatic at birth.
* *Diagnosis:* IgM turns positive after 1 week and may remain positive for years. IgG follows the same course but remains positive for life.

Treatment

Maternal infection is treated with spiramycin, which reduces the fetal infection rate. Although widely used in France, spiramycin has not received FDA approval in the United States. It can be obtained from Rhone-Poulenc Pharmaceuticals or via the spiramycin program of the FDA Division of Special Pathogens and Immunologic Drugs.[1,2]

Refer to a specialist for treatment and ultrasound monitoring of the fetus. For congenital infection, treat with pyrimethamine, sulfadiazine, and folinic acid. Seek specialist advice.

References

1. American College of Obstetrician Gynecologists (2000). Perinatal viral parasitic infections. ACOG Policy Bull. 20. Washington, DC: American College of Obstetricians and Gynecologists.

2. Piper J, Wen T (1999). Perinatal cytomegalovirus and toxoplasmosis: challenges of antepartum therapy. *Clin Obstet Gynecol* 42(1):81–94.

Syphilis

* *Maternal:* risk of congenital infection is 50% in primary and secondary syphilis, 40% in latent infection, and 10% in tertiary syphilis. Maternal disease is detected by routine antenatal serological screening.

- *Fetal:* clinical features include stillbirth, intrauterine growth restriction (IUGR), nonimmune hydrops, rhinitis, skin rash, hepatosplenomegaly, "mulberry molars," "saber shins," saddle-nose deformity, interstitial keratitis, eighth nerve deafness, and peg-shaped incisors.
- *Diagnosis* is based on serology or positive dark-field microscopy or staining for treponemes in samples from the placenta or umbilical cord.
- *Treatment:* maternal infection is treated with penicillin. Neonates should be treated for neurosyphilis (cannot be excluded).

Parvovirus B19

- *Maternal:* presents with fever, malaise, polarthralgia, coryza, and rash. May be mistaken for rubella. See Management of rash contact in pregnancy (p. 711).
- *Fetal:* anemia leading to nonimmune hydrops. Fetal loss is 9%.
- *Diagnosis:* serology in the mother. Fetal infection can be diagnosed by amniotic fluid sampling, fetal blood sampling, or postmortem.
- *Treatment:* intrauterine blood transfusion. One-third of cases resolve without transfusion.

Varicella zoster

- *Maternal:* presents with a vesicular rash. There is an increased risk of complications, e.g., pneumonitis. See Management of rash illness in pregnancy (p. 711).
- *Fetal:* Primary VZV infection during the first half of pregnancy has been associated with limb hypoplasia, cicatricial lesions, psychomotor retardation, cutaneous scars, chorioretinitis, cataracts, cortical atrophy, microcephaly, microphthalmus, and IUGR. The risk of developing the syndrome is 1% if the fetus is at <20 weeks and 2% at 13–20 weeks.
- *Diagnosis* is usually clinical. It may be confirmed by VZV PCR of skin lesions in the mother.
- *Treatment:* acycloviracyclovir PO or IV for the mother. Use varicella zoster immune globulin (VZIG) for the neonate if the mother develops chickenpox within 5 days of delivery.

Rubella

Congenital rubella syndrome is rare since the introduction of vaccination.
- *Maternal:* presents with rash illness. See Management of rash illness in pregnancy (p. 711).
- *Fetal:* infection is more severe in early pregnancy, with >85% chance of being affected by either multiple defects or spontaneous abortion in the first 2 months. Clinical features include "blueberry muffin" skin, cataracts, glaucoma, microphthalmia, sensorineural deafness, patent ductus arteriosus (PDA), atrioventricular (AV) septal defects, pulmonary artery stenosis, microcephaly, meningoencephalitis, IUGR, hepatosplenomegaly, interstitial pneumonitis, and thrombocytopenia.
- *Diagnosis* is based on maternal serology.
- *Treatment:* none

Cytomegalovirus

- *Maternal:* infection is usually asymptomatic but may present with an infectious mononucleosis–like syndrome. It occurs in 1–2% of seronegative women during pregnancy; a small number of cases are due to viral reactivation.
- *Fetal:* infection of the neonate may occur in utero or, more commonly, perinatally. Clinical features include IUGR, microcephaly, periventricular calcifications, sensorineural deafness, blindness with chorioretinitis, mental retardation, hepatosplenomegaly, thrombocytopenic purpura, and hemolytic anemia. Incidence of sequelae is 25% for primary infection and 8% with recurrent infection; ~1% die at or soon after birth. 15% appear normal, but hearing defects or mental retardation become apparent in later life.
- *Diagnosis:* detection of CMV in the urine within the first week of life confirms the diagnosis.
- *Treatment:* there is little information regarding the use of ganciclovir in the setting of congenital CMV infection.

Herpes simplex

Maternal

Primary infection presents with a vesicular genital rash, and 15% of pregnant women with a history of genital HSV infection experience recurrent lesions at delivery. Around 2% of pregnant women with a history of recurrent HSV infection are asymptomatically shedding at the time of delivery.

Fetal

HSV is usually acquired intrapartum but may be acquired in utero. From 75 to 90% of infants with neonatal HSV are born to infected asymptomatic mothers who have no known history of genital HSV. Oral-labial herpes presents a greater risk of postnatal HSV acquisition than genital HSV. Clinical features include skin lesions, chorioretinitis, microcephaly, hydranencephaly, and microphthalmia.

While primary HSV infections in the first trimester are associated with higher rates of spontaneous abortion and stillbirth, infection later in pregnancy appears more likely to be associated with preterm labor or growth restriction. Of greatest concern is the risk of primary infection acquired at birth, which could lead to herpetic meningitis.

Diagnosis

This is usually clinical in the mother. It may be confirmed by serology or PCR.

Treatment

During the first and second trimesters, treat the mother with PO or IV acyclovir. During the third trimester or for genital lesions at the time of delivery, consider Caesarean section.

Infants born to women with active lesions should be isolated and closely observed during the first month of life for features of neonatal HSV infection.

Maternal infections associated with neonatal morbidity

Pelvic inflammatory disease

Pelvic inflammatory disease (PID) is associated with chlamydial infection in over 50% of cases, and gonorrhea in around 14%. Many cases are asymptomatic. Pregnant women with PID should be treated with IV antibiotics, as it is associated with an increase in preterm delivery and maternal and fetal morbidity (e.g., ophthalmia neonatorum).

Listeria monocytogenes

Pregnant women are 20 times more likely to contract listeriosis than other adults; ~33% of all cases of listeriosis occur during pregnancy. Acquisition is mainly by the ingestion of contaminated food.

Pregnant patients are often asymptomatic or present with a flu-like febrile illness. These mild symptoms notwithstanding, listeriosis can still lead to premature delivery, neonatal sepsis, and stillbirth. Placental transfer of the organism can cause amnionitis with spontaneous septic abortion or premature labor with delivery of an infected baby.

Fetal infection may cause sepsis, meningoencephalitis, or disseminated infection with microabscesses. Neonatal infection has a mortality of around 50%, particularly in early-onset sepsis (p. 699). Late-onset infection typically presents as meningitis at 3–4 weeks of age.

Management

Prevention is by avoidance of potentially contaminated foods. Treatment is with ampicillin (or TMP-SMX in those with serious penicillin allergies; it has not been approved for use in pregnancy).

Other

- Malaria
- Varicella zoster and herpes simplex (pp. 343 and 341)
- Hepatitis B (p. 359).
- Group B streptococcus (p. 199)
- Chorioamnionitis (p. 718)
- Leptospirosis (p. 292)
- *Ureaplasma urealyticum* (p. 302)
- *Mycoplasma hominis* (p. 302)

Management of rash contact in pregnancy

See also recommendations from the Centers for Disease Control and Prevention (CDC) Website at www.cdc.gov.

Contact with a non-vesicular rash

The important infective causes are measles, rubella, and parvovirus B19. Intervention is indicated for other possible causes in the absence of the development of symptoms in the pregnant woman.

All pregnant women with contact with a nonvesicular rash illness should be investigated for asymptomatic parvovirus B19 infection and for asymptomatic rubella infection unless there is satisfactory evidence of past rubella infection (vaccine or natural infection). A significant contact is defined as being in the same room for a significant period of time (>15 minutes) or face-to-face contact.

Rubella

A mother is extremely unlikely to be susceptible to rubella if she has had at least two previous positive rubella antibody tests or at least two doses of rubella vaccine documented, or one vaccine dose followed by one positive rubella antibody test. She should be reassured, but told to see her physician if a rash develops.

If rubella susceptibility is possible, a serum sample should be taken and tested for rubella-specific IgG and IgM.

- If IgG-positive and IgM-negative, the mother can be considered immune with no evidence of recent primary infection. If IgG levels are low, it is worth repeating the test. There are rare occasions when IgG may precede IgM positivity in primary infection.
- If IgM and IgG are negative, the patient is susceptible.
- If IgM is detected, further advice should be sought. The control of rubella in the United States means that *most* rubella-specific IgM-positive results don't reflect recent rubella. Unless seroconversion has been demonstrated, further specialist testing is required.

Parvovirus B19

All women should be investigated for asymptomatic infection. This should not be delayed pending the development of symptoms, as asymptomatic infection is just as likely as symptomatic infection to infect and damage the fetus, and active management of the infected fetus reduces the risk of poor outcome.

Maternal serum should be taken as soon after rash contact as possible and tested for parvovirus B19–specific IgG and IgM.

- If IgM but not IgG is detected, tests should be repeated on another fresh serum sample.
- If IgG is detected and IgM is not present, the mother can be reassured.
- If both IgG and IgM are negative, another sample should be taken 1 month after the last contact. If these remain negative, the mother can be reassured that she has not been infected but informed that she is susceptible. If the mother is found to have developed asymptomatic infection, she should be managed as detailed in Management of rash illness in pregnancy (p. 711).

Measles

If epidemiological and clinical features suggest the source patient has measles, passive prophylaxis with IM human normal immunoglobulin should be considered. This should be given as soon as possible after exposure and certainly within 6 days. It attenuates maternal illness, but does not confer any benefit on the fetus.

If the mother has received two doses of measles vaccine the probability of becoming infected is very low. If vaccination history is negative or uncertain, serum should be taken for an urgent measles IgG and results awaited before giving human normal immunoglobulin (HNIG).

If IgG-positive within 10 days of contact, no further action is required. If measles IgG is not present, HNIG should be given and serological tests repeated at 3 weeks. There is no point in giving HNIG if the contact was more than 10 days prior to presentation.

Contact with a vesicular rash

Pregnant women who are exposed to varicella or herpes zoster in pregnancy should seek medical attention as soon as possible. Contact is considered significant if the mother was in the same room for 15 minutes or more, or had face-to-face contact of any duration.

Patients can be reassured that they are protected if they themselves have a history of varicella or herpes zoster.

If there is an uncertain or absent history of infection, the mother's susceptibility should be determined urgently by VZV IgG testing. VZIG should be offered to VZV IgG-negative women within 10 days of exposure (or within 10 days of rash onset in cases of continuous household exposure, e.g., an infected child in the house). The 10-day administration window allows ample time for antibody testing before proceeding with administration of VZIG.

Around 50% of women who receive VZIG following household exposure will develop chickenpox; another 25% are infected subclinically. However, disease is attenuated (the risk of fatal varicella is estimated to be about five times higher in pregnant than in nonpregnant adults, with fatal cases concentrated late in the second or early third trimester) and the risk of fetal infection reduced.

If contact was before the infectious period (i.e., more than 48 hours before chickenpox rash onset or before the appearance of shingles vesicles), VZIG is not indicated.

References

1. Health Protection Agency. *Rashes in pregnancy—HPA Guidelines—information and advice*. http://www.hpa.org.uk/infections/topics_az/pregnancy/rashes/default.htm (accessed August 19, 2008).

2. Department of Health. *Green Book*. http://www.dh.gov.uk/PolicyAndGuidance/HealthAndSocialCareTopics/GreenBook/fs/en (accessed August 19, 2008).

Management of rash illness in pregnancy

Rubella, parvovirus B19, and varicella zoster virus are the infections of most relevance because of their potential impact on the fetus and neonate. With the exception of varicella, these infections do not have a specific impact on the fetus beyond 20 weeks' gestation.

Investigation is recommended at any gestation: age calculation may not be accurate, and achieving an accurate diagnosis is helpful in guiding the advice given to the mother regarding contact with other pregnant women and neonates (e.g., antenatal clinics).

Other infections (enterovirus, infectious mononucleosis, syphilis, streptococcus, meningococcus) are managed as usual in the mother, and the neonate should be followed up.

If investigation is commenced some weeks after rash or contact, it may not be possible to confirm or refute a possible diagnosis.

Patients presenting with a nonvesicular rash

All pregnant women with a nonvesicular rash illness compatible with rubella or parvovirus B19 should be investigated simultaneously for both infections regardless of previous history, immunization, or prior testing.

Rubella infection

Although more recent estimates are not available, some data indicate that up to 10% of women of childbearing age in the United States are susceptible to rubella.[1]

Risk of adverse fetal outcome is 90% at a gestational age of <11 weeks and 20% at 11–16 weeks, falling to a minimal risk of deafness at 16–20 weeks and no increased risk after this time.

Management of pregnant women with proven primary or symptomatic reinfection with rubella varies with the gestation at which infection took place and the individual circumstances of the woman. The only available intervention is termination of the pregnancy.

There is a low but significant risk to the fetus in maternal asymptomatic reinfection within the first 16 weeks of gestation. It may be that further fetal investigation by virus detection (to ascertain whether infection has occurred) is warranted. Such investigations are, however, invasive and risk adverse outcome.

Parvovirus B19

Fetal infection at <20 weeks' gestation is associated with a 9% excess fetal loss and 3% rate of hydrops fetalis (of which ~50% die).

For maternal parvovirus B19 infection diagnosed during pregnancy, the fetus should be scanned by ultrasound 4 weeks after the onset of illness or date of seroconversion, and then at 1- to 2-week intervals until 30 weeks' gestation. If findings suggest development of hydrops fetalis, the patient should be referred to a fetal-medicine unit for consideration of fetal blood sampling and intrauterine transfusion (which improves outcome). Termination is not recommended.

Patients presenting with a vesicular rash

Around 10% of young pregnant women are susceptible to varicella zoster virus infection and are at risk of severe disease, particularly in the late second and early third trimester. The case fatality rate for women developing varicella in pregnancy is 1 in 1000.

They must be advised to consult their general practitioner at the first sign of chickenpox. Those with suspected chickenpox should avoid contact with others who might be at risk (other pregnant women and neonates).

Diagnosis

If clinical diagnosis cannot be made with some certainty, confirm varicella infection by virus, antigen, or virus detection in vesicle fluid and urgent serological testing for VZV IgM.

Management

Women presenting within 24 hours of onset of the first observable lesion should be offered 7 days of aciclovir/acyclovir or aciclovir/valacyclovir treatment. Antivirals are not recommended in those presenting over 24 hours after rash onset (there is no evidence that they alter the clinical course in uncomplicated cases).

Uncomplicated cases can be managed at home with daily review, but those in whom fever persists and fresh vesicles are appearing 6 or more days after initial presentation should be referred to the hospital. Also consider hospitalization for those patients who are approaching term, have a bad obstetric history, are smokers, have chronic lung disease, or have poor social circumstances, or if the managing physician is unable to monitor the patient closely.

Severe disease includes pneumonitis, neurological symptoms other than headache, hemorrhagic rash and bleeding, severe extensive rash or numerous mucosal lesions, and significant immunosuppression. Urgent hospital review is indicated. Those with severe disease should be referred to specialist isolation facilities under the joint care of an obstetrician, infectious disease specialist, and pediatrician. Treatment is with IV aciclovir/acyclovir for at least 5 days.

The fetus

Consequences of primary maternal varicella in the first 20 weeks include spontaneous miscarriage in the first trimester and the risk of congenital varicella syndrome (~1% in the first 12 weeks, and 2% between weeks 13 and 20 of pregnancy).

Features include dermatomal skin scarring, eye defects (chorioretinitis, cataract, microophthalmia), limb hypoplasia, and neurological abnormalities (microcephaly, cortical atrophy, mental retardation, bladder and bowel dysfunction).

- *Infection before 20 weeks' gestation:* perform a specialist ultrasound at 5 weeks postinfection (or 16–20 weeks' gestation) looking for polyhydramnios, microcephaly, hyperechogenic liver foci, and hydrops fetalis. A neonatal eye examination should be performed at birth.
- *Infection after 20 weeks' gestation:* congenital varicella syndrome does not occur, but maternal infection up to 1 week from delivery may lead to herpes zoster in an otherwise healthy infant. There are occasional reports of mild fetal damage up to 28 weeks' gestation.
- *Infection from 1 week before to 1 week after delivery* may lead to severe neonatal varicella. Such infants should be given prophylactic VZIG, with aciclovir/acyclovir if maternal disease onset was 4 days before to 2 days after delivery. See p. 700 for management of disease exposure in neonates.

References

1. Health Protection Agency. *Rashes in pregnancy—HPA Guidelines—information and advice*. http://www.hpa.org.uk/infections/topics_az/pregnancy/rashes/default.htm (accessed August 19, 2008).

2. Department of Health. *Green Book*. http://www.dh.gov.uk/PolicyAndGuidance/HealthAndSocialCareTopics/GreenBook/fs/en (accessed 19 August 2008).

Prevention of congenital and perinatal infection

General points

Any strategy aimed at preventing congenital or perinatal infection should start well before conception with education and general public health measures, e.g., vaccination against diseases such as rubella that are associated with congenital and perinatal disease, and in some countries, screening for group B *Streptococcus* (GBS) carriage.

In terms of infection history and rash contact advice, physicians should ask all pregnant women at the initial visit whether they have previously had chickenpox or shingles, and if they have not, to advise that they make immediate contact if they develop a rash in pregnancy or have contact during pregnancy with someone with a rash.

In the United States, maternal screening includes evaluating for evidence of immunity to the following:

- Rubella: nonimmune women should be vaccinated postpartum. Vaccination in pregnancy is not recommended.
- Syphilis: to prevent congenital syphilis in the neonate
- Hepatitis B: identification of maternal infection allows a course of active and passive immunization to be undertaken in at-risk neonates after birth, in an attempt to prevent infection.
- HIV

Pregnancies complicated by congenital infection should be referred to specialists in maternal–fetal medicine ("high-risk" obstetrics). Amniocentesis is the method of choice for fetal sampling in those cases of possible congenital infection in which such invasive investigations may be warranted. Maternal investigations for possible infective causes in cases of fetal hydrops, fetal brain lesions, unexplained severe growth restriction, or in uterodemise are recommended.

Certain interventions may prevent or reduce neonatal acquisition, or treat infections in neonates exposed in utero. These are detailed below.

Infants in whom congenital infection is suspected and those born preterm where infection may have played a role need follow-up with a pediatric neurologist.

Preventing neonatal varicella

Give VZIG to the following infants:

- Those whose mothers develop varicella from 7 days before to 7 days after delivery, as they will not be protected by maternal antibody

- Those who are VZV antibody-negative (i.e., born to susceptible uninfected mothers) and are exposed to varicella or herpes zoster in the first 7 days of life
- Those born before 28 weeks' gestation or weighing less than 1 kg who are exposed to varicella or herpes zoster, as transfer of maternal IgG antibodies may be inadequate. Some infants beyond 28 weeks' gestation at birth may become VZV antibody-negative if they are >60 days old or have had repeated blood samples, despite a maternal history of varicella or zoster; serological testing is recommended.

Intravenous acyclovir should be
- Given urgently to those infants developing varicella despite VZIG
- Considered as prophylactic treatment in those infants whose mothers develop varicella from 4 days before to 2 days after delivery (there is a high risk of fatal outcome despite VZIG prophylaxis).

Mothers with varicella can breast-feed, but if they have lesions close to the nipple they should express milk from the affected breast until the lesions have crusted. This milk can be fed to the baby if they are covered by VZIG and/or acyclovir.

If other children in the family have varicella and the mother has had varicella (or is VZV antibody-positive), there is no reason to prevent a new baby from going home. If the mother is susceptible, contact with siblings with varicella should be delayed until the new baby has reached 7 days of age.

Preventing neonatal HIV

Neonatal HIV transmission is a significant problem, particularly in resource-poor countries with a high prevalence of maternal HIV. Maternal transmission can occur in utero by passage of virus across the placenta, during delivery from blood and placental fluids, and through breast milk.

Transmission can be reduced through delivery through Caesarean section, avoidance of breast-feeding (advice that may be impractical in certain developing countries), and maternal treatment with antiretrovirals. See HIV prevention (p. 747) for more details.

Preventing neonatal hepatitis B

In contrast to adult infection, most (90%) neonates infected with hepatitis B perinatally go on to become chronic carriers. All infants born to HBsAg-positive mothers should receive IM hepatitis B immune globulin within 12 hours of birth, along with their first dose of hepatitis B vaccine (into the *other* thigh).

This strategy is effective in 90% of cases; a Cochrane review reported the relative risk of developing hepatitis B infection at 0.08 compared to no intervention.[1] The second and third vaccine doses are given at 1 and 6 months with testing to confirm immunity at 1 year.

Prevention and treatment of other neonatal infections

Prevention of other infections requires a combination of good maternal health (aiming to reduce the chance of uterine or intrapartum transmission) and a low threshold for investigating and treating at-risk neonates whe~~ ~~infection develops, if severe disease is to be avoided.

Specific interventions are indicated in certain cases of group B strept~~o~~coccal infection (p. 199), neonatal HSV infection (p. 710), toxoplasmos~~is~~ (p. 468), and neonatal CMV infection (p. 352).

Reference

1. Lee C, Gong Y, Brok J, Boxall EH, Gluud C (2006). Hepatitis B immunisation for newborn infan~~t~~ of hepatitis B surface antigen-positive mothers. *Cochrane Database of Systematic Reviews* Issue Oxford: Update Software.

Chorioamnionitis

Chorioamnionitis is inflammation of the chorion and amnion, the mem~~-~~ branes surrounding the fetus. Early recognition of maternal chorioamnio~~-~~ nitis is important, as it is associated with early-onset bacterial infections ~~of~~ the neonate with consequent neonatal morbidity and mortality.

Etiology

Usually, chorioamnionitis is associated with a bacterial infection. Organism~~s~~ residing in the vagina and cervix ascend into the uterus, initiating infectio~~n~~ of the fetal membranes and amniotic fluid. Ascending infection may b~~e~~ facilitated by poor urogenital hygiene and certain sexual practices.

Villitis is seen in around 6% of placentas after delivery (not necessaril~~y~~ due to infection). Conservative estimates place the incidence of infectiv~~e~~ chorioamnionitis at around 1% of all deliveries. Chorioamnionitis (whic~~h~~ may be clinically silent) greatly increases the risk of preterm labor. The ris~~k~~ of developing chorioamnionitis is highest following premature rupture ~~of~~ the membranes (PROM) or prolonged labor.

Maternal mortality is rare. More significant is the impact on the neonate~~.~~ The risk of neonatal infection increases with the time from membran~~e~~ rupture.

Although bacterial vaginosis is an important cause of premature labor~~,~~ overt neonatal infection is uncommon.

Clinical features

These include fever (>37.8°C), maternal tachycardia, less commonly, feta~~l~~ tachycardia (>160 beats/min), purulent amniotic fluid or vaginal discharge~~,~~ uterine tenderness, and raised maternal WBC count. The presence of a~~t~~ least two of these features is associated with an increased risk of neonatal sepsis.

Mothers with genuine chorioamnionitis may be asymptomatic. Epidura~~l~~ anesthesia during labor may be associated with a low-grade fever that ca~~n~~ prompt suspicion of maternal chorioamnionitis. The reasons for this are not clear.

Diagnosis

Diagnosis is usually made clinically by the above criteria in the intrapartum period. Antenatal screening examinations may have detected GBS carriage.

ssociated with an increased risk of chorioamnionitis. Asymptomatic mothers presenting with premature labor or PROM should have silent horioamnionitis excluded (e.g., amniotic fluid examination).

- *Amniotic fluid examination:* amniotic fluid may be obtained by amniocentesis if appropriate (risk of rupturing fetal membranes if intact). It can be examined for WBC count, pH, glucose, cytokine levels, and microscopy and microbiological culture performed. Certain centers perform PCR to detect common causes of infection.
- *Blood tests:* WBC count (may be raised in mothers who have been given steroids), CRP, blood cultures if febrile
- *Histology:* diagnosis may be confirmed or refuted only on histological examination of the placenta, fetal membranes, and umbilical cord for evidence of inflammation and infection.

Neonates born to mothers with suspected chorioamnionitis should be assessed for evidence of sepsis.

Management

For mothers presenting with PROM and no obvious infection, a balance needs to be struck between avoiding the complications of prematurity and those of chorioamnionitis. Subclinical infection may be a precipitant of PROM.

Mothers are usually given steroids to promote fetal maturation prior to delivery. In the absence of clinical infection, there is no evidence that prophylactic antibiotics improves outcome, but they are normally given along with steroids. Mother and fetus must be assessed regularly for signs of distress or the onset of chorioamnionitis.

For mothers presenting with acute chorioamnionitis, delivery must be expedited. If signs of fetal distress develop, emergency delivery may be necessary. Antibiotics should *not* be withheld with the intention of obtaining neonatal cultures.

Mothers in preterm labor or with PROM at less than 36 weeks' gestation should receive prophylactic antibiotics, as should mothers in labor at term with risk factors for fetal GBS infection.

The standard drug treatment of the mother with chorioamnionitis includes clindamycin and an aminoglycoside. Ampicillin or penicillin may have already been given to some mothers as prophylaxis against GBS infection of the neonate. Ampicillin covers GBS, *Haemophilus* species, most enterococci strains, and *Listeria* species.

The infant should be assessed and treated for any evidence of infection.

Puerperal sepsis

Any infection following delivery is classified as postpartum or puerperal infection. *Puerperal pyrexia* is defined as a maternal temperature of >38°C on more than one occasion on the first 14 days after delivery; 90% of infections are genital or urinary in origin.

Etiology

Sources of infection include endometritis (most common), wound infections, perineal cellulitis (usually seen around day 2 after delivery), mastitis, pneumonia (a complication of anesthesia), retained products of conception, UTIs, and septic pelvic phlebitis (pregnant women are at increased risk of thrombosis).

Risk factors include Caesarean delivery, PROM, frequent cervical examination, internal fetal monitoring, pre-existing pelvic infection, diabetes, and obesity.

The uterine cavity is normally sterile until rupture of the amniotic sac and the organisms isolated in endometritis are those normally present in the bowel, vagina, perineum, and cervix. Uterine infections are most likely after prolonged rupture of the membranes and after instrumental delivery. Genital tract infections may be polymicrobial and include *E. coli*, GAS, GBS, *Bacteroides*, and *Clostridium* species.

Clinical features

The source of infection may be indicated by the history. Was the delivery vaginal (with or without instruments?) or Caesarean? Did premature rupture of the membranes occur? Was there intrapartum fever?

Patients may be febrile or hypotensive and may have symptoms and signs indicative of the causative infection. Look for signs of UTI, deep vein thrombosis (DVT), wound infection, respiratory symptoms (pneumonia or septic pulmonary embolus), abdominal pain and tenderness on bimanual examination with foul-smelling vaginal discharge (suggestive of endometritis, although GAS infections are associated with odorless lochia), and evidence of mastitis.

Diagnosis and management

Investigations

Obtain CBC, urinalysis, blood cultures, and urine cultures, swab and culture any wounds or discharges, and swab for *Chlamydia* from the cervix and lochia.

Pelvic ultrasound may help detect pelvic abscesses or infected hematomas. Contrast abdominal CT may be required if non–pregnancy-related abdominal sources of infection are suspected.

Management

Provide fluid resuscitation and respiratory support, if required. Antibiotic therapy should be guided by the likely source of infection. Avoid use of tetracyclines if the mother is breast-feeding.

Mild cases of endometritis may be managed by broad-spectrum PO antibiotics (e.g., amoxicillin-clavulanate); moderate to severe cases require intravenous therapy. Mastitis should respond to PO dicloxacillin or cephalexin; mothers should continue to express milk to prevent blockage and breast engorgement.

Check for abscess development. Treat UTI or pyelonephritis as indicated. Septic pelvic thrombosis requires anticoagulation and broad-spectrum antibiotics. Infected wounds may need surgical debridement or drainage in combination with antibiotic therapy.

If the patient fails to respond, check the culture results and appropriateness of antibiotic therapy; exclude pelvic and abdominal collections and abscesses (wound, breast). If sensitivities are not available, consider adding gentamicin and changing to a third-generation cephalosporin.

Early surgical referral is essential if there is evidence of spreading skin infection despite antibiotic therapy. Consider synergistic gangrene. Urgent surgical debridement may be required.

If GBS, *Chlamydia*, or *N. gonorrhoea* is cultured, inform the pediatrician or family practitioner so infection can be excluded in the child.

Primary immunodeficiency

Most of these rare conditions are inherited as single-gene disorders and present in early infancy or childhood. They can be divided into three groups:
- Antibody-deficiency syndromes
- Selective T-cell deficiencies
- Mixed T- and B-cell defects

Antibody-deficiency syndromes

The lifetime prevalence of severe antibody deficiency syndromes is ~16/million of the population in the West. Partial antibody deficiency occurs in about 1/700 Caucasians, most of whom are healthy.

X-linked agammaglobulinemia

This presents with recurrent infections during the first 2 years of life. Affected children have very few B cells and low levels of circulating IgG.

Patients are prone to infections with the following pathogens: *H. influenzae*, *S. pneumoniae*, *Mycoplasma* spp., *Ureaplasma* spp., *Campylobacter jejuni*, *Giardia lamblia*, and enteroviruses.

Treatment is with intravenous immunoglobulin (IVIG). Prognosis is relatively good, with >90% survival at 30 years.

Common variable immunodeficiency (CVID)

Peak incidence is in early childhood and late adolescence. Serum Ig levels are variable, but IgA is virtually absent, IgG is <2 g/L, and IgM is <0.2 g/L (but may be normal or raised). There is often a family history of selective IgA deficiency and/or autoimmune disease.

CIVD is associated with major histocompatibility complex (MHC) haplotype HLA A1, B8, C4A*QO, DR3 in 50% of patients. One-third of patients are severely lymphopenic with CD4+ T-cell counts of <0.4 10⁹/L, low numbers of B cells, and a relative increase in CD8+ T cells; 70% of patients have features such as inflammatory bowel disease, splenomegaly, lymphadenopathy, autoimmune diseases, and malignancies.

Treatment is with IVIG. Prognosis is relatively good, with ~70% survival at 30 years.

Thymoma with hypogammaglobulinemia

Thymoma occurs in patients >40 years and is associated with or followed by hypogammaglobulinemia. Clinical features are similar to CVID but prognosis is poorer; patients usually die within 15 years of symptom onset.

Selective IgA deficiency

Complete absence of IgA occurs in ~1/700 Caucasians. Most people are healthy and only ~5% suffer from recurrent respiratory tract infections. This deficiency may be a mild variant of CVID and is also associated with the MHC haplotype HLA A1, B8, C4A*QO, DR3.

There is a small increase of IgA deficiency in celiac disease, Still's disease, rheumatoid arthritis, and epilepsy patients, but this may be drug related, e.g., sulfasalazine, gold, penicillamine, or antiepileptics.

IgG subclass deficiencies

The clinical significance of IgG subclass deficiencies is debatable. IgG2 deficiency is the most common type and may be associated with recurrent respiratory tract infections or be asymptomatic.

Selective IgM deficiency

Complete deficiency is very rare. Most cases are associated with rare conditions, e.g., Wiskott–Aldrich or Bloom's syndromes, or are secondary to lymphoma.

Functional immunoglobulin deficiency

This is defined as the complete or partial failure to produce antibodies to specific proteins, peptides, or polysaccharides in the presence of normal total Ig levels. The mechanism is unknown. Only functional IgG deficiency is clinically important.

Selective T-cell deficiency

These conditions are very rare. Infections associated with T-cell deficiency include herpes simplex virus (HSV), varicella zoster virus (VZV), cytomegalovirus (CMV), adenovirus, papilloma virus, rotavirus, *Mycobacterium* spp., *Cryptococcus neoformans*, *Toxoplasma gondii*, *Candida* spp., *Aspergillus* spp., *Pneumocytis jiroveci*, *Cryptosporidium* spp., and *Strongyloides* spp.

Children remain relatively healthy unless the condition is also associated with macrophage dysfunction or antibody deficiency.

Thymic aplasia (Di George syndrome)

This is caused by fetal malformation of the third and fourth branchial arch during gestation. Severely affected infants usually die from associated cardiac abnormalities. Those that survive have a few circulating T cells (<10%) and remain healthy. Severely affected infants are prone to recurrent infections, especially life-threatening CMV and VZV disease.

Treatment is with a thymus transplant.

Purine nucleoside phosphorylase (PNP) deficiency

This autosomal recessive condition is characterized by T-cell deficiency, susceptibility to severe CMV and VZV infections, autoimmune blood dyscrasias, lymphoma, and neurological disease. Most patients present in infancy. Bone marrow transplantation is the best treatment.

Severe combined immunodeficiency (SCID)

SCID is due to rare mutations in genes that influence the maturation of lymphocytes, e.g., adenosine deaminase deficiency, X-linked SCID, lymphocyte MHC class II deficiency, reticular dysgenesis, and multiple interleukin deficiency.

Infections are usually much more severe than those seen in primary hypogammaglobulinemia and selective T-cell deficiency, probably because macrophage function is affected. Infants present with failure to thrive, diarrhea, *Pneumocystis jiroveci* pneumonia, and or mucocutaneous or systemic candidiasis. Immunization with live vaccines, e.g., polio or BCG, may cause fatal infection.

Most patients die within 2 years unless they undergo hematopoietic stem cell transplantation.

Secondary immunodeficiency

Secondary immunodeficiency is defined as a defect in the components or function of the immune system, occurring as a result of another disease or condition. It may affect humoral immunity, cell-mediated immunity, or both. HIV infection, drugs, and lymphoreticular malignancies are the most important causes (Table 4.16).

Table 4.16 Causes of secondary immunodeficiency

Cause	Examples	Humoral immunity	Cell-mediated immunity
Viruses	HIV	√	√
	Rubella	√	
Drugs	Corticosteroids		√
	Cyclophosphamide		√
	Azathioprine		√
	Cyclosporin/tacrolimus		√
	Mycophenylate		√
	Anti-T-cell antibodies		√
	Gold	√	
	Penicillamine	√	
	Sulphasalazine	√	

Table 4.16 (Contd.)

Cause	Examples	Humoral immunity	Cell-mediated immunity
	Phenytoin	√	
	Methotrexate		√
	Bleomycin		√
	Vincristine	√	√
	Cis-platinum		√
Malignancy	Chronic lymphocytic leukemia	√	
	Myeloma	√	
Metabolic	Renal failure	√	√
	Liver failure	√	√
	Trauma	√	√
	Vitamin A deficiency	√	
	Vitamin B_{12} deficiency	√	
	Zinc deficiency		√
Ig loss	Nephrotic syndrome	√	
	Protein-losing enteropathy	√	
	Dystophia myotonica	√	

Infections in asplenic patients

The spleen, the largest lymphoid organ in the body, performs a wide range of immunological functions that protect the body from severe infections. The relation between an absent or hypofunctioning spleen and severe infection has long been recognized; it is termed post-splenectomy sepsis (PSS) or overwhelming post-splenectomy infection (OPSI).

Asplenia is usually acquired (due to surgical removal of the spleen for traumatic or therapeutic reasons) but may rarely be congenital. A number of conditions may also lead to functional hyposplenism.

Etiology

The following organisms are associated with PSS:
• *S. pneumoniae*
• *H. influenzae*
• *N. meningitidis*
• *Capnocytophaga canimorsis*
• *Salmonella* spp.

- *Plasmodium falciparum*
- *Babesiosis*
- *Erlichiois*
- *Bartonella bacilliformis*

Clinical features

The risk of PSS is highest in the first few years after splenectomy.

PSS has a short prodrome with fever, chills, pharyngitis, muscle aches, vomiting, and diarrhea. In adults there is usually no obvious site of infection, whereas in children meningitis is common. Deterioration is usually rapid and occurs over hours with septic shock, DIC, seizures, and coma.

Diagnosis[1]

The diagnosis is clinical; all asplenic patients with fever should be considered to have and PSS and be managed for PSS.

The presence Howell–Jolly bodies (nuclear remnants) on the blood film confirms hyposplenism, but they may not always be present.

Management[1]

Asplenic patients should be given a supply of prophylactic antibiotics for self-administration at the first sign of serious illness.

If the patient presents acutely with PSS, they should receive immediate treatment with IV antibiotics, e.g., ceftriaxone + vancomycin.

Prevention[1]

For use of prophylactic antibiotics, some guidelines recommend that lifelong oral penicillin V be given to patients with an absent or dysfunctional spleen, whereas others recommend prophylaxis from ages 0 to 5, or for 1 year following splenectomy.

Immunization against *S. pneumoniae*, *N. meningitis*, *H. influenzae*, and influenza virus is recommended for all apslenic patients.

Reference

1. Davies JM (2002). Updated guideline. The prevention and treatment of infection in patients with an absent or dysfunctional spleen. *Clin Med* 2:440–443.

Neutropenic sepsis

Neutropenia is associated with an increased risk of bacteremia and severe infection. Although *neutropenia* is defined as an absolute neutrophil count $<0.5 \times 10^9$ cells/L, many experts believe that the risk of infection increases when the neutrophil count falls below 1×10^9 cells/L. In very immunocompromised patients, signs of infection may be absent, and the first and only sign of infection may be fever ($>38°C$).

Febrile neutropenia is a medical emergency, and appropriate antimicrobial therapy should be started immediately, as the mortality of neutropenic patients with untreated gram-negative sepsis approaches 40%.

Classification

Febrile neutropenia can be divided into four categories:
- Microbiological documented infections (MDI) with bacteremia
- MDI with isolation of a significant pathogen from a well-defined site of infection, e.g., urine, respiratory, abscess
- Clinically documented infection without microbiological proof
- Unexplained fever without clinical or microbiological proof

Etiology

In the 1970s, gram-negative rods were the predominant pathogen.

In the 1980s, gram-negative bacteria became the predominant pathogens, mainly as a result of fluoroquinolone prophylaxis.

In the late 1990s, an increase in gram-negative pathogens was again seen; the reasons for this are not clear.

Evaluation of the febrile neutropenic patient

The following factors should be considered:
- Underlying disease (e.g., solid tumor or hematological malignancy) and stage
- Previous history of infection
- Clinical features: fever, symptoms and signs of infection, systemic upset, metabolic instability
- Neutrophil count: at time of onset and during previous 30 days, expected neutrophil count kinetics and duration of neutropenia
- Lymphocyte count: at time of onset and previous 30 days
- Platelet and fibrinogen levels

A number of studies have been performed to try to stratify patients into high- and low-risk patients, using clinical and laboratory parameters.

Management

Initial studies used a combination β-lactam/aminoglycoside regimen. More recent studies have shown that monotherapy with β-lactam active against *Pseudomonas* spp. (e.g., ceftazidime, piperacillin-tazobactam, cefepime, or meropenem) was associated with a lower rate of clinical failures and adverse events and a trend toward better survival.

The choice of antimicrobial regimen should follow local antimicrobial policy and be based on local microbiological data.

If clinical findings suggest a possible gram-positive infection, e.g., line infection, a glycopeptide should also be started. Microbiologically documented infections should be treated with appropriately tailored antimicrobial therapy.

Neutropenic patients who remain febrile after 24–48 hours of therapy should be evaluated for treatment failure:
- Persistence of fever >39°C and chills 24–48 hours after starting therapy
- Relapse of fever >38°C after at least 24 hours of defervescence
- Progression of sepsis syndrome
- Development of DIC, ARDS, multiorgan failure
- Persistence of positive cultures despite 24 hours of therapy

- Relapse of primary infection
- Appearance of a new infection

Consider alternative causes of fever:
- Drug-resistant organisms (bacteria, viruses, fungi, protozoa)
- Drug reactions
- Infusion of blood products
- Graft vs. host disease.

Empirical anti-gram-positive therapy

Despite a lack of evidence of benefit, many centers add empirical gram-positive cover after 48 hours of antibiotic therapy. The IATG-EORTC (International Antimicrobial Therapy Group of the European Organization for Research and Treatment of Cancer) Trial XIV showed that there was no difference in time to defervescence in patients receiving piperacillin-tazobactam who were randomized to vancomycin or placebo.[1]

Empirical antifungal therapy

This has been shown to be of benefit in patients with persistent febrile neutropenia. The IATG-EORTC showed that although there were no differences in defervescence and survival between patients who received and did not receive antifungal therapy, there were no deaths from fungal infection in patients receiving amphotericin, and the number of documented fungal infections was higher in the placebo group.[2]

Alternative antifungal regimens

- Lipid amphotericin preparations (p. 74) are as effective and less toxic but much more expensive than conventional amphotericin B.
- Voriconazole has been evaluated and did not meet criteria for non-inferiority to liposomal amphotericin B.
- Caspofungin and micafungin have been evaluated and found to be non-inferior to liposomal amphotericin B.
- Posaconazole is used as prophylaxis against fungal infection in certain high-risk hosts, but because of PO formulation only is not typically used in febrile neutropenia.

Adjunctive therapies

- Granulocyte-colony-stimulating factor (G-CSF)
- Granulocyte-macrophage-colony-stimulating factor (GM-CSF)
- Granulocyte infusions
- Infusion of immunoglobulins

References

1. Cometta A, Kern WV, deBock R, et al. (2003). Vancomycin versus placebo for treating persistent fever in patients with neutropenic cancer receiving piperacillin-tazobactam monotherapy. *Clin Infect Dis* 37(3):382–389.

2. Hughes WT, Armstrong D, Bodey GP, et al. (2002). 2002 guidelines for the use of antimicrobial agents in neutropenic patients with cancer. *Clin Infect Dis* 34(6):730–751

Infections in transplant recipients

The advent of immunosuppression has resulted in a marked growth in organ transplantation over the last 30 years. Apart from medical and surgical issues related to function and rejection of transplanted organs, infections are the most important problem.

Most infections occur during the first 4 to 6 months after transplantation. The following risk factors have been identified:

- Pretransplant factors (underlying medical conditions, lack of immunity, prior latent infections, colonization with nosocomial organisms, prior medications)
- Transplantation factors (type of organ, trauma of surgery)
- Immunosuppression (medication, chemotherapy, irradiation)
- Allograft reactions (graft vs. host disease)

Sources of infection

The sources of infection can be divided into three categories.

Host factors (endogenous)

- Reactivation of viruses (HSV, VZV, CMV)
- Barrier disruption causing invasive disease (mucositis, IV catheters)
- Colonization with resistant flora (gram-negatives, vancomycin-resistant enterococci [VRE], yeasts)
- Reactivation of fungi (*Aspergillus*)
- Reactivation of parasites (*Toxoplasma, Strongyloides*)

Environmental factors (exogenous)

- Importance of positive pressure ventilation (*Aspergillus* spores)
- Opportunistic pathogens (*Legionella, P. jirovecii, Listeria*)

Organ transplant/blood products

- Viral (CMV, HBV, HCV, HIV, HHV-6, HHV-7, TTV, parvo, HTLV-1)
- Bacterial (organ contamination, TB)
- Unknown (variant Creutzfeldt–Jakob disease [vCJD], pig retroviruses)

Clinical features

The clinical manifestations are variable and depend on a number of factors, including prior immune status of the host, reason for transplant (e.g., viral hepatitis, diabetic nephropathy), type of transplant (solid organ or hematopoietic stem cell [HSCT]), preconditioning treatment, time after transplantation, degree of immunosuppression, likelihood of exposure, and infecting pathogen.

Hematopoietic stem cell transplant-associated infections

Pre-engraftment, profound neutropenia is associated with ablation of humoral and cell-mediated immunity. Infections during this period may include bacteremia (gram-positive and gram-negative) HSV, candidemia, and invasive fungal disease.

During the post-engraftment period up until 100 days post-HSCT, B- and T-cell immunity starts to recover. The most common infections are caused by gram-positive and gram-negative bacteria, fungi, CMV, PCP, and other viruses (RSV, parainfluenza, adenovirus, JC, BK).

From 100 days to 1 year post-HSCT, B- and T-cell function continues to recover but may take 18–36 months to fully recover. The most common infections are caused by VZV and encapsulated bacteria.

Solid-organ transplant-associated infections

In the early postoperative period, standard postoperative infections (VAP, line infection, wound infection, UTI) with nosocomial pathogens predominate. Between the second and sixth postoperative months, immunosuppression is established, and a wide range of bacterial, viral, fungal, and protozoal infections may occur.

After 6 months, patients with good allograft function on a stable immunosuppressive regime have the same risk of bacterial infections as that of a minimally immunosuppressed patient in the community. In contrast, patients with rejection are at increased risk of opportunistic infections such as those seen prior to 6 months.

Pretransplantation screening

Pretransplantation screening of the donor, recipient, and/or blood products is performed in order to try and prevent or predict transplant-related infections.

Recipient screening
- Ongoing or active infection
- Serological testing for HBV, HCV, HIV, HSV, VZV, EBV, CMV, T. pallidum, T. gondii
- In endemic areas consider T. cruzi, Histoplasma, Strongyloides

Donor screening
- Serological testing for HBV, HCV, HIV, T. pallidum, T. gondii (cardiac)
- Culture of cadaveric organs, perfusates, transport medium
- If living donor, take clinical and epidemiological history and consider tuberculin testing and fungal serology
- In endemic areas, consider screening for malaria, T. cruzi

Blood products
- Screening for HBV, HCV, HIV, T. pallidum
- Leukodepleted blood reduces the risk of CMV.

Post-transplantation surveillance

Post-transplantation surveillance is performed in order to guide pre-emptive therapy and monitor response to treatment:
- CMV disease by PCR
- Surveillance cultures for multi-drug-resistant pathogens

Prevention of infection

Routine immunizations for people with chronic diseases, e.g., pneumococcal, influenza immunization, should be given prior to transplantation.

Prophylatic antimicrobials are commonly given in the first few months after transplantation, e.g., TMP-SMX, antivirals (acyclovir, valacyclovir, ganciclovir or valganciclovir), and antifungals (nystatin, fluconazole, or voriconazole). Protocols differ between different transplant centers.

HIV epidemiology

There are an estimated 33 million people living with HIV/AIDS, with 2.7 million new infections and 2.1 million deaths in 2007. The majority of new infections occur in young adults (aged 15–24 years old) in developing countries. Sub-Saharan Africa bears the brunt of the epidemic, but there are growing epidemics in Asia, notably in India and China, which may eclipse the African epidemic in the next decade.

Although the introduction of highly active antiretroviral therapy (HAART) has dramatically reduced morbidity and mortality in North America and western Europe, most patients who require HAART in the developing world do not have access to it.

HIV transmission

HIV may be transmitted via a number of routes:
- Sexual transmission
- Perinatal transmission: intrapartum, peripartum, breast-feeding
- Blood transfusion
- Intravenous drug use or sharing needles
- Occupational transmission: needlestick injury or mucocutaneous exposure.

The risk of transmission differs with the route of infection (Table 4.17).

Table 4.17 HIV transmission rates

Exposure	Risk/10,000 exposures
Blood transfusion	9,000
Intravenous drug use	67
Receptive anal intercourse	50
Needlestick injury	30
Receptive vaginal intercourse	10
Insertive anal intercourse	6–7
Insertive vaginal intercourse	5

HIV natural history

The natural history of HIV infection is divided into the following stages (Fig. 4.2):
- *Primary infection:* diagnosis is based on a plasma HIV RNA level >10,000 copies/mL + indeterminate or negative serology or recent seroconversion.
- *Acute retroviral syndrome* (2–3 weeks): clinical features include fever (96%), adenopathy (74%), pharyngitis (70%), rash (70%), myalgia

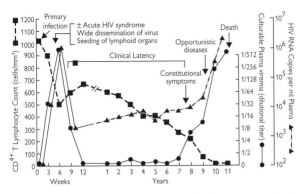

Fig. 4.2 Typical course of HIV infection. Reproduced with permission from Fauci AS Patales G, Stanley S, Weuoman D (1996). Immunopathogenic mechanisms of HIV infection. *Ann Intern Med* 124(7):654–663.

Table 4.18 CD4 count and HIV complications

CD4 count	Complications
>500/mm³	Acute retroviral syndrome, candida vaginitis, persistent generalized lymphadenopathy (PGL), Guillain–Barré syndrome, myopathy, aseptic meningitis
200–500/mm³	Pneumococcal and other bacterial pneumonia, pulmonary tuberculosis, herpes zoster, oropharyngeal candidiasis, cryptosporidiosis, Kaposi sarcoma, oral hairy leukoplakia, cervical intraepithelial neoplasia, cervical cancer, B-cell lymphoma, anemia, mononeuritis multiplex, idiopathic thrombocytopenic purpura (ITP), Hodgkin's lymphoma, lymphocytic interstitial pneumonitis (LIP)
<200/mm³	*Pneumocystis jiroveci* pneumonia (PCP), disseminated histoplasmosis, disseminated cocciodiodomycosis, miliary/extrapulmonary TB, progressive multifocal leukoencephalopathy (PML), wasting syndrome, peripheral neuropathy, HIV-associated dementia, cardiomyopathy, vacuolar myopathy, progressive radiculopathy, non-Hodgkin's lymphoma (NHL)
<100/mm³	Disseminated herpes simplex, toxoplasmosis, cryptococcosis, chronic cryptosporidiosis, microsporidiosis, esophageal candidiasis
<50/mm³	Disseminated cytomegalovirus (CMV), disseminated *Mycobacterium avium* complex (MAC), primary central nervous system lymphoma (PCNSL)

(54%), diarrhea (32%), headache (32%), nausea and vomiting (27%), hepatosplenomegaly (14%), weight loss (13%), thrush (12%), and neurological symptoms (12%). This is accompanied by rapid decline in CD4 T-lymphocyte count and high concentrations of HIV RNA in the plasma.
- *Recovery and seroconversion* (2–4 weeks): characterized by recovery of CD4 cell count and reduction in plasma HIV viral load to a set point
- *Asymptomatic chronic HIV infection* (average 8 years): associated with gradual decline in CD4 cell count
- *Symptomatic HIV infection/AIDS* (average 1–3 years): occurs when the CD4 count declines to <200/mm³ and the viral load begins to rise

Death usually occurs 10–11 years after infection in untreated individuals.

Complications of HIV infection

As the CD4 count declines, the complications shown in Table 4.18 may occur.

HIV classification

There are two commonly used classification systems.

CDC 1993 revised classification

This categorizes patients according to clinical categories (A, B, C) and CD4 count categories (1,2,3). Patients in categories A3, B3, and C1 to C3 are defined as having AIDS (Table 4.19).

World Health Organization classification

This categorizes patients into four clinical stages, regardless of CD4 cell count. Patients with clinical stage 4 are defined as having AIDS (Table 4.20).

Table 4.19 CDC 1993 revised classification of HIV

	A (asymptomatic, acute HIV, PGL)	B (symptomatic)	C (AIDS indicator conditions)
CD4 ≥500/mm³	A1	B1	C1
CD4 200–499/mm³	A2	B2	C2
CD4 <200/mm³	A3	B3	C3

Table 4.20 WHO classification of HIV

Stage	Symptoms
1	Asymptomatic
	Persistent generalized lymphadenopathy (PGL)
	Performance scale 1: asymptomatic, normal activity
2	Weight loss, <10% of body weight
	Minor mucocutaneous manifestations (seborrheic dermatitis, prurigo)
	Fungal nail infections, recurrent oral ulcerations, angular cheilitis
	Herpes zoster, within the last 5 years
	Recurrent upper respiratory tract infections (e.g., bacterial sinusitis)
	And/or performance scale 2: symptomatic, normal activity
3	Weight loss, >10% of body weight
	Unexplained chronic diarrhea, >1 month
	Unexplained prolonged fever (intermittent or constant), >1 month
	Oral candidiasis (thrush)
	Oral hairy leukoplakia
	Pulmonary tuberculosis, within the past year
	Severe bacterial infections (e.g., pneumonia, pyomyositis)
	And/or performance scale 3: bedridden, <50% of the day during the last month
4	HIV wasting syndrome, as defined by CDC*
	Pneumocystis jiroveci pneumonia
	Toxoplasmosis of the brain
	Cryptosporidiosis with diarrhea, >1 month
	Cryptococcosis, extrapulmonary
	Cytomegalovirus (CMV) disease of an organ other than liver, spleen, or lymph nodes
	Herpes simplex virus (HSV) infection, mucocutaneous >1 month, or visceral any duration
	Progressive multifocal leukoencephalopathy (PML)
	Any disseminated endemic mycosis (e.g., histoplasmosis, coccidioidomycosis)
	Candidiasis of the esophagus, trachea, bronchi, or lungs
	Atypical mycobacteriosis, disseminated
	Non-typhoid *Salmonella* septicemia
	Extrapulmonary tuberculosis
	Lymphoma
	Kaposi sarcoma (KS)
	HIV encephalopathy, as defined by CDC†
	And/or performance scale 4: bedridden, >50% of the day during the last month

* HIV wasting syndrome: weight loss of >10% of body weight, plus either unexplained chronic diarrhea (>1 month) or chronic weakness and unexplained prolonged fever (>1 month).

† HIV encephalopathy: clinical finding of disabling cognitive and/or motor dysfunction interfering with activities of daily living, progressing over weeks to months, in the absence of a concurrent illness or condition other than HIV infection that could explain the findings.

Initial evaluation of HIV patient

All newly diagnosed HIV patients should be carefully evaluated to determine the clinical stage of disease, coexistent infections, and laboratory abnormalities:

- Full blood count
- Biochemistry profile: renal and liver function tests
- Fasting blood glucose and serum lipids
- Serology for HIV (if laboratory confirmation not available), hepatitis A, B, and C, CMV, syphilis, and *T. gondii*
- Urinalysis
- Cervical smear in women
- Testing for *C. trachomatis* and *N. gonorrhoeae* is optional but should be considered for those at high risk.
- Tuberculin skin test (unless previous history of TB or positive test)
- Chest X-ray

CD4 T-cell count

This is an indicator of immunocompetence and is a string predictor of progression and survival. It is checked at baseline to assess the need for antiretroviral therapy. Once treatment starts, the CD4 count usually rises by 100–150 cells/mm^3 per year, with an accelerated response in the first 3 months. During treatment, it is monitored every 3–6 months.

Plasma HIV RNA

Numerous studies have shown an association between decrease in plasma viremia and improved survival. Baseline viral load may be a consideration regarding when to start treatment. It should be measured immediately before and 2–8 weeks after initiation of treatment. Its main role is in monitoring the response to therapy. HIV viral load should be checked every 3–4 months in patients on a stable antiretroviral regimen or earlier if clinically indicated.

HIV drug resistance testing

For patients with HIV-RNA >100,000 copies/mL, genotypic drug resistance testing is recommended, regardless of whether the patient starts antiretroviral therapy. If treatment is deferred, this should be repeated prior to starting therapy. In antiretroviral naive patients, a genotypic assay is generally preferred. Drug resistance testing should also be performed in the setting of virological failure to assist with choosing new drugs.

HLA-B*5701 screening

The abacavir hypersensitivity reaction (ABC HSR) is a multi-organ clinical syndrome that occurs in 5–8% of patients within 6 weeks of starting abacavir therapy. Several studies have shown an association between the HLA allele HLA-B*5701 and ABC HSR. For this reason, all patients should be screened for this allele prior to starting abacavir therapy, and those who are HLA-B*5701-positive should not be given the drug.

Co-receptor tropism assays

During acute or recent infection, most patients harbor a CCR5 tropic (R5) virus. In untreated patients, the virus shifts to using CXCR4 (R4 tropic) or both (dual/mixed tropic). The CCR5 inhibitors (maraviroc and vicriviroc) are a new class of drugs that prevent HIV entry into target cells by binding to CCR5. Co-receptor tropism assays should be performed prior to considering therapy with CCR5 receptor antagonists.

HIV skin complications (1)

Skin manifestations are common in HIV-infected patients and may be caused by bacteria, fungi, viruses, parasites, or drugs.

Bacillary angiomatosis

This is caused by *Bartonella henselae* and *Bartonella quintana* (see *Bartonella* species, p. 299).

Lesions start as red or purple papules that expand into nodules or pedunculated masses. They appear vascular and may bleed with trauma.

Skin biopsy shows vascular proliferation, inflammation, and typical organisms on Warthin–Starry silver stain. Serology (immunofluorescence assay [IFA] or enzyme immunosorbent assay [EIA]) may be used to support the diagnosis.

Treatment is with oral erythromycin or doxycycline for >3 months.

Cutaneous candidiasis

This is usually caused by *Candida albicans*.

Lesions are moist, red, and scaly and may have satellite lesions. It may also cause intertrigo, balanitis, glossitis, angular cheilitis, paronyhchia, and nail dystrophies.

Diagnosis is usually clinical but may be confirmed by KOH preparation or wet mount.

Treatment may be topical (e.g., ketoconazole, miconazole, clotrimazole, or nystatin) or systemic (e.g., fluconazole).

Cryptococcosis

This is caused by *Cryptococcus neoformans* (see *Cryptococcus neoformans*, p. 426) as part of disseminated disease.

Lesions are nodular, popular, follicular, or ulcerated and may resemble molluscum. They usually occur on the face, neck, and scalp.

Skin biopsy with Gomori methenamine silver stain shows typical budding yeasts and positive culture. Serum cryptococcal antigen is usually positive. Lumbar puncture should be performed in patients with positive cultures or cryptococcal antigen to exclude cryptococcal meningitis (see *Cryptococcus neoformans*, p. 426).

Treatment is with oral fluconazole 400 mg/day for 8 weeks followed by 200 mg/day for nonmeningeal disease and combination amphotericin and 5FC for cryptococcal meningitis.

See the IDSA Guidelines (www.idsociety.org) for further details.

Dermatophyte infections

This is caused by a variety of fungi, e.g., *T. rubrum*, *T. mentagrophytes*, *T. tonsurans*, *T. soudanense*, *M. canis*, and *E. floccosum*.

It may present with fungal nail infections (onychomychosis), athlete's foot (tinea pedis), or ringworm (tinea corporis, tinea cruris, tinea capitis).

Diagnosis is confirmed by skin scrapings for KOH preparation and culture.

Treatment is with oral terbinafine or itraconazole for nail infections, or with topical agents (e.g., clotrimazole, ketoconazole, miconazole, terbinafine) for skin infections.

Drug eruptions

Common causes include antibiotics (e.g., TMP-SMX and β-lactams), anticonvulsants, and non-nucleoside reverse transcriptase inhibitors (NNRTIs) (see Non-nucleoside reverse transcriptase inhibitors, p. 91).

Lesions occur within 2 weeks of a new drug and present as an itchy, morbilliform, exanthematous eruption ± fever. More severe forms include urticaria, toxic epidermal necrolysis, Stevens–Johnson syndrome, hypersensitivity reactions (especially abacavir and nevirapine), and anaphylaxis.

Treatment of uncomplicated cases is with antihistamines and topical antipruritics and topical corticosteroids. For severe reactions, discontinue the drug and administer supportive care.

Folliculitis

Folliculitis is usually caused by *S. aureus*. Other causes include *Pityrosporum ovale* (intrafollicular yeast), *Demodex folliculorum* (intrafollicular mite), and eosinophilic folliculitis (unknown cause).

Lesions are itchy, follicular papules and pustules on the face, trunk, and extremities. Folliculitis occurs at a CD4 count of 50–250 cells/mm^3. It often relapses and remits. It may recur with immune reconstitution.

Diagnosis is clinical and confirmed by skin biopsy.

Treatment is of the underlying cause.

Herpes simplex

This is caused by herpes simplex virus (see Herpes simplex virus, p. 341).

Lesions begin as papules, which develop into vesicles and ulcerate and crust. They are usually found on the lip, in the mouth, or in the genital region. Recurrences are common.

Diagnosis is usually clinical but may be confirmed by PCR, HSV antigen detection, viral culture or Tzanck prep.

Treatment is with oral valacyclovir for 7–10 days. Severe or disseminated disease may require intravenous acyclovir (see Antivirals for HSV and VZV, p. 79).

Herpes zoster (shingles)

Shingles is caused by reactivation of varicella zoster virus (see Varicella zoster virus, p. 343). This affects 5% of healthy adults but is 15–25 times more common in HIV-infected adults.

The rash is usually preceded by a painful prodrome in the region of a dermatome. This is followed by the development of a dermatomal vesicular rash.

Diagnosis is usually clinical but may be confirmed by PCR, HSV antigen detection, viral culture, or Tzanck prep.

Treatment is with oral valacyclovir for 7–10 days. Severe or dissemi-nated disease may require intravenous acyclovir (see Antivirals for HSV and VZV, p. 79).

HIV skin complications (2)

Kaposi sarcoma

KS is caused by human herpes virus 8 (HHV-8, see Human herpes virus type 8, p. 737). It can occur in the general population but is 20,000 times more common in HIV-infected individuals.

Lesions are purple to brown-black macules, papules, nodules, and patches that occur on the legs, face, mouth, and genitalia. Complications include lymphedema and visceral involvement.

Diagnosis is clinical but may be confirmed by biopsy.

HAART is associated with lesion regression, decreased incidence, and prolonged survival. Local injection of vinblastine reduces lesion size. Extensive disease is treated with chemotherapy, e.g., anthracyclines or paclitaxel (more toxic).

Prurigo nodularis

The cause is unknown.

Lesions are hyperpigmented, hyperkeratotic papules and nodules that usually occur on the chest. They are usually intensely itchy, resulting in excoriation, ulceration, and scars.

Diagnosis is usually clinical but may be confirmed by biopsy.

Treatment is with topical steroids, occlusive dressings, antihistamines, or phototherapy. Refractory cases may benefit from thalidomide.

Scabies

Scabies is caused by *Sarcoptes scabiei*.

Lesions are small, red papules that are intensely itchy; sometimes there are burrows. They occur in the finger webs, wrist, periumbilical area, axilla, thighs, buttocks, genitalia, legs, and feet. A severe, crusted form (Norwegian scabies) may occur in immunocompromised patients.

Diagnosis is clinical and confirmed by microscopic examination of the mite.

The patient and all close contacts should be treated simultaneously with permethrin cream 5%, or lindane 1%, or ivermectin (severe or refractory cases). Pruritis may respond to antihistamines. Bedding and clothing must be washed in hot water or dry cleaned.

Seborrheic dermatitis

The cause is unknown, but *Pityrosporum* is often recovered from lesions.

Lesions are erythematous plaques with greasy scales and indistinct mar-gins. They usually occur on the scalp and face, behind the ears, and on the sternum, axillae, and sometimes pubic area.

Diagnosis is clinical.

Treatment is with a weak topical steroid, e.g., hydrocortisone 2.5% ± ketoconazole 2% cream. Scalp lesions may be treated with various shampoos, e.g., tar-based, selenium sulfide or zinc pyrithione containing, or ketoconazole shampoo.

HIV oral complications

A number of oral complications may occur in HIV-infected patients.

Apthous ulcers

The cause is unknown. Differential diagnosis includes HSV, CMV (see *Cytomegalovirus*, p. 351), and drug-induced ulcers.

Diagnosis is clinical. Biopsy is recommended for nonhealing ulcers.

Treatment is with topical lidocaine solution, Orabase®, or Aphthasol® (amlexanox oral paste 5%). Refractory cases may require oral prednisolone, colchicine, dapsone, pentoxifylline, or thalidomide.

Oral candidiasis (thrush)

Thrush is caused by *Candida* species, usually *C. albicans* (see *Candida* species, p. 417).

Lesions are white, painless plaques on the buccal and pharyngeal mucosa or the tongue. Risk factors include CD4 <250 cells/mm^3 and use of antibiotics and corticoteroids.

Diagnosis is clinical but may be confirmed by KOH preparation. Culture is only indicated for speciation and drug susceptibility testing, e.g., for refractory cases.

Treatment is with oral clotrimazole, nystatin, or fluconazole. Most cases respond in 7–14 days, unless there is prior azole exposure and CD4 count <50 cells/mm^3. Refractory cases may require itraconazole suspension, amphotericin suspension, or intravenous echinocandin.

Oral hairy leukoplakia

This is caused by Epstein–Barr virus (see Epstein–Barr virus, p. 347) and is found almost exclusively in HIV-infected patients with low CD4 counts.

It presents as unilateral or bilateral adherent white frond-like patches on lateral margins of the tongue.

Diagnosis is usually clinical; biopsy is rarely required.

Treatment is not usually required as it is usually asymptomatic. It responds to HAART. Occasionally, patients are treated for pain or cosmetic reasons, with topical podophyllin, surgical excision, cryotherapy, or antivirals.

Salivary gland enlargement

This may be due to HIV-related lymphoid proliferation.

It presents with unilateral or bilateral parotid enlargement. It is usually asymptomatic but may present with pain or xerostomia.

Diagnosis is by fine needle aspiration (FNA) for microbiology, cytology, and decompression. Occasionally, biopsy is required to exclude a tumor.

Treatment is by FNA for decompression of fluid-filled cysts.

Other conditions

The oral cavity may be involved in a number of conditions, e.g.:

- Herpes simplex virus infections
- Kaposi sarcoma
- Leishmaniasis (p. 478)
- Syphilis (p. 642)

HIV cardiovascular complications

The main concern is the increased risk of cardiovascular disease due to metabolic complications of HAART, e.g., hyperlipidemia.

Dilated cardiomyopathy

The cause is unknown, but hypotheses include mitochondrial toxicity from zidovudine, HIV infection of myocardial cells, L-carnitine deficiency, and selenium deficiency.

Incidence is declining; previously it was 30–40% in patients with AIDS (pre-HAART), now it is 3–15%.

Clinical features include congestive cardiac failure, arrhythmias, cyanosis, syncope, and sudden death.

Diagnosis is by echocardiogram, which shows ejection fraction ≤50% ± arrhythmias on ECG.

Treatment is with HAART and an angiotensin-converting enzyme (ACE) inhibitor. Diuretics, e.g., furosemide or spironolactone, are given for persistent symptoms. Digoxin may be given for refractory cases. Other options include treatment of hypertension and hyperlipidemia, discontinuation of alcohol and cocaine, and discontinuation of azathioprine. Some clinicians recommend supplements of L-carnitine or selenium (if deficient).

Endocarditis

HIV has no effect on the incidence of endocarditis, apart from in intravenous drug users in whom it is more common. Endocarditis is associated with increased mortality in patients with AIDS (30%).

Myocarditis

The cause is unclear in most cases. HIV may have a direct effect; 20% are associated with infections, e.g., cryptococcis, CMV, EBV, HSV, TB, and *T. gondii*.

Pericardial effusion

The cause is unknown. Pericardial effusion occurs in ~10% of untreated HIV patients. Incidence has been declining in the HAART era. Most cases are small. There is a high mortality in patients with AIDS.

Pericarditis

Causes include mycobacteria, pyogenic bacteria, lymphoma, Kaposi sarcoma, viruses, and fungi. Aspiration and pericardial biopsy may yield a diagnosis. The effect of HAART is unknown.

Pulmonary hypertension

The cause is unknown, but HHV-8 has been implicated. Clinical features are similar to those of primary pulmonary hypertension with exertional dyspnea, fatigue, cough, hemoptysis, chest pain, and syncope.

CXR shows enlarged pulmonary vessels and right ventricular and right atrial hypertrophy. Echocardiography shows a dilated right atrium and ventricle ± tricuspid regurgitation. Cardiac catheterization shows an increased pulmonary artery pressure, increased right atrial pressure, and normal pulmonary capillary pressure.

Treatment is difficult, as the condition is usually progressive. Some studies report improvement with HAART; others show no benefit. Other options include epoprostenol, diuretics, oral anticoagulant, sildenafil, and antiviral therapy (controversial).

HIV pulmonary complications

HIV infection may be associated with a number of pulmonary complications, some of which are considered AIDS-defining illnesses.

Pneumocystis jiroveci pneumonia (PCP)

This fungus, formerly called *Pneumocystis carinii,* is the most common cause of infection in HIV-infected patients. It is a ubiquitous environmental organism, transmitted by inhalation. PCP may be due to acquisition of a new infection or reactivation of previous infection.

PCP is associated with a CD4 count <200 cells/mm^3. Incidence in the West is low because of HAART and PCP prophylaxis. It remains a common AIDS presentation in developing countries.

Clinical features include progressive dynspea, fever, chills, malaise, chest pain, and weight loss. Examination reveals crepitations or wheeze but may be normal in 50%. Hypoxia is common. It may desaturate on exercise.

Chest X-ray shows diffuse interstitial/alveolar infiltrates; 25% are normal in early disease. CXR signs may be highly variable.

Induced sputum is diagnostic in ~60%. Bronchoalveolar lavage is diagnostic in >95%. Molecular diagnostic tests look promising.

TMP-SMX is the treatment of choice. Alternatives include clindamycin and primaquine; dapsone, atovaquone, and intravenous pentamidine. If there is a partial pressure of arterial oxygen (PaO$_2$) <7 kPa or alveolar–arterial (A–a) gradient >3.5 KPa, give prednisolne.

Secondary prophylaxis should be given to all patients who have had PCP and be continued until the CD4 count is >200 cells/mm^3 for ≥3 months.

Pneumonia

Pneumonia is an acute infection of the lung that presents with fever, dyspnea, and cough ± sputum production.

It may be caused by a wide variety of pathogens: pyogenic bacteria (*S. pneumoniae, H. influenzae, P. aeruginosa, S. aureus*), PCP, TB, cryptococcosis, cytomegalovirus, or *Aspergillus* spp.

Onset and duration of symptoms are short in influenza and bacterial pneumonia, longer in PCP and TB.

A high CD4 count is usually correlated with "normal" pathogens, e.g., *S. pneumoniae*, TB, *S. aureus*, and influenza. A CD4 count <200 cells/mm^3 is associated with opportunistic pathogens, e.g., *Pneumocystis jiroveci*, *C. neoformans*, histoplasmosis, coccidiodomycosis, *Nocardia* spp., and *Rhodococcus equi*.

CXR may appear show typical or atypical appearances or may even be normal in patients, e.g., with PCP and TB. Intrathoracic lymphadenopathy suggests TB, atypical mycobacteria, lymphoma, or Kaposi sarcoma.

Injection drug use is associated with *S. aureus* pneumonia.

For prophylaxis, TMP-SMX reduces the incidence of PCP and bacterial pneumonia. Influenza vaccination appears to reduce the risk of influenza. The effects of pneumococcal vaccination are variable.

For laboratory diagnosis, expectorated sputum is used for TB diagnosis. Induced sputum is better for PCP. Bronchoscopy has a yield of ~95% for PCP. Tests to consider in patients who are not responding to treatment are *Legionella* urinary antigen, serum cryptococcal antigen, and *H. capsulatum* serum or urinary antigen. Also consider bronchoscopy and CT thorax.

Treatment is of the underlying cause.

For secondary prophylaxis, patients who present with AIDS-defining pulmonary infections, e.g., PCP, should be treated with TMP-SMX until their CD4 count is consistently >200 cells/mm^3.

Lymphoid interstitial pneumonitis (LIP)

LIP is a diffuse interstitial lung disease characterized by a polyclonal lymphoid cell infiltrate in the alveolar septae. It occurs in <1% of HIV-infected adults but up to 40% of HIV-infected children.

Clinical features are fever, dyspnea, weight loss, pleuritic pain, and arthralgia. Adults may be asymptomatic. Chest examination shows bibasal crepitations. Children may have clubbing and adenopathy.

CXR shows bilateral reticulonodular shadowing. High-resolution CT scan shows ground-glass shadowing and pulmonary nodules.

Diagnosis is established by lung biopsy in adults. In children, persistence of abnormalities for >2 months and exclusion of other infectious causes is considered diagnostic.

Treatment is with oral prednisolone. Optimal duration of treatment is unknown; 6–12 months is usually given. The condition may improve with institution of HAART.

It resolves after 6–12 months in some patients. Others may require lifelong low-dose steroids.

Pneumothorax

In HIV-infected patients, the most common cause is *Pneumocystis jiroveci* (PCP), and a spontaneous pneumothorax should prompt investigation for PCP. Pneumothorax may also occur in TB, pulmonary cryptococcosis, and lymphoid interstitial pneumonitis. Iatrogenic causes include central line insertion, thoracocentesis, and bronchoscopy. Risk factors include male sex, smoking, patients on inhaled pentamidine, patients with bullae on CXR, ventilated patients, and injection drug users.

It presents with pleuritic chest pain, dyspnea, and cough. On examination there is hyperresonance to percussion and reduced breath sounds.

The diagnosis is confirmed on CXR, which shows a rim of air around the lung.

Treatment is with aspiration or chest drain insertion.

PCP-associated pneumothorax is associated with higher mortality.

Reference

National Institutes of Health. Guidelines for the prevention and treatment of opportunistic infections in HIV-infected adults and adolescents (2008). Available from http://aidsinfo.nih.gov/Guidelines/Default.aspx?MenuItem=Guidelines.

HIV gastrointestinal disease

Gingivitis/periodontitis

Gum inflammation and bleeding are caused by oral anaerobic bacteria There are four phases: linear gingival erythema, necrotizing gingivitis, necrotizing periodontis, and necrotizing stomatitis.

Diagnosis is clinical. Orthopantogram may show bony loss.

Treatment is with routine dental care plus antiseptic mouthwash. A dental opinion should be sought regarding curettage and debridement. Antibiotics, e.g., metronidazole, are given for necrotizing stomatitis.

Oropharyngeal candidiasis

This is usually caused by *Candida albicans*. Diagnosis is clinical. Treatment is with oral fluconazole.

Esophageal candidiasis

This is caused by a number of *Candida* spp. It usually occurs in patients with a CD4 count <100 cells/mm^3.

Clinical features are dysphagia, odynophagia, and retrosternal pain.

Diagnosis is clinical but upper GI endoscopy may be performed if there is atypical presentation or a poor response to treatment.

Treatment is with fluconazole for 14–21 days.

Secondary prophylaxis may be considered in patients with >3 episodes in 1 year.

Following multiple treatments with azoles, patients may develop azole-resistant *Candida* esophagitis. In this situation, intravenous echinocandin therapy may be necessary.

Nausea and vomiting

These are often due to medications (especially antiretrovirals, antibiotics, opiates). They may also be due to abacavir hypersensitivity, nevirapine hepatotoxocity, or lactic acidosis. Other causes include adrenal insufficiency, uremia, hypercalcemia, CNS lesions, and GI disease.

Investigations include lactate level, ultrasound or CT abdomen, and CT brain.

Treat the underlying cause. If the condition is due to drugs, consider changing them. Otherwise, use symptomatic treatment.

Diarrhea

Diarrhea is usually caused by drugs (especially protease inhibitors). But it may also be due to a number of pathogens, e.g., *Salmonella* spp., *Shigella* spp, *Campylobacter* spp., *E. coli*, *S. aureus*, or viruses.

Chronic diarrhea may be due to *Cryptosporidium*, *Microsporidium*, *M. avium* complex (MAC), *Cyclospora*, *Isospora*, *G. lamblia*, *E. histolytica*, or HIV enteropathy.

Clinical features include fever, abdominal cramps, diarrhea, tenesmus, and PR bleeding.

For diagnosis, send blood cultures and stool to the lab for microscopy, ova, cysts, and parasites. Test for *C. difficile* toxin. Take blood cultures for MAC and *Salmonella* spp. CT abdomen may be helpful to determine the cause of an acute abdomen. Colonoscopy is helpful for the diagnosis of CMV colitis; it also helps to rule out Kaposi sarcoma and lymphoma.

Treat the underlying cause. If diarrhea is due to drugs, consider changing them. Otherwise, use symptomatic treatment.

HIV liver disease

Deranged liver function tests

These are common in HIV-infected patients and may be due to a variety of causes:

- Drug toxicity e.g., NNRTIs (especially nevirapine), protease inhibitors, TMP-SMX, TB drugs, statins, paracetamol
- Alcohol toxicity or substance abuse
- Viral hepatitis (acute infection, flare of chronic disease, drug resistance)
- Opportunistic infections, e.g., MAC, CMV, TB.

Lactic acidosis/hepatic steatosis

Hyperlactatemia is defined as a venous lactate level >2 mmol/L. It can occur with any nucleoside reverse transcriptase inhibitor (NRTI) but is most commonly caused by d4T, ddl, or both.

The mechanism is NRTI-mediated inhibition of DNA polymerase gamma, leading to depletion of mitochondrial DNA.

It can be asymptomatic or associated with a symptomatic and sometimes fatal acidosis. Asymptomatic elevations in lactate occur in 8–20% of patients on prolonged HAART. Symptomatic hyperlactatemia occurs in 0.5–1/100 patient-years of NRTI exposure.

For diagnosis, patients who have symptoms compatible with lactic acidosis (nausea, vomiting, abdominal pain) or abnormal liver function tests or amylase should have their lactate levels measured. A lactate level >5 mmol/L is considered diagnostic.

For treatment, stop the NRTIs and switch to another drug class. Substitution of abacavir, 3TC (lamivudine), FTC (emtricitabine), or TDF (tenofozir) may be possible in patients who are not seriously ill.

Prognosis is related to lactate level: 7% if lactate 5–10 mmol/L, >30% if lactate 10–15 mmol/L, and >60% if lactate >15 mmol/L.

Viral hepatitis

All patients who develop deranged liver function tests should be screened for the hepatitis viruses.

Patients may acquire an acute hepatitis (e.g., HAV or HEV) transmitted via the feco-oral route. Patients with HIV may be chronically infected with other blood-borne viruses such as HBV or HCV.

All patients should be advised to avoid or limit their intake of alcohol. They should also be vaccinated against HAV and HBV if nonimmune when their CD4 count is >200 cells/mm^3.

For treatment of HBV, patients who do not require HAART should receive treatment with pegylated interferon-A; alternatives are entecavir or adefovir. In patients who require HAART, treatment with two agents active against HBV is recommended, e.g., tenofovir and emtricitabine.

For treatment of HCV, patients who require treatment should be given pegylated interferon and ribavirin. Sustained virological response rates are lower for genotype 1 (14–29%) than for genotypes 2 and 3 (44–73%).

Cholangiopathy

This syndrome of biliary obstruction is caused by infection-associated strictures. There are four types: papillary stricture and stenosis, sclerosing cholangitis-like, papillary stenosis + sclerosing cholangitis, and extrahepatic strictures.

Causes include *Cryptosporidium parvum* (most common), *Microsporidia*, *Cyclospora cayetanensis*, and CMV; 20–40% of cases are idiopathic. The CD4 count is usually <100 cells/mm^3.

Clinical features include right upper quadrant pain, fever, and diarrhea (if there is intestinal involvement).

Liver function tests show cholestatic derangement. Ultrasound shows dilated bile ducts. Diagnosis is confirmed by ERCP.

Treatment is sphincterotomy for papillary stenosis. Endoscopic stenting is used for isolated bile duct stricture. Ursodeoxycholic acid has been used experimentally in cholangiopathy without stenosis. Use pathogen-specific therapy, if possible.

Average survival in the HAART era is 9 months; it is worse if ALP >1000 IU/L.

Pancreatitis

Pancreatitis is a well-recognized complication in HIV-infected patients.

There are a number of causes: drugs (especially ddI or ddI plus d4T). It may also occur as a complication of protease inhibitor (PI)-associated hypertriglyceridemia or NRTI-induced lactic acidosis. Opportunistic infections such as CMV, MAC, TB, crypotosporidiosis, toxoplasmosis, and cryptococcosis have also been implicated.

Diagnosis is based on an amylase >3 times the upper limit of normal. A CT scan should be performed to stage the disease, detect complications, and exclude other diagnosis.

Treatment is supportive: fluids, antibiotics, and analgesia.

Prognosis is related to the APACHE II score.

HIV-associated nephropathy

This is the leading cause of end-stage renal disease (ESRD) in HIV-infected patients. Risk factors include black race, male gender, and a family history of renal disease.

This condition is usually a late manifestation of HIV disease (CD4 count <200 cells/mm³). Proteinuria may be massive and predates renal insufficiency. Rapid progression to ESRD occurs if not treated.

For diagnosis, protenuria (nephrotic range) is common. Renal ultrasound shows normal to large echogenic kidneys. Renal biopsy is diagnostic.

HAART improves renal survival. Blood pressure should be maintained <125 mmHg systolic using an ACE inhibitor. Corticosteroids may be given as rescue therapy (or as a bridge to HAART).

HIV neurological complications

Peripheral neuropathy

Peripheral neuropathy is another relatively common complication of HIV therapy. There are a number of possible causes:

- *Distal sensory neuropathy (DSN):* pain and numbness in glove-and-stocking distribution. CD4 count is usually <200 cells/mm³.
- *Antiretroviral toxic neuropathy (ATN):* same as DSN but associated with ddI, ddC, and d4T. It is more common in older patients with diabetes. It can occur at any CD4 count.
- *Tarsal tunnel syndrome:* pain and numbness in anterior part of soles of feet
- *HIV-associated neuromuscular weakness syndrome:* ascending paralysis with arreflexia ± cranial nerve or sensory involvement. It is usually associated with d4T and has poor survival.
- *HIV-associated myopathy* (AZT myopathy): pain, aching, and weakness of proximal muscles. It is associated with AZT and raised creatinine kinase (CK) level. It can occur at any CD4 count.
- *Polyradiculitis:* rapidly evolving weakness and numbness in legs with bladder and bowel incontinence. It may be caused by CMV or HSV. CD4 count is <50 or >500 cells/mm³.
- *Vacuolar myopathy:* stiffness, weakness, and numbness in legs followed by bowel and bladder incontinence. Need to exclude vitamin B_{12} deficiency and HTLV-1 infection. CD4 count is <200 cells/mm³. Physiotherapy, methionine, or HAART may be helpful.
- *Inflammatory demyelinating polyneuropathies:* weakness in arms and legs with minor sensory component. It can occur at any CD4 count. Treatment is with plasmapheresis, IVIG, and/or HAART.
- *Mononeuritis/mononeuritis multiplex:* asymmetrical mix of motor and sensory defects occurring over weeks. CD4 count is variable. Treat with steroids if CD4 count is >200 cells/mm³. Consider treating for CMV if CD4 count is <50 cells/mm³.

Central nervous system manifestations

Central nervous system involvement may be due to HIV itself, opportunistic infections, or malignancies.

- *Cryptococcal meningitis* (8–10% of all AIDS patients) presents with fever, headache, visual changes, stiff neck, cranial nerve deficits, and seizures. It progresses over 2 weeks. CD4 count is <100 cells/mm³. CSF is India ink positive in 60–80%; CSF culture is positive in 95–100%. Cryptococcal antigen is >95% sensitive and specific.
- *HIV-associated dementia* (HAD, 7%) presents with a triad of cognitive, motor, and behavioral dysfunction over weeks to months. Afebrile. CD4 count <200 cells/mm³. Elevated B₂ microglobulin. Neuropsychological tests show subcortical dementia.
- *Toxoplasmosis* (2–4%) presents with fever, reduced conscious level, focal neurological deficits, and seizures. The CD4 count is <200 cells/mm³. MRI scan shows ring-enhancing lesions. Toxoplasma IgG is falsely negative in 5%; 85% respond to empiric therapy in 7 days. Brain biopsy makes the definitive diagnosis.
- *Primary CNS lymphoma* (2%): clinical presentation is afebrile with altered mental status, focal neurological deficits, and seizures with progression over 2–8 weeks. CD4 count is <200 cells/mm³. Suspect this if the patient has no response to anti-toxoplasma therapy. Thallium 201 SPECT scanning is 90% sensitive and specific.
- *Progressive multifocal leukoencephalopathy* (PML, 1–2%) presents with impaired speech, vision, and motor function. There is no fever or headache. CD4 count is usually <100 cells/mm³. MRI shows multifocal lesions in the subcortical white matter. CSF or brain biopsy is positive for JC virus (p. 386).
- *CNS tuberculosis* (0.5–1%) presents with fever, headache, meningism, impaired conscious level, and focal neurological deficits. CD4 count is <100 cells/mm³. CT/MRI scan shows meningeal enhancement, hydrocephalus, and tuberculomas. ZN smear is positive in 20%. CXR shows active TB in 50%. The gold standard for diagnosis is a positive CSF culture for *M. tuberculosis*.
- *CMV encephalitis* (>0.5%) presents with fever, lethargy, delirium, disorientation, headache, neck stiffness, photophobia, and cranial nerve deficits. CD4 count is <100 cells/mm³. Patients may have CMV retinitis. CSF is CMV PCR positive. Definitive diagnosis is made by brain biopsy.
- *Neurosyphilis* (0.5%) has various clinical presentations: meningitis-like, tabes dorsalis, general paresis of the insane, meningovascular strokes/myelitis, and ocular manifestations (iritis, uveitis, optic neuritis). It occurs at any CD4 count. Diagnosis is a positive CSF VDRL test (60–70%).

HIV-associated malignancies

Malignancies are generally more common in HIV-infected patients than in HIV-uninfected patients. Certain malignancies are particularly associated with HIV infection.

Kaposi sarcoma

KS is caused by HHV-8. It is the most common HIV-associated malignancy. The rate is 20,000-fold higher in HIV-positive than in HIV-negative individuals, and 300-fold higher than in other immunosuppressed patients.

It is more common in men who have sex with men (MSM) and more common in women.

KS presents with purple, brown to black macules, nodules, and papules on the face, mouth, legs, and genitals. Visceral involvement affects the lungs and GI tract. HAART is associated with a decreased incidence and regression of lesions.

Treatment may be local, e.g., vinblastine injections, or systemic, e.g., liposomal anthracycline.

Non-Hodgkin's lymphoma

From 50 to 80% of patients are EBV-positive. The CD4 count is <100cells/mm^3, and it is 200–600 times more common in patients with HIV than in the general population. Most cases are high-grade diffuse, large-cell, or Burkitt-like lymphomas. They usually present with advanced disease, sparse lymph nodes, and constitutional B symptoms.

Diagnosis is made by biopsy of the brain, lymph nodes, or bone marrow. CT is better than endoscopy for assessing GI involvement.

Treatment is with HAART plus chemotherapy. Initial response rates are 60–80%, but median survival is <1 year.

Primary CNS lymphoma

See HIV neurological complications (p. 745).

Primary effusion lymphoma

This is caused by HHV-8 and EBV. It is very rare, accounting for <0.14% of non-Hodgkin's lymphomas in patients with AIDS. It presents with serous effusions (pleural, pericardial, peritoneal, joint spaces).

Diagnosis is made by examining the effusions.

Treatment is with HAART plus chemotherapy.

Cervical cancer

Cervical cancer is associated with human papilloma virus (HPV) types 16, 18, 31, 33, and 35. Cervical intraepithelial neoplasis (CIN) and invasive cervical cancer are both more common in HIV-positive than in HIV-negative women. The frequency and severity of cervical dysplasia increase with progressive immune compromise.

The CDC recommends a gynecological examination and Pap smear at baseline at 6 months and then yearly in HIV-infected women.

HIV prevention

Almost three decades after the start of the HIV epidemic, it has reached every country of the world. Although HIV was initially described in MSM, 80% of infections are now transmitted heterosexually, and >50% of HIV-infected people are now women. Mother-to-child transmission accounts for >90% of HIV-infected children worldwide. Intravenous drug use is also fueling transmission in central and eastern Europe and certain countries in Asia.

The epidemic continues unabated, especially in Sub-Saharan Africa and Southeast Asia. In developed countries, advances in antiretroviral therapy have resulted in significant reductions in morbidity and mortality. However, complacency and recurrence of high-risk behavior among some populations have resulted in a resurgence of sexually transmitted diseases and a recent increase in HIV incidence in these populations.

Prevention of perinatal transmission

The three major factors associated with perinatal HIV transmission are high maternal plasma HIV viral load, prolonged rupture of membranes, and breast-feeding. A number of studies have been performed to try to prevent perinatal transmission and have shown the following:

- Antiretroviral therapy of the mother during pregnancy and labor reduces maternal viremia and HIV transmission.
- Antiretroviral therapy of the child (in utero and after birth) reduces HIV transmission.
- Delivery by Caesarean section has led to a decline in HIV transmission.
- Continuation of antiretroviral therapy in mothers who choose to exclusively breast-feed is beneficial.
- There are concerns about the use of single-dose nevirapine in the developing world because of the potential for development of NNRTI resistance.

Prevention of sexual transmission

A number of factors have been identified as important in sexual transmission: plasma HIV RNA level, genital HIV RNA level, acute infection vs. advanced disease, degree of immunosuppression, genital ulcers, inflammatory STIs, cervical ectopy, uncircumcised status, host genetics, and levels of cytokines and chemokines. Interventions to reduce sexual transmission include the following.

- *Reduction of HIV RNA level:* studies in Africa have shown that antiretroviral therapy reduces the risk of HIV transmission between serodiscordant couples by >80%.
- *HSV-2 suppression:* treatment with valacyclovir was associated with reduction in plasma and genital HIV-1 levels and reduced incidence of HIV transmission. However, use of acyclovir was not associated with reduced HIV acquisition in two other studies.[1]
- *Male circumcision:* several ecological studies and three randomized controlled trials have shown that male circumcision is associated with a 60–70% reduction in rates of HIV acquisition.[1] Circumcision also reduced the frequency of genital ulcer disease and HIV acquisition by female sexual partners. Modeling studies now suggest that male circumcision in Sub-Saharan Africa could potentially prevent 5.7 million infections and 2 million deaths over the next 20 years, if the intervention could be delivered safely and cost-effectively.
- *Microbicides:* whereas circumcision is a method that can protect men from HIV, there is an urgent need to develop female-controlled

methods of protection. Numerous studies have investigated the effectiveness of female condoms, diaphragms, and microbicides but have failed to show benefit. In some studies, the use of microbicides has been associated with an increased risk of HIV acquisition.

• Post-exposure prophylaxis following sexual exposure (PEPSE)[2] is recommended when the individual presents within 72 hours after anal and or vaginal intercourse with a known HIV positive source or a source from a group or area of high HIV prevalence.

HIV vaccines

Despite billions of dollars spent and over 20 years of research, an effective vaccine for the prevention of HIV remains elusive. Specific characteristics of the virus that hinder vaccine development include the extreme genetic variability in circulating viral isolates worldwide, biological properties of HIV that impede immune attack, and a high mutation rate that allows for rapid escape from adaptive immune responses.

References

1. Padian NS, Buvé A, Balkus J, et al. (2008). Biomedical interventions to prevent HIV infection: evidence, challenges and the way forward. *Lancet* 372:585–599.

2. Fisher M, Benn P, Evans B, et al. (2006). UK guideline for the use of post-exposure prophylaxis for HIV following sexual exposure. *Int J STD AIDS* 17:81–92.

Immunizations

Routine childhood immunizations

Childhood immunizations are available to all children in the U.S., regardless of ability to pay. Many programs such as Vaccines for Children, as well as state health departments, provide free immunizations. The introduction of immunization has resulted in dramatic declines in certain diseases, e.g., meningitis caused by *H. influenzae* type B and *N. meningitidis* serogroup C. Routine childhood immunization schedules vary from country to country. The U.S. routine childhood immunization schedule for ages 0–6 is summarized in Table 4.21, and for ages 7–18 in Table 4.22.

In September 2008, the human papillomavirus vaccine (HPV) was introduced into the routine immunization schedule for girls. Unlike other childhood immunizations, the HPV vaccine is used to prevent the development of cervical cancer, rather than a childhood infectious disease.

Routine immunization schedules can be found online at http://www.cdc.gov.

Nonroutine immunizations

Some children who may be at increased risk of certain diseases (e.g., tuberculosis and hepatitis B) may be given additional vaccines (see Table 4.23).

Further information

Further information on immunizations is available from the Centers for Disease Control and Prevention: http://www.cdc.gov/mmwr/preview/mmwrhtml/mm5551a7.htm

Table 4.21 Recommended immunization schedule for persons aged 0–6 years: United States, 2007

Vaccine ▼ / Age ▶	Birth	1 month	2 months	4 months	6 months	12 months	15 months	18 months	19–23 months	2–3 years	4–6 years
Hepatitis B[1]	HepB	HepB			HepB					HepB Series	
Rotavirus[2]			Rota	Rota	Rota						
Diphtheria, Tetanus, Pertussis[3]			DTaP	DTaP	DTaP		DTaP				DTaP
Haemophilus influenzae type b[4]			Hib	Hib	Hib[4]	Hib					
Pneumococcal[5]			PCV	PCV	PCV	PCV				PCV / PPV	
Inactivated Poliovirus			IPV	IPV		IPV					IPV
Influenza[6]						Influenza (Yearly)					
Measles, Mumps, Rubella[7]						MMR					MMR
Varicella[8]						Varicella					Varicella
Hepatitis A[9]						HepA (2 doses)				HepA Series	
Meningococcal[10]										MPSV4	

Legend:
- ■ Range of recommended ages
- ■ Catch-up immunization
- ■ Certain high-risk groups

See footnote1 (at 2 months for Diphtheria, Tetanus, Pertussis)

This schedule indicates the recommended ages for routine administration of currently licensed childhood vaccines, as of December 1, 2006, for children aged 0–6 years. Additional information is available at http://www.cdc.gov/nip/recs/child-schedule.htm. Any dose not administered at the recommended age should be administered at any subsequent visit, when indicated and feasible. Additional vaccines may be licensed and recommended during the year. Licensed combination vaccines may be used whenever any components of the combination are indicated and other components of the vaccine are not contraindicated and if approved by the Food and Drug Administration for that dose of the series. Providers should consult the respective Advisory Committee on Immunization Practices statement for detailed recommendations. Clinically significant adverse events that follow Immunization should be reported to the Vaccine Adverse Event Reporting System (VAERS). Guidance about how to obtain and complete a VAERS form is available at http://www.vaers-hhs.gov or by telephone, 800-822-7987

Table 7.22 Recommended immunization schedule for persons aged 7–18 years, United States, 2007

Vaccine ▼	Age ► 7–10 years	11–12 YEARS	13–14 years	15 years	16–18 years
Tetanus, Diphtheria, Pertussis[1]	See footnote 1	Tdap	Tdap		
Human Papillomavirus[2]	See footnote 2	HPV (3 doses)	HPV Series		
Meningococcal[3]	MPSV4	MCV4		MCV4[3] MCV4	
Pneumococcal[4]		PPV			
Influenza[5]		Influenza (Yearly)			
Hepatitis A[6]		HepA Series			
Hepatitis B[7]		HepB Series			
Inactivated Poliovirus[8]		IPV Series			
Measles, Mumps, Rubella[9]		MMR Series			
Varicella[10]		Varicella Series			

Legend:
- ■ Range of recommended ages
- ▨ Catch-up Immunization
- ▨ Certain high-risk groups

This schedule indicates the recommended ages for routine administration of currently licensed childhood vaccines, as of December 1, 2006, for children aged 7–18 years. Additional information is available at http://www.cdc.gov/nip/recs/child-schedule.htm. Any dose not administered at the recommended age should be administered at any subsequent visit, when indicated and feasible. Additional vaccines may be licensed and recommended during the year. Licensed combination vaccines may be used whenever any components of the combination are indicated and other components of the vaccine are not contraindicated and if approved by the Food and Drug Administration for that dose of the series. Providers should consult the respective Advisory Committee on Immunization Practices statement for detailed recommendations. Clinically significant adverse events that follow Immunization should be reported to the Vaccine Adverse Event Reporting System (VAERS). Guidance about how to obtain and complete a VAERS form is available at http://www.vaers-hhs.gov or by telephone, 800-822-7987

Source: Centers for Disease Control and Prevention (2007). CDC recommended immunization schedules for persons aged 0–18 Years—United States, 2007. MMWR Morb Mortal Wkly Rep 55(51):Q1–Q4.

Table 4.23 Additional childhood vaccines

Age of child	Vaccine	Diseases protected against
At birth, for babies who are more likely to be exposed to TB	BCG	Tuberculosis
At birth, for babies whose mothers are hepatitis B positive	Hep B	Hepatitis B

Notifiable diseases (ND)

The statutory requirement for the notification of certain infectious diseases (e.g., cholera, diphtheria, smallpox and typhoid) started toward the end of the 19th century. Since then, the list of diseases has expanded considerably (Table 4.24).

The prime purpose of the notifications system is to detect possible outbreaks or epidemics. Accuracy of diagnosis is secondary, and a clinical suspicion of a notifiable infection is all that is required. If a diagnosis later proves incorrect, it can always be changed or canceled.

State-by-state regulations may vary, so consultation of local or state health departments is important regarding reporting rules.

Table 4.24 Notifiable diseases

Acute encephalitis	Paratyphoid fever
Acute poliomyelitis	Plague
Anthrax	Rabies
Cholera	Relapsing fever
Diphtheria	Rubella
Dysentery	Scarlet fever
Food poisoning	Smallpox
Leprosy*	Tetanus
Leptospirosis	Tuberculosis
Malaria	Typhoid fever
Measles	Typhus fever
Meningitis	Viral hemorrhagic fever
Meningococcal septicemia	Viral hepatitis
Mumps	Whooping cough
Ophthalmia neonatorum	Yellow fever

* Leprosy should be notified directly to the CDC.

Bioterrorism

Biological warfare has a long and unpleasant history. Around 400 BCE the Scythians were attempting to poison their arrows with blood and manure, and in the 14th century the Tarter catapulted the corpses of plague victims into the city of Kaffa with the intention of initiating an outbreak. The years after the Second World War saw a race to develop more effective biological agents, before various treaties later led to the limitation and even destruction of biological weapons stockpiles by many nations (UK 1957, USA 1973).

Today around 17 countries are suspected of having biological weapons programs. The threat of biological warfare is seen as issuing not primarily from states but from independent organizations and terrorists. The term *deliberate release* refers to any intentional spread of a biological or chemical agent. This release may be overt (e.g., a prior warning, or the release may be apparent, either from the use of an explosive device or because a suspicious substance is obviously visible) or covert (the release not becoming apparent until the first cases of disease arise).

Only two proven deliberate releases have more recently affected a large number of people: contamination of restaurant salads with *S. typhimurium* in Oregon in 1984 and dissemination of *Bacillus anthracis* via the U.S. mail in 2001.

Organisms with the potential to be used as weapons agents

The ideal biological-weapon agent has low visibility and high potency, is accessible with a long shelf-life, is relatively easy to deliver, and shows limited epidemic spread. A small amount of agent may be capable of killing a large number of people (particularly in a metropolitan environment) and creating a disproportionate level of fear and disruption—a key part of their attractiveness to terrorist organizations.

Category A agents

Those organisms that are easily disseminated or transmitted from person to person, with high mortality rates and the potential for major public health impact and requiring special action for public health readiness, are as follows:

- Anthrax (p. 204): pulmonary anthrax presents with a severe febrile illness or sepsis with respiratory failure (massive mediastinal lymphadenopathy). The organism may be identified in blood cultures or sputum.
- Smallpox (p. 389): individuals previously vaccinated lose protection after 10–20 years. Vaccination provides moderate protection if given within 2–4 days of exposure. Disease may develop 1–3 weeks after exposure.
- Botulism (p. 214): toxin may be inhaled or food-borne. Antitoxin is available.
- Plague (p. 263): inhaled as aerosol, causing pneumonic plague
- Tularemia (p. 266)
- Viral hemorrhagic fevers (p. 403)

Category B agents

These are moderately easy to disseminate, have moderate morbidity rates and low mortality rates, and require enhancement of both diagnostic capacity and disease surveillance. They include glanders (p. 251), melioidosis (p. 250), brucellosis (p. 261), psittacosis (p. 305), and Q fever (p. 298).

Recognizing an attack

In the absence of issued warnings or a very obvious release (e.g., explosive device), the first indicator of an outbreak may be a cluster of symptomatic cases. Such clusters may present acutely or over a period of days or weeks. Isolated fatalities due to undiagnosed febrile illness are not uncommon. Prompt epidemiological inquiry is essential. Features indicative of deliberate release include the following:

- An unusually large number of patients over a short time period
- Cases that are linked by epidemiological or geographical features
- Signs or symptoms that are unusual or very severe
- Unknown cause or an identified cause unresponsive to normal therapy or unusual in the United States or where acquired

Remember that symptoms may also be due to radiological or chemical contamination.

Responding to an attack

Consider the risk of transmission to or contamination of staff and other patients. It may be appropriate to isolate affected patients and to use personal protective equipment. Decontamination of potentially exposed individuals is vital for suspected releases of *Bacillus anthracis*.

Expert advice must be sought locally and the health protection unit informed. Empirical antibacterial prophylaxis is indicated for possible exposure to certain bacterial agents such as anthrax, plague, and tularemia (ciprofloxacin) or brucella, burkholderia, and Q fever (e.g., doxycycline).

National agencies have stockpiles of suitable antibiotics for such emergencies. Early cases should be managed according to the best available advice until more detailed epidemiological information and laboratory tests are available. In the United States, management of all incidents is led by the police with involvement of other emergency and health services as appropriate.

All microbiological testing of suspect material must be done in *specialist* laboratories.

More information

The CDC Web site has extensive information on the management of deliberate-release incidents, including clinical and diagnostic algorithms, antibiotic protocols, and guidelines for dealing with suspicious packages.

See http://www.cdc.gov.

Index